Orthokeratology

To all those who have worked tirelessly and altruistically over the last 40 years to develop the science and art of orthokeratology to the present status as an exciting and rapidly growing part of global vision correction.

For Butterworth-Heinemann

Publishing Director: Caroline Makepeace
Development Editor: Kim Benson
Project Manager: Derek Robertson
Design: George Ajayi

Orthokeratology
Principles and Practice

John Mountford Dip App Sc, FCLSA, FAAO

Optometrist and Contact Lens Specialist, Brisbane, Australia

David Ruston BSc FCOptom DipCLP FAAO

Managing Director, Optometric Educators Ltd, Contact Lens Practitioner and Optometrist, London, UK

Trusit Dave PhD MCOptom FAAO

Director, OptiMed Ophthalmic Medical Instruments, Eyetech Optometrists, Coventry, UK

Foreword by

Edward S Bennett OD MSEd

Executive Director of the RGP Lens Institute; Associate Professor of Optometry and Co-Chief of the Contact Lens Clinic, University of Missouri School of Optometry, St Louis, Missouri, USA

BUTTERWORTH
HEINEMANN

EDINBURGH LONDON NEW YORK OXFORD PHILADELPHIA ST LOUIS SYDNEY TORONTO 2004

BUTTERWORTH-HEINEMANN
An imprint of Elsevier Limited

ISBN 0 7506 4007 3

British Library Cataloguing in Publication Data
A catalogue record for this book is available from the British Library

Library of Congress Cataloging in Publication Data
A catalog record for this book is available from the Library of Congress

Note
Medical knowledge is constantly changing. As new information becomes
available, changes in treatment, procedures, equipment and the use of drugs
become necessary. The authors/contributors and the publishers have taken
great care to ensure that the information given in this text is accurate and up
to date. However, readers are strongly advised to confirm that the
information, especially with regard to drug usage, complies with the latest
legislation and standards of practice.

Printed in China

The
publisher's
policy is to use
paper manufactured
from sustainable forests

Contents

Foreword   vii

1. History and general principles   1
   John Mountford

2. Corneal topography and its measurement   17
   Trusit Dave

3. Overnight and extended wear of rigid
   gas-permeable (RGP) lenses   49
   Trusit Dave

4. Design variables and fitting philosophies of
   reverse geometry lenses   69
   John Mountford

5. Patient selection and preliminary
   examination   109
   David Ruston and John Mountford

6. Trial lens fitting   139
   John Mountford

7. Corneal and refractive changes due to
   orthokeratology   175
   John Mountford

8. Computerized modeling of outcomes and lens
   fitting in orthokeratology   205
   John Mountford

9. Lens delivery, aftercare routine and problem-
   solving   227
   David Ruston, Trusit Dave and John Mountford

10. A model of forces acting in
    orthokeratology   269
    John Mountford

11. The future   303
    John Mountford

Index   311

Foreword

There are many benefits to gas permeable rigid lenses, including quality of vision and eye health, not to mention their uses in presbyopia and keratoconus. However, one of their most exciting applications is in the rapidly growing area of orthokeratology. Although orthokeratology has been a process that has been available for over 40 years, it has only been in the last decade that the interest has greatly escalated. This has been the result of several new developments including:

- a better understanding of how orthokeratology results in myopia reduction and how to predict the specific amount of reduction
- sophisticated lens designs which can often reduce the patient's baseline myopic correction without the need for a series of lenses
- overnight therapy and retainer wear to allow the patient the convenience of not wearing lenses during their waking hours, and
- introduction of corneal topography instrumentation and orthokeratology software to assist in lens design and monitoring of corneal change.

The individual most responsible for these developments has been the 'father' of modern orthokeratology, John Mountford. Along with Helen Swarbrick, he has increased our understanding of the relationship between orthokeratology lens design and the concurrent changes in the tear layer and corneal tissue resulting in myopia reduction. Lacking from the rapid growth of ortho-keratology, however, has been a contemporary clinical text that describes such important topics as patient selection, corneal topography, lens design and fitting, aftercare and problem solving. *Orthokeratology*, authored by John Mountford and noted orthokeratology specialists Trusit Dave and David Ruston, provides this information and more.

It is quite evident that the ability to improve a patient's unaided vision and, therefore, their quality of life via orthokeratology is one of the most exciting developments in the eyecare field today. It is important for every practitioner seriously to consider incorporating orthokeratology into everyday practice. Not only is this a great practice-builder, but the opportunity to improve patients' ability to function without correction – and without surgery – makes eyecare practice much more fulfilling for the orthokeratologist.

The important new text will provide any practitioner, ranging from the practicing ortho-keratologist to the novice clinician, with the important information to successfully implement orthokeratology into their practice.

Edward S. Bennett OD, MSEd, 2004
Executive Director of the RGP Lens Institute;
Associate Professor of Optometry and
Co-Chief of the Contact Lens Clinic,
University of Missouri School of Optometry,
St. Louis, Missouri, USA

Chapter 1

History and general principles

John Mountford

CHAPTER CONTENTS

The practitioners 2
The academics 4
The computer programmers 5
The material companies 5
Terminology 6
Aims and objectives of this book 12
References 13

Appendix
The first meeting of the International
  Orthokeratology Society, 13 October
  1962 14

Orthokeratology is, all of a sudden, a "hot topic" once again. However, it has been in a constant state of evolution for 40 years. In 1962, George Jessen caused a degree of controversy at the International Society of Contact Lens Specialists conference in Chicago when he first described his "orthofocus" procedure. The report of the meeting was reprinted in full in *Contacto* (Nolan 1995) and makes for interesting and delightful reading. The amazing thing is to read Newton Wesley's almost prophetic comments on the research that would need to be done to place the technique on a solid scientific basis. The research that he outlined 40 years ago is just starting to be carried out now. The National Eye Research Foundation has kindly given permission for a full reprint of the paper to be included in the appendix to this chapter.

The name "orthokeratology" was coined by Wesley at the meeting, and was adopted as the recognized term for the procedure. Kerns (1976) defined orthokeratology as "the reduction, modification or elimination of a refractive error by the programmed application of contact lenses." Modern marketing has attempted to put a different spin on the process by using alternative descriptors, but there is something special about orthokeratology having such a long history that demands some respect from the profession.

Orthokeratology was discovered and developed by optometrists, and is the one area of contact lens practice to which we can claim total ownership in terms of research and development. It is ours. As a sign of respect for all those practitioners who spent a lifetime dedicated to the development of the procedure, this textbook will only use the term "orthokeratology" to describe the design, fitting, and science behind the process of applying contact lenses with the deliberate intention of altering the refractive state of the eye.

Traditional orthokeratology did not have the advantages that are currently available, like corneal topography, computer-aided design and computer numeric-controlled (CNC) lathes: the successes were totally due to individual practitioner skill and experience. Hindsight is always 20/20, but it is amazing to realize that a great deal was accomplished in those early days, and the reader is encouraged to take the time to review the work of those early pioneers. Coon (1982) was the first to publish a thorough review of the literature on the various techniques and philosophies in his study of the Tabb method. Carney (1994) also published an excellent analysis of the traditional techniques, whilst Mountford (1997) reviewed the controlled studies of Kerns, Coon, Brand, and Polse.

These three controlled studies led to the sudden and prolonged demise of published articles on orthokeratology (Bara 2000). Interviews with practitioners who were actively involved in the procedure as background information for the chapter in Phillips & Speedwell's *Contact Lenses* made it clear that there were strong disagreements between what they had achieved in practice and what was reported in the studies (Mountford 1997). As a result, the developments continued to be made, as they still are today, by practitioners. The advancement in orthokeratology has also been accelerated by active academic involvement, along with the support of the two major companies that produce the materials from which the lenses are made. The following brief history therefore deals mainly with the individuals involved and their contributions to this ever-evolving emerging science. The reader will find references throughout this book that cite the practitioners' published works as well as those of the academics.

THE PRACTITIONERS

The first report of a new development in orthokeratology was published in 1989 by Wlodyga & Bryla. Richard Wlodyga is an experienced and well-read practitioner. He basically adapted an earlier concept that was described by Fontana, and started the reverse geometry revolution in orthokeratology.

Fontana described a "one-piece bifocal" lens, with the central 6.00 mm optic zone being cut 1.00 D flatter than the peripheral section of the lens, which was fitted on-*K*. The lens had a major advantage over its contemporaries in that centration was better. The common problem with traditional orthokeratology was control of lens centration. Superior decentration was responsible for induced with the-rule astigmatism (Kerns 1976), and the addition of a relatively steeper peripheral area on the lens tended to decrease the problem.

There are some who consider the Fontana lens to be a true reverse geometry lens, but it was, in fact, a recessed optic lens. With the lathing technology available at the time, it was simply impossible to produce a true reverse curve lens. The difference between the two design concepts is shown in Figure 1.1.

Wlodyga made the logical assumption that if a lens was made with a very flat base curve or back optic zone radius (BOZR), the first back peripheral radius (BPR$_1$) would need to be more than 1.00 D steeper than the base. His initial concept was to make a lens with a 3.00 D steeper secondary curve in order to control centration, and he needed someone who was prepared to make it for him. He eventually found Nick Stoyan, who produced specialty rigid lenses in his Californian laboratory

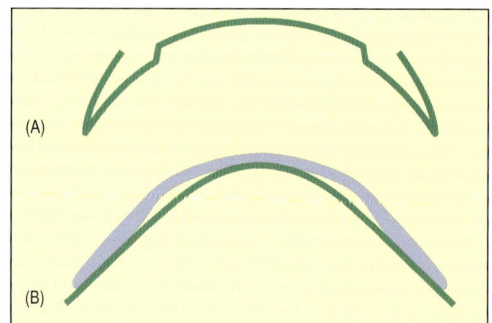

Figure 1.1 The difference in construction between (A) "recessed optic," as described by Fontana, and (B) a true reverse geometry lens.

(Contex). Stoyan had always had a reputation as an innovator and manufacturer of extremely high-quality lenses. His perfectionist nature made him one of the first to use the new CNC lathes that offered much better quality in terms of finish and reproducibility. The relationship forged between Wlodyga and Stoyan is what originally set modern orthokeratology on course.

The Contex OK-3 was a 9.6 mm total diameter (TD) lens with a 6.00 mm back optic zone diameter (BOZD), 3.00 D steeper reverse curve (forming the tear reservoir or TR) and an aspheric peripheral curve that was 0.50 mm wide. If the lens diameter was altered, the optic zone (BOZD) and peripheral curve (PC) remained constant, with the TR width being varied. This was the first three-zone orthokeratology lens, and Stoyan was granted a patent for the design and use of the lens for orthokeratology. Siviglia had earlier been granted a patent for a lens with a 1.50 D steeper than BOZR lens for use in postrefractive surgery conditions, but no mention of orthokeratology was made in the patent documents, so Stoyan can still rightfully claim precedence in the area.

Wlodyga and Stoyan were recognized for their contribution to the field by being awarded the Founders Award at the first Global Orthokeratology Symposium in 2002.

The fitting philosophy of the Contex lens was based on central and temporal keratometry readings, with the initial lens being fitted 1.50 D (0.30 mm) flatter than the flat-*K* reading. The accepted methodology of a series of progressively flatter lenses was then fitted until the maximum refractive change had been achieved. A totally unforeseen result of the new design was that the refractive changes were, on average, twice that achieved with the traditional techniques, and in half the time. The epithet "accelerated orthokeratology" was used to describe the technique. The range of lenses available eventually encompassed BOZDs from 6.00 to 8.00 mm in 0.50-mm steps and reverse curves from 1.00 to 15.00 D steeper than the BOZR.

Sammi El Hage applied topography data to the design and fitting of the lens. The BOZR was based on the Jessen factor, where the liquid lens provided the refractive correction, i.e., the higher the degree of myopia, the flatter the lens is fitted.

The rest of the lens construction was described in terms of a polynomial equation, even though the basic design could still be described as a three-zone lens. The technique was named controlled keratoreformation (CKR).

The major problem with both the CKR and Contex three-zone lenses continued to be centration, or the lack of it. Variations to the total diameter (TD) and reverse curves were made and prism ballast applied, to little effect. Tom Reim totally redesigned reverse geometry lenses, and used a wider peripheral alignment curve to control centration. The reverse curve was narrow (0.60 mm) and steep, and the alignment curve extended to 1.00 mm in width, with a fixed relationship to the corneal surface. The lens was called the Dreimlens and the process renamed "advanced orthokeratology."

At approximately the same time, Mountford redesigned the Contex lenses and added a wide (1.10 mm) tangent periphery in order to control centration better (see Ch. 4). Jim Day (Fargo Lens) varied the Dreimlens concept by dividing the alignment curves into two sections, eventually settling on a hyperbolic alignment zone. He also developed the fitting philosophy that matched the lens back surface area to that of the cornea, and, like Reim and El Hage, used a variation of the Jessen factor as a means of determining the BOZR and refractive change required. Further variations on the Dreimlens theme were developed by Roger Tabb (Nightmove), John Reinhart and Jim Reeves (R&R), George Glady (Emerald and Jade), Nick Stoyan (Contex E series) and Jim Edwards with the WAVE design.

Jerry Leggerton developed the Corneal Refractive Therapy (CRT) design, and changed the reverse curve construction to that of a sigmoid curve, which effectively blends the BOZR to the peripheral curve, which is a tangent. The sigmoid curve is used to alter the sagittal height of the lens, thereby exerting greater control over the fit. Tangents were also used by Mountford and Noack for the Contex T, Ideal series, and BE. The BE is the only four- or five-zone reverse geometry lens that does not base the fitting on the Jessen factor, but instead uses modeled squeeze film forces in the postlens tear layer to determine the optimal tear layer profile for the lens, and thereby the back surface construction.

All these designs have different fitting philosophies, but the fact is that they all do the same job, and no one design is inherently superior to the other, as the underlying mechanisms that make orthokeratology "work" are similar (see Ch. 10). What is different about them is the fitting philosophy, and whether it is keratometry- or topography-based.

Stuart Grant introduced the concept of overnight orthokeratology. Since the lenses required approximately 8 h/day to cause an effective change, he reasoned that the new extended-wear materials should be used and the lens slept in overnight, so that patients could be correction-free for their waking hours. This had major benefits over day-wear orthokeratology for obvious reasons, and became the common form of treatment in Australia as early as 1994. Overnight orthokeratology was a revolutionary concept.

Russell Lowe, a Melbourne-based optometrist, improved the fitting process by taking repeated topography readings on each individual patient and calculating the mean and standard deviation of error of the instrument. This lead to a marked improvement in first-fit success, and by extension, a logical method of refining the fit to correct for adverse outcomes. In the author's opinion, this application of routine experimental procedure to clinical practice was a major step forward.

Finally, no review of the practitioners involved in the development of modern orthokeratology would be complete without referring to Dr Kame.

The late Roger Kame was a universally highly respected clinician who was in constant demand for conferences and continuing education events due to his superb lecturing skills, and his ability to make complex problems easily understood. Along with Todd Winkler, he published the first textbook on accelerated orthokeratology, and coined the term "reverse geometry lenses." In an interview with the author a few years ago, he described his growing interest in the "new" orthokeratology, and his trepidation at being seen to be involved in what was then considered to be a "fringe" practice. However, as his battle with cancer later showed, his courage and determination knew no limits, and he started publicly lecturing on his

experiences with orthokeratology. By being the first mainstream researcher and clinician to do so, he not only raised the profile of orthokeratology, but also increased the growing acceptance of the procedure. The inaugural Roger Kame Memorial Award was presented to Professor Brien Holden at the 2002 Global Orthokeratology Symposium in Toronto, Canada.

THE ACADEMICS

Anecdotes are not science, and anecdotal reports are not proof. Practitioners are limited in their ability to perform research in practice due to the difficulties in ensuring control and the influence of bias. For a procedure like orthokeratology to become accepted, it must be able to prove its claims by subjecting them to independent scrutiny, and that means academic control. Fortunately, many academics have become involved in this type of research, and have added immensely to the science of the subject.

Doug Horner and Sarita Soni (Indiana) were conducting research into the visual and refractive effects of radial keratotomy in the early 1990s when a practitioner told them of his experiences with accelerated orthokeratology. They included a group of orthokeratology patients in their study, and expanded the research to include studies of the short-term corneal response to the lens. They also wrote a chapter on the topic for Bennett & Weissman's *Contact Lens Practice* textbook. Sarita Soni is still deeply involved in orthokeratology research today.

Joshua Joe, Harue Marsden, and Tim Edrington (Southern California) fell under the influence of Roger Kame and studied the changes in visual acuity, refraction and corneal eccentricity with the Contex OK–3.

In Hong Kong, Lui and Edwards performed the first controlled study of orthokeratology with reverse geometry lenses and compared the results to those of a control group fitted with standard contour lenses. Under the leadership of Pauline Cho, the Hong Kong Poly-U continues to do excellent research into the differences in performance between lens designs, corneal topography, and its influence on the outcomes and myopia control with orthokeratology.

Helen Swarbrick, Gunther Wong, and Dan O'Leary from the University of New South Wales published the results of a breakthrough study that showed that the refractive changes were mainly due to epithelial thinning. Helen continues to be involved in orthokeratology research, with Masters student Ram Sridharan studying the changes in corneal shape, thickness, refraction, and visual acuity to short-term exposure to lens wear.

Ahmed Alharbi studied the long-term predictability and safety as well as the refractive and corneal changes to overnight orthokeratology as part of his PhD thesis. In Melbourne, Christa Bara studied the effects of changes in the depth of the postlens tear layer at the BOZD on the refraction, visual acuity, and topography of a group of subjects, and in New Zealand, Helen Owens and Jennifer Craig are involved in evaluating the endothelial curvature changes and the effect, if any, of corneal bending on the outcome.

The Cornea and Contact Lens Research Unit (CCLRU) has recently become involved in orthokeratology research, with Nina Tahhan leading a group examining the differences in results between lens designs.

Joe Barr at Ohio State led the group consisting of Nicholls, Marsich, Nguyen, and Bullimore that published the first study on the efficacy of overnight orthokeratology, and is involved in the LOOK study with Marjorie Rah, John Mark Jackson, Ed Bennett, and Harue Marsden.

As Editor of *Contact Lens Spectrum*, Joe Barr has been at the forefront of promoting education and awareness of the rapid changes occurring in the field. Along with Ed Bennett, Pat Caroline, and Craig Norman, he organized the highly successful Global Orthokeratology Symposium in Toronto in August 2002.

In Canada, Des Fonn's group is studying the topographical thickness changes across the corneal surface, and in the UK, Trusit Dave is supervising research into methods of measuring the apical clearance of lenses in situ as well as the ocular aberrations induced by reverse geometry lenses. Nathan Efron's Eurolens group at Manchester has also started orthokeratology research – a most welcome development!

One of the frustrations of writing this book has been knowing about the research being undertaken, and some of the results being generated, yet being unable to put anything in print due to confidentiality agreements. However, many academics freely made available the results of their research prior to publication, and the author's thanks goes to Helen Swarbrick, Gavin Boneham, and especially Pauline Cho for their generous assistance.

Orthokeratology research is also being done in China, with numerous papers being published in the *Chinese Journal of Optometry and Ophthalmology*. The difficulties associated with translation have prevented their wider availability, but where applicable, the results of the studies have been included in the text.

The result of all this research effort will be improved designs and, hopefully, the ability to improve the predictability of orthokeratology, as well as a much better understanding of the anatomical, physiological, and visual changes that occur. There are a lot of unanswered questions in a host of areas in orthokeratology, requiring a prolonged research effort to resolve. The areas that require future research are outlined in the final chapter.

THE COMPUTER PROGRAMMERS

The design and fitting of reverse geometry lenses require the use of advanced mathematics, which is not usually accessible to the private practitioner. Specialized computer programs are required for the calculations, and the outstanding architects of these advanced tools are undoubtedly Don Noack and Tom Geimer. Don Noack wrote the complex platform that is used to fit BE lenses, and the Free Design program, and Tom Geimer wrote Ortho-Tools. These are an excellent teaching and learning resource, and an outline of both programs is covered in Chapter 8.

THE MATERIAL COMPANIES

As stated before, for a new procedure to become really accepted, it must first prove itself to be effective at the hands of objective researchers, and secondly, gain Food and Drug Administration (FDA) approval so that it is available in the US market. Also, the FDA stamp of approval has a high international standing, and can affect the acceptance of the process in other markets. The funding for this research and the costs involved in gaining FDA approval are usually borne by the companies that manufacture the materials from which the lenses will be made. Both Polymer Technology Corporation and Paragon Vision Sciences have been at the forefront of these efforts, both by developing the high-*Dk* materials required (Boston XO and Paragon HDS 100), and also by sponsoring much of the research currently underway. They have also been heavily involved in the FDA approval process. They are deeply committed to marketing orthokeratology worldwide, and were major sponsors of the Global Orthokeratology Symposium.

TERMINOLOGY

The International Standards Organization (ISO) has compiled a complete list of terms that describe in full every aspect of contact lens design. Unfortunately, these terms have been largely ignored by orthokeratology lens designers and manufacturers, and substituted by other names for the various curves in order to differentiate their particular design from all the others. This leads to unfortunate and unnecessary confusion. The following section is a glossary of common terms used in orthokeratology, with reference to the ISO 8320 (British Standards Institute 1995) edition.

Back optic zone radius (BOZR)

The radius of curvature of the back optic diameter of a lens with a single refracting surface is called the BOZR. It is given the common misnomer of "base curve" or back central optic radius, which actually denotes the back central optic radius of a multifocal lens. ISO measures BOZR in millimeters, but American labs and practitioners usually denote the radius in its equivalent dioptric power. This is done by dividing 337.5 by the BOZR in millimeters.

Back optic zone diameter (BOZD)

This is defined as the diameter over which the BOZR acts. Other terminologies used are the back optic zone (BOZ) or simply OZ. The BOZDs of four- and five-zone lenses range from a minimum of 5.50 mm to 6.50 mm, with 6.00 mm the most common.

First back peripheral radius (BPR$_1$)

The curve immediately adjacent to the BOZR is BPR$_1$. In orthokeratology terms, it is commonly known as either the "tear reservoir (TR) curve" or "reverse curve (RC)." It is usually measured by its degree of steepening compared to the BOZR, and expressed in diopters, i.e., 3.00 D steeper than BOZR. Other lens-specific terms are return curve (CKR) and sigmoid curve (CRT). The majority of manufacturers do not disclose the value of the reverse curve.

First back peripheral diameter (BPD$_1$)

This denotes the width of the BPR$_1$. Equivalent terms are TR width and RC width. In the majority of four- and five-zone lenses, this value is fixed and is commonly between 0.50 and 1.00 mm wide, depending on the design.

Second and third back peripheral radii (BPR$_2$ and BPR$_3$)

In standard lens designs, these curves represent that part of the lens commonly referred to as the "edge lift." However, in orthokeratology designs, these curves represent curves that are designed to come into near-alignment with the corneal surface and effect control over lens centration. They are usually referred to as the "alignment curves (AC)" or zones. A four-zone lens will have a single AC that is usually 1.00 mm wide, and spherical, aspheric, or hyperbolic in construction. Tangents (flats) can also be used as alignment zones. Synonyms are "anchor zone" (CKR) and "landing zone" (CRT). Alternatively, a five-zone lens has two ACs, with the first being slightly steeper than the second. The total width is still approximately 1.00 mm, with each curve being half of the total.

Fourth back peripheral radius (BPR$_4$)

This is the final curve on the back surface of a reverse geometry lens and is commonly referred to as the "edge lift" or peripheral curve (PC). It is commonly 0.30–0.50 mm wide on the majority of lenses.

In general, the nomenclature of a four-zone lens is the BOZR, RC, AC, and PC, whilst a five-zone lens consists of BOZR, RC, AC$_1$, AC$_2$, and the PC. Alternatively, lenses such as the CRT have BOZR, sigmoid curve, tangent, and PC, whilst the BE has BOZR, RC$_1$, RC$_2$, tangent, and PC. The construction of a five-zone lens is shown in profile in Figure 1.2.

Tear reservoir

As stated above, the TR is used to describe the steepening of the RC with respect to the BOZR. It

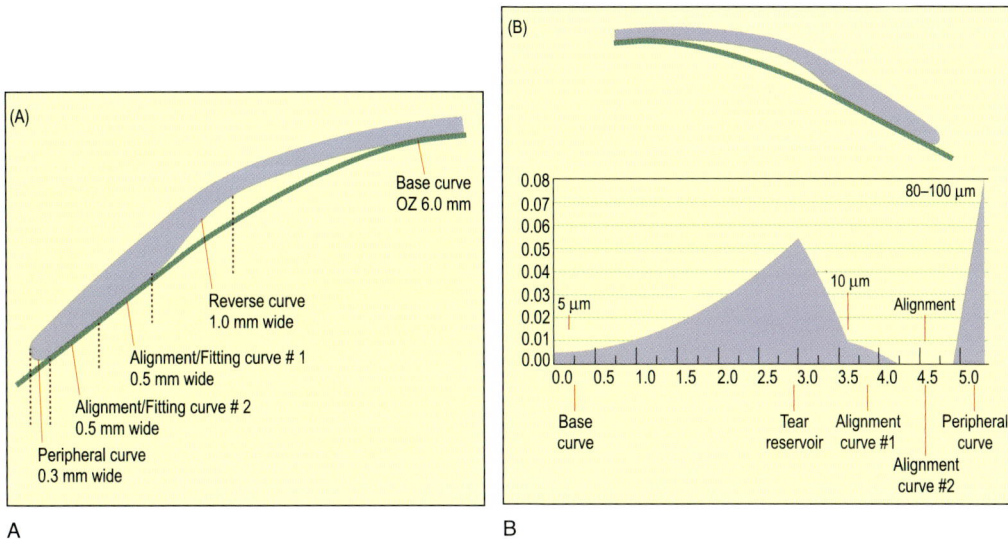

Figure 1.2 Construction of a five-zone lens. (A) Clearances and widths of the zones on the lens back surface; (B) side profile of the lens on the eye, with its associated tear layer profile. Courtesy of Patrick Caroline.

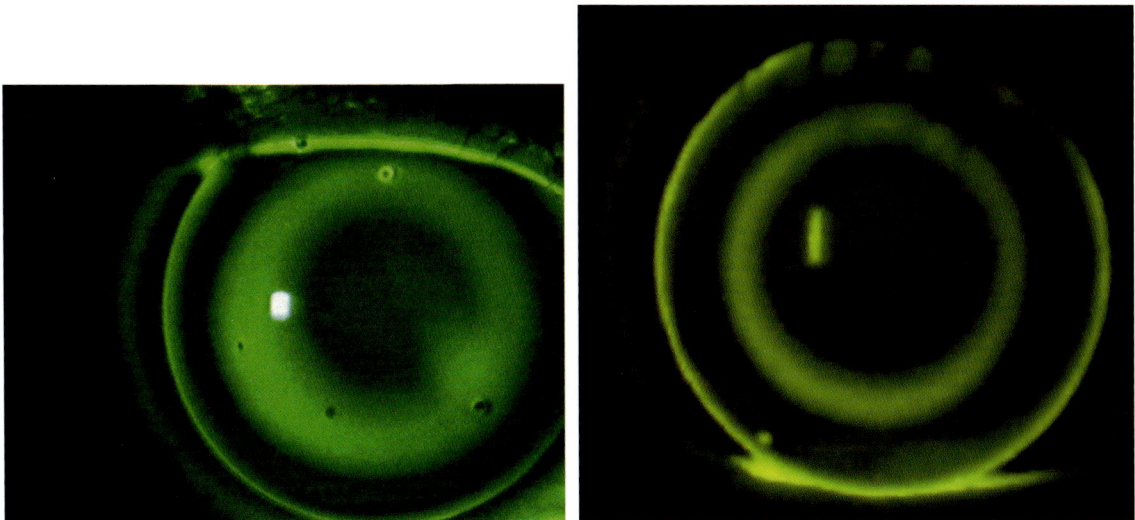

Figure 1.3 The fluorescein patterns of (A) a three-zone lens showing a deep and wide tear reservoir and (B) a four-zone lens with a narrow and deep tear reservoir.

is also used to describe the appearance of the annulus of tears at the BOZD/RC junction. The earlier Contex three-zone lenses, for example, usually showed deep and wide tear reservoirs, whilst the newer four- and five-zone lenses exhibit narrow and deep reservoirs (Fig. 1.3).

Central touch zone

Reverse geometry lenses, when fitted correctly, show an area of "central touch" over the pupil zone. The term "touch" may be a misnomer, as the tear layer present under the lens at the apex is less than the 20 μm that is usually accepted as the minimal thickness at which fluorescein becomes visible under a lens. However, the area and centration of the touch with respect to the pupil center are used as a means of determining the relative accuracy of the lens fit.

Corneal sag and elevation

The sagittal height (z) of the cornea is the vertical distance from a line joining the common point of

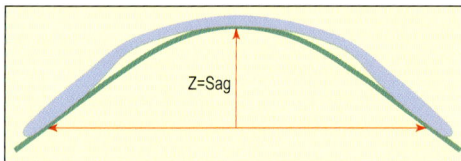

Figure 1.4 The sagittal height (z) of the cornea from the chord over which it is measured.

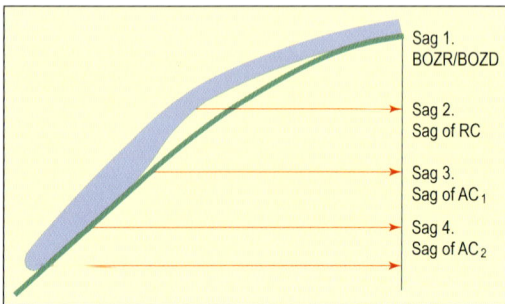

Figure 1.5 The sag height of a reverse geometry lens is equal to the sags of the individual curves over their respective diameters. BOZR, back optic zone radius; BOZD, back optic zone diameter; RC, reverse curve; AC, alignment curve.

interest on the corneal surface (the chord) to the apex of the cornea (Fig. 1.4). This term is then linked to the sag height of the lens (see later). Topographers, however, measure elevation, which is the measurement from the corneal apex to the chord of reference. The two terms result in identical measurements, and are basically synonyms.

Lens sag

A contact lens prescription is usually written as a means of specifying the radii and diameters of the varying curves that make up the design. Lens sag is simply the sagittal height of each of the individual zones of the lens added together (Fig. 1.5). As can be seen from the diagram, the sag of the lens is equal to the sag of the BOZR/BOZD, plus the sag of the RC over its width, and the sags of the alignment curves. The sag of a lens is commonly only measured to the diameter that represents the common chord of contact between the lens and the corneal surface (see Ch. 4).

Jessen factor

Jessen's original orthofocus technique consisted of making the radius of the BOZR equal to the refractive change required, using the general rule of 0.20 mm difference in radii being clinically equivalent to 1 D. Therefore, a 3.00 D refractive error would result in the lens being fitted with the BOZR 3.00 D (0.60 mm) flatter than the flat-K reading. All current four- and five-zone lenses, with the exception of the BE, use a variation of the Jessen factor as a means of determining the refractive change required and the BOZR of the lens. The variation is an extra increase in flattening of the BOZR as a "compression factor" and ranges from zero to 1.00 D.

Clearance factor

The term was originally coined by Noack to describe the difference in tear layer thickness between the apex of the cornea and the maximum tear layer depth at the edge of the BOZD. A lens with an apical clearance of 5 μm and a tear layer thickness of 65 μm at the BOZD would therefore have a clearance factor of 60 μm. Clearance factor is also used to describe the tear layer thickness at various points away from the corneal apex, such as at the RC/AC interface (Fig. 1.2B).

Cone angles

Cone angles are used to describe a tangent periphery. A tangent is a flat or straight line and does not have a radius of curvature. Instead, the angle that the tangent makes with the optic axis is termed the cone angle (see Ch. 4 for the construction of tangents). Tangents are used in some orthokeratology lens designs to control lens centration.

Bull's eye

The term "bull's eye" is used to describe the fluorescein pattern of an ideally fitting reverse geometry lens. However, it is most commonly used to describe the appearance of the post-

wear topography map of an ideal response to the wear of the lens (Fig. 1.6). The map shows a well-centered area of central corneal flattening, surrounded by a zone of steepening and little or no change in the peripheral corneal shape.

Smiley face

A "smiley-face" topography plot results when the lens fit is effectively too flat. The lens decenters superiorly, with the resulting topography difference map showing a crescent-shaped area of steepening within the pupil zone, and the area of apical flattening decentered upwards (Fig. 1.7). This is an unacceptable outcome of lens wear, and the fit must be adjusted.

Central island

A "central island" postwear topography plot indicates that the lens is effectively too steep. The difference map shows a perfectly centered area of central corneal steepening that is approximately 2.00 mm in diameter, surrounded by a

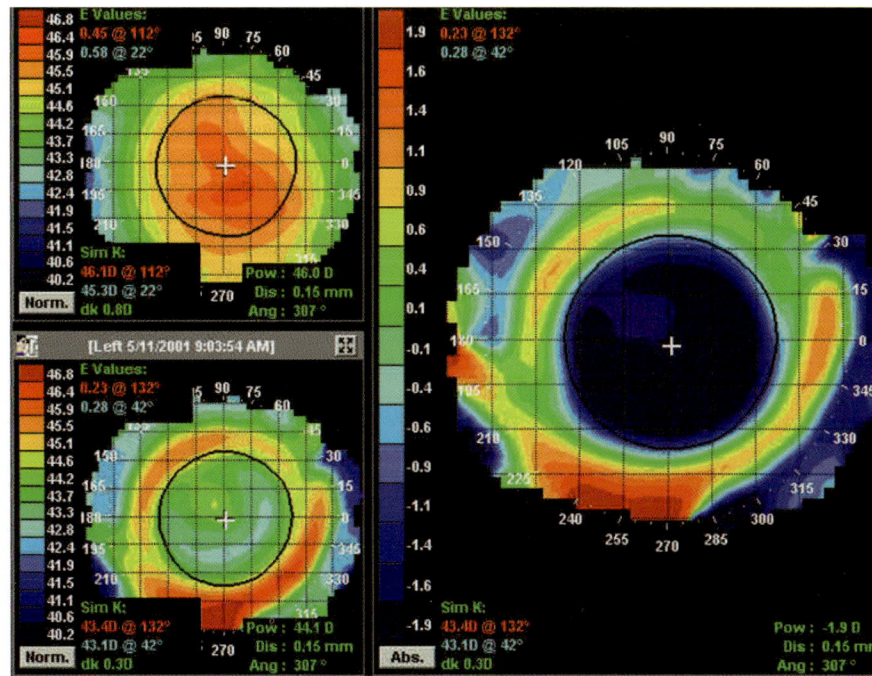

Figure 1.6 A bull's eye topography plot. The top left is prefit and bottom left is postwear, with the subtractive difference shown on the right-hand side.

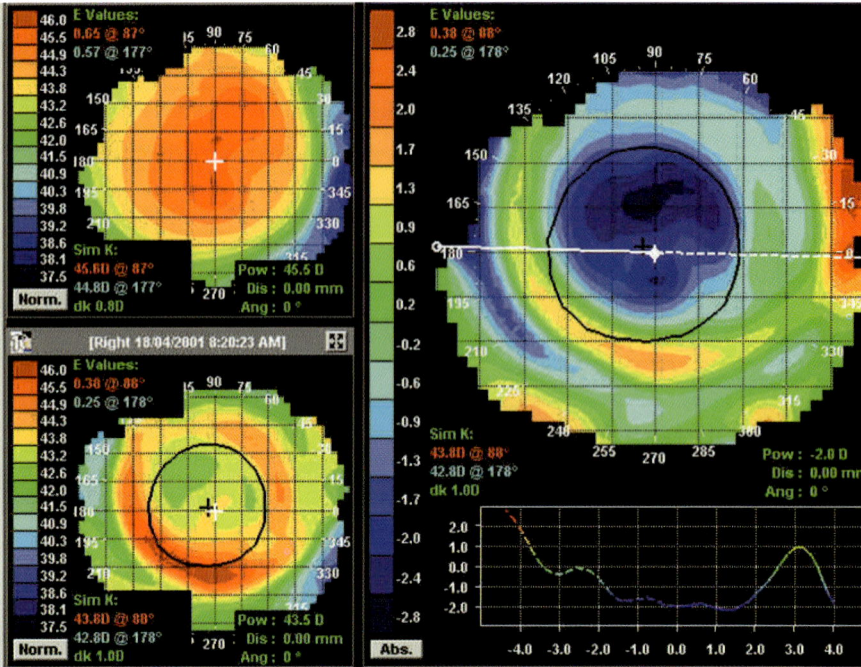

Figure 1.7 A smiley-face topography plot. Note the inferior crescent of steepening, and the off-center position of the flattened zone.

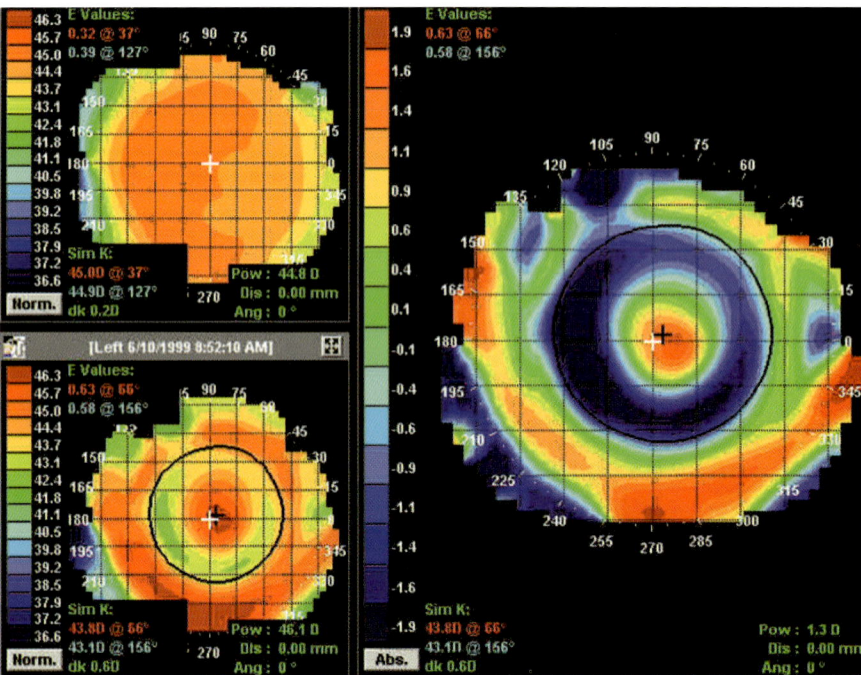

Figure 1.8 A central island topography plot.

"moat" of marked flattening, which is followed by the annulus of steepening (Fig. 1.8). The peripheral cornea usually shows an area of distortion from a tight alignment zone. The best corrected visual acuity (BCVA) is adversely affected by central islands, and they must be resolved in order for a

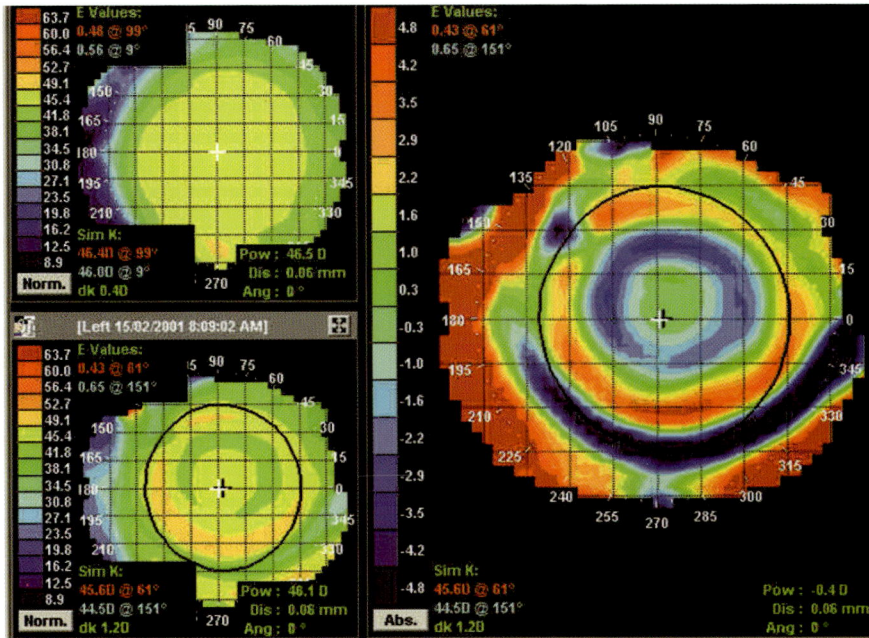

Figure 1.9 A smiley-face pattern with a fake central island.

correct outcome to occur. Clinical experience shows that there are two types of central island. In some cases, the island is flatter than the original corneal apex, but still steeper than the surrounding corneal area. These types may resolve within the first week of lens wear, and should be considered to be incomplete bull's-eye plots. In other cases, however, the island is appreciably steeper than the original corneal curve. These will not resolve with time, and require a refit of the lens.

Smiley face with fake central island

A lens that is excessively flat will decenter and cause a smiley-face pattern as well as central corneal staining. The resulting distortion of the topographer mires leads to inaccuracies in the reconstruction algorithm, resulting in the appearance of a steep island. In these cases, the plots will show both a smiley face and a central island (Fig. 1.9). It is the decentration of the area of paracentral steepening that confirms the diagnosis of a flat-fitting lens, with the central island simply indicating that the lens is excessively flat.

A full description of the topography outcomes following lens wear is given in Chapter 6.

Treatment zone diameter

The area of effective corneal flattening is called the treatment zone (T×Z). It is defined as the chord at which there is no change from the original corneal surface when the *refractive power* subtractive map is used. The cursor is moved from the center to the nasal side until the dioptric change is equal to zero, and the distance noted. The process is repeated for the temporal side. The addition of the two values is the T×Z.

Ring jam

Disruption of the epithelial surface (or tear film) leads to distortion and "crowding" of the topographer mires. This can occur centrally and, in the case of an extremely tight alignment curve, in the peripheral cornea. Excessive distortion of the mires, leading to either gaps in the continuity of the image, or adjacent mire reflections actually coming into contact with each other, leads to a breakdown in the ability of the reconstruction algorithm to determine the correct localized curvature accurately. The reconstructed map therefore shows areas of marked steepening or

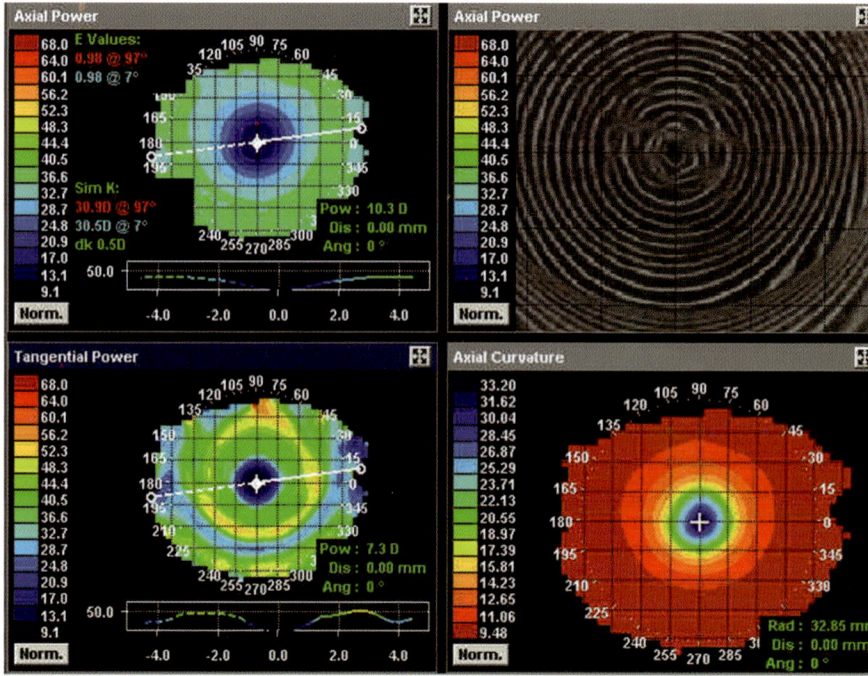

Figure 1.10   Ring jam. Note the distortion of the central mires. The map shows a small area of marked central flattening, which is a totally inaccurate representation of the data.

flattening with respect to the adjacent corneal area, and is a totally inaccurate representation of the surface (Fig. 1.10). This phenomenon is commonly called "ring jam."

Night therapy

Night therapy is the use of orthokeratology lenses only at night, with no lens wear required for the normal waking hours. It is also known as "night-wear orthokeratology."

In other areas, the usual nomenclature used to describe the corneal response to lens wear and the associated pathological terminologies are still used in orthokeratology. The simple fact is that the ISO definitions are relatively clumsy terms, and the simple expediency of using terms such as RC, AC, and so on does tend to make communications between practitioners more immediate, without the necessity to "translate" what is meant. It would appear that the above terms have become entrenched in orthokeratology circles in preference to the ISO equivalents, but as long as a common language is used, confusion should be minimal.

AIMS AND OBJECTIVES OF THIS BOOK

The problem with writing a book on this subject is trying to get specific information about each of the designs, as most manufacturers and designers treat their lenses as intellectual property and proprietary information. To describe the lenses in the manufacturer's terms would simply lead to an "advertorial" on each, which is of little value. The approach, therefore, has been to describe the underlying mathematical principles involved in the construction and fitting of orthokeratology lenses in a generic manner, with specific mention of the designs as needed.

There are basic underlying concepts, such as sag fitting, surface area matching and lens construction, that are common to all the different lens types. The aim of this book is therefore to demonstrate these underlying principles from the initial mathematical basis through to the actual application of fitting. If the concepts and formulae in the text are applied, it is possible for practitioners not only to design their own lenses, but also to be able to resolve any fitting difficulties that occur when proprietary lens designs are used.

There is a pronounced emphasis on the role of corneal topography throughout the text. The authors are convinced, from both a scientific and clinical viewpoint, that topography is essential to the correct fitting and aftercare of the orthokeratology patient. The keratometer simply cannot supply the information required to fit the lenses accurately or monitor the changes, and should be treated as inferior technology. The authors consider that the practice of orthokeratology without topography may be unethical. Topography-based orthokeratology is the "gold standard" of practice and every patient deserves to receive this level of service.

Wherever possible, the results of controlled research have been used to specify factors such as refractive change and visual acuity improvements. There are anecdotal remarks, but they are mainly concerned with the approaches to problem-solving that have been found to work in practice. Anecdotal remarks concerning fitting, aftercare, problem-solving, and other areas were only included when all authors agreed on the statement, with further corroboration sought from other experts in the field as required.

The author, like most optometry students of the 1970s, was taught that orthokeratology was a strange American pastime that "really didn't work." In 1992, Harris & Stoyan published a report on the "new" accelerated technique which caught the author's eye. A project was planned to fit 20 volunteers with the lenses, prove that it didn't work, and publish the results. Of the 20 volunteers, 11 achieved unaided acuity of 6/5 (20/15) in both eyes. The question then arose: why didn't it work on the other nine? One could simply have published a paper on the results and moved on, but there is something indescribable about the experience of having a patient remove a lens and read the 6/5 line unaided, with a look of absolute amazement, that is somehow addictive. Ten years on, and we still don't know all the answers to the myriad of questions that orthokeratology raises. Why does it work? How does it work? What changes in the cornea? What are the physiological, visual and physical effects, the limits, the dangers? How is it *controlled*?

What is known is that the attempt to answer these and other questions leads to areas of study concerning the mathematical basis of corneal shape, lens design, and corneal topography that have had a massive effect on all other areas of contact lens practice. Trying to understand orthokeratology and its lens designs opens new vistas to the possibilities of advanced lens designs for other applications such as postgraft and refractive surgery cases that were not available before. All this benefits the patient. There is no more satisfying specialty than orthokeratology.

REFERENCES

Bara C (2000) Mechanism of action of the reverse geometry gas permeable contact lens in orthokeratology. M.Sc. Thesis, University of Melbourne

British Standards Institute (1995) Contact lens standards. ISO 8320

Carney L G (1994) Orthokeratology. Chapter 37. In Rubin M, Guillon M (eds) Contact lens practice. Chapman and Hall Medical, London

Coon L (1982) Orthokeratology, Part 1: Historical perspectives. Journal of the American Optometric Association 53: 187–195

Harris D, Stoyan N (1992) A new approach to orthokeratology. Contact Lens Spectrum 7(4): 37–39

Kerns R (1976) Research in orthokeratology, Part 7. Journal of the American Optometric Association 48: 1541–1553

Mountford J A (1997) Orthokeratology. In: Phillips A J, Speedwell L (eds) Contact lenses: a textbook for students and practitioner, vol. 4. London, Butterworths

Nolan J (1995) Flashback: the first ortho-K meeting. Contacto 38(4): 9–14

Soni P S, Horner D J (1993) Orthokeratology. In: Bennett E S, Weissman B A (eds) Clinical contact lens practice. J B Lippincott, Philadelphia, pp 49-1–49-7

Wlodyga R J, Bryla C (1989) Corneal molding; the easy way. Contact Lens Spectrum 4(58): 14–16

The first meeting of the International Orthokeratology Society, 13 October 1962

Transcript supplied by Joseph Nolan, OD, FIOS

As chairman of this first meeting, Dr. George N. Jessen called the session together at 7.30 p.m. After some introductory remarks, he reported on his experience with the techniques of "ortho-focus." In his opinion there were many instances in which hyperopia, myopia, and astigmatism of the cornea could be changed towards emmetropia by attempting to mold the cornea with a contact lens.

His technique was to fit steeper in the hyper-ope and flatter in the case of myopia. Dr. Jessen also stated that he feels in most patients with ammetropia of a noninflammatory nature the eyelids are largely responsible for the myopic pressure exerted on the eye.

The eyelid pressure can increase the intraocular pressure to 40–60 mmHg as compared with 6–7 mmHg increase due to the extrinsic ocular muscles upon strong convergence. Myopes who continue to progress after being fit with contact lenses are those who still squint, despite the lenses.

Those who do not progress have their eyes wide open. Most younger people have astigmatism with-the-rule, while most older people have against-the-rule. Why? Is this due to the change in eyelid condition due to the pressure as muscle tissue ages and tone decreases or the increased scleral rigidity? The lids do not bend the cornea as much as previously.

One millimeter of bend or change in corneal radius equals 6 D. Those who have done scleral buckling in retinal surgery have changed the eye as much as 4, 5, and 6 mm, proving that the eye is malleable.

Jessen started using the "ortho-focus" technique following a request from a friend – a recruiting officer for the Merchant Marine Academy. Some of the applicants for the academy qualified except for visual acuity of 20/40 or 20/50. What could be done to correct the acuity? Some were corrected by ortho-optics. On another occasion, a potential football player and also an applicant to the academy had a −3.00 D correction and an acuity of 20/400. He had to have 20/25 unaided. What could be done?

Jessen did not promise but went ahead and fitted the boy flatter than K and plano correction. After 3 months of wear, he had obtained the needed 20/25 acuity. Jessen wrote the Navy telling them of what he was doing. They did not object. The boy is now attending the academy. Whenever he has to take a test he wears his "ortho-focus" for 2 or 3 days, then takes his test and has 20/20 acuity. The boy was certified before and after the original fitting by an ophthalmologist.

Jessen said he finds it easier to work with hyperopes and astigmats than with myopes. The hyperopes and astigmats are fitted with spherical bases steeper than K. He can then get a swelling of the cornea into the lens and they see very well. The myope is more difficult and should be fitted younger. Jessen cited the case of Dr. Joseph Cinefro's son. He put on "ortho-focus" lenses when he manifested 0.50 D of myopia. Lenses should be put on as young as possible: 7, 8, or 9 years of age.

A typical example is a child who fails an eye test at school. Parents tell him they don't want glasses on their child. Jessen is then able to offer them this alternative of "ortho-focus" contacts and hold a normal curvature like braces on the teeth, or the child can be fitted with glasses. It is the parents' choice to make.

A −2.00 D myope can be fitted 2.00 D flatter than K with plano correction. A plus 2.00 D hyperope would be fitted with 2.00 D steeper than K with plano correction. An astigmat could be fitted with a Cycon with prism, of opposite curves, or the astigmatic cornea could be fitted with a spherical lens.

Jessen said we are finally approaching the possibility of wiping out low refractive errors. He did not think it would be possible to correct high amounts of myopia or correct aphakic patients. He estimated that 90% of ammetropic patients had less than 3.00 D. He concluded his talk by saying that we now have a good chance of correcting these conditions. He then opened the meeting for discussion.

Dr. Robert Koetting asked: why don't we try to correct the high myope, or the patient with the large refractive error? Dr. Jessen answered by stating that these are pathological: those that have −12 to −15 D have signs of chorioretinitis – they show large myopic crescents. He did not think that correction should be attempted on such patients. Koetting said we should investigate the factors involved in changing the cornea so that we can proceed on a sound basis.

Another fitter stated that whenever he fitted a patient and the cornea became steeper, especially in the center, that they experienced discomfort. Jessen replied that all he knew was that when his hyperopic patients, when fitted with a deCarle bifocal with a steep central zone, removed their lenses, they invariably saw better without correction than they previously did. They are confident the phenomenon is due to their contact lenses.

It was suggested that we as fitters should do some basic research, rather than wait 10 years for results to explain what happened 10 years before. We could establish where the corneal swelling with clarity ends and swelling with cloudiness begins. He estimated it would take about a year to conduct this study, that such a study could be sponsored by the National Eye Research Foundation.

Physiologists and men at the universities should partake in this study and also study the chemistry of the aqueous and the cornea that might cause one cornea to be more malleable than another.

Dr. Jessen stated that Dr. Schick of Indiana University is conducting basic research on myopia and contact lenses. [Dr. Schick replied, but the first few sentences are not discernible.] Dr. Schick asked Dr. Jessen how he could dare to change a pilot's corneas when the lives of 100 passengers are entrusted to his care? Dr. Jessen said that the pilot wears his glasses on the field and in the airplane and contact lenses only prior to testing unaided visual acuity – to achieve a temporary flattening of the cornea. Following his answer, there was a heated discussion concerning the laws and regulations as opposed to what is right. A pilot with normal acuity with glasses can be every bit as good as a pilot with 20/20 without glasses.

Dr. Sharp asked Dr. Schick: "What can we do then as an alternative?" Dr. Shick said: "There must be a better way." Dr. Sharp again asked, "What way?" Dr. Middleton then interrupted: "By the way, what are we discussing here? Morality or contact lenses?"

There was much laughter at this broadside. He chided the group that Dr. Schick was entitled to be heard. Furthermore, like it or not, when we attempt to change the corneal contour we are dealing with physiology. He continued with remarks illustrating his point. He then turned the discussion over to Dr. Schick who continued with remarks illustrating his point.

Dr. Schick said that most of our errors are not due to corneal changes. How do we know we are working on the right thing when we work on the cornea? What is the cause of the error? By reducing hydraulic pressure in the eyes, the myopia might be reduced. By increasing this pressure, the eyeball length could increase.

Dr. Newton K. Wesley then rose to his feet and began to speak. He told of coining the title of "orthokeratology" as opposed to the term "ortho-focus." He told of always having been afraid of corneal distortion, that his own left eye had been diagnosed as keratoconic and his right eye had not. He then wore a scleral lens 3 h and in that short time developed keratoconus in his right eye. His ophthalmologist stated that it would have developed in any event.

But how could it develop in 3 h? Wesley reminded the group that fluid lenses distort the eye tremendously. He also cited the Indian tribe that deliberately reshaped the skull, thereby influencing the shape and growth of the brain. He then discussed the particular patients fitted with Feinbloom tangent cone lenses: a –4.00 D myope who then went to –11.00 D while wearing the lenses. Dr. Wesley took away the lenses and a month elapsed before the eye returned to normal.

He also spoke of another patient, Dave Pattis, who wore scleral fluid lenses day and night for 3 years. He developed pannus, opacities, and his vision went from 20/20 to 20/200 – his Rx went from –5 D to about –13.00 D. Upon removal of the lenses, his eyes returned to normal and were free of irregularities and his Rx was again –5.00 D 1 month later.

Dr. Wesley continued by saying we have all fitted flatter in keratoconus cases. He gave an example of where he, Dr. Zekman, and Evelyn Corral molded keratoconic eyes before and after fitting with contacts. The change in curvature averaged 1.50 D flatter than the original curves after using base curves of 4–5 D flatter. If we could do this with weak and diseased eyes, the chances are that we could do the same with normal eyes. "Is there one amongst you who has not distorted an eye in fitting?" Wesley asked. Remember that microlenses were 2.50–6.00 D flatter than K. This is the history of contact lenses – not just a few hundred cases, but hundreds of thousands and millions of patients.

He agreed with all that was said about basic research, but he wanted to know how much we can change the corneal curve and how we change it. What about the changes in corneal structure, not just curvature? The changes in acuity – not the letters, but the flares, dispersion, and polyopia. The pressure changes – does the pressure go up, go down or does it stay the same? The amount of edema: what happens to the corneal topography; hyperopic and myopic control; amblyopia? There are many subjects we can cover.

He told of his strong interest in myopia, that it was one of the reasons he went into optometry. When you consider that myopia can be a change of the front or back surface of the crystalline lens, you are going to have to prove which one of the surfaces change if you say that this is the cause of the myopia. Or, you must say they stay the same

and that the myopia is caused by something else. You will also have to be able to measure accurately the distance from the fovea to the front of the eye, from the front of the cornea to the back of the cornea, from the front to the back of the crystalline lens. You must be able to measure these distances, because a change in one of these distances causes the myopia. We also have index myopia – we must establish indices – we do not even have instrumentation to measure myopia in any of these forms except for the keratometer.

Continuing, Wesley said that the variables of measurement have to be established – that is basic research. He agreed with all the statements made by Schick and Koetting that this basic research must be done. Individual cases do not prove anything – where were the controls? We have too many records which prove that controls were not established. He gave an example of orthodonture, that the changes are made very gradually.

Turning the discussion to creating a new name for the group, he suggested Society of Orthokeratology as opposed to Ortho-Focus. He then suggested we should set up certain research projects, especially in the problem of myopia.

A general discussion followed on the choice of title for the group as to its correctness in describing what is accomplished by fitting using this concept.

Dr. Schick was elected president. The following men were named but no particular office was given to them. Dr. Charles May, Dr. Middleton, Dr. Victor Arias, and Dr. Koetting. Dr. Jessen agreed to be secretary. Dr. Middleton suggested that Dr. Wesley be a counselor to the society, but he should not be part of a committee. The assembled members agreed to annual dues of $5.00 per year. Jessen duly recorded each name.

The meeting concluded with a statement of our aim: that we are dedicated to the prevention and correction of ammetropia and attendant visual problems.

Editor's note: This manuscript was adapted from two tape recordings, transcribed by Dr. Sharp. Some sections of the tape were not discernible, could not be transcribed, or background noise made individual dialogue impossible to ascertain.

Chapter 2

Corneal topography and its measurement

Trusit Dave

CHAPTER CONTENTS

Introduction 17
Historical overview 18
Computer-assisted videokeratography 19
Design factors 24
Algorithms in videokeratoscopy 29
Corneal power displays 33
Summary 44
References 45

INTRODUCTION

The cornea is the most powerful refractive surface of the eye, accounting for almost two-thirds of its total optical power. Measurement of its shape has an important role in a variety of optometric and ophthalmological techniques, such as contact lens fitting and refractive surgery. Furthermore, evaluating sequential changes in corneal topography with time has an important role in monitoring corneal pathologies, contact lens-induced changes, refractive surgery, and orthokeratology. More recently, with the development of modern-day computer systems, researchers have been able to process large amounts of information and this has enabled the reconstruction of the cornea using detailed models.

Currently, most eye-care practitioners use the keratometer to determine central corneal curvature. There are numerous limitations when this method is applied to techniques such as screening for keratoconus and surgical or nonsurgical keratoreformation. The principal reasons are that the keratometer does not resolve peripheral corneal power, only paracentral. The keratometer is often described as an instrument that derives central corneal curvature; this loose term is an incorrect description. Furthermore, in deriving the corneal curvature, the keratometer assumes that the cornea is spherical. Therefore, greater errors in paracentral curvature arise with surfaces of increasing asphericity.

Numerous methods have been proposed in order to calculate the topography of the cornea. However, the success of these methods depends

Table 2.1   Expected accuracy of central radius of curvature measurements as derived by Stone (1962)

Actual corneal radius	7.84 mm
Measurement of cornea assuming accuracy of ± 0.02 mm	7.82–7.86 mm
Nearest contact lens fit	7.80 or 7.85 mm
Actual lens radius assuming accuracy of ± 0.02 mm	7.78–7.82 mm or 7.83–7.87 mm
Maximum error between cornea and lens	0.06 mm

ultimately on their accuracy, repeatability, and ease of use. The accuracy of an instrument may be defined according to the tolerance that is expected when the instrument is to be used for a clinical function. For purposes such as contact lens fitting, Stone (1962) has stated that the radius of curvature should be measured within ± 0.02 mm. Table 2.1 shows how the expected accuracy of radius of curvature was derived by Stone (1962).

In addition, repeatability may be defined as the ability of an instrument to reproduce the same measurement on two independent occasions when no change in the structure to be measured has taken place.

HISTORICAL OVERVIEW

The first development in the assessment of gross corneal topography was the keratoscopic disk by Placido in 1880. This simple hand-held instru-

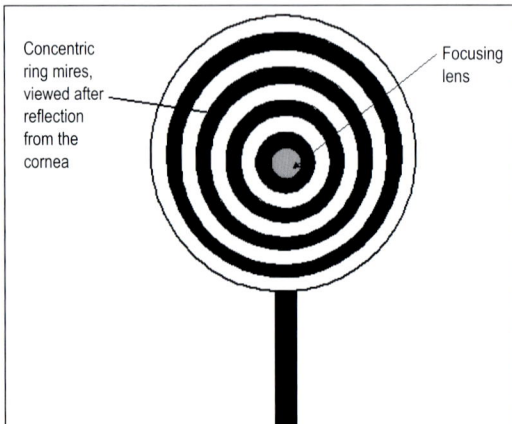

Figure 2.1   Placido disk concentric ring target.

ment was used for observation rather than actual measurement of corneal contour (Fig. 2.1). The following valuable information may be derived from the Placido disk:

- corneal toricity
- the approximate location of the principal meridians
- gross changes in shape
- localized surface irregularities
- the approximate position of the corneal apex with respect to the line of sight.

Information of this nature would be of great use in clinical practice, particularly if a hard copy could be made, such as a photographic recording. Gullstrand (Ludlum et al 1967) was one of the first investigators to introduce the photokeratoscope. Many new designs have emerged – all of which have attempted to measure a larger area of the cornea by using various shaped targets. Gullstrand used a plane object surface, which prevented larger areas of corneal surface being measured. Nevertheless, he found that the normal individual had a smooth corneal surface that flattened away from the corneal apex. Later, using a flat object of tangential design, measurements of up to 7 mm in diameter were obtained (Fincham 1953). Knoll et al (1957) used a hemispherical or cylindrical object surface that enabled an area of 10 mm of corneal surface to be measured. The advantage of using an object of hemispherical design was that the size of the target was much reduced, thus making the instrument less bulky (Fig. 2.2).

Ludlum et al (1967) considered the limitations of photokeratoscopes at that time. Three suggestions were made from their study:

- The image plane (located behind the cornea) should be flat. This point is particularly important with respect to the design of a target for the following reason: if the image lies on a curved image plane, then there will be one point of focus on the flat plane of the photographic film. Ludlum et al (1967) found that, for an ellipsoidal target surface, the image from a spherical reflecting surface lay on a flat plane.
- The analysis of the data should be detailed and accurate. Numerous methods have been adopted to calculate the parameters describing

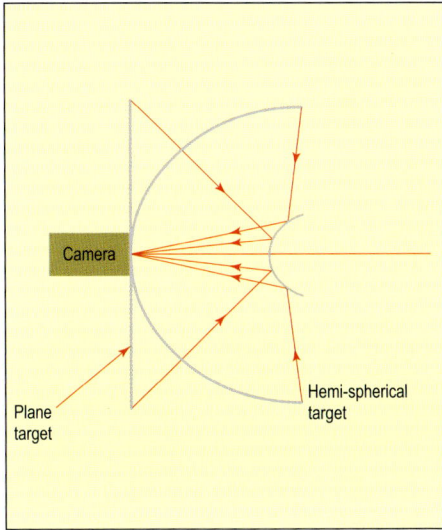

Figure 2.2 The difference in area of corneal surface measured for a plane target and a hemispherical target.

the corneal profile; the various techniques are discussed later in this chapter.

- There should be accurate and reproducible alignment of the patient's line of sight with that of the instrument. Accurate alignment is necessary in order to position the vertex normal of the cornea (that point on the corneal surface that is perpendicular to the keratoscope axis when the subject is viewing the fixation target) relative to the line of sight.

More recently, computers have been used to analyze the data supplied from the photographic image of the corneal surface. Known as computer-assisted videokeratoscopes, these instruments have been used for clinical applications such as contact lens fitting and corneal screening for refractive surgical procedures.

Bibby (1976) stated the technical requirements for reliable topography measurement as follows:

1. The units to describe corneal topography must be independent of the shape being measured.
2. The instrument should measure the total area of interest.
3. All information should be acquired simultaneously.
4. The technique should have high accuracy and reproducibility.

If one accepts the above technical requirements, then it is possible to assess the suitability of other techniques. Thus, applying the first requirement, instruments such as the keratometer only measure central radius of curvature and assume that the surface being measured is spherical. This is not true for the cornea that has been shown to be best approximated to a conic section (Bibby 1976, Guillon et al 1986). Furthermore, keratometry does not fulfill the second requirement, because only the central 3 mm of the corneal surface is measured. In order to resolve larger areas of the cornea, the keratometer requires the use of an accessory device (the topogometer), which involves repeated measurement, and the additional inaccuracy of asking the patient to alter fixation to another point.

Various modern corneal topographic systems are now available. A description of some of the more widely used systems will now be presented.

COMPUTER–ASSISTED VIDEOKERATOGRAPHY

Computer-assisted videokeratography combines the principle of keratoscopy with computerized image analysis and data processing using personal computers (Gormley et al 1988). Examples of commercially available systems and their respective technical details are summarized in Table 2.2.

With the development of computer hardware in terms of processing speed and storage capacity, the number of points analyzed on the corneal surface has increased dramatically. The number of rings and points of analysis are chosen in order to provide adequate resolution of the corneal surface (Table 2.2). Images obtained from the videokeratoscopes are digitized and topographic data points are extracted in polar coordinates. Various forms of presentation of these data are available, such as color-coded dioptric maps, Placido images, wire mesh and solid models and elevation maps, to mention but a few.

A significant amount of research has taken place regarding the accuracy of modern computer-assisted keratoscopic devices on test surfaces (Hannush et al 1989, 1990, Koch et al 1989, 1992).

Table 2.2 The principal features of currently available commercial topography systems. The orthokeratology pluses and minuses represent the authors' experience in the use of these topographers for orthokeratology (OK).

Topographer	Type	Points analyzed	Coverage	Alignment	Maps/modules	OK positive attributes	OK negative attributes
ATLAS (Carl Zeiss), formerly known as the Mastervue system (www.humphrey.com)	Placido/slope			Manual focus, autocapture	Simulated ablation module, elevation maps, Healing trend/STARS™ display, corneal irregularity measure, contact lens-fitting module	Good repeatability and accuracy on eyes. Easy access to R_0 and Q. Q-value is for flat meridian. STARS display	Relatively small corneal coverage (7–8 mm). Lack of central smoothing can lead to false central islands
Dicon CT 200 Paradigm Medical Instruments, Inc. (www.paradigm-medical.com)	Large Placido/slope			Autofocus, autoalignment	Axial, instantaneous, difference maps, bull's-eye peak elevation (targets suspect areas), VISX cap program, change and trend analysis, irregularity indices	Relatively good repeatability. Off-center fixation points. Easy access to R_0 and eccentricity (flat meridian)	Some dispute exists as to the compatibility of e-valves from this instrument and that used by ortho-k programs
Euclid ET-800 (Euclid Systems Corporation)	Moiré fringe/elevation	300 000	Complete corneal coverage (16 × 22 mm)	Autofocus and capture following manual alignment	Moiré raw data map, sagittal depth (elevation) maps, spherical difference map, ellipsoidal difference map, axial curvature, instantaneous curvature maps	Theoretically a very good instrument. Total corneal coverage. Raw elevation, R_0 and eccentricity	Not yet widely used in orthokeratology
EyeMap EH-290 (Alcon) (www.alconlabs.com)	Large Placido/slope with 23 rings	8000+	0.46–10 mm	Fully automated (centering/focusing/capture)	Absolute, relative maps in axial and instantaneous curvature. Advanced contact lens software, keratoconus detection, corneal statistical information	Relatively accurate, poor repeatability on autofocus. Gives R_0 as a mean value, and P (shape factor) values	Care in patient placement before capture is essential in order to maximize the area of coverage
EyeSys Corneal Analysis System (EyeSys Technologies, Houston, TX)	Large Placido/slope with 10 rings (20 interfaces)			Autofocus, manual capture	Axial and instantaneous maps, elevation and semimeridian eccentricity maps. Sagittal height difference from a reference surface, Holladay diagnostic summary 2000 and axial difference maps. Pro-Fit contact lens-fitting software	Very good large Placido instrument. Easy access to smoothed R_0 value and eccentricity. STARS useful for tracking regression effects	Care in patient placement before capture is essential in order to maximize the area of coverage

Table 2.2   contd.

Topographer	Type	Points analyzed	Coverage	Alignment	Maps/modules	OK positive attributes	OK negative attributes
Keratograph/CTK corneal topographer (Oculus) (www.oculususa.com)	Large Placido/slope with 22 rings	22 000 measuring points		Manual alignment, autofocus and capture	Fluo-image, Fourier analysis and Zernike analysis, elevation or height map, refractive map or 3D animation. Keratoconus detection and classification software is also standard	Relatively accurate and repeatable. R_0 available from maps; eccentricity also available	Care in patient placement before capture is essential in order to maximize the area of coverage
Keratron (EyeQuip, a division of Alliance Medical Marketing) (www.eyequip.com)	Placido cone/slope with 28 border rings. Second far mires cone available for deep-set eyes	7168 points measured; 70 000 analyzed	0.33–10.7 mm	Patented infrared automated image capture system	Instantaneous, axial and Gaussian curvature; multiple K reading formats; pupil outline/center and decentration. Difference mapping: subtract maps from one another in curvature or height format. Comparison mapping; move axis mapping (map from vertex, pupil center, or any location). Height mapping, 3D maps, meridian profile (view any meridian in profile). Maloney indices: keratometry for abnormal corneas, corneal irregularity indices. Pupil measurement: edge detection, diameter and offset	Highly accurate and repeatable instrument. R_0 eccentricity and elevation values available for flat and steep meridian in CL module	The R_0, eccentricity, and elevation are only available from the CL module section. It can be time-consuming getting all the data out. The instrument would benefit greatly if a statistical output was given, as with the Medmont. Another problem is that the subtractive maps will commonly show what appear to be central islands. These are due to the lack of smoothing as the apex is reached, and the arc–step develops tangent normals that have an infinite radius
KR-8000P (Topcon corporation) (www.topcon.com)	Large Placido/slope (infrared) with 10 rings			Autoalignment, autofocus, and autocapture	Axial, instantaneous, refractive, and axial difference maps. Keratometric data and peripheral keratometric maps and a contact lens-fitting module. The KR-8000P also provides keratometric and autorefraction data	Basic topographer. Some useful features include the fact that the infrared rings do not induce reflex lacrimation. It is fully automatic in terms of alignment, It produces autorefraction data simultaneously	Not enough maps such as elevation maps, spherical difference maps. Not as much versatility as some of the more costly topographers. Little data on accuracy and repeatability

Table 2.2 *contd.*

Topographer	Type	Points analyzed	Coverage	Alignment	Maps/ modules	OK positive attributes	OK negative attributes
Medmont E300 (Medmont Pty Ltd, Australia)	Placido/ slope, 32 rings	15 120	0.25–11 mm	Automated image capture, manual focus using 3D focusing target. The best four frames are automatically captured and displayed. The advanced analysis software corrects defocused, off-centered images and compensates for errors due to misalignment	Axial, instantaneous, elevation, raw image. Subtractive axial, instantaneous, refractive power and elevation maps. 3D imaging of maps. Pupil detection. Statistical analysis of raw data of repeated readings	Highly accurate and repeatable topographer. Has automatic statistical data on R_0, elevation, eccentricity, Q, flat- and steep-K available for any specified chord or axis. Gives the mean and SD values of four repeated readings. Large area of corneal coverage	Poor availability. Production of this instrument is far below demand, and practitioners do not like to wait for months for delivery
Orbscan II (Bausch & Lomb)	Scanning slit and large Placido. Dual elevation and slope		Complete corneal coverage	Manual alignment and autocapture	Axial, instantaneous, difference, elevation, sphere difference maps. Posterior corneal curvature maps, pachymetry maps (also difference)	Has poor accuracy and repeatability	Not suitable for orthokeratology in its current state
PAR CTS (PAR Vision Systems)	Stereo photogrammetry (measures elevation)		Complete corneal coverage	Manual alignment and focus		Not currently widely used in orthokeratology	

Table 2.2 contd.

Topographer	Type	Points analyzed	Coverage	Alignment	Maps/modules	OK positive attributes	OK negative attributes
PAR CTS (PAR Vision Systems)	Stereo photogrammetry (measures elevation)		Complete corneal coverage	Manual alignment and focus		Not currently widely used in orthokeratology	
TMS-2N (TOMEY) (www.tomey.com)	Cone-type/ slope Placido/ slope 28 or 34 rings	7168– 8500	Within 0.19–10 mm	Automatic alignment, focus and capture	Axial, instantaneous, height. Spherical difference map (enhanced elevation). Various map options also available such as single, multiple, difference, meridional, 3D, and numeric. Klyce statistics, keratoconus screening, and contact lens-fitting module also available	One of the original topographers. The new version is totally automatic	The practitioner cannot monitor the patient during the capture process. The R_0 and eccentricity values are time-consuming to track down. Also, a "global" eccentricity value is given, and not the eccentricity along the flat meridian

R_0, apical radius; Q, asphericity.

The results show an acceptable level of accuracy and reproducibility. Hannush et al (1989) found measurements to be within 0.5 D in 76% of the readings on human corneas for rings 2 through to 13 for the Topographic Modeling System 1 (TMS-1). In a study by Koch et al (1992), the mean absolute differences between the keratometer and the EyeSys in terms of power were 0.19 D and 0.21 D for the steep and flat meridians, respectively. Tsilimbaris et al (1991) found a clinically significant difference between the EyeSys and Javal keratometer when measuring astigmatic eyes with a cylinder greater than 1.50 D. A mean difference of 0.84 D was found, but only 18 eyes were measured. Tsilimbaris et al (1991) suggested that a possible explanation could be poor focusing on one of the two astigmatic meridians.

Antalis et al (1993) compared the EyeSys (CAS) and the TMS-1 in terms of central corneal curvature in 18 eyes with a variety of corneal conditions. The average differences for the two instruments were −0.2 ± 0.7 D for the flat central meridian and −0.7 ± 0.9 D for the steep central meridian. Correlation coefficients for the two instruments were 0.9901 and 0.9937 for the flat and steep meridians, respectively. Both instruments were also found to correlate relatively well with the keratometer (correlation coefficient, $r = 0.9617$ and 0.9844 respectively). However, the use of correlation coefficients to compare the agreement of instruments is not an appropriate statistical test as it merely shows the level of association. Bland & Altman (1986) suggested that a plot of the difference of the two readings versus their respective means is a more accurate method.

Jeandervin & Barr (1998) compared the repeatability and accuracy of four commercially available topographers (Alcon Eyemap, EH-290, EyeSys 2000, and Humphrey ATLAS) in 10 optometry students. Two independent repeat measurements of the right eye were taken to evaluate repeatability, whereas precision was evaluated using four calibration spheres. Although there was no statistically significant difference for the four topographers, the EyeSys had the greatest repeatability, followed by both Humphrey instruments. Greatest accuracy was observed with the ATLAS topographer.

With respect to the precision of Placido systems for abnormal corneas, McMahon et al (2001) compared the test–retest reliability of three commercially available Placido ring video-keratoscopes in subjects with keratoconus. Nine subjects (16 eyes) had up to four images per eye generated in random order from the EyeSys II, Dicon CT-200, and Keratron. The short-term variability was 0.61–3.31 for the Dicon, 0.94–1.51 for the EyeSys, and 0.58–2.85 for the Keratron with respect to axial curvature. For measurements of instantaneous curvature, the variability was 1.07–6.82 for the Dicon, 0.79–1.77 for the EyeSys, and 1.23–3.03 for the Keratron. The authors concluded that their results supported the notion that Placido devices have reduced repeatability when measuring corneal irregularities.

Unfortunately, there are limitations of the keratoscopic approach in the analysis of corneal shape. Firstly, as already stated by Ludlum et al (1967), the image of the target mires should lie on a flat plane. Even with the modification of the target plane, it is not possible to achieve this for all corneas because of the large variety of normal corneal shapes. Thus, there could be errors induced from poor focus of different rings. Secondly, it has been shown that slight decentration of the alignment and focus results in large errors in actual measurement (Nieves & Applegate 1992). Thus, various modifications in the design of instruments have a role in reducing errors due to poor focus and misalignment.

DESIGN FACTORS
Working distance

Working distance, mire size, and the size and position of the reflected mire image are all intimately related. For example, as working distance decreases, the influence of instrument alignment error will increase (Nieves & Applegate 1992, Antalis et al 1993); however, the influence of facial anatomical factors is reduced, so enabling a larger area of the cornea to be measured. Using a micron positioner (a device used to position a test surface accurately with respect to the videokeratoscope axis), Nieves & Applegate (1992) determined the effect of working distance on the accuracy of measurements found with the TMS and EyeSys videokeratoscopes for two acrylic spheres ($r = 7.1153$ mm and $r = 7.9497$ mm). The results showed that the EyeSys (which has a larger working distance) consistently measured the sphere to a higher degree of accuracy than the TMS-1 for both frontal plane (x- and y-axis) and axial (z-axis) misalignment. Applegate (1992) pointed out that the working distance chosen by the manufacturers of the EyeSys (Model I) and TMS-1 probably represents two extremes of realistic values.

As a general rule, instruments that use large working distances, which are less susceptible to focusing error, will also have large Placido designs (Fig. 2.3). Conversely, smaller Placido designs (often referred to as cone designs) will be associated with smaller working distances. With the improvement in autoalignment and focusing systems, manufacturers are tending to use smaller cone-type Placido rings that permit greater corneal coverage.

Defining a reference point for corneal modeling

Irrespective of manufacturer design, all videokeratoscopes at present use the same alignment

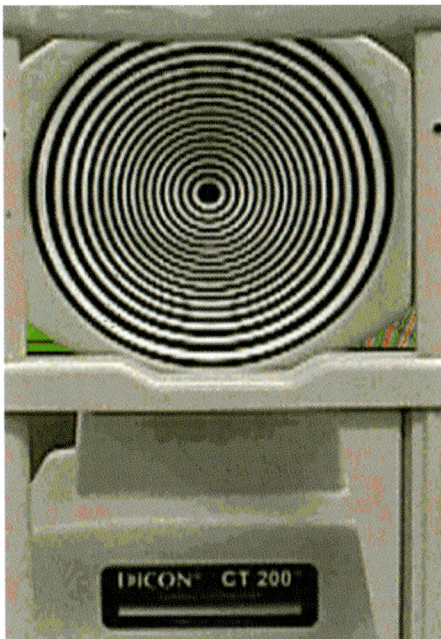

Figure 2.3   Large Placido mire.

principle (Mandell 1992). The subject views a luminous fixation point, the image of which is viewed by the practitioner on the monitor. At this point, the subject's line of sight is coaxial with the instrument axis. Finally, the practitioner must then center the reflected image of the luminous markers with respect to a reference marker on the monitor. The final stage of alignment fulfills one of the assumptions and criteria for videokeratoscopy – that the instrument axis should be perpendicular to the cornea. The consequence of the alignment procedure is that the instrument axis may be perpendicular to an undefined point on the cornea. Figure 2.4 shows the point of alignment with the cornea when the conventional procedure of alignment is performed.

Although, after alignment, the optic axis of the instrument is perpendicular at a point on the cornea and is directed therefore towards the instantaneous (tangential) radius of curvature, measurements are performed from an eccentric and unknown point. The point on the cornea from where measurements are performed with present videokeratoscopes is unique. Mandell (1992) suggested that from a clinical and functional viewpoint, the ideal reference point would be the intersection of the line of sight with the corneal surface. Manufacturers of most videokeratoscopic systems are now able to locate the entrance pupil on dioptric maps. Mandell (1992) described a simple modification to conventional videokeratoscope alignment where measurements are centered about a unique point on the corneal surface where the line of sight and the instrument axis intersect. This point is not as peripheral on the cornea as with conventional alignment procedures. Figure 2.5 summarizes the modification as described by Mandell (1992).

Figure 2.4 shows that, from the videokeratoscope view, the monitor reference pattern will be displaced away from the center of the entrance pupil. The reason for this is that the instrument requires the optic axis of the instrument to be perpendicular to the corneal surface. In Figure. 2.5, the subject is asked to view an eccentric target so that the monitor reference pattern of the videokeratoscope is placed in the center of the entrance pupil as viewed in the monitor. Once this has been accomplished, the luminous fixation marker is then aligned with the monitor reference pattern. After alignment in this manner, the line of sight and the optic axis of the videokeratoscope intersect at a unique point on the cornea and measurements are centered about a point where the line of sight intersects the cornea.

More recently, Hubbe (1994) evaluated the effect of alignment of the EyeSys CAS in five corneas and three aspheric test surfaces of varying radius with the line of sight directed at 2.5°, 5°, and 10° below the videokeratoscope axis (the instrument axis was still perpendicular to the surface under test). Hubbe (1994) found that a 5° deviation from the fixation source, a significant difference between opposing semimeridians in the aspheric surfaces and patient corneas ($P < 0.05$), occurred. Furthermore, the color-coded maps mimicked the appearance of keratoconus. Hubbe (1994) concluded that accurate alignment with the line of sight is important as misalign-

ment can induce errors in the subsequent calculations to determine corneal topography.

Focusing systems

User errors can only be attributed to alignment inaccuracy. The importance of accurate z-axis (i.e., along the instrument axis) alignment has been shown to be critical in the accurate measurement of corneal topography (Mandell 1992, Nieves & Applegate 1992). Mandell (1992) found that the impact of z-axis alignment error on corneal radius derivation was greater with instruments that operated at shorter working distances. Using the EyeSys and the TMS videokeratoscopes (the EyeSys has a longer working distance than the TMS), Mandell (1992) found that the effect of z-axis defocus was greater with the TMS than the EyeSys. Nieves & Applegate (1992) confirmed these results in a similar study using the same instruments.

Manufacturers also attempted to redesign instruments in order to minimize errors due to z-axis misalignment. The MasterVue Smart Topography system (now known as the ATLAS topographer) incorporated a dual-camera system that enabled the operator to view a magnified image of the centrally reflected rings as well as the overall cornea. Theoretically, z-axis errors reduce because of the smaller depth of focus obtained using the second higher-magnification camera. Figure 2.6 shows how the dual-camera system operates.

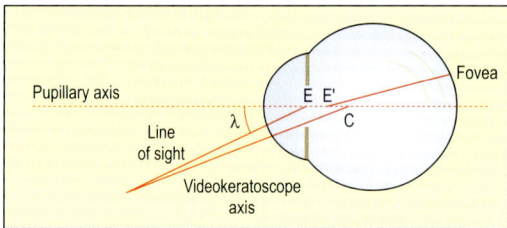

Figure 2.4 The position of the various reference points and axes after alignment has been performed. *E* and *E'* are entrance and exit pupils, respectively, *C* is the center of curvature of the cornea. The videokeratoscope axis is aligned with an unknown point on the cornea. Reproduced with permission from Mandell (1992).

Image editing

The ability to edit captured Placido ring images forms an important aspect of corneal topographic accuracy. Facial contours can interfere with the Placido mires. Figure 2.7 illustrates how a digitally captured Placido image, if unedited, would result in errors in the nasal area of the image. The Humphrey topographer provides two chin-rests so that patients can turn their face in order to reduce nasal shadowing. Practitioners performing procedures such as orthokeratology must take the time to analyze these Placido images and make the appropriate corrections to the computer digitization. Other factors such as long lashes are

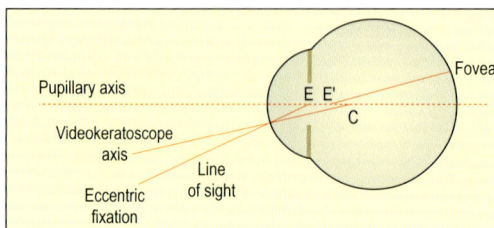

Figure 2.5 Alignment proposed by Mandell (1992) in order to align the videokeratoscope axis with the line of sight at the corneal surface. For abbreviations, see Figure 2.4.

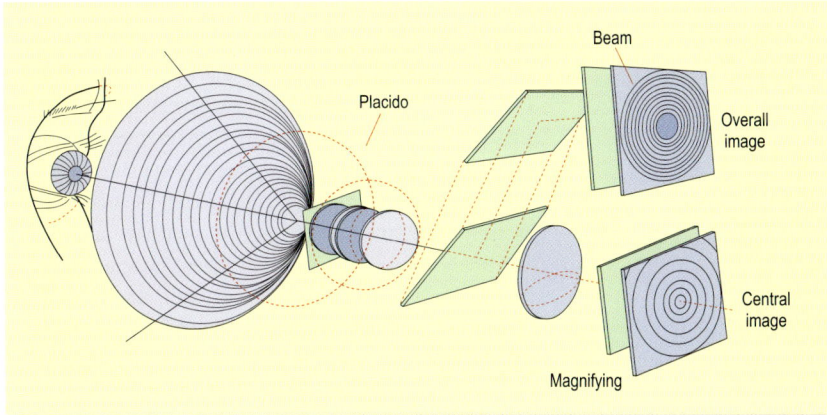

Figure 2.6 The MasterVue dual-camera system used to obtain accurate z-axis alignment (reproduced from MasterVue literature).

also frequently responsible for loss of data in the superior area of the cornea. Variability in the tear film due to excessive lipids can also interfere with the shape of the reflected Placido mires. Asking the patient to blink several times to dissipate some of the lipids can help but, rather than introduce further inaccuracies, practitioners would be wise simply to delete any suspect areas.

Rasterstereography and scanning slit topography systems

Rasterstereography was initially used for the measurement of corneal topography by Bonnet & Cochet (1962). The principle involves projecting a grid of light on to the corneal surface. As the cornea is transparent, the technique involves rendering the cornea opaque. Originally, talcum powder (with the use of a suitable anesthetic) was used to form a real image of the target. The use of talcum powder to make the cornea opaque was the major drawback of this technique.

More recently, this method has attracted more popularity as talcum powder has been replaced with sodium fluorescein. The mechanics have been concisely described by Arffa et al (1989): a projected grid of light is used to illuminate the cornea and then viewed at a specific angle from the projection source (Fig. 2.8). The whole system is incorporated on a Zeiss stereo photo slit lamp. Image acquisition involves focusing the slit lamp on the corneal surface; when in focus, a flash is triggered which provides the required intensity for image analysis. The flashlight passes through the cobalt blue excitation filter causing the projected grid pattern to fluoresce. The image is then

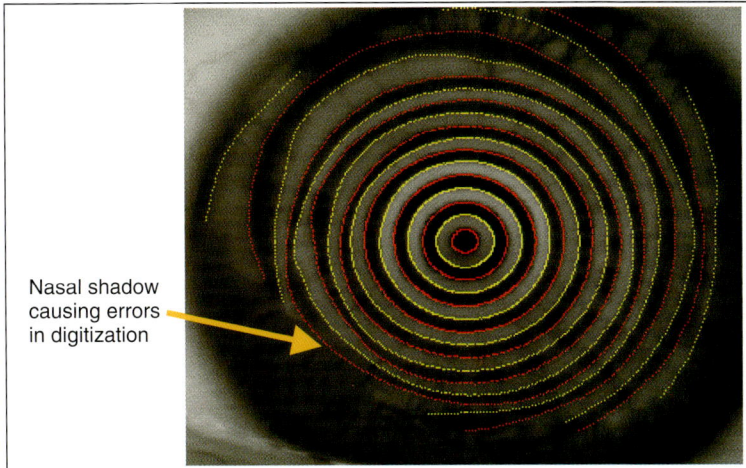

Figure 2.7 Incorrect digitization induced by nasal shadow. If unedited, this image will result in poor accuracy of the measurement of the cornea.

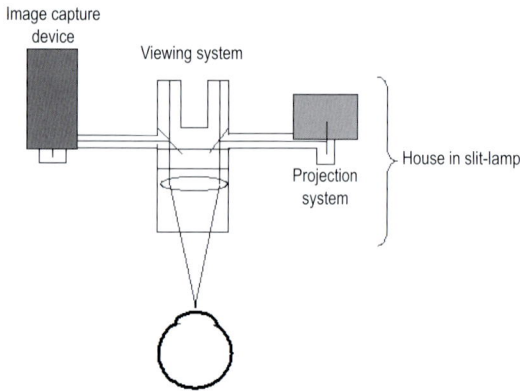

Figure 2.8 The design of the apparatus similar to that used by Arffa et al (1989).

viewed by the video camera through a yellow barrier filter so that the residual blue light is absorbed. The resulting image is then digitized and analyzed using suitable computer software.

The shape of the corneal surface is then determined by the distortion and separation of the projected grid. The computer calculates the elevation of the corneal surface by comparing the displacement of the projected grid lines on the cornea to the position of the grid lines when projected on a flat plane. A two-dimensional matrix of approximately 3000 elevation points is created for each image. From this, a three-dimensional display of the corneal surface is produced.

The accuracy of elevation measurements is dependent on the magnification used on the slit lamp. At ×16, one can visualize the entire cornea and elevation accuracy is approximately 10 μm. At higher magnifications, even more accuracy is possible. Furthermore, the accuracy is also dependent on the length of the profile examined. Arffa et al (1989) found that, for a length of 8 mm of the corneal profile, the accuracy was 0.11 D, but for only 5 mm the accuracy was reduced to 0.5 D. This was determined in a laboratory using matt-finished steel balls; no aspheric test surfaces were used in their analysis.

With respect to alignment, any section of the projected grid may be analyzed and used as a reference point. Generally, the apex of the cornea is chosen as the reference point. A commercially available device has been developed (the PAR Technology corneal topography system). Studies (Belin et al 1992, Belin & Zloty 1993) indicate that the instrument is both highly accurate and reproducible in determining the topography of spheres. An 8-mm test area was used on non-calibrated steel balls of 20, 18, and 12 mm diameter, from which standard deviations of 0.03, 0.02, and 0.01 D, respectively, were found. In contrast to the study by Arffa et al (1989), smaller test areas did not result in significant reductions in the accuracy of elevation measurements. No tests were performed on mechanically measured aspheric test pieces.

Belin & Zloty (1993) assessed the accuracy of the PAR system using decentered spheres, whole cadaver eyes before and after epithelial removal, lamellar keratectomy, and laser photoablation. Four spheres were used (37.49, 42.21, 48.05, and 55.76 D), the effect of decentration (0.5 mm in the x-, y-, and z-axes) and the size of the optical zone (5, 6 and 8 mm) were assessed, and the best fitting sphere determined. The principle of derivative of rasterstereogrammetry is elevation. Therefore, in theory, there is no need for accurate alignment with the apex of a surface as it will be that point with the greatest elevation or that point with the smallest radius of curvature. Belin & Zloty (1993) found an average error of 0.04 D when decentering by 0.5 mm; the maximum error was 0.1 D for the 37.49 D sphere with a 5.0 mm optical zone. They concluded that the effect of misalignment and optical zone diameter had little effect on the results obtained.

A study by Schultze (1998) compared the elevation accuracy of three Placido-based systems with the PAR rasterstereogrammetry system using test surfaces representing the normal cornea (aspheric surfaces) and surfaces mimicking myopic ablation. The 'normal' surface was rotationally symmetric whilst the simulated photorefractive keratectomy (PRK) surface had a 5.5-mm diameter central zone with a 1-mm blend radius. The Placido systems evaluated were the Alcon EH–290, Humphrey ATLAS, and Keratron

Table 2.3 Accuracy of elevation measurement for artificial surfaces using four topographers

Topographer	Asphere error (μm)	Simulated PRK error (μm)
EH-290	14.3 ± 5.2	10.6 ± 4.5
ATLAS	3.7 ± 0.7	29.5 ± 1.8
Keratron	1.2 ± 0.4	28.0 ± 2.1
PAR	1.8 ± 0.1	4.7 ± 0.3

PRK, photorefractive keratectomy.

(Alliance Medical). Table 2.3 summarizes the results.

The topographers showed similar accuracies for both the Placido and rastersterogrammetry-based systems for aspheric surfaces for all but the EH–290, which resulted in the greatest error. The simulated PRK surfaces however resulted in increased measurement error for the Placido-based systems.

Another topographer utilizes similar principles – the Euclid topographer (Euclid System Corp.). As with the PAR system, sodium fluorescein is used to allow the formation of a real projected image on the cornea. Two identical sinusoidal wave patterns are projected on to the eye from specific angles and captured using a charge-coupled device (CCD) camera. Two-dimensional Fourier transforms are applied to calculate the phase shift of the projected wave pattern. Elevation points are calculate directly for over 300 000 data points on the corneal surface in terms of x, y, and z coordinates (details of the topographer are supplied in Table 2.2).

Another system, the Orbscan (Bausch & Lomb) uses a modified approach to derive true elevation data of the corneal surface. Using a scanning slit beam, 40 slit sections are captured across the cornea. Then, using three-dimensional ray tracing, the profile of the cornea is determined. The various sections are "stitched" together to produce an entire corneal map.

The initial system (Orbscan I) was found to provide useful data, such as topography, and corneal pachymetry. Subsequently, a new version, the Orbscan II (Bausch & Lomb), has both scan-

ning slit and Placido measurement. The principal reason for including the Placido rings was to increase sensitivity of normal corneal measurement whilst retaining the benefits of scanning slit to be able to measure more distorted corneas (which Placido-based systems cannot effectively measure).

Rasterstereography and scanning slit topography are accurate techniques for measuring corneal curvature. They utilize a real image as opposed to a virtual image like that used in reflective methods such as keratometry and keratoscopy. The analysis of a reflected image on highly distorted corneas can cause significant distortion of the image such that analysis is almost impossible. On the other hand, a projected target is considerably less affected (Belin & Zloty 1993). Therefore, non-Placido-based systems are advantageous in patients with significant distortion such as in advanced keratoconus and postkeratoplasty.

ALGORITHMS IN VIDEOKERATOSCOPY

Problem outline

To appreciate the basic problems involved in corneal shape measurement, it is worth considering what actually occurs when capturing the reflected image of a known target source (Fig. 2.9).

Essentially, a target source of known dimensions and shape (housed in a faceplate) illuminates the cornea. Owing to the reflective properties of the cornea, a virtual image of the target source forms behind the cornea. As the shape of the reflecting surface dictates the appearance of the reflected image, reverse ray tracing from the image plane to the target source would enable calculation of the reflecting surface

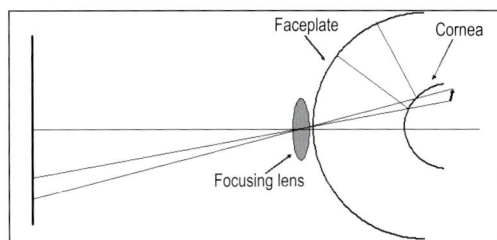

Figure 2.9 The principles of videokeratoscopy.

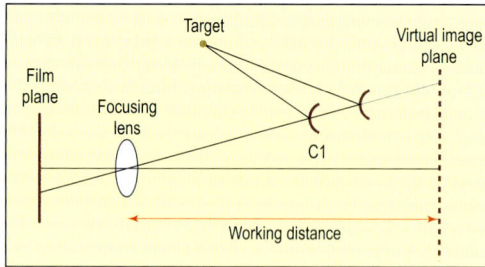

Figure 2.10   How two corneal surfaces of different radii of curvature (C_1 and C_2) can result in the reflected mire image lying at the same point on the photographic film. When the system is in focus, the working distance is always constant and spans from the focusing lens to the virtual image behind the cornea. Therefore, the two surfaces cannot be differentiated at the film plane. After Wang et al (1989).

parameters. Unfortunately, the problem is not as simple as may initially appear.

Reconstruction of a 3D surface from a 2D photograph

In order to define the corneal profile, three parameters are required – the value of x, y, and z coordinates of the corneal surface. The image captured in videokeratoscopy is two-dimensional. In order to determine the corneal profile, the two-dimensional image must be converted into a three-dimensional surface. Unfortunately, the two-dimensional image in videokeratoscopy has insufficient information to enable a point-by-point localization of the reflected mires in three-dimensional space.

Wang et al (1989) concisely illustrated this problem (Fig. 2.10). Thus, the instantaneous radius of curvature at a point on the corneal surface cannot be uniquely determined from measurements of the film plane unless assumptions are made. All that can be stated is that there is a surface that intercepts the reflected ray path. Furthermore, the distance from the focusing lens to the virtual image (and therefore the focal plane) is constant. A unique relationship for corneal curvature can only be determined if the object and image distances are known. However, assumptions must be made, as the object distance is not known (i.e., the distance from the target to the cornea).

The effect of continuous targets and meridional skew

A common assumption made in some video-keratoscopes using concentric rings is that light commencing at one meridian from the object plane lies in the same meridian at the film plane. This does not apply to targets which consist of point sources, as each point can be easily located in the image plane, therefore any skewing of the image can be easily detected as the target is not continuous like a ring. Assuming that there is no meridional skew could lead to errors in the reconstruction of the corneal surface. Klein (1997) calculated the skew ray error for ellipsoidal and keratoconic corneas and corneas that have undergone decentered PRK. Negligible error was found for ellipsoidal and centered PRK corneas. However, for keratoconic and decentered PRK significant errors were found in corneal curvature. Thus, skew ray error induces significant error in abnormal, asymmetric corneas.

Data resolution in videokeratoscopy

Before making any assumptions in reconstructing the corneal profile, the reflected rings are digitized. The accuracy of the reconstruction will therefore ultimately depend on the resolution of the digitization procedure.

Maguire et al (1987a) calculated the effect of frame resolution on corneal position accuracy and the subsequent error that could occur for a 40-D surface (Table 2.4). The EyeSys corneal analysis system measures ring separation to subpixel resolution (Hodd & Ruston 1993). Andersen et al

Table 2.4 The influence of frame resolution on the localization accuracy of the cornea and measurement error for a 40-D surface (after Maguire et al 1987a)

Frame resolution (lines per frame)	Localization accuracy at the cornea (μm)	Measurement error with 40 D surface (D)
500	30	1.2
1000	15	0.6
2000	7.5	0.3

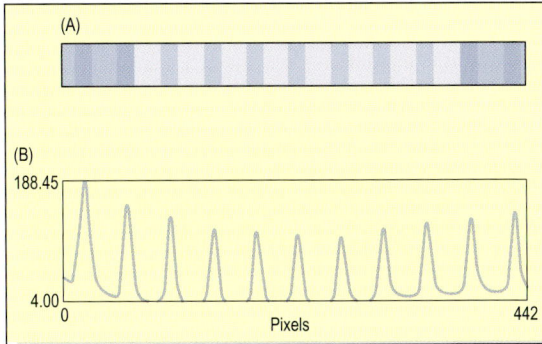

Figure 2.11   (A) The image of a target ruler and (B) the light intensity profile. The location of the ruler lines can be resolved to subpixel resolution from the intensity profile. Reproduced from Dave (1995).

(1993a) have described a similar procedure, where the distribution of light intensity is measured and plotted as a function of pixel distance. The location of the ring was given by the peak of the intensity distribution of the digitized image (Fig. 2.11).

Algorithms used in the reconstruction of the corneal profile

Having captured and digitized the reflected mire image, the corneal profile must be reconstructed. As described earlier, there are numerous difficulties in reconstructing a three-dimensional surface from a two-dimensional image but, by making certain assumptions, these difficulties may be overcome. In general, the following assumptions are made for the various reconstruction techniques:

- The working distance from the target to the image is constant.
- The instrument axis is perpendicular to the corneal surface.
- The light from one meridian of the target is reflected in the same meridian in the film plane. The assumption here is that there is no circumferential tilt of the corneal surface. For point targets, this assumption is not required.
- The position of the image at the film plane (camera) is unique for a particular surface.
- The image plane lies on a flat plane.

The various methods of reconstructing the corneal surface have generally taken three forms:

the calibration method, one-step curve fitting, and the multiple-arc technique.

Calibration method

The classical method of calibration involves taking photographs of reflected target rings from steel balls of known radii. The separations of adjacent ring images are measured and a set of calibration graphs are constructed that plot ring image separation for various spherical surfaces against the radius or power of that surface (Mandell & St Helen 1968, Townsley 1970). Then, for actual subjects, ring separations are measured again and radius values are obtained from the calibration graphs. The calibration method assumes that the cornea is spherical between adjacent rings. Errors result in this technique because it is assumed that the instantaneous center of curvature for the various reflected rings lies on the optic axis of the instrument; although this applies to a spherical surface, it does not apply to an aspheric cornea where the instantaneous radius of curvatures lie on an evolute (Bennett 1968).

Knoll (1961) found an error in radius of curvature of ±0.2 mm using spherical surfaces for the calibration method. Stone (1962) also found a comparable error of ±0.25 mm, again, with spherical surfaces. Calculating peripheral radius of curvature of nonspherical surfaces such as the cornea using a calibration method based on spherical surfaces unnecessarily introduces and biases the derived radius to that of a spherical surface.

One-step curve fitting

Originally proposed by El Hage (1971, 1972), this method attempts to fit a polynomial curve of the form, $x = A_0 + A_1y + A_2y^2$ . . . to the cornea with the origin (0, 0) at the corneal apex. Differential equations were used to derive the polynomial equation matching the corneal surface. The order of the polynomial used was dependent on the number of rings in the keratoscope target. Furthermore, the keratoscope used was unusual in design in that a stop was placed at the principal focus of the camera lens to ensure that reflected light would return parallel to the instrument axis. Designing the keratoscope in this manner enabled El Hage

(1972) to simplify the differential equation used to calculate the polynomial function describing corneal shape. Using spheres and conic surfaces, El Hage (1972) found an error of 0.02 mm in terms of sagittal depth measurements at the periphery of the curve.

More recently, Edmund (1985) derived a method where the size of reflected rings from hypothetical conic sections was found by calculation and compared with the size of reflected rings from a photograph of a surface. The corneal profile is fitted to a conic curve by comparing the reflected ring size using least squares.

The disadvantage of one-step curve fitting is that the cornea is modeled on a specific mathematical function. Because of such approximations it is likely that the derived profile will be relatively insensitive to local corneal variation.

The multiple-arc technique

Originally devised by Townsley (1967), Doss et al (1981) ascribed the name to this method of calculating the corneal profile. The model considers that a meridional section of the cornea can be composed of several multiple arcs between corneal reflection points. A smooth curve would be guaranteed by the fact that each adjacent arc would share a common tangent where they meet (Fig. 2.12).

Klyce (1984) improved the algorithm by adding a separate algorithm for the calculation of central corneal elevation (previously Doss et al (1981) preset the central radius of curvature to 7.80 mm and thereby biased the profile). Further, Klyce (1984) also made an allowance for the centers of curvature to lie on a point other than the optic axis of the instrument. One fundamental assumption made in the calculations was that the height of the point of reflection at the cornea was

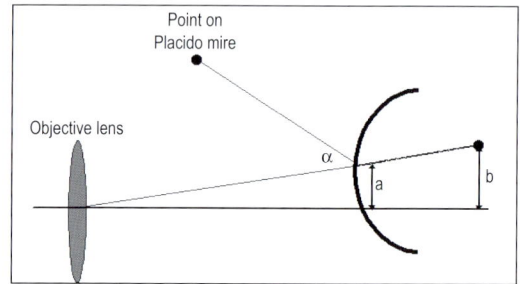

Figure 2.13 The incorrect assumption that the reflection height at the corneal surface (A) equals that in the image plane (B). Wang et al (1989) avoided this assumption by calculating angle α.

equal to that at the image plane (Fig. 2.13). More recently, Wang et al (1989) modified this approach to avoid making this latter assumption. Andersen et al (1993a, b) derived a similar technique based on locating the angular subtense of the targets at the image plane using a reference sphere and then using these values to derive the corneal coordinates using other algorithms.

Earlier version of the multiple arc technique were not suitable to resolve the topographic details of a nonspherical surface (Wang et al 1989). The fact that the image height is assumed to be equal to the height at which reflection from the corneal surface occurs is a significant source of error (Wang et al 1989). Wang et al (1989) corrected this source of error by calculating the value of the angular subtense of the reflected mires (Figure 2.11); using an angle avoided making the above assumption. Further, they compared the accuracy of the old and new methods for a spherical and aspheric surface ($r_0 = 7.33$, $e = 0.5$). They found that the new method significantly improved the accuracy of the algorithms for an aspheric surface. There was very little difference in the accuracy in calculating the radius of curvature for a spherical surface.

Placido-based systems primarily derive the slope of the corneal surface. Unlike rasterstereographic and scanning slit systems (which primarily derive corneal height data), certain assumptions need to be made. From a contact lens fitting and surgical perspective, accurate corneal height data are preferable. Nevertheless, Placidobased systems are still more popular with practitioners and certainly the results of various studies show little difference between Placido systems and

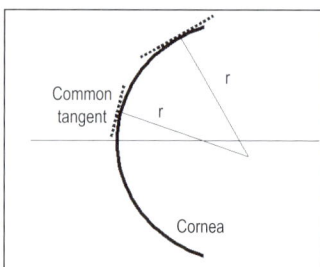

Figure 2.12 The multiple arc technique. r, radius of curvature of the arc.

height-deriving systems in terms of measurement accuracy when measuring normal corneas. Some studies have in fact shown that Placido systems offer greater sensitivity and accuracy for normal corneas. However, when one measures distorted or irregular-shaped corneas, Placido-based systems are generally regarded as providing less accurate data, possibly due to increased smoothing of the digitized mires. The choice of topography systems therefore depends on the principal use of the system. For orthokeratology, the most important information required is the prefit corneal apical radius and eccentricity data (or corneal height data over fixed chord length).

Sagittal and tangential maps

When light from an off-axis, oblique point reflects from a curved surface, two focal points arise. These points are the tangential and sagittal points of focus when the meridian contains the instrument axis and point of interest (known as the meridional plane). They arise due to the aberration effects of oblique astigmatism. Tangential radius represents the radius of curvature of the corneal surface that contains the target mires. It represents the "true" corneal shape. The sagittal radius represents the radius of the corneal surface perpendicular to the reflected mires. Sagittal measurements are useful for the analysis of the optical effects of corneal topography. Figure 2.14 illustrates the difference between the tangential and sagittal radius.

Sagittal or axial maps have limitations as the radius of curvature at each point on the corneal surface is biased to the optic axis. This invariably results in a poor representation of corneal shape as the true locus of curvature of the cornea lies on an evolute. Axial maps are useful in observing the optical effect of corneal shape. Tangential maps offer a better representation of corneal shape, as they are not biased to the optic axis. For more information, see the section on qualitative descriptors of corneal topography, below.

CORNEAL POWER DISPLAYS

Depending on the method used, corneal power can be displayed in four ways for the same corneal radius. The problem arises because videokeratoscopes derive corneal radius: power measurements are simply calculated as a transformation. The four measures are shown in Figure 2.15.

$$F = \frac{(n-1)}{r} \qquad \text{Equation 2.1}$$

where n is the refractive index of the cornea and r the local radius of the spherical arc. This formula only holds for paraxial rays.

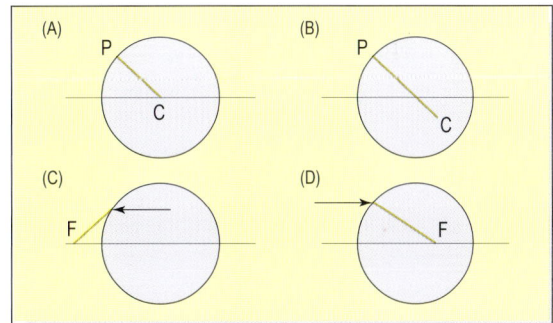

Figure 2.15   The four powers derived from radius of curvature measurements. The power measured in Figure 2.15(A) describes the power as defined by the optic axis. The power is dependent on the refractive index of the cornea and r is the sagittal radius of curvature of the cornea (see Equation 2.1). Figure 2.15(B) shows the corneal power as defined by the tangential radius and refractive index of the cornea (see Equation 2.1). Figure 2.15(C) and 2.15(D) show the posterior and anterior corneal power. Videokeratoscopes measure total corneal power as defined in Figure 2.15(A) and 2.15(B), depending on whether sagittal or tangential power is required.

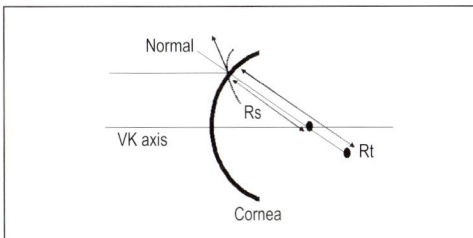

Figure 2.14   Sagittal and tangential radius of curvature for an aspheric surface. VK, videokeratoscope.

Klein (1993) suggested that the use of this method was incorrect as it was being applied to nonparaxial zones of the cornea.

Classification of corneal topography

Modern corneal topography yields a high-resolution analysis of the cornea. With such a large volume of numeric information, numerous investigators have developed qualitative and quantitative displays in order to summarize measurements.

Anatomical classification

Since the early investigations by Javal and Helmholtz, a basic model of corneal topography has been established (Miller 1980). This classical model of the corneal contour was of a surface comprising two distinct zones – a central spherical area (known as the corneal cap) measuring 4–5 mm in diameter, and a peripheral zone that flattens progressively towards the limbus. The central zone is responsible for forming the fovea. More recently, the cornea has been described more

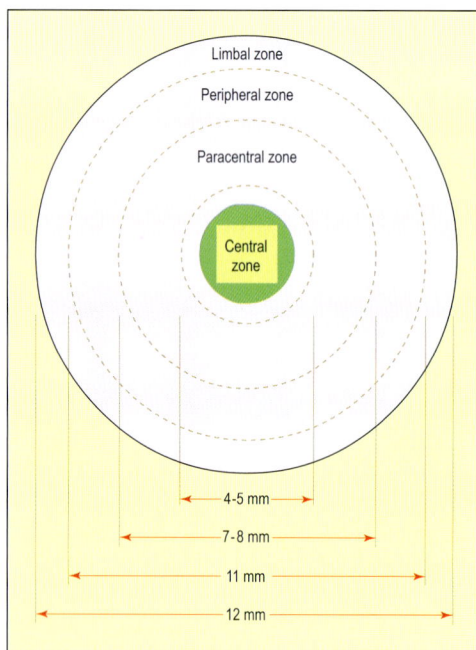

Figure 2.16   The anatomical zones on the corneal surface as described by Waring (1969).

specifically in terms of four anatomical zones (Waring 1969). These zones are the central, paracentral, peripheral, and limbal zones (Fig. 2.16).

The center of the cornea shown in Figure 2.16 is known as the geometric center. The significance of the geometric center is only for localization. The geometric center should not be confused with the corneal apex, which represents the point of maximum curvature on the cornea. The position of the corneal apex is independent of the geometric center of the cornea and has been shown to lie, on average, approximately 0.5 mm temporally (Mandell and St Helen 1965, Edmund 1987). In reality, classification of the cornea in terms of anatomical zones is inappropriate, as the cornea is a smooth surface whose curvature changes in a continuous manner. Waring (1969) suggested that classification of the cornea into anatomical zones is of use when designating locations on the cornea.

Qualitative descriptors of corneal topography

The earliest qualitative descriptor of corneal topography was the Placido disk, where the image of a ring-shaped target provided the user with information regarding the degree of corneal toricity, corneal apex position, and peripheral corneal shape. More recently, with the development of computerized videokeratoscopes, investigators have been able to create more sophisticated qualitative descriptors. Some of these descriptors are described below.

Classification of topography with sagittal (axial) maps

Maguire et al (1987a) and Gormley et al (1988) have described the use of color isoptor contour maps in order schematically to present data obtained from topographical systems. A variety of colors is used to denote the sagittal power distribution across the entire cornea (Fig. 2.17).

Practitioners should remember that the pattern observed depends on the range of the color-coded scale and the step size. An absolute scale (as in the EyeSys topography system) is useful, as it remains constant from one examination to

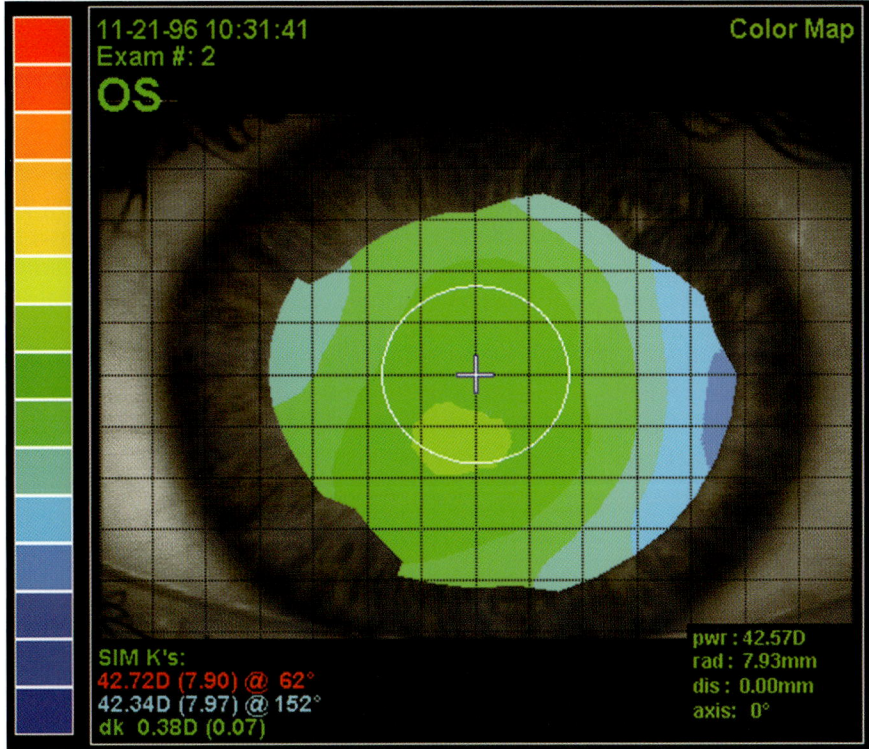

the next. Thus, for comparative purposes it represents a useful plot. Unfortunately, sagittal maps and tangential maps are fixation-dependent. Thus, map appearance and curvature values vary considerably depending on patient fixation and corneal asymmetry.

Numerous patterns may be used to describe certain forms of corneal topography. Bogan et al (1990) further simplified these by describing them as round, oval, symmetrical bowtie, asymmetric bowtie, and irregular. In their classification scheme, Bogan et al (1990) used the shapes formed by color-coded contour maps in the paracentral and central corneal zones to define specific patterns (Fig. 2.18). The paracentral and central areas of the cornea were used because they are the most important optically and because these are the areas measured most accurately by the Corneal Modeling System (Hannush et al (1989).

After observing the patterns from 216 eyes, Bogan et al (1990) defined these shapes as follows:

- Round: these patterns represent an approximately spherical cornea, as the change in power in the central/paracentral zone would not be significant.
- Oval: the ratio of the shortest to longest diameter at the color zone is less than two-thirds. This would represent an approximately spherical cornea; there is no detectable difference between oval and round patterns in terms of refraction and keratometry. One possible reason for this could be that keratometry only measures the central 3–4 mm of the cornea and this may not be a large enough area to detect any differences in astigmatism for the two patterns. Round and oval patterns accounted for 43.4% of the patterns observed by Bogan et al (1990).

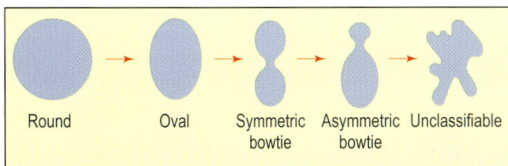

Figure 2.18 The five patterns observed in color-coded topographic maps of normal eye, as described by Bogan et al (1990).

- Symmetric bowtie: this pattern represents regular astigmatism. For a pattern to be classified as a symmetric bowtie there must be a central constriction in the outline of the color zone from the color-coded contour maps. Bogan et al (1990) found a statistically significant difference in the level of astigmatism between symmetric bowtie patterns and the round or oval patterns.
- Asymmetric bowtie: these patterns are very similar to symmetric bowtie patterns in that there is an area of constriction in the bowtie. However, the constriction is not centered with respect to the bowtie (Fig. 2.18). Statistically significant differences between symmetric and asymmetric pattern astigmatism have been found and are attributed to factors such as eccentric fixation, corneal apex position, contact lens wear, and radial asymmetry in the rate of change of peripheral curvature. Bowtie patterns accounted for 49.6% of patterns observed by Bogan et al (1990).
- Irregular: no clear pattern can be identified according to the above criteria. Bogan et al (1990) found 7.1% of subjects with this type of pattern; however, no sign of corneal disease in these people was observed. It is possible that tear film disturbances could cause this type of irregularity.

Tangential (instantaneous) maps

As defined in Figure 2.14, the tangential radius of curvature illustrates the localized curvature of the cornea in the meridional plane (the plane that contains the corneal point of interest and the videokeratoscope axis). Figure 2.19 shows axial (sagittal) and tangential maps for a subject who has had a corneal graft.

Currently, most topography devices have the facility to display sagittal and tangential maps. Tangential and axial maps assume that, during the alignment of the videokeratoscope, the normal to the corneal point of interest lies within the meridional plane. If this were true, radius of curvature measurements in pathological conditions such as keratoconus would be accurate. In practice, this condition does not normally occur and therefore tangential maps provide only limited fixation axis independence.

Mean curvature and Gaussian maps

Sagittal and tangential maps are somewhat simplified, as they calculate corneal topography on a meridian-by-meridian analysis. Videokeratoscope algorithms bias calculations by assuming that the normal to each point on the corneal surface lies in the meridional plane. The normal to the point of interest may not necessarily lie in the meridional plane, especially for irregular corneas (as shown in Fig. 2.20). From differential geometry, this point will have specific direction in which there is a maximum and minimum curvature, the difference being the local cylinder. Note that this is not the same as the sagittal and tangential curvature (which lie in the meridional plane). The Gaussian curvature is defined as the geometric mean of the maximum and minimum curvature (see Equation 2.2).

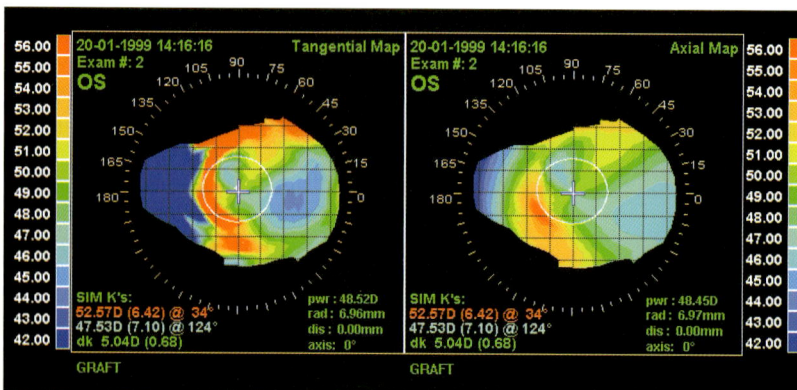

Figure 2.19 Sagittal and tangential maps in a patient post keratoplasty.

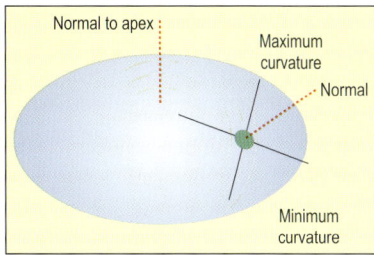

Figure 2.20
Three-dimensional smooth surface: each point has a unique direction in which there is a maximum and minimum curvature.

$$r_g = \sqrt{r_{max} \times r_{min}} \qquad \text{Equation 2.2}$$

where r_g is the Gaussian curvature, and r_{max} and r_{min} the maximum and minimum curvature of a specific point on the corneal surface.

Barsky et al (1997) computed the axial, tangential, and Gaussian curvature for a keratoconic cornea for conventional alignment and when the videokeratoscope is aligned with the corneal apex. They found significant variations in the color maps and apical powers for both axial (sagittal) and tangential curvatures (more so with axial curvature). Gaussian curvature maps, however, produced curvature values that were identical. This illustrates one major drawback in conventional tangential and sagittal measurement – they are fixation-specific and dependent on corneal symmetry. The Orbscan system (Bausch & Lomb) has the facility to display arithmetic mean power maps. These maps, like Gaussian curvature maps, are also not dependent on fixation or corneal symmetry. They show the local curvature of the cornea and are useful in determining the exact location and effect of surface irregularities (Fig. 2.21).

Elevation maps

Elevation maps display the sagittal height (in μm) of the cornea from a fixed, flat reference plane. This map, like the Gaussian and mean power maps, is also independent of fixation and corneal asymmetry (Fig. 2.21). These maps are useful clinically to evaluate true corneal shape. The drawback of elevation maps is that subtle variations in elevation are not easily discernible by viewing the map alone. In order to reveal idiosyncracies in corneal height data, the general shape of the cornea needs to be removed. One method is to remove the spherical component of the corneal topography. These spherical difference elevation maps are useful to view the difference between corneal irregularities from a spherical surface. In essence, these maps effectively enhance the ability to view departures from a smooth spherical surface. Figure 2.22 shows a spherical difference elevation map of an orthokeratology patient. The corneal elevation/depression (in μm) is subtracted from the elevation data of a 9 mm spherical surface. The 9 mm reference sphere is chosen as it matches the axial radius of curvature 1 mm

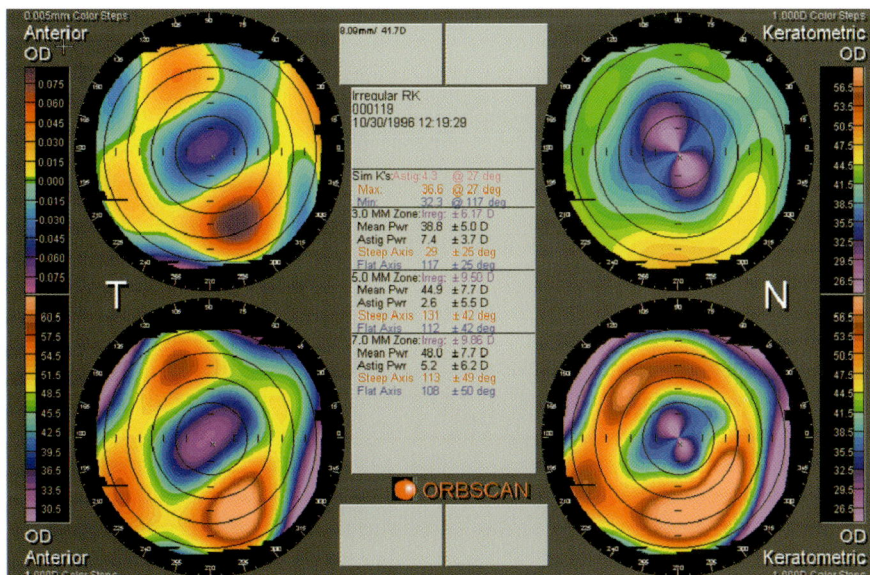

Figure 2.21 Irregular radial keratotomy (RK) performed on a patient. The axial map (top right) fails to illustrate much of the detail regarding the corneal shape. The tangential map (bottom right) only shows the localized area of steepening following the procedure (often referred to as the RK knee). The anterior elevation and mean power map (left, top and bottom respectively) are of similar appearance and show the points of greatest elevation on the corneal surface.

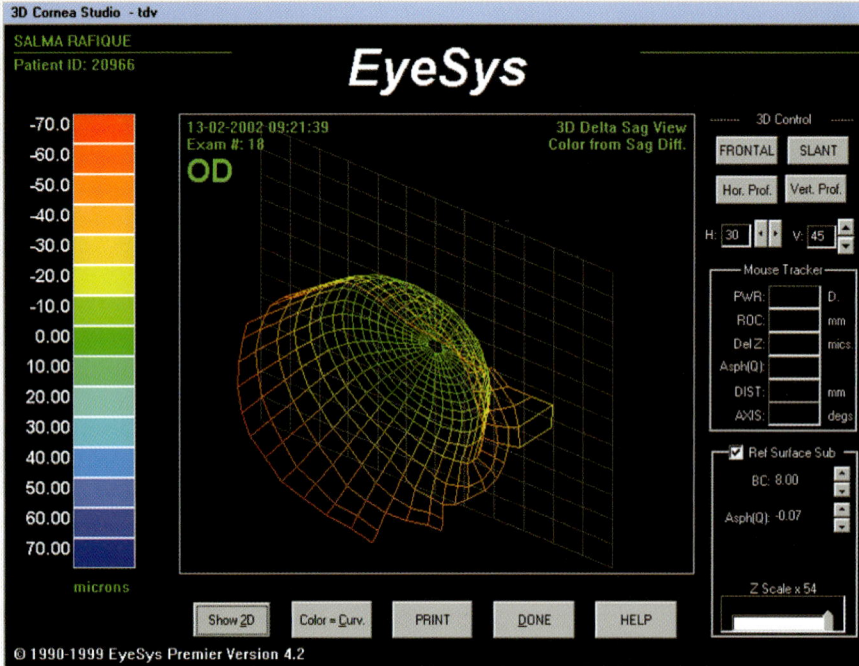

Figure 2.22 Spherical difference elevation map of a patient who has undergone orthokeratology treatment with a Contex OK704CYF lens.

temporally from the map center. The flat plateau in the center (green) demonstrates that the central cornea postorthokeratology is spherical followed by depression (or relative steepening). Spherical difference elevation maps therefore show the radial difference between a best-fit sphere and the cornea. Ellipsoidal difference height maps are even more advantageous as corneal shape is better described according to ellipses (rather than spheres); in fact, a useful feature would be to view the difference between pretreatment elevation and posttreatment elevation. Ellipsoidal difference elevation maps are available in the Euclid ET–800 topographer (Euclid Systems Corporation).

The surface regularity index and surface asymmetry index

Computer algorithms may be derived in order to calculate indices that complement the data from contour maps. Two such indices, the surface regularity index (SRI) and the surface asymmetry index (SAI), have been assessed in two clinical studies by Dingledein et al (1989) and Wilson & Klyce (1991).

The SRI determines the central corneal optical quality; it is a measure of localized surface regularity. The lower the value of this index, the smoother the surface. Thus, for a perfectly smooth surface a theoretical value of zero would be found. However, in practice this is not possible due to instrument errors. Wilson & Klyce (1991) found a high correlation between the SRI and best-corrected spectacle acuity ($r = 0.8$, $P < 0.001$) in 31 eyes that met their criteria for inclusion. Clinically, the SRI may be used to differentiate between reduced visual acuity due to factors other than corneal topography.

The SAI determines the asymmetry of the central corneal surface power. The value represents the centrally weighted summation of differences in corneal power 180° apart over 128 equally spaced meridians. For a perfectly regular surface, such as a sphere, a theoretical value of zero would be found. Again, due to instrument errors, this is not the case. Dingledein et al (1989) found a reasonable correlation between SAI and best spectacle corrected visual acuity ($r = 0.76$, $P < 0.001$) in 39 eyes with keratoconus, compound myopic astigmatism, epikeratophakia, and two corneas from patients with 20/20 vision. The differences in values of SAI for normals and those with keratoconus with best-corrected spectacle acuity of 20/20 were statistically significant ($P < 0.001$). In a more recent study by Wilson & Klyce (1991), a relatively low correlation was found between this index and best-corrected spectacle acuity ($r = 0.62$, $P < 0.005$). This discrepancy may be due to the relatively small sample sizes. Clinically, the SAI may be used as a quantitative indicator for monitoring changes in corneal topography. The derivation of these indices is described by Wilson & Klyce (1991). They suggest that the incorporation of these indices would be a useful tool when combined with color-coded maps for the assessment of corneal topography.

Quantitative descriptors of corneal topography

For purposes such as contact lens fitting and surgical modification of the corneal surface, accurate knowledge of the corneal surface parameters is essential. Qualitative assessment is of use only to summarize the enormous amount of data derived from corneal topographic systems. Quantitative descriptors in the form of mathematical functions may be useful to describe the corneal surface whilst allowing the practitioner to retain the concrete information provided from videokeratoscopy. The cornea may be described mathematically in one of three ways: curvature, position, and slope. However, there is no agreement as to the appropriate method of describing corneal shape. Some of these mathematical descriptors are discussed below.

Corneal radius and shape

The radius of curvature of the anterior corneal surface and its refractive index determine the power of that surface. The smaller the radius, the greater the refracting power of that surface. The apical radius of the cornea defines the size of the corneal profile. Guillon et al (1986) showed a variety of corneal shapes within the normal population. Therefore, mathematical descriptors that show a continuous change in curvature would more accurately model the shape of the cornea. It appears that descriptions have taken two separate forms: certain researchers have provided precise descriptions using complex polynomial formulae

(Howland et al 1992), whereas others have approximated corneal contour to conic sections (Townsley 1970, 1974, Bibby 1976, Guillon et al 1986). Generally, the results of these studies have shown that modeling the corneal surface in terms of second-order polynomials (conics) is acceptable. The family of second-order polynomial curves used as descriptors of the cornea are known as conics. Mathematically, they are defined as follows:

$$\frac{x^2}{a^2} + \frac{y^2}{b^2} = 1 \qquad \text{Equation 2.3}$$

where a and b are the semimajor and semiminor axes respectively. x is the sagittal depth at a chord length of y.

The family of surfaces and curves that may be derived from a cone (a solid surface produced by the revolution of either of two straight lines meeting at a point about the other) are defined below:

- Conicoids: on rotating conic sections about an axis of symmetry, one produces surfaces known as conicoids.
- Conic sections: these two-dimensional sections are defined according to two factors – the apical radius of curvature and a term known as the eccentricity (e). Baker (1943) derived an equation to describe a conic section:

$$y^2 = 2r_0x - px^2 \qquad \text{Equation 2.4}$$

where x and y are the Cartesian coordinates (the origin is conveniently placed at the corneal apex), r_0 is the apical radius of curvature, and p is an index of peripheral flattening (the shape factor) and indicates the level of asphericity. For example, $p < 0$, hyperbola; $p = 0$, parabola; $0 < p < 1$, oblate (flattening) ellipse; $p = 1$, sphere; $p > 1$, prolate (steepening) ellipse. Bennett (1968) has shown a direct relationship between p and e where

$$p = 1 - e^2 \qquad \text{Equation 2.5}$$

The advantage of Baker's and Bennett's notation is that the formula is simplified and it is capable of describing all conic sections. A simple mathematical relationship can be shown to link Equations 2.3 and 2.4, as shown in Equation 2.6.

$$r_0 = \frac{b^2}{a} \text{ and } p = \frac{b^2}{a^2} \qquad \text{Equation 2.6}$$

Manufacturers of topography systems have used this information to produce numeric maps (as in the EyeSys topographer). These maps display apical radius, eccentricity, and peripheral sagittal radii of curvature. Known as numeric maps, they provide the orthokeratologist with sufficient information to derive the initial trial lens.

Unfortunately, there may not be sufficient repeatability within instruments and between instruments to derive the same eccentricity value consistently within the same cornea. The reason for this is that, although systems may be accurate for nonbiological surfaces, the Placido ring reflection off the corneal surface may result in difficulty in consistently imaging the rings from the peripheral cornea. As a result, variability in *e*-values will occur. Another factor that may be responsible for a lack of agreement between different instruments is that some topography systems derive *e*-values within a specific zone, such as the Keratron (Optikon, Italy).

High-order polynomial descriptors

The corneal surface is a complex shape. In order to describe it mathematically high-order polynomial expressions may be used. A study by Howland et al (1992) attempted to describe corneal shape in precisely this manner. Using the corneal TMS (Computed Anatomy Inc., New York), fourth-order polynomial expressions from the Taylor series were fitted to corneal surface coordinates. From the expressions, the mean corneal curvature (MCC) at any point on the surface was computed and compared with the measured curvature derived from the TMS.

Howland et al (1992) concluded that polynomials captured gross features of curvature but did not resolve sufficient detail. However, from their study they suggested that the use of polynomial fitting could form a classification scheme for describing corneal topography.

The use of corneal topography in orthokeratology

The principal application of corneal topography for eye-care practitioners is contact lens fitting, corneal screening, and refractive surgery. Most topography systems now have contact lens modules that use information acquired from topography measurement in order to determine the initial lens for rigid lens fitting. Practitioners may also specify the level of apical clearance or even design custom lenses for patients. Szczotska (1997) clinically evaluated the EyeSys Pro-Fit software (version 3.1) in terms of its efficiency in fitting RGP lenses to 22 normal subjects. Comparing the EyeSys fitting to manually fitted patients showed identical success rates (77%) with no subsequent modification of lens fit. However, EyeSys-based fitting reduced chair time by 51.4%. The author concluded that EyeSys-based rigid gas-permeable (RGP) lens fitting improved efficiency in normal eyes.

Corneal topographical analysis has proved to be invaluable and essential to the practice of orthokeratology. As with refractive surgery, practitioners involved with any procedure introducing a change to the corneal shape must have access to a topographical device. The primary aim of using such a device is twofold: firstly, to be able to record baseline data that will enable the practitioner to choose a suitable trial lens and secondly, so that any change in corneal shape can be accurately documented. The use of difference maps has greatly enhanced the understanding of lens-induced changes that occur in orthokeratology.

Difference maps and application of topography to orthokeratology

Figure 2.23A shows an example of a difference map. All difference maps show three maps: the top left (in Fig. 2.23A) is the pretreatment sagittal topography plot, the lower left the posttreatment sagittal plot, and the right map shows the point-by-point difference in sagittal radius from pre- to posttreatment. The increments on the numeric scale on the right can be set to diopters or in millimeters depending on practitioner preference. It shows the change in corneal curvature from pre- to posttreatment.

As well as being an objective measure of the change induced during orthokeratology, difference maps can also inform the practitioner of the effect of the fit of the contact lens on the corneal surface. Figure 2.23A shows a difference map

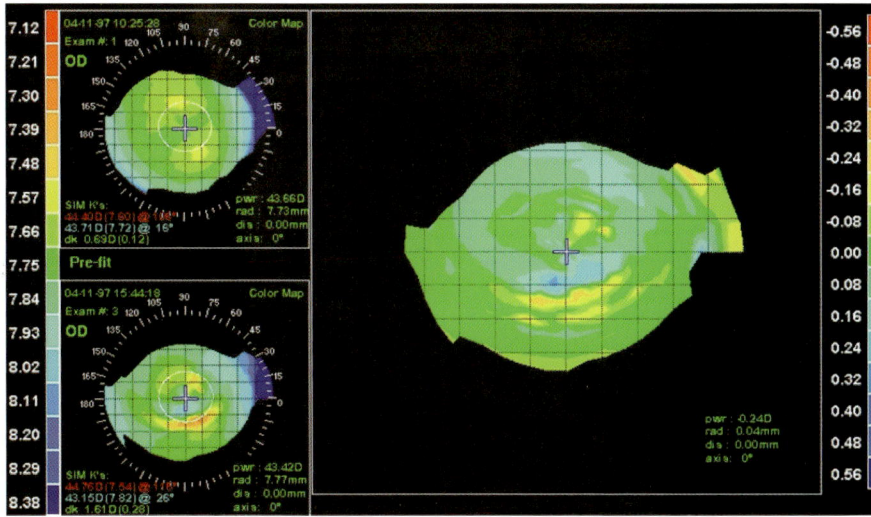

Figure 2.23 (A) The use of difference maps shows the corneal response to a high-riding OK 704C lens (Contex Inc, California). The left-hand map shows the difference between pre- and posttreatment. The superior flattening and inferior steepening is a classic sign of a flat high-riding lens.

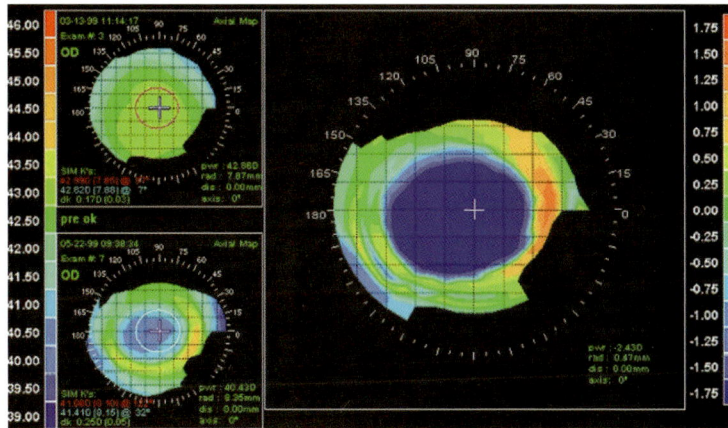

Figure 2.23 (B) An ideal response to orthokeratology. The top left map shows a sagittal map before treatment whereas the lower map shows the sagittal map posttreatment. The difference map shows that the lens has flattened the cornea centrally by 2.22 D with little change in the peripheral cornea.

where the relative inferior steepening implies that the fitted lens displaced upward and hence flattened the superior cornea whilst secondarily inducing inferior steepening. Lenses inducing such a change in topography generally have a sag that is less than the sag of the cornea at an equivalent chord diameter (i.e., the lens is too flat). Conversely, Figure 2.23B shows an ideal response to orthokeratology where the lens has remained centered and induced a smooth central area of flattening without inducing corneal distortion. Note that the change in refractive error is of the order of 2.00 D. Figure 2.23C shows an area of central steepening; lenses inducing this type of topographic change are usually too steep.

As will be discussed in Chapter 3, lens binding following overnight wear is common. However, in nearly all cases lenses tend to become mobile after a period of eye opening. Unfortunately, lenses may occasionally bind and induce corneal distortion. The topographic hallmark of binding-induced distortion is a sharp ring of localized steepening (Fig. 2.24). This area of steepening (usually red in color) corresponds to epithelial indentation at the site of lens binding. In most cases, binding occurs in the superior area of the cornea.

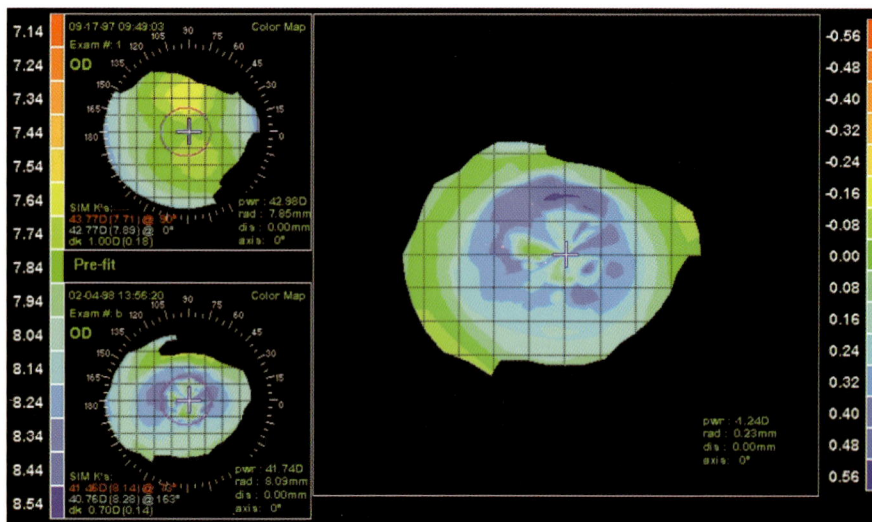

Figure 2.23   (C) Localized central steepening is observed in the difference plot (right). The map represents the difference in corneal topography before and after overnight wear with an OK 704CF (Contex, Sherman Oaks, California) trial lens.

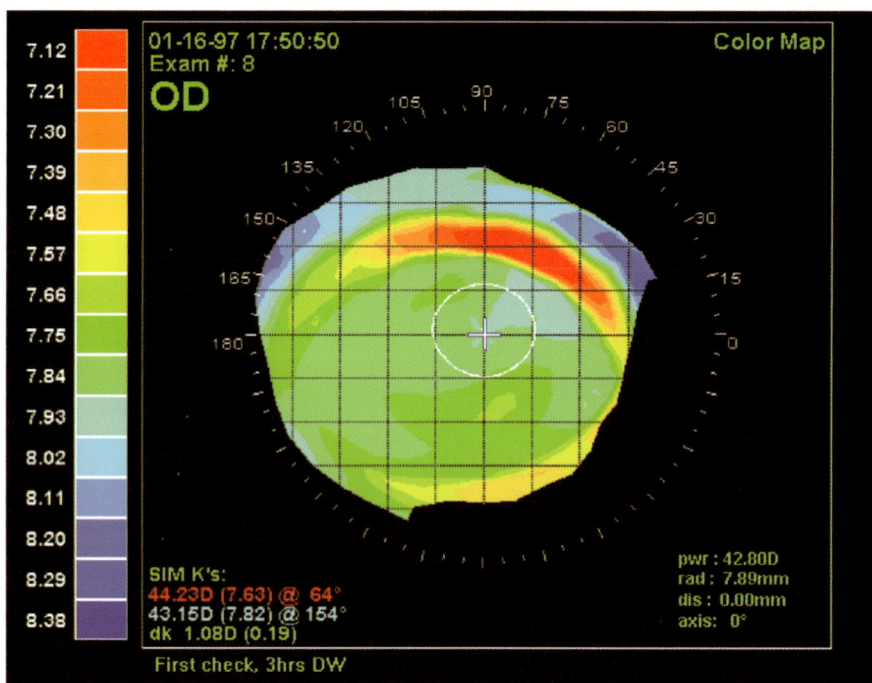

Figure 2.24   Topographic sagittal map of a cornea upon removal of a bound lens. The red area superiorly indicates the primary site of lens binding.

The modern approach to orthokeratology lens fitting is based on matching the corneal sag to the sag of the contact lens for reverse geometry lenses. Current programs used to perform such calculations require the use of the apical radius of the cornea and the corneal eccentricity. Almost all modern topography systems display these parameters. However, the practitioner must be aware whether the mean (global) corneal eccentricity is derived or whether the eccentricity over a specific zone or meridian is derived, as this can result in significant discrepancies with respect to the final predicted lens.

Currently, there are no publications directly relating to the accuracy of corneal topographic systems in predicting accurate orthokeratology

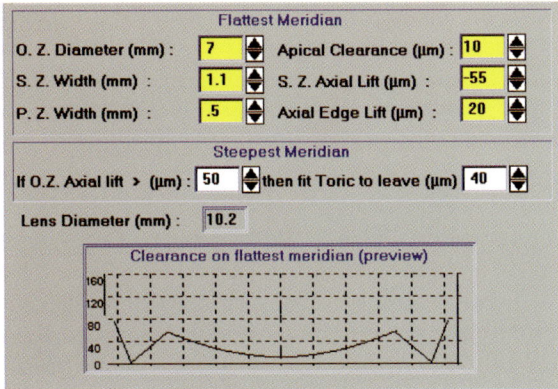

Figure 2.25 (A) The Keratron tear layer profile design section. The required tear layer profile is shown and the subsequent predicted sodium fluorescein pattern is shown in Figure 2.25(B). (B) The predicted sodium fluorescein pattern for the tear layer profile shown in Figure 2.25(A).

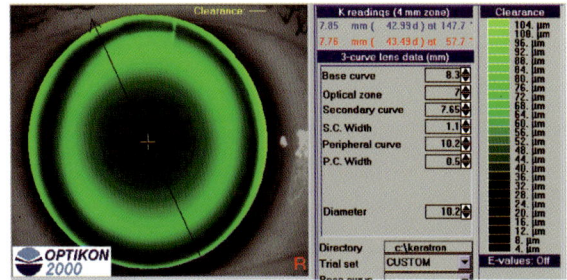

lenses. However, the Keratron topographer has the facility for the practitioner to perform sagittal-based fitting on tricurve lenses. All that needs to be entered into the contact lens module of the software is the lens/corneal clearance at the back optic zone diameter (BOZD), the tear reservoir, and the lens edge in order to produce a required tear layer profile (Fig. 2.25A). The computer then derives the contact lens curves that produce the required tear layer profile and subsequently the predicted sodium fluorescein pattern is displayed (Fig. 2.25B). It must be stated that, although in principle this appears to be a logical way of designing a lens, the practitioner's choice of tear reservoir height and back optic zone radius (BOZR) would not then be determined in a scientific manner. The Keratron therefore has no advantages over other topographic systems provided one uses a computer program to design the lenses (as is generally the case).

Which topographer is most suitable?

Most orthokeratologists would agree that it is essential to have a topographic device when embarking on orthokeratology treatment. There are numerous devices available in the market place, so which one is most appropriate? Ideally, one requires a device that is accurate and repeatable. Dave et al (1998a) showed that the EyeSys (model II) topographer exhibited progressively poorer repeatability in the peripheral cornea. Furthermore, the variability of repeatability was also dependent on the corneal meridian such that greatest repeatability was found in the temporal meridian and poorest repeatability in the superior and nasal corneal meridians. The authors suggested that this meridional dependence was due to the ocular adnexa (lids, tear film, etc.) and not simply a factor associated with the videokeratoscope. In another study by Dave et al (1998b), the accuracy of the EyeSys corneal topographer was assessed using various aspheric (P-values of 0.8 and 0.5) and spherical surfaces. They found that the EyeSys topographer had a high level of accuracy and repeatability. However, the accuracy reduced with increasingly flattening surfaces, i.e., as the P-values decreased (Tables 2.5 and 2.6). However, as expected, the repeatability was exceptionally high and constant for all surfaces

Table 2.5 Accuracy of measuring aspheric surfaces using the EyeSys topographer (after Dave et al 1998b)

P-value	Bias (mm)	SD (mm)
Overall	0.022	0.0422
1	0.0003	0.0134
0.8	0.0167	0.028
0.5	0.049	0.056

Table 2.6 Repeatability of the EyeSys topographer for spherical and aspheric surfaces (after Dave et al 1998b)

Meridian	Bias (mm)	SD (mm)
Temporal	0.01	0.01
Nasal	0.01	0.01
Superior	0.01	0.01
Inferior	0.01	0.01

Table 2.7 Accuracy and precision (precision values in brackets) of four topographers in measuring six artificial surfaces (after Tang et al 2000)

Test surface	Keratron (μm)	Medmont (μm)	TMS (μm)	PAR-CTS (μm)
Sphere	2 (<0.0)	2 (0.5)	3 (2.9)	2 (12)
Asphere	1 (1.1)	2 (0.2)	9 (2.2)	2 (8.8)
Multicurve	2 (0.4)	9 (0.8)	93 (1.1)	27 (20)
5.0 Bicurve	115 (28.9)	93 (9.8)	16 (12.3)	33 (9.2)
6.5 Bicurve	78 (<0)	34 (4)	3 (5.7)	44 (14.5)
8.5 Bicurve	28 (0.3)	29 (1.8)	40 (4.6)	19 (15.5)

TMS, Topographic Modeling System.

measured, thus confirming that the biological structure of the cornea and adnexa reduce repeatability of topographers in a clinical environment.

Another requirement for topographic devices is that the device will not exhibit any bias towards any type of surface structure, i.e., it should be able to measure a normal nontreated eye with the same accuracy as any eye that has undergone treatment. In an interesting study by Tang et al (2000), the accuracy (root mean square error) and precision (maximum standard error) of four topographers using six test surfaces were determined. The surfaces comprised a sphere, asphere, multicurve, and three bicurve surfaces. The results are summarized in Table 2.7.

The Medmont exhibited greatest accuracy and precision in measuring the aspheric surface. This surface represented the "normal" cornea. The TMS showed greatest accuracy in measuring bicurve surfaces (symbolizing the profile of the cornea postrefractive surgery and orthokeratology) followed by the Medmont and Keratron;

however, the Medmont had the greatest precision in measuring bicurve surfaces. This study indicates that the algorithms and design of different topographers result in bias towards different surfaces. For orthokeratology it is most important to determine pretreatment corneal shape (or sag) and therefore the practitioner must choose a topographer that has the highest accuracy and precision in measuring the "normal" cornea.

Orthokeratology fitting is considerably different from fitting conventional geometry rigid lenses. The apical clearance in conventional lenses is of the order of 15–20 μm; however, orthokeratology lenses are fitted to have an apical clearance of the order of 2–6 μm (mode of 4 μm). Therefore, in order to fit a lens within 4 μm one requires a precision of 2 μm. Hough & Edwards (1999) utilized a well-known formula used to derive sample size for clinical trials (see Equation 2.7). Knowing the standard error (precision) of fitting required and the repeatability of the topographer, one can derive the number of readings required to achieve this defined precision.

$$n = \frac{\sigma^2}{e^2} \qquad \text{Equation 2.7}$$

where σ is the standard deviation of repeatability of the topographer and e the standard error or precision required.

Cho et al (2002) utilized this formula to determine the number of measurements required for four topographers (Dicon CT200, Humphrey ATLAS 991, Medmont E300, Orbscan II) for orthokeratology fitting with a precision of 3 μm. The authors found that the Dicon required 64 repeat readings, Humphrey 12, Medmont two, and Orbscan 552. Practitioners can themselves determine the number of repeat readings required by their topographer by deriving the standard deviation of repeatability for elevation over a 9 mm chord and inputting the value into Equation 2.7.

SUMMARY

Eye-care practitioners have always been aware of the need to understand the topographical nature of the corneal surface. Within the last decade, researchers in this field have made a number of significant improvements to older systems. Data are now stored as digitized images on computer disks to enable easy access and to eliminate errors such as shrinkage and distortion that occurred with older photographic storage media. Accurate localization of the target rings (using techniques which allow the reflected Placido rings to be located accurately) from digitized images has also aided the increase in accuracy compared to instruments where ring images were located manually. The improvement of target design (by having a greater number of rings and by modifying the spatial arrangement of the rings) has permitted greater detailed analysis of the cornea. Representation of the data has now evolved into detailed mathematical descriptors and schematic color-coded topographical maps. Modern topography devices use sophisticated algorithms that no longer bias corneal curvature to spherical surfaces, thereby improving their accuracy. However, with our greater understanding, we have also discovered limitations of current display options such as sagittal and tangential maps as computed curvature measurements are dependent on fixation and corneal symmetry. Investigators have shown that Gaussian curvature, elevation maps, and mean curvature maps permit independence of fixation axis. Currently, the Orbscan system allows practitioners to view these types of curvature maps, enabling greater localization of corneal abnormalities.

There are numerous applications for the use of topographical systems in areas such as contact lens fitting (Hodd & Ruston 1993, McCarey et al 1993), diagnosis and monitoring of keratoconus (Maguire & Bourne 1989, Maguire & Lowry 1991, Wilson et al 1991), monitoring of corneal shape after refractive surgery (Maguire et al 1987b; McDonnell et al 1989), corneal grafting, and postoperative management of cataract patients. Practitioners involved in orthokeratology must make use of modern-generation videokeratoscopes so that changes in corneal shape can be accurately documented and the necessary prescreening performed. The development of topography systems will undoubtedly be in the area of computer software.

REFERENCES

Andersen J, Koch-Jensen P, Osterby O (1993a) Corneal topography: image processing and numerical analysis of keratoscopy. Acta Ophthalmologica 71: 151–159

Andersen J, Koch-Jensen P, Osterby O (1993b) Corneal topography: photokeratoscopy including the central region. Acta Ophthalmologica 71: 145–150

Antalis J J, Lembach R G, Carney L G (1993) A comparison of the TMS-1 and the Corneal Analysis System for the evaluation of abnormal corneas. CLAO Journal 19: 58–63

Applegate R A (1992) Optical and clinical issues in the measurement of corneal topography. Ophthalmic and Visual Optical Technical Digest

Arffa R C, Warnicki J W, Rehkopf P G (1989) Corneal topography using rasterstereography. Refractive Corneal Surgery 5: 414–417

Baker T Y (1943) Ray tracing through non-spherical surfaces. Proceedings of the Physics Society 55: 361–364

Barsky B A, Klein S A, Garcia D D (1997) Gaussian power with cylinder vector field representation for corneal topography maps. Optometry and Vision Science 74: 917–925

Belin M W, Zloty P (1993) Accuracy of the PAR corneal topography system with spatial alignment. CLAO Journal 19: 64–68

Belin M W, Litoff D, Strods S J, Winn S S, Smith R S (1992) The PAR technology corneal topography system. Refractive Corneal Surgery 8: 88–96

Bennett A G (1968) Part I Aspherical contact lens surfaces. Ophthalmic Optician: 1037–1040

Bibby M M (1976) Computer assisted photokeratoscopy and contact lens design. Optician 171(4423): 37–44

Bland J M, Altman D G (1986) Statistical methods for assessing agreement between two methods of clinical measurement. Lancet 1: 307–310

Bogan S J, Waring I G O, Ibrahim O, Drews C, Curtis L (1990) Classification of normal corneal topography based on computer-assisted videokeratography. Archives of Ophthalmology 108: 945–949

Bonnet R, Cochet D (1962) New method of topographical ophthalmometry – its theoretical and clinical applications. American Journal of Optometry 39: 227

Cho P, Lam A, Mountford J, Ng L (2002) The performance of four different corneal topographers on normal human corneas and its impact on orthokeratology lens fitting. Optometry and Vision Science 79(3): 175–183

Dave T N (1995) Evaluation of videokeratoscopy. PhD thesis. Aston University, Birmingham, UK

Dave T N, Ruston D M, Fowler C W (1998a) Evaluation of the EyeSys model II computerized videokeratoscope. Part I: clinical assessment. Optometry and Vision and Science 75: 647–655

Dave T N, Ruston D M, Fowler C W (1998b) Evaluation of the EyeSys model II computerized videokeratoscope. Part II: the repeatability and accuracy in measuring convex aspheric surfaces. Optometry and Vision Science 75: 656–662

Dingledein S A, Klyce S D, Wilson S E (1989) Quantitative descriptors of corneal shape derived from computer-assisted analysis of photokeratographs. Refractive Corneal Surgery 5: 372–378

Doss J D, Hutson R L, Rowsley J J, Brown D R (1981) Method for calculation of corneal profile and power distribution. Archives of Ophthalmology 99: 1261–1265

Edmund C (1985) The central–peripheral radius of the normal corneal curvature. A photokeratoscopic study. Acta Ophthalmologica 63: 670–677

Edmund C (1987) Location of the corneal apex and its influence in the stability of the central corneal curvature. A photokeratoscopy study. American Journal of Optometry and Physiological Optics 64: 846–852

El Hage S G (1971) Suggested new methods for photokeratoscopy: a comparison for their validities. Part I. American Journal of Optometry and Physiological Optics 48: 897–912

El Hage S G (1972) Differential equation for the use of the diffused ring keratoscope. American Journal of Optometry and Physiological Optics 49: 422–436

Fincham E F (1953) New photokeratoscope utilizing a hemispherical object surface. Medical and Biological Illustration 3: 87

Gormley D J, Gersten M, Koplin R S, Lubkin V (1988) Corneal modelling. Cornea 7: 30–35

Guillon M, Lyndon D P, Wilson C (1986) Corneal topography: a clinical model. Ophthalmology and Physiological Optics 6: 47–56

Gullstrand A, Ludlum P (1966) Photographic-ophthalmometric and clinical investigations of corneal refraction. American Journal of Optometry 43: 43

Hannush S B, Crawford S L, Waring G O, Gemmill M C, Lynn M J, Nizam A (1989) Accuracy and precision of keratometry, photokeratoscopy, and corneal modeling on calibrated steel balls. Archives of Ophthalmology 107: 1235–1239

Hannush N B, Crawford S L, Waring G O, Gemmill M C, Lynn M J, Nizam A (1990) Reproducibility of normal corneal power measurements with a keratometer, photokeratoscope and video imaging system. Archives of Ophthalmology 108: 539–544

Hodd N F B, Ruston D M (1993) The EyeSys corneal analysis system: its value in contact lens practice. Optometry Today 33(17): 12–22

Hough T, Edwards K (1999) The reproducibility of videokeratoscope measurements as applied to the human cornea. Contact Lens and Anterior Eye 22: 91–99

Howland H C, Glasser A, Applegate R (1992) Polynomial approximations of corneal surfaces and corneal curvature topography. Ophthalmic and Visual Optics Technical Digest 3: 34–36

Hubbe R E (1994) The effect of poor fixation on computer-assisted topographic corneal analysis. Ophthalmology 101: 1745–1748

Jeandervin M, Barr J (1998) Comparison of repeat videokeratography: repeatability and accuracy. Optometry and Vision Science 75(9): 663–669

Klein S A (1993) Improvements for video-keratography. Ophthalmic and Visual Optics Technical Digest

Klein S A (1997) Axial curvature and the skew ray error in corneal topography. Optometry and Vision Science 74: 931–944

Klyce S D (1984) Computer-assisted corneal topography. Investigations in Ophthalmology and Visual Science 25: 1426–1435

Knoll H A (1961) Corneal contours in the general population as revealed by the photokeratoscope. American Journal of Optometry and Archives of the American Academy of Optometry 38: 389–397

Knoll H A, Stimson R, Weeks C L (1957) New photokeratoscope utilizing a hemispherical object surface. Journal of the Optical Society of America 47: 221

Koch D, Foulks G N, Moran C T, Wakil J S (1989) The corneal EyeSys system: accuracy analysis and reproducibility of first-generation prototype. Refractive Corneal Surgery 5: 424–429

Koch D D, Wakil J S, Samuelson S W, Haft E A (1992) Comparison of the accuracy and reproducibility of the keratometer and the EyeSys corneal analysis system model I. Journal of Cataract and Refractive Surgery 18: 342–347

Ludlum W M, Wittenburg S, Rosenthale J, Harris G (1967) Photographic analysis of the ocular dioptric components. American Journal of Optometry and Archives of the American Academy of Optometry 44: 276–296

Maguire L J, Bourne W M (1989) Corneal topography of early keratoconus. American Journal of Ophthalmology 108: 107–112

Maguire L J, Lowry J C (1991) Identifying progression of subclinical keratoconus by serial topography analysis. American Journal of Ophthalmology 112: 41–45

Maguire L J, Singer D E, Klyce S D (1987a) Graphic presentations of computer-analyzed keratoscope photographs. Archives of Ophthalmology 105: 223–230

Maguire L J, Klyce S D, Singer D E, McDonald M B, Kaufman H E (1987b) Corneal topography in myopic patients undergoing epikeratophakia. American Journal of Ophthalmology 103: 404–416

Mandell R B (1992) The enigma of the corneal contour. CLAO Journal 18: 267–273

Mandell R B, St Helen R (1965) Position and curvature of the corneal apex. American Journal of Optometry 46: 25–29

Mandell R B, St Helen R (1968) Stability of the corneal contour. American Journal of Optometry and Archives of the American Academy of Optometry 12: 797–806

McCarey B E, Amos C F, Taub L R (1993) Surface topography of soft contact lenses for neutralizing astigmatism. CLAO Journal 19: 114

McDonnell P J, McClusky D J, Garbus J J (1989) Corneal topography and fluctuating visual acuity after radial keratotomy. Ophthalmology 96: 665–670

McMahon T T, Anderson R J, Joslin C E, Rosas G A (2001) Precision of three topography instruments in keratoconus subjects. Optometry and Vision Science 78(8): 599–604

Miller D C J (1980) A proposed new division of corneal division of corneal functions. New York, Raven Press

Nieves J E, Applegate R A (1992) Alignment errors and working distance directly influence the accuracy of corneal topography measurements. ARVO abstracts. Investigations in Ophthalmology and Visual Science

Schultze R L (1998) Accuracy of corneal elevation with four corneal topography systems. Journal of Refractive Surgery 14(2): 100–104

Stone J (1962) The validity of some existing methods of measuring corneal contour compared with suggested new methods. British Journal of Physical Optics 19: 205–230

Szczotska L B (1997) Clinical evaluation of a topopographic based contact lens fitting software. Optometry and Vision Science 74: 14–19

Tang W, Collins M J, Carney L, Davis B (2000) The accuracy and precision performance of four videokeratoscopes in measuring test surfaces. Optometry and Vision Science 77: 483–491

Townsley M (1967) New equipment and methods for determining the contour of the human cornea. Contacto 11: 72

Townsley M (1970) New knowledge of the corneal contour. Contacto 14: 38–44

Townsley M (1974) The graphic presentation of corneal contours. Contacto 18: 24–32

Tsilimbaris M K, Vlachonikolis I G, Siganos D, Makridakas G, Pallikaris I G (1991) Comparison of keratometric readings as obtained by Javal ophthalmometer and corneal analysis system (EyeSys). Refractive Corneal Surgery 7: 368–373

Wang J, Rice D A, Klyce S D (1989) A new reconstruction algorithm for improvement of corneal topographical corneal analysis. Refractive Corneal Surgery 5: 379–387

Waring G O (1989) Making sense of keratospeak. Proposed conventional terminology for corneal topography. Refractive Corneal Surgery 5: 362–367

Wilson S E, Klyce S D (1991) Quantitative descriptors of corneal topography. Archives of Ophthalmology 109: 349–353

Wilson S E, Lin D T C, Klyce S D (1991) Corneal topography of keratoconus. Cornea 10: 2–8

Chapter **3**

Overnight and extended wear of rigid gas-permeable (RGP) lenses

Trusit Dave

CHAPTER CONTENTS

Introduction   49
Hypoxia   50
Physiological signs   51
Composition   51
Tonicity and pH   51
Clinical complications   60
References   65

INTRODUCTION

Almost since the advent of contact lenses, both clinicians and scientists have been baffled as to the variability of the individual subjective response to overnight or extended-wear contact lenses. This is highlighted by reports in the literature. For example, Dick (1957) published a clinical case study of a patient who successfully wore polymethyl methacrylate (PMMA) lenses continuously for 3 months. Furthermore Sloan (1965) reported the results of a clinical trial involving 50 patients wearing PMMA lenses over 7 years. However, in light of the developments in polymer science and greater knowledge of the corneal response to oxygen deprivation, our chances of successfully fitting patients with rigid gas-permeable (RGP) lenses have increased significantly.

The applications of RGP lenses for overnight and extended wear became apparent to investigators in the 1980s after the publication of a landmark study by Holden & Mertz (1984). The study showed that the oxygen transmissibility (Dk/t) of any contact lens should be no less than 87×10^{-9} $(cm^2/s)(mlO_2/ml \times mmHg)$ (or 87 Barrers) in order to limit corneal swelling to that found after sleep without a contact lens. The inherent properties of modern-day RGP materials make them ideal for extended wear. However, as with soft lenses, they can induce adverse reactions. Furthermore, these reactions are more prevalent with extended wear. The most commonly reported complications have been lens binding (Polse et al 1987, Swarbrick 1988), 3 and 9 o'clock staining, and corneal warpage (Holden et al 1988). However, the use of purely overnight-wear RGP lenses (as opposed to daytime wear) offers the orthokeratologist a number of advantages:

- Patients do not have adaptation problems. The absence of the blink reflex and reduced lens movement allows the patient to be comfortable.
- Overnight wear of RGP lenses does not result in significant lens deposition (Bennett et al 1986, Elie 1986). This is partly due to the fact that lenses are only worn during sleeping hours and due to the properties of modern contact lens materials.
- Rigid lenses offer superior handling compared to soft lenses (Key & Mobley 1989).

Unfortunately, no clinical studies relating to overnight wear of RGP lenses were found whilst compiling this review. However, important publications describing the complications of extended-wear RGP lenses will be discussed. The major complications of extended-wear RGP lenses arise because of the effects of oxygen depletion (hypoxia), lens adherence, and ocular infection. Each of these factors will now be considered in detail.

HYPOXIA

Basic physiology

Corneal tissue undergoes more metabolic activity than any other structure in the body. This high level of metabolic activity is principally responsible for maintaining corneal transparency. Oxygen, being a major requirement for any metabolic process, is derived from both the anterior and posterior surfaces of the cornea. Under normal circumstances, the cornea produces energy using aerobic respiration. This process effectively converts glucose into high levels of energy and basic waste products. When hypoxic stress is placed on the cornea (oxygen deprivation), the metabolic cycle used to convert glucose into energy is impeded. Instead, anaerobic respiration begins, producing less energy and a less basic waste product known as lactic acid. The presence of lactic acid encourages water to permeate the cornea by a process known as osmosis (where water moves from a low concentration to a high concentration). The inabil-

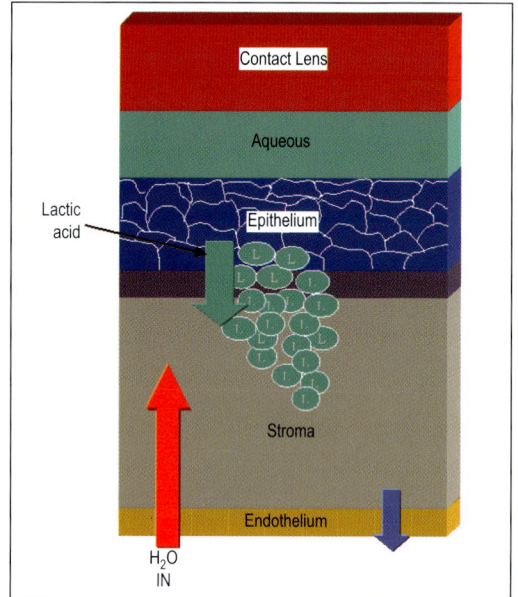

Figure 3.1   The effect of corneal hypoxia.

ity of the endothelial pump to remove water at the same rate at which it enters the cornea results in corneal edema (Fig. 3.1).

As well as the accumulation of lactic acid, carbon dioxide also builds up in the corneal stroma. Eventually, the pH of the cornea reduces (an acid shift). It is thought that 30% of corneal acidosis is because of the accumulation of carbon dioxide (hypercapnia).

Oxygen transmissibility and corneal edema

In a landmark study, the minimum oxygen transmissibility required of a contact lens in order to restrict overnight corneal swelling to 4% was

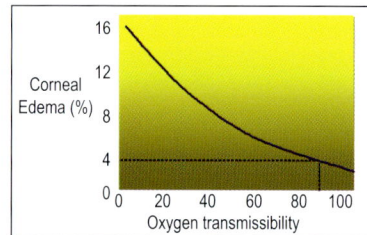

Figure 3.2   The relationship between oxygen transmissibility and corneal edema for extended wear (reproduced with permission from Holden & Mertz 1984© Association for Research in Vision and Ophthalmology).

derived (Holden & Mertz 1984). These authors discovered that a transmissibility of 87×10^{-9} (cm $\times$ ml O_2)/(s $\times$ ml $\times$ mmHg) was needed in order to achieve the same level of swelling following sleep (Fig. 3.2). Furthermore, a transmissibility of 24×10^{-9} (cm $\times$ ml O_2)/(s $\times$ ml $\times$ mmHg) was required for the daily wear of contact lenses. At present, none of the conventional soft contact lenses meet the "holy grail" oxygen transmissibility requirement of 87×10^{-9} (cm $\times$ ml O_2)/(s $\times$ ml $\times$ mmHg) required to limit corneal swelling to 4%. Therefore, use of these materials for extended wear poses a risk in compromising corneal health. Only the modern silicone hydrogels and rigid lenses are able to meet the physiological requirement for overnight wear.

The oxygen delivery through a rigid contact lens is not solely dependent on the material or lens design. The tear pump, lid tension, and rapid eye movements also play an important role in the transmission of oxygen (Koetting et al 1985). The tear pump is known to provide 16–19% tear exchange (Polse 1979). However, during sleep or overnight wear, the tear pump cannot exert its effect. Tear stagnation plays an important role in the mechanism of ocular infection (Fletcher et al 1993a,b). Overnight wear of both hydrogel and rigid lenses reduces tear flow beneath a contact lens; the principal advantage of rigid lenses is that in the open-eye situation the pump will exert a greater effect and thus resolve edema at a faster rate (Holden et al 1988).

PHYSIOLOGICAL SIGNS

The ocular effects of extended-wear RGP lenses will be discussed in terms of the morphological changes that occur to anatomical structures of the eye and also with respect to recognized ocular conditions.

Changes in the tear film following extended wear

As the tear pump is not active during the closed-eye situation, tear stagnation is present within overnight wear of RGP lenses. Tear flow beneath a contact lens is an important factor in the pathogenesis of contact lens-related ocular inflammation. Tear stagnation results in decaying debris and bacteria becoming trapped between the posterior surface of the contact lens and the corneal epithelium (Mertz & Holden 1981, Zantos 1984). In addition, there is no doubt that the layers of the tear film are disturbed following contact lens insertion. Various investigators have demonstrated that one factor associated with *Pseudomonas* infection in contact lens wearers is an absence of the mucous layer of the tear film during contact lens wear (Fleiszig et al 1994a). In an eye not wearing a contact lens, *Pseudomonas* binding to the epithelium is inhibited by the mucous layer.

Changes to tear biochemistry following contact lens wear have been explored in detail and are beyond the scope of this chapter. However, some of the more fundamental changes associated with extended wear will be discussed.

COMPOSITION

Closed-eye lens wear has been associated with increased levels of inflammatory cells (Wilson et al 1989). The number of polymorphonuclear leukocytes (PMNs), however, is dependent on the level of adaptation of the contact lens wearer. Thakur & Willcox (2000) compared the number of PMNs and the levels of inflammatory mediators in tears following sleep in a noncontact lens-wearing (NCLW) group, a nonadapted group (NACLW), and an adapted group (ACLW). Significantly higher levels of PMNs were found in the NACLW group compared with other groups. Furthermore, a significantly higher level of PMN chemoattractants was observed in the ACLW group compared to the neophyte and nonlens-wearing groups.

Changes in the concentration of certain protein in the tears can also be an indicator of inflammation. Typically, studies have analyzed the concentration of immunoglobulin A (IgA) in tears and ascertained that lower levels are found in adapted contact lens wearers – suggesting that the eye is a state of subclinical inflammation (Vinding et al 1987). Many more chemical changes occur in the tear film from the open- to closed-eye situation and with the introduction of a contact lens. However, this area is more of academic interest.

TONICITY AND PH

When an unadapted subject inserts a contact lens (soft or rigid), reflex lacrimation dilutes the tear film, resulting in tears of lower osmolarity. However, once adaptation is complete, tear osmolarity is generally found to be higher. The most obvious reason for this would be reduced stimulation of tears due to reduced corneal sensitivity. Other explanations also exist, such as increased aqueous evaporation and deposits on the lens.

There is as yet little agreement as to the nature of pH shift in eyes wearing RGP lenses. Various studies have presented conflicting results. For example, Norn (1988) demonstrated a reduced pH shift in all lens types whereas Carney & Hill (1976) reported no change.

Epithelium (microcysts)

One of the first results of reduced oxygen levels at the anterior corneal surface is decreased cell production (Hamano et al 1983). A number of studies have shown that a reduction in the number of epithelial cells due to hypoxia results in epithelial cell enlargement, epithelial thinning, and, somewhat surprisingly, increased cell life (Bergmanson et al 1985, Holden et al 1985a, Lemp & Gold 1986). Epithelial thinning may be explained by the fact that there is reduced epithelial mitosis in the presence of a rigid lens. Therefore, with cell loss exceeding cell production there would be a natural reduction in epithelial thickness (Ren et al 1999, Landage 2000, Bergmanson 2001). The effect of lid tension through the contact lens may induce squeeze pressure on the epithelial cells. Ren et al (1999) found increased epithelial cell flattening following RGP lens wear in rabbits.

An alteration in cell production causes the formation of epithelial microcysts (Fig. 3.3). Bergmanson (1987) suggested that microcysts represent an extracellular accumulation of broken-down cellular material in the basal epithelial layers of the corneal epithelium. Clinically, they appear as tiny translucent dots within the epithelium that are best detected with a slit lamp with high illumination and partial retroillumination (Zantos & Holden 1978). The numbers of microcysts show a correlation to the oxygen permeability (Dk) of the lens (Holden et al 1985a), the modality of wear (Holden et al 1985a), and the duration of wear (Fonn & Holden 1988).

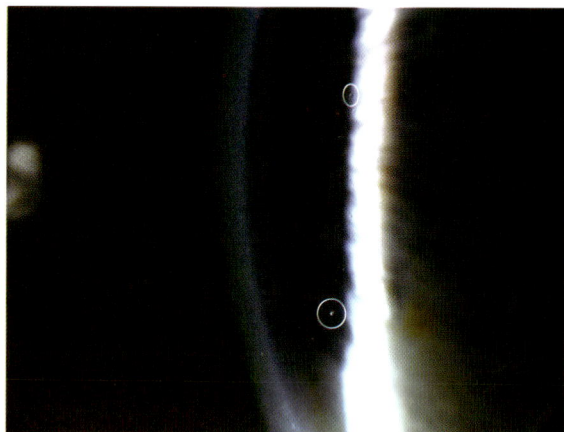

Figure 3.3   Epithelial microcysts.

Table 3.1   The relationship between the number of microcysts and lens modality

Lens type/Dk/wear	Number of microcysts
Soft DW	5
Soft EW	28
RGP (very low Dk) EW	23
RGP (low Dk) EW	17
RGP (medium Dk) EW	3
RGP (high Dk) EW	0

Dk, oxygen permeability; DW, daily wear; EW, extended wear; RGP, rigid gas-permeable.

Holden et al (1985a) counted the number of microcysts for various Dk lenses (low, medium, and high), lens type (RGP and soft) and usage (daily or extended wear). Table 3.1 summarizes the results.

A change in the metabolic activity of the cornea and those events that lead to tissue acidosis can compromise epithelial integrity. Metabolic corneal staining is generally induced by epithelial decompensation and microcysts that have broken through the epithelium (Fig. 3.4). Epithelial decompensation is clinically visible as diffuse punctate epithelial staining. In circumstances of extreme hypoxia, large full-thickness breaks may be observed (Efron 1999). This is because of the loosening of tight junctions and reduction in the

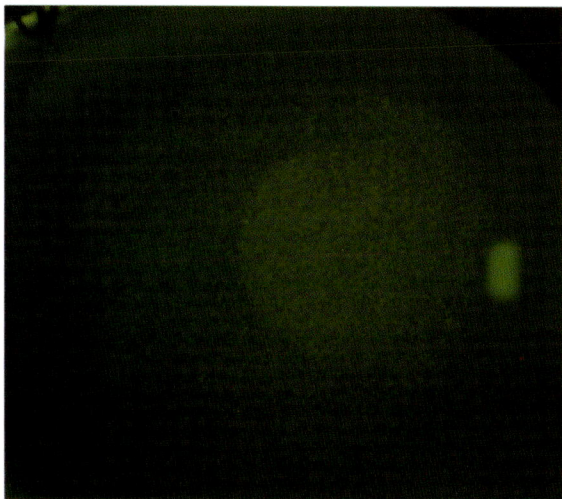

Figure 3.4 Metabolic epithelial staining.

number of hemidesmosomes (Bergmanson 1987, Madigan et al 1987, Madigan & Holden 1992).

In one of the largest studies ever to investigate contact lens-related complications, Hamano et al (1985) recorded the prevalence of clinically significant corneal erosion and/or punctate staining in 66 218 patients. They found a prevalence of only 0.5% for the RGP lens-wearing group, 1.3% in the PMMA group, and 0.9% in the soft contact lens group.

Interestingly, the magnitude of the figures correlates with the level of oxygen transmissibility of the lenses in question, thus providing further indirect evidence that corneal hypoxia results in epithelial decompensation. It should be noted that epithelial microcysts are also found in the noncontact lens-wearing patients; however, they are significantly less.

Polse et al (1987) conducted an extended-wear comparative prospective study over 6 months with 27 RGP wearers and nine soft lens wearers (oxygen transmissibility (Dk/L) 19.58 and 20.5 respectively). The incidence of epithelial microcysts was 22% for the RGP group and 56% for the soft lens group. It is interesting to note that both lenses had approximately the same degree of oxygen transmissibility; one explanation for this may be the effect of the tear pump that would be operational in the open-eye situation.

Later, in 1988, Polse et al evaluated the effects of extended wear in a group of 35 subjects who wore RGP lenses of mean transmissibility of 37×10^{-9} (cm × ml O_2)/(s × ml × mmHg) for a period of 6 months. Subjects attended for six morning visits at monthly intervals to assess slit-lamp findings, corneal thickness, and refraction. Corneal swelling was found to be $5.9 \pm 3.3\%$ and microcysts were found in 6.5% of subjects. It is important to note that these rather modest complications were observed in subjects wearing lenses with a transmissibility of only 37×10^{-9} (cm × ml O_2)/(s × ml × mmHg). Currently, manufacturers can produce lenses with a Dk/L that exceeds the Holden–Mertz criterion for physiologically acceptable extended wear (87×10^{-9} (cm × ml O_2)/(s × ml × mmHg)).

In another study, Key & Mobley (1989) studied the corneal response to extended-wear RGP lenses using the Paraperm EW lens (Dk 56) over 12 months in 372 subjects. Key & Mobley (1989) found mild 3 and 9 o'clock staining in 12.3%. MacKeen et al (1992) looked at 202 eyes over 12 months for extended wear using Menicon SF-P RGP lenses. Subjects wore lenses for an average of 6.2 days before cleaning. No significant complications were observed. Sigband & Bridgewater (1994) conducted a 3-month extended-wear trial on 81 subjects wearing FluroPerm 151 lenses (Paragon Vision Sciences, Arizona). The authors observed no physiological or pathological complications. Fifteen subjects discontinued due to poor comfort.

The epithelial effects of 24-h RGP lenses of varying transmissibility were determined in a study by Ichijima et al (1992). Rigid lens materials with transmissibility of 0, 33, 56, and 64×10^{-9} (cm × ml O_2)/(s × ml × mmHg) were placed on rabbit eyes for 24 h, after which the corneal epithelium was studied using the Tandem scanning confocal microscope (TSCM) and confirmed with scanning electron microscopy. TSCM showed no superficial epithelial cells but only the deeper exposed wing cells with the PMMA lens ($Dk/L = 0$). The lens with a transmissibility of 33×10^{-9} and 56×10^{-9} (cm × ml O_2)/(s × ml × mmHg) resulted in partial superficial epithelial cell desquamation. However, no epithelial swelling was detected with the 56×10^{-9} lens. The highest-transmissibility lens ($Dk/L = 65$) resulted in no epithelial swelling or epithelial desquamation.

Another objective study was conducted by Ichijima et al (2000), in which the concentrations of glucose and lactate were measured in the corneal epithelium, stroma, and aqueous humor using an enzyme assay. Lenses of four different transmissibilities (27, 43, 70, and 125×10^{-9} (cm $\times$ ml O_2)/(s $\times$ ml $\times$ mmHg)) were worn by eight rabbits in the right eye (the left eye was a control) for 1 month of continuous wear. The authors discovered that RGP lens-induced hypoxia is associated with an alteration in glucose-lactate metabolism. Extended wear of low-Dk/L lenses (27–70) resulted in increasing levels of lactate in the epithelium (as measured at day 7 and 1 month) and decreasing levels of lactate in the stroma and aqueous humor. However, the 125×10^{-9} lens showed no increase in epithelial lactate levels. The use of modern high-Dk materials is mandatory when performing overnight orthokeratology. Most modern orthokeratology lenses are made from materials with Dks of over 100 Barrers.

In summary, there is now widely accepted scientific proof that high-oxygen-transmissibility RGP lenses induce a reduced microcystic response compared to lower-transmissibility lenses. Furthermore, the incidence of microcysts increases with modality of wear, i.e., increased number of microcysts with extended wear (Holden et al 1987). More sensitive techniques such as TSCM have confirmed that ultrahigh-Dk lenses cause little or no effect on the corneal epithelium (Ichijima et al 1992). However, from a clinical standpoint the most sensitive test of corneal hypoxia available to practitioners is observation of epithelial microcysts. Generally, it is recommended that if more than 30 microcysts are observed, clinical intervention is required (Efron 1999). The aim of treatment is to increase the oxygen transmission to the cornea; this may be achieved through increasing the Dk, reducing lens thickness, increasing the effectivity of the tear pump, reducing wearing time, and reducing the number of nights of wear.

Stroma

The principal effect of corneal hypoxia is corneal edema. The mechanism of edema formation was discussed earlier in this chapter. However, other factors also play a role in lens-induced corneal edema. As well as hypoxia, hypercapnia, increased temperature, increased humidity and hypotonicity are known to induce edema (Sweeney & Holden 1991). However, of these factors, hypoxia is thought to be responsible for approximately 50% of all corneal edema (Sweeney & Holden 1991).

The long-term effects of edema and corneal acidosis were described by Holden et al (1985a). They found that, in a sample of extended-wear soft contact lens wearers who wore their lenses for 5 years, corneal edema reversed within a few days. However, stromal thinning continued for up to 10 days and was permanent. This thinning was attributed to the acidic shift in the cornea. Most clinicians unfortunately do not have a quantitative method of deriving corneal swelling, as with the studies discussed so far. However, the degree of corneal edema may be estimated by detecting subtle changes in the cornea using the slit lamp. In order to observe edema in a clinical setting, practitioners must detect striae. There is a general relationship where one stria approximately equates to 5% edema and endothelial folds around 10% edema (Woods 1989). Naturally, practitioners would also consider any other clinical indicators such as microcysts where the presence of microcysts indicates that normal corneal metabolism is being impeded.

Kamiya (1986), using the Menicon EX lens in 44 subjects worn on an extended-wear schedule for 1 year, found no signs of edema or ocular infection. In an important comparative study, Polse et al (1987) found approximately equal levels of corneal swelling (7.8% for the RGP sample and 7.3% for the soft lens sample). The oxygen transmissibility of both soft and RGP lenses was also similar (20.5 and 19.58 respectively). Using a lens originally designed for extended wear (Paraperm EW, Dk 52), Key & Mobley (1989) found 8% corneal swelling that recovered to normal after 2 h. Kok et al (1992) confirmed these findings in a study where Quantum lenses (Dk 92) were worn on an extended-wear basis by 32 subjects (62 eyes). They also found corneal thinning over the first 6 months and corneal flattening over the first 3 months.

Corneal thickness was also measured by Iskeleli et al (1996) in a group of 57 eyes using the Hoya Hard EX contact lens (Dk 125). Lenses were worn on average for a period of 5.28 ± 1.43 days over a 6-month period. Corneal thickness was measured at 1, 3, and 6 months. They found no statistically significant difference in corneal thickness at 1 month. However, a significant decrease in corneal thickness was observed at 3 and 6 months ($P < 0.001$). No serious complications were found in the course of the study and all 29 subjects continued RGP extended wear. The authors concluded that RGP extended wear provides an alternative to soft lens extended wear.

Generally, one may conclude that high-transmissibility lenses will result in less overnight edema. This statement can be substantiated by the work of Hideji et al (1989), who measured the corneal swelling following RGP lenses of various Dk values against high and low hydrogels and elastomer lenses before and after 24-h wear in rabbits. Greatest swelling was observed with PMMA lenses (21.6 ± 5.4%); conversely, least swelling was observed with the Menicon SF-P (or super EX) lens (Dk 116) (swelling = 2.9 ± 4.0%) – a value similar to that following overnight eye closure. The corneal swelling after elastomer lenses was also found to be similar to that found with the Menicon SF-P lens. With respect to modern-day orthokeratology, where lenses are worn only overnight and not during the day, there will be a greater rate of recovery and less hypoxic stress on the cornea. The very-high-Dk materials available today (up to 210) mean that there is less chance of observing the levels of corneal edema found in the aforementioned studies.

Swarbrick et al (1998) measured corneal and epithelial thickness in 11 eyes after orthokeratology treatment performed on a daily wear basis. Subjects wore OK704 lenses (Dk = 88, Contex Inc., Sherman Oaks, CA) for 28 days. The authors found central epithelial thinning (7.1 ± 7.1 μm) and mid-peripheral thickening approximately 2.5 mm from the corneal center (13.0 ± 11.1 μm) by day 28 (Figs 3.5 and 3.6). These measurements were found to be statistically significant. The authors proposed that the epithelium was either redistributed or compressed. Proposed mechanisms for the stromal changes were postlens tear forces, lens-induced edema, and pressure exerted by the steeper secondary curve on the lens. Unfortunately, the low subject numbers and the accuracy and repeatabil-

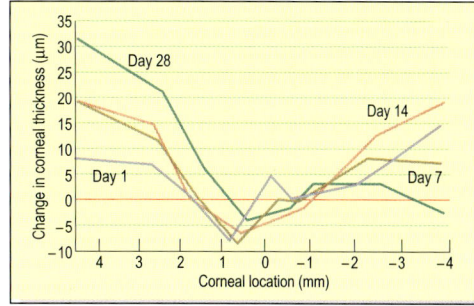

Figure 3.5   Change in corneal thickness following daily wear of reverse geometry lenses. Positive values represent thickness measurements performed on the nasal cornea. Reproduced with permission from Swarbrick et al (1998) © The American Academy of Optometry.

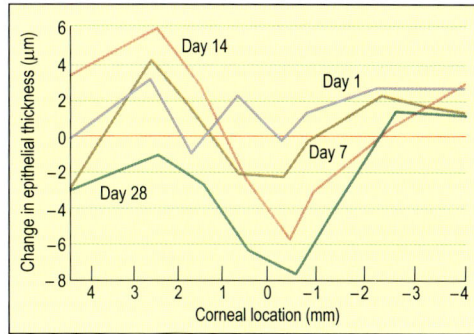

Figure 3.6   Changes in epithelial thickness following orthokeratology. Reproduced with permission from Swarbrick et al (1998) © The American Academy of Optometry.

ity of the pachometer mean that further clinical studies need to be performed.

Endothelium

Essentially, two complications occur to the endothelium following extended wear of contact lenses; these are endothelial blebs and polymegathism.

The bleb response

Zantos & Holden (1977) were the first investigators to observe changes to the endothelium. The endothelial mosaic was found to contain localized dark areas similar to the appearance of cell "drop-out" among groups of endothelial cells. Zantos & Holden (1977) referred to this appearance as endothelial blebs. This response can occur within minutes of inserting a contact lens (Zantos & Holden 1977). The number of endothelial blebs usually follows a chronological cycle: the greatest number of blebs is observed at 20–30 min and reduces to equilibrium at 45–60 min. The equilibrated level lasts for the duration of contact lens wear (Zantos & Holden 1977).

Vannas et al (1984) performed histological studies of the endothelial bleb response. They found that blebs were not associated with cell loss but rather with individual endothelial cell edema. Fluid was also found between cells. The appearance of dark areas when viewed using the slit lamp therefore represents an optical phenomenon (which is concisely described by Efron (1999)). Individual cell edema causes the posterior endothelial cell wall (in contact with the aqueous) to bow. The anterior cell wall does not bow because it is in contact with the comparatively rigid Descemet's membrane. The principle of specular microscopy relies on light being reflected from the posterior endothelium to the microscope (the observation system). A change in configuration of the reflecting surface (in this case, the bowed posterior endothelium) changes the direction of the reflected path of light and thus it is not detected by the microscope (Fig. 3.7).

In order to investigate the etiology of blebs, Holden et al (1985b) assessed the effects of five stimuli on the corneal endothelium and corneal thickness. The stimuli were:

1. silicone elastomer contact lens
2. silicone elastomer contact lens in combination with anoxia
3. anoxia alone
4. thick hydroxyethylmethacrylate (HEMA) contact lens
5. gas mixture of 9.8% carbon dioxide, 20.5% oxygen, and the balance nitrogen.

The resultant effect common to the stimuli that induced blebs was the ability of these stimuli to reduce the pH in or near the corneal endothelial layer, i.e., there was a local acidic shift. As discussed above, acidic shift in the cornea may be induced by hypoxia or by hypercapnia.

Clinically, the presence of endothelial blebs has no known adverse effects. Indeed, blebs have been detected in the noncontact lens-wearing eye – more so upon waking (Khodadoust & Hirst 1984). The diurnal variation in the appearance of blebs may again be accounted for by the fact that the cornea is mildly hypoxic upon waking. If, however, a repetitive exaggerated bleb response is observed, practitioners should increase the lens transmissibility in an attempt to reduce lens-induced hypoxia, which will otherwise lead to an acidic shift in the cornea.

Polymegathism

Polymegathism describes a variation in endothelial cell size (Fig. 3.8). Scientifically, the severity of polymegathism is measured using an index known as the coefficient of variation (COV) of cell size (see below).

$$COV = \frac{\text{Standard deviation of cell area in a given field}}{\text{Mean area of cells in a given field}}$$

The COV value has greater meaning when compared before and after lens wear in an individual subject. Furthermore, the COV is somewhat confusing in that the same value is possible for different mean cell areas (Doughty 1990). Other terms used to describe the endothelium are:

- endothelial cell density (number of cells per square millimeter)
- % hexagonal cells (polygonality).

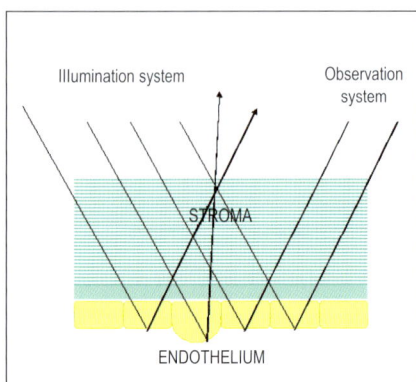

Figure 3.7   Demonstration of why blebs are not visible with specular reflection. Adapted from Efron (1999).

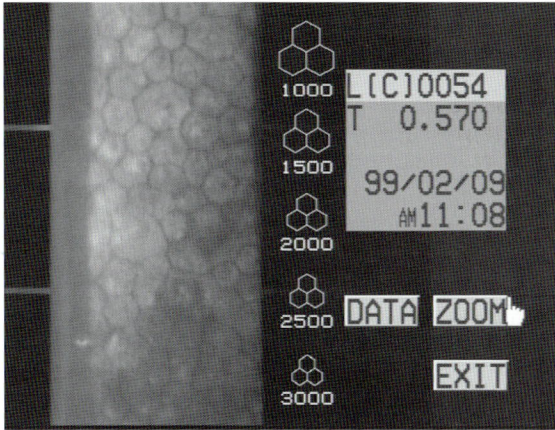

Figure 3.8 Endothelial polymegathism. Courtesy of Topcon Corporation, Tokyo, Japan.

Endothelial cell density changes throughout life (Yee et al 1985, Esgin & Erda 2000), therefore clinical studies must account for these age-related changes. MacRae et al (1985) conducted an age-matched controlled clinical trial involving three groups of lens wearers:

- daily-wear soft contact lenses for an average of 6.3 years
- long-term (> 20 years) users of hard contact lenses
- former users of hard contact lenses who had worn them for an average of 9.6 years but who had discontinued them for an average of 4.3 years.

They found no significant difference in endothelial cell densities but discovered that there was a significant variation in cell size (polymegathism) and cell shape (polymorphism). Furthermore, the authors also found that the endothelial changes were similar in soft and hard contact lenses.

The effect of extended-wear rigid lenses with Dks of 71 and 92 was assessed in 16 patients by Nieuwendaal et al (1991). Subjects wore lenses for between 7 and 24 months. Morphometric analysis revealed no significant change in cell size or shape. The authors attributed this to the high Dk of the lenses used in the study.

Conflicting evidence exists with respect to the change in endothelial cell density and contact lens wear. For example, some investigators (McMahon et al 1996, Setaelae et al 1998) found a significant reduction in endothelial cell density in PMMA wearers compared to control groups. Conversely, Chang et al (2001) found no change in endothelial cell density in daily wear soft contact lens wearers. Interestingly, Esgin & Erda (2000) found an increase in endothelial cell density in 97 unadapted eyes wearing high-Dk (92) daily-wear rigid lenses: the increase was dependent on the subjects' initial endothelial cell densities. Thus, subjects with cell densities less than the age-related norm observed significant increases in endothelial cell density within the first 3 months of lens wear. The authors explained this phenomenon as an adaptation to a new oxygen environment by cell migration and mitotic activity.

However, virtually all the studies agree that extended-wear lenses and low-Dk daily-wear lenses induce a change in cell shape and size. Bergmanson (1992) conducted a histopathological examination of the polymegethous human corneal endothelium. He found that the polymegethous endothelial cells had normal organelles and thus presumably functioned normally. However, ultrastructural examination of the lateral cell walls showed that they adopted a new oblique rather than straight appearance. Bergmanson used this clinical finding to interpret the pleomorphic changes observed with the specular microscope.

His thesis is that apparently shrunken cells observed with the specular microscope do not actually change in terms of their volume (Fig. 3.9). The cells' anterior face will have increased in size (the posterior face of the cell is viewed with the specular microscope).

Bergmanson (2001) concluded that the functional consequence of polymegethism has yet to

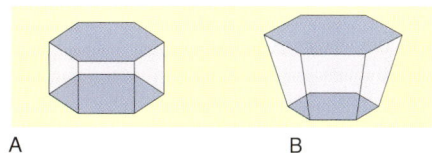

A   B

Figure 3.9 (A) Graphic representation of a normal endothelial cell. (B) Polymegethous cell, where the inferior face (that viewed by the specular microscope) has shrunk but the superior face has increased its surface area.

Table 3.2 Summary of some complications found in various studies (see text for further explanation)

Study type	D (months)	n	Lens worn or Dk/L	Complications			Success rate (%)
				Cornea	Conjunctiva	Limbus	
Kamiya (1986) Single sample, prospective	12	44	Menicon® EX	Mean curvature flattening 0.36 D in first week Corneal astigmatic change 0.98 D Refractive astigmatism change 1.06 D No corneal edema No vascularization	3 patients showed a mild superior tarsal papillary reaction No CLPC	No infiltrates	70
Polse et al (1987) Comparative prospective	6	RGP 27 Soft 9	RGP 19.58 Soft 20.5	**Corneal swelling** **Other** Microcyst incidence Epithelial stain	**RGP group** 7.8% 2–13% incidence of: adherence, corneal compression, trapped debris, limbal and central epithelial keratitis 22% 10%	**Soft group** 7.3% 1 case of CLPC 1 case of non-infectious infiltrative keratitis 56%	% subjects on EW after study 74 RGP 33 soft
Polse et al (1988) Single sample, prospective	6	35	Mean Dk/L = 37 Measurements conducted in morning on six monthly visits	Mean swelling = 5.9% (± 3.3%) 10% adherence 20% limbal keratitis 6.5% microcysts			RGP EW is acceptable with current test lens for many patients
Key & Mobley (1989) Single sample, prospective	12	372	Paraperm ® EW	Mild 3 and 9 o'clock stain (12.3%) Edema (incidence 1.5%) Corneal swelling 8% recovering to near normal after 2 h Adherence (10%) Corneal flattening (mean 0.128 D)	Hyperemia (3.1%)	No neovascularization	83
MacRae et al (1991) Meta-analysis	Evaluation of other studies 1980–1988	22 739	Soft DW Soft EW RGP EW	12-month studies showed that RGP EW had 1/3 of adverse reactions of EW soft contact lenses. Also the severe abrasion/keratitis rate was 1/4 of that of EW soft contact lenses Overall, the total number of abrasion/keratitis and corneal ulcers was 159			

Table 3.2 *contd.*

Study type	D (months)	n	Lens worn or *Dk/L*	Complications			Success rate (%)
				Cornea	Conjunctiva	Limbus	
MacKeen et al (1992) Multicenter prospective	12	202 eyes	Menicon ® SF-P	24 patients had problems with lens adherence; there were no other complications Average wear time 6.2 days before cleaning			66% rated comfort and satisfaction as very good. 72 eyes failed to complete the study; of these, 43% failed due to discomfort
Sigband & Bridgewater (1994) Multicenter prospective	3	162 eyes	FluoroPerm 151	132 eyes completed the study without any physiological or pathological complications. 30 eyes discontinued due to poor comfort			81.5% successfully completed the trial. The authors attributed the high success rate to the high oxygen permeability and lens surface characteristics
Kok et al (1992)	3–24	62 eyes	Quantum (*Dk* 92)	Significant decrease in corneal thickness over 6 months (*P* < 0.05) Significant changes in corneal curvature (*P* < 0.05) over 3 months, notably in the vertical meridian No other complications			61% remained on EW 29% changed to daily wear 10% unavailable for follow-up

RGP, rigid gas-permeable; CLPC, contact lens papillary conjunctivitis; DW, daily wear; EW, extended wear.

be demonstrated. However, although there is no proof that polymegethism reduces recovery from edema, there does appear to be some correlation (McMahon et al 1996).

The complications of extended RGP lens wear and many of the studies discussed so far are summarized in Table 3.2.

CLINICAL COMPLICATIONS

Almost all orthokeratology patients are treated with the overnight wear of contact lenses. The changes induced by a contact lens in a closed-eye environment to ocular metabolism and physiology mean that the eye is at greater risk of infection compared to a nonlens-wearing eye. However, there is no evidence to suggest that extended-wear high-*Dk* RGP lens wear leads to any more serious complications than modern soft lenses. In fact, when one considers the fact that lenses are physically worn no more than daily wear lenses – as opposed to continuously with extended wear – the whole prospect of overnight wear appears to be safer. Nevertheless, one needs to be aware of potential complications and advise all patients of potential risks. Therefore, each type of complication associated with extended-wear contact lenses will be briefly reviewed (see Table 3.2 for summary).

Lens adherence

Lack of lens mobility, zero blinking, and the forces exerted by the eyelid during eye closure are factors thought to be associated with RGP lens binding or adherence. A number of investigators have found lens adherence in extended-

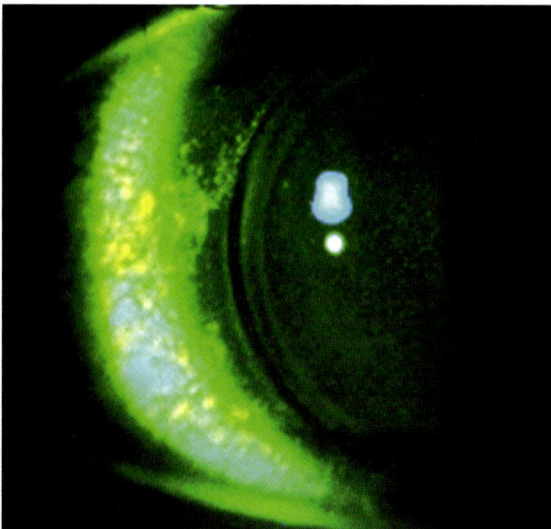

Figure 3.10 Corneal indentation ring following rigid gas-permeable lens extended wear. Note also the relative inferior nasal position of the ring stain.

wear RGP subjects (Zantos & Zantos 1985, Polse et al 1987, Swarbrick & Holden, 1987, 1989, Kenyon et al 1988, Swarbrick 1988). Reported rates of adherences vary from between 20 and 50% in overnight RGP lens wear with conventional geometries (Swarbrick & Holden 1987, Kenyon et al 1988). The lens typically occupies an inferior nasal position – sometimes bound to the conjunctiva. Few subjective symptoms are reported from subjects; this is probably because of the fact that the lens is immobile (Swarbrick & Holden 1989). However, studies have demonstrated that signs of adherence usually disappear after 1–2 h of eye opening (Kenyon et al 1988, Swarbrick & Holden 1989).

Examination of the cornea with sodium fluorescein shows the presence of an epithelial indentation ring corresponding to the edge of the lens (Fig. 3.10).

Etiology

Clinicians have long known that rigid lens adherence has been a patient-dependent response. Investigators have also shown that binding is a patient-dependent response (Swarbrick & Holden 1989). Swarbrick & Holden (1996) attempted to find which ocular characteristics were associated with RGP lens adherence.

The authors selected a sample of 22 subjects who had previously worn RGP lenses overnight in a previous clinical trial. The authors measured the following ocular characteristics at controlled times:

- Corneal curvature
  - Central
  - Peripheral
  - Toricity
  - Corneal eccentricity
- Tear film
  - Tear break up time (TBUT)
  - Tear volume (phenol red thread test)
  - Tear meniscus height
- Eyelid
  - Vertical palpebral aperture size
  - Lid tension (subjective observer grading)
  - Tarsal conjunctival grade
- Corneal thickness

- Ocular rigidity (by differential, two-weight Schiötz tonometry).

The overall frequency of lens adherence was found to be 44% (± 30.6). Of the above ocular characteristics, four factors were found to influence the frequency of overnight RGP adherence. Lower levels of ocular rigidity, tighter lids, thinner corneas, and lower levels of corneal toricity were likely to influence lens adherence.

In a previous study by Swarbrick (1988), a possible etiology for lens binding was proposed. Swarbrick suggested that overnight wear of RGP lenses resulted in thinning of the postlens tear film because of lid closure. The resultant postlens tear film was composed of a thick viscous mucous layer that induces lens adherence.

Swarbrick & Holden (1996) suggested that these four ocular factors (ocular rigidity, tighter lids, thinner corneas, and lower levels of corneal toricity) might exacerbate tear thinning by molding corneal tissue toward the posterior contact lens surface. Although three of the four factors may explain how the thin tear film may facilitate lens adherence, the role of corneal toricity appears to be more difficult to explain. Moreover, other studies have found conflicting results in that greater levels of corneal toricity are associated with lens adherence. The degree of corneal toricity in subjects in the Swarbrick & Holden (1996) study was limited (0.06–1.20 D) and hence the authors' conclusion that further investigation is necessary.

The incidence of lens adherence following overnight orthokeratology would appear to be similar to that encountered with conventionally designed lenses (British Orthokeratology Society 2001); i.e., in the region of 30–60%. Swarbrick & Holden (1996) compared the effect of lens fit using conventionally designed lenses on lens adherence. In three separate studies involving 11 subjects, the effect of peripheral fit (loose versus tight), lens diameter (8.7 versus 9.6 mm) and central fit (steep versus flat) was investigated. None of the lens design factors except central fit had any effect on the frequency of lens adherence. Flat-fitting lenses induced a statistically significant increase in frequency of lens adherence (incidence of 84% for flat and 49% for steep lenses).

Although flat-fitting lenses appear to have induced greater levels of binding in the Swarbrick & Holden study, lenses were not fitted as flat as reverse geometry lenses. In addition, the design of reverse geometry lenses differs considerably in that there is a secondary steeper (reverse) curve and the lenses are significantly larger (of the order 10–11.5 mm). The net effect of the reverse curve effectively increases the sag of the lens, unlike a conventionally flat fitting lens that will have reduced sag. Orthokeratology lenses are fitted to match corneal sag. Whilst many orthokeratologists order lenses with fenestrations, the effect of fenestrating does not appear to have any effect on lens adherence, although lenses may unbind more easily on awakening (John Mountford, personal communication).

Noninfectious ocular inflammation

Contact lens-induced sterile infiltrative keratitis (CL-SIK) describes the presence of stromal infiltrates without any corneal infection. Localized conjunctival and limbal hyperemia may also be visible adjacent to the sterile corneal infiltrate. The presence of infiltrates without any significant epithelial break indicates that there is some form of ocular inflammation. Tear stagnation and hypoxia/hypercapnia may be responsible for the ocular inflammation during extended contact lens wear.

It is now known that associated with the stagnated tear film is an increased level of IgA and albumin; the activation of plasminogen and complement, and higher levels of PMN or white blood cells (Swarbrick & Holden 1997). This state of subclinical inflammation could easily develop into a "full-blown" inflammation in the presence of bacterial endotoxins (Fig. 3.11 illustrates the mechanism of this "full-blown" inflammation).

The use of extended-wear RGPs and soft contact lenses may induce corneal hypoxia. As blood vessels dilate under hypoxic conditions, inflammatory cells will be able to leak from the blood vessels and produce what we as practitioners clinically diagnose as infiltrates. In a recent study, the relative incidence of CL-SIK was compared in RGP, PMMA, soft contact lenses, and extended-wear soft contact lenses (Stapleton et al

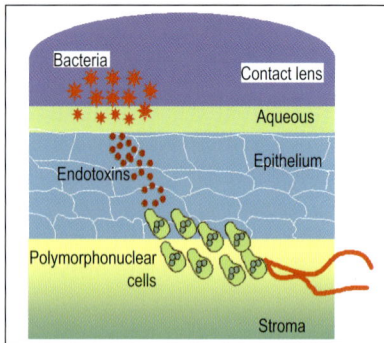

Figure 3.11   The mechanism of ocular inflammation.

1992). With the relative risk of RGP lenses set at 1, the relative risks of the other modalities were found to be as shown in Table 3.3.

Thus, RGP lenses appear to offer a lower risk of ocular inflammation compared to soft contact lenses for daily wear. Unfortunately, the study did not compare the incidence of inflammation with extended wear of RGP lenses.

Microbial infection

Contact lens-induced microbial infiltrative keratitis (CL-MIK) describes the appearance of stromal infiltrates with microbial infection. Microbial keratitis is an ocular emergency and is therefore the most serious complication of contact lens wear.

Numerous studies have been conducted highlighting the incidence of microbial keratitis in the contact lens-wearing population. Table 3.4 gives a summary of recent studies highlighting the incidence of CL-MIK.

Table 3.3 Relative risk of contact lens-induced sterile infiltrative keratitis (CL-SIK) in terms of lens modality

Lens modality	Relative risk (to DW RGP lenses)
DW RGP	1
DW PMMA	1
DW SCL	2.1
EW SCL	2.4

DW RGP, daily-wear rigid gas-permeable; PMMA, polymethyl methacrylate; SCL, soft contact lens; EW, extended wear.

Table 3.4 Incidence of contact lens-induced microbial keratitis

Study	DW soft	EW soft	DW RGP
Poggio et al (1989)	4.1 per 10 000	20.9 per 10 000	
MacRae et al (1991)	5.2 per 10 000	18.2 per 10 000	6.8 per 10 000
Stapleton et al (1993) (relative risk compared with RGP daily wear)	4.2 per 10 000	36.8 per 10 000	
Nilsson & Montan (1994)	2.17 per 10 000	13.3 per 10 000	1.48 per 10 000
Cheng et al (1999)	3.5 per 10 000	20 per 10 000	1.1 per 10 000

DW, daily wear; EW, extended wear; RGP, rigid gas-permeable.

Although few studies have concentrated on the incidence of CL-MIK in extended-wear RGP lenses, it can be seen from Table 3.4 that DW RGP lenses exhibit the lowest incidence of CL-MIK.

A recent study by Ren et al (2002) determined the effects of oxygen transmissibility and lens type on the corneal epithelium during extended wear. Of 178 subjects taking part in the double-masked study, 27 wore a relatively high oxygen-permeable soft disposable hygrogel lens for 6 nights extended wear (control), 33 wore a silicone hydrogel lens for 6 nights extended wear, 66 wore a silicone hydrogel for 30 nights continuous wear and 52 wore a high-Dk RGP lens for 30 nights continuous wear. Amongst other factors, the investigators assessed *Pseudomonas aeruginosa* binding to exfoliated epithelial cells at baseline, 1, 3, 6, 9, and 12 months.

The silicone hydrogels resulted in significantly less *Pseudomonas* binding than the control lens, with no significant difference in binding with 6-night versus 30-night EW. A remarkable adaptive recovery was found after 6 months with all soft lens wearers, with a gradual return to prelens *Pseudomonas* binding levels. Thirty-night continuous wear of the hyper-Dk RGP lens produced no significant increase in *P. aeruginosa* binding over 1 year.

The two most serious organisms involved in CL-MIK are *Acanthamoeba* (an ameba) and *P. aeruginosa* (Gram-negative): these will now be discussed in greater detail.

Acanthamoeba

Acanthamoeba is an abundant free-living genus of ameba. It can survive in diverse conditions and feeds on bacteria, fungi, other protozoa, and blue/green algae (Dryden & Wright 1987). Therefore, it comes as no surprise that it is usually found in greatest numbers where other microorganisms are present. When *Acanthamoeba* is in its active form it is referred to as a trophozoite. When in an environment of little nourishment, *Acanthamoeba* has the ability to encyst. The cyst form is extremely resistant to drying, temperature extremes, and damage by chemicals. The cyst has a double cell wall (which is probably what makes it so resistant) and has a polygonal structure (Illingworth & Cook 1998). In the cyst form it may survive for many years until a food source becomes available, when it will revert to its trophozoite form.

The mode of infection appears to be accidental. Humans are generally exposed to *Acanthamoeba* while swimming in pools, lakes, and domestic tapwater (Illingworth & Cook 1998). It is generally recognized that infection to an eye wearing contact lenses is as a result of contamination of the lens during cleaning (i.e., rinsing in tapwater) and inadequate disinfection systems. There is a higher incidence with daily wear hydrogel lenses (Moore et al 1987) but other modalities of wear have also been associated with the infection, such as RGP lenses (Koenig et al 1987). With regard to the actual binding of the ameba to the cornea, specific binding sites may be present. Furthermore, different strains of *Acanthamoeba* may bind more effectively to the corneal epithelium (Illingworth & Cook 1998).

The clinical presentation of *Acanthamoeba* is variable. However, patients are often reported to complain of photophobia, pain, and tearing. It is often said that patient symptoms are disproportionate to the clinical signs. The earliest sign may take the form of fine epithelial erosions, microcystic edema, and patchy anterior

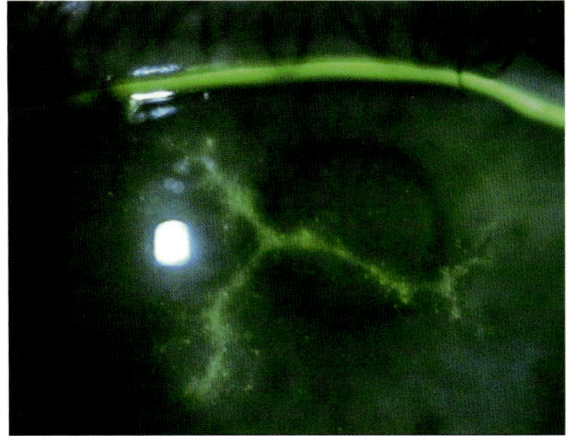

Figure 3.12   Dendritic-type epithelial erosion in *Acanthamoeba* keratitis. Courtesy of John Mountford.

stromal infiltrates (Key et al 1980, Moore & McCulley 1989, Berger et al, 1990). In such a situation the practitioner must consider the patient's symptoms first. Furthermore, the literature shows publications of case histories where no corneal staining was observed during the onset of infection (Bacon et al 1993). Another common finding is the presence of a dendritic-type keratitis, as shown in Figure 3.12 (Johns et al 1987).

If such a finding is observed in a contact lens wearer associated with symptoms of severe pain, then the practitioner should not discount the presence of acanthamebal infection. Possibly the most pathognomonic sign of *Acanthamoeba* is that of a radial pattern of perineural infiltrates (Moore et al 1986). The etiology of these infiltrates is unknown; clinicians should not rely on this finding as *Acanthamoeba* keratitis may occur with perineural infiltrates. Many texts also associate acanthamebal infection with a ring-type infiltrate (with or without an overlying epithelial defect), as shown in Figure 3.13. This infiltrate can occur in the early or late stage of the disease (Theodore et al 1985).

In terms of prevention, practitioners should advise contact lens wearers to replace lens cases on a regular basis and not use any type of homemade saline. Patients should never use tapwater for rinsing lenses and must be advised to adhere to cleaning and disinfection regimes.

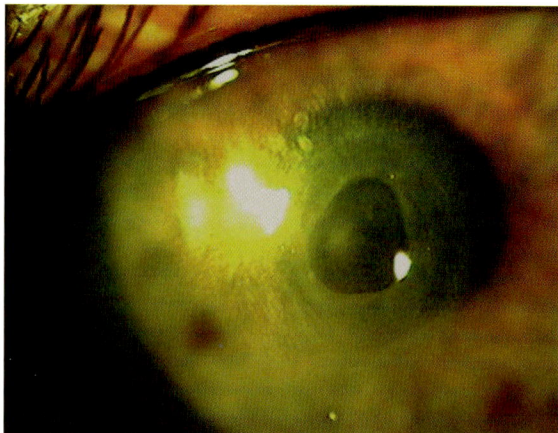

Figure 3.13   Ring-type infiltrate as seen in *Acanthamoeba* keratitis.

Pseudomonas aeruginosa

Pseudomonas aeruginosa is a rod-shaped Gram-negative bacteria. The term "Gram-negative" refers to the fact that it does not stain with the Gram staining procedure. Generally, Gram-positive bacteria such as *Staphylococcus aureus* produce less severe corneal ulcers compared to Gram-negative bacteria such as *Pseudomonas*. However, severe corneal infections have been associated with the Gram-positive *Bacillus* bacterium (Donzis et al 1988). *Pseudomonas* infection of the cornea produces a severe and potentially devastating infection. *Pseudomonas* is a widespread microorganism found in soil, water, plants, and sewage.

The mode of infection has been a subject of great interest to academics and clinicians alike. Fleiszig et al (1992) found that increased adherence of *Pseudomonas* to the corneal epithelium was associated with extended-wear hydrogel lenses. In a separate study, Fleiszig & Efron (1992) found that in a group of 45 weekly extended-wear RGP lens-wearing subjects (Boston Equalens II and Quantum II), the conjunctival flora was significantly altered before and after the trial. They found an increase in potentially pathogenic microorganisms, including Gram-negative bacteria.

Fletcher et al (1993) observed that *Pseudomonas* smooth lipopolysaccharide (a component of Gram-negative bacterial cell walls) was responsible for the adherence of *Pseudomonas* to contact lenses and the corneal epithelium. Nevertheless, the corneal epithelium in the absence of contact lenses is remarkably resistant to *Pseudomonas* infection. The reason for the greater risk in the presence of contact lenses lies in the protective tear film. Fleiszig et al discovered that, in the absence of a contact lens, *Pseudomonas* could not infect the cornea due to the protective barrier formed by the mucous layer overlying the corneal epithelium (Fleiszig et al 1994a). Epithelial cell polarity also has an impact on the likelihood of infection. Fleiszig et al (1998) found that the top of the cell was the most resistant surface of the epithelium (that surface in contact with the tear film). The lateral and basal surfaces were found to be more prone to infection. Thus, any break in the epithelium may also increase susceptibility to infection.

The fact that *Pseudomonas* can also infect an intact corneal epithelium led to Fleiszig et al (1998) concluding that stagnation of cytotoxic bacteria against the corneal epithelium may promote the pathogenesis of infection. Therefore, immobile soft lenses may facilitate *Pseudomonas* infection. More recently it has been discovered that *Pseudomonas* can cause infection in one of two ways: firstly, by inducing cell death (cytotoxicity) and secondly, by invading the host epithelium where damage is largely induced via the host's immune system (Fleiszig et al 1994b, 1996).

Clinically, the corneal infection presents in an acute manner; there is a large, rapidly developing ulcer with dense stromal infiltrates. Damage to corneal tissue occurs not only as a result of cytotoxicity but as a result of the host immune system due to PMNs releasing lysosomal enzymes.

REFERENCES

Bacon A S, Dart J K, Ficker L A et al (1993) *Acanthamoeba* keratitis. The value of early diagnosis. Ophthalmology 100: 1238–1243.

Berger S T, Monino B J, Hoft R H et al (1990) Successful medical management of *Acanthamoeba* keratitis. American Journal of Ophthalmology 110: 395–403

Bergmanson J P G (1987) Histopathological analysis of the corneal epithelium after contact lens wear. American Journal of the Optometric Association 58: 812

Bergmanson J P G (1992) Histopathological analysis of the corneal endothelial polymegethism. Cornea 11: 133–142

Bergmanson J P G (2001) Effects of contact lens wear on corneal ultrastructure. CLAE 24: 115–120

Bergmanson J P G, Ruben M, Chu L W F (1985) Epithelial morphological response to soft hydrogel contact lenses. British Journal of Ophthalmology 69: 373–379

British Orthokeratology Society (2001) Annual discussion meeting.

Carney L G, Hill R M (1976) Tear pH and the hard contact lens patient. International Contact Lens Clinic 3: 27

Chang S W, Hu F R, Lin L L (2001) Effects of contact lenses on corneal endothelium – a morphological and functional study. Ophthalmologica 215(3): 197–203

Cheng K H, Leung S L, Hoekman H W, Beekhuis W H, Mulder P G, Geerards A J, Kijlstra A (1999) Incidence of contact-lens-associated microbial keratitis and its related morbidity. Lancet 17 (9174): 181–185

Dick R B (1957) Contact lenses in constant use for a three month period: a case report. American Journal of Optometry and Physiological Optics 35: 248–250

Donzis P B, Mondino B J, Weissman B A (1988) *Bacillus* keratitis associated with contaminated contact lens care systems. American Journal of Ophthalmology 105: 195–197

Doughty M J (1990) The ambiguous coefficient of variation: polymegathism of the corneal endothelium and central corneal thickness. ICLC 17: 240

Dryden R C, Wright S J L (1987) Predation of cyanobacteria by protozoa. Canadian Journal of Microbiology 33: 471–481

Efron N (1999) Contact lens complications. Butterworth-Heinemann, Oxford, pp. 75–80

Elie R (1986) Gas permeable extended wear lenses: an excellent solution for aphakic patients. CLAO Journal 12(1): 51–53

Esgin H, Erda N (2000) Endothelial cell density of the cornea during rigid gas permeable contact lens wear. CLAO 26(3): 146–150

Fleiszig S M J, Efron N (1992) Conjunctival flora in extended wear of rigid gas permeable contact lenses. Optometry and Vision Science 69(5): 354–357

Fleiszig S M J, Efron N, Pier G B (1992) Extended wear enhances *Pseudomonas aeruginosa* adherence to human corneal epithelium. Investigative Ophthalmology and Visual Science 33: 2908–2916

Fleiszig S M J, Zaidi T S, Pier G B (1994a) Ocular mucous and *Pseudomonas aeruginosa* adherence. Advances in Experimental Medicine and Biology 350: 359

Fleiszig S M J, Zaidi T S, Fletcher E L (1994b) *Pseudomonas aeruginosa* invades corneal epithelial cells during experimental infection. Infection and Immunity 62: 3485

Fleiszig S M J, Zaidi T S, Preston M J (1996) The relationship between cytotoxicity and epithelial cell invasion by corneal isolates of *Pseudomonas aeruginosa*. Infection and Immunity 64: 2288

Fleiszig S M J, Lee E J, Wu C et al (1998) Cytotoxic strains of *Pseudomonas* can damage the intact corneal surface in vitro. CLAO Journal 24(1): 41–47

Fletcher E L, Fleiszig S M J, Brennan N A (1993a) Lipopolysaccharide in adherence of *Pseudomonas aeruginosa* to the cornea and contact lenses. Investigative Ophthalmology and Vision Science 34(6): 1930

Fletcher E L, Weissman B A, Efron N (1993b) The role of pili in the attachment of *Pseudomonas aeruginosa* to unworn hydrogel contact lenses. Current Eye Research 12: 1067

Fonn D, Holden B A (1988) Rigid gas-permeable vs. hydrogel contact lenses for extended wear. American Journal of Optometry and Physiological Optics 65(7): 536–544

Hamano H, Hori M, Hamano T et al (1983) Effects of contact lens wear on mitosis of corneal epithelium and lactate content of aqueous humor of rabbit. Japanese Journal of Ophthalmology 27: 451–458

Hamano H, Kitano J, Mitsunaga S (1985) Adverse effects of contact lens wear in a large Japanese population. Contact Lens Association Ophthalmology Journal 11: 141

Hideji I, MacKeen D L, Hamano H, Jester J V, Cavanagh H D (1989) Swelling and deswelling of rabbit corneas in response to rigid gas permeable, hydrogel and elastomer contact lens wear. CLAO Journal 15(4): 290–297

Holden B A, Mertz G W (1984) Critical oxygen levels to avoid corneal edema for daily and extended wear contact lenses. Investigations in Ophthalmology and Visual Science 25: 1161–1167

Holden B A, Sweeney D F, Vannas A, Nilsson K T, Efron N (1985a) Effects of long-term extended contact lens wear on the human cornea. Investigations in Ophthalmology and Visual Science 26: 1489–1501

Holden B A, Williams L, Zantos S G (1985b) The etiology of transient endothelial changes in the human cornea. Investigations in Ophthalmology and Visual Science 26: 1354–1359

Holden B A, Grant T, Kotow M (1987) Epithelial microcysts with daily and extended wear of hydrogel and rigid gas permeable contact lenses. Investigations in Ophthalmology and Visual Science 28 (suppl): 372

Holden B A, Sweeney D F, La Hood D, Kenyon E (1988) Corneal deswelling following overnight wear of rigid and hydrogel contact lenses. Current Eye Research 7(1): 49–53

Ichijima H, Petroll W M, Jester J V, Ohashi J, Cavanagh H D (1992) Effects of increasing *Dk* with rigid contact lens extended wear on rabbit corneal epithelium using confocal microscopy. Cornea 11(4): 282–287

Ichijima H, Imayasu M, Ren D H, Cavanagh H D (2000) Effects of RGP lens extended wear on glucose-lactate metabolism and stromal swelling in the rabbit cornea. CLAO Journal 26(1): 30–36

Illingworth C D, Cook S D (1998) *Acanthamoeba* keratitis. Surveys in Ophthalmology 42: 493–508

Iskeleli G, Oral A Y, Celikkol L (1996) Changes in corneal radius and thickness in response to extended wear of rigid gas permeable contact lenses. CLAO 22(2): 133–135

Johns K J, O'Day D M, Head W S et al (1987) Herpes simplex masquerade syndrome: acanthamoeba keratitis. Current Eye Research 6: 207–212

Kamiya C (1986) Cosmetic extended wear of oxygen permeable hard contact lenses: one year up. Journal of the American Optometric Association 57(3): 182–184

Kenyon E, Polse K A, Mandell R B (1988) Rigid contact lens adherence: incidence, severity and recovery. Journal of the American Optometric Association 59: 168–174

Key J E, Mobley C L (1989) Paraperm EW lens for extended wear. Contact Lens Association of Ophthalmology Journal 91: 1125–1128

Key S N, Green W R, Willaert E et al (1980) Keratitis due to *Acanthameoba castellanii*. A clinicopathologic report. Archives of Ophthalmology 98: 475–479

Khodadoust A A, Hirst L W (1984) Diurnal variation in corneal endothelial morphology. Ophthalmology 91: 1125

Koenig S B, Solomon J M, Hyndiuk R A et al (1987) *Acanthamoeba* keratitis associated with gas permeable contact lens wear. American Journal of Ophthalmology 103: 832

Koetting R A, Castellano C F, Nelson D W (1985) A hr lens with extended wear possibilities. Journal of the American Optometric Association 56(3): 208–211

Kok J H, Hilbrink H J, Rosenbrand R M, Visser R (1992) Extended-wear of high oxygen-permeable quantum contact lenses. International Ophthalmology 16(2): 123–127

Ladage P M (2000) Basal epithelial cell turnover following RGP extended contact lens wear in the rabbit cornea. Investigations in Ophthalmology Visual Science 41: S75

Lemp M A, Gold J B (1986) The effects of extended-wear hydrophilic contact lenses on the human corneal epithelium. American Journal of Ophthalmology 101: 274–277

MacKeen D L, Sachdev M, Ballou V, Cavanagh H D (1992) A prospective multicenter clinical trial to assess safety efficacy of Menicon SF-P RGP lenses for extended wear. CLAO Journal 18(3): 183–186

MacRae S M, Matsuda M, Yee R (1985) The effect of long-term hard contact lens wear on the corneal endothelium. CLAO Journal 11(4): 322–326

MacRae S, Herman C, Stulting R D et al (1991) Corneal ulcer and adverse reaction rates in premarket contact lens studies. American Journal of Ophthalmology 111: 457

Madigan M C, Holden B A (1992) Reduced epithelial adhesion after extended contact lens wear correlates with reduced hemidesmosome density in the cat cornea. Investigations in Ophthalmology and Visual Science 33(2): 314–323

Madigan M C, Holden B A, Kwok L S (1987) Extended wear of contact lenses can compromise corneal epithelial adhesion. Current Eye Research 6(10): 1257–1260

McMahon T T, Polse K A, McNamara N (1996) Recovery from induced corneal edema and endothelial morphology after long-term PMMA contact lens wear. Optometry and Vision Science 73: 184

Mertz G W, Holden B A (1981) Clinical implications of extended wear research. Canadian Journal of Optometry 43: 203–205

Moore M B, McCulley J P (1989) *Acanthamoeba* keratitis associated with contact lenses: six consecutive cases of successful management. British Journal of Ophthalmology 73: 271–275

Moore M B, McCulley J P, Kaufman H E, Robin J P (1986) Radial keratoneuritis as a presenting sign in acanthamoeba keratitis. Ophthalmology 104: 1310–1315

Moore M B, McCulley J P, Newton C et al (1987) *Acanthamoeba* keratitis: a growing problem in soft and hard contact lens wearers. Ophthalmology 94: 1654–1661

Nieuwendaal C P, Kok J H C, De Moor A M, Costing J, Venema H W (1991) Corneal endothelial cell morphology under permanent wear of rigid contact lenses. International Ophthalmology 15(5): 313–320

Nilsson S E, Montan P G (1994) The annualized incidence of contact lens-induced keratitis in Sweden and its relation to lens type and wear schedule: results of a three-month prospective study. Contact Lens Association Ophthalmology Journal 20: 225

Norn M S (1988) Tear fluid pH in normals, contact lens wearers and pathological cases. Acta Ophthalmologica 66: 485

Poggio E C, Glynn R J, Schein O D et al (1989) The incidence of ulcerative keratitis among users of daily-wear and extended wear soft contact lenses. New England Journal of Medicine 321: 779

Polse K A (1979) Tear flow under hydrogel contact lenses. Investigations in Ophthalmology and Visual Science 18(4): 409–413

Polse K A, Sarver M D, Kenyon E, Bonnano J (1987) Gas permeable hard contact lens extended wear: ocular and visual responses to a 6-month period of wear. Contact Lens Association of Ophthalmology Journal 13: 31–38

Polse K A, Rivera R K, Bonanno J (1988) Ocular effects of hard gas-permeable-lens extended wear. American Journal of Optometry and Physiological Optics 65(5): 358–364

Ren D H, Petroll W M, Jester J V, Cavanagh H D (1999) The effect of rigid gas permeable contact lens wear on proliferation of rabbit corneal and conjunctival epithelial cells. CLAO Journal 25: 136–141

Ren D H, Yamamoto K, Ladage P M, Molai M, Li L, Petroll W M, Jester J V, Cavanagh H D (2002) Adaptive effects of 30-night wear of hyper-O(2) transmissible contact lenses on bacterial binding and corneal epithelium: a 1-year clinical trial. Ophthalmology 109(1): 27–39

Setaelae K, Vasara K, Vesti E, Ruusuvaara P (1998) Effects of long-term contact lens wear on the corneal endothelium. Acta Ophthalmologica Scandinavica 76(3): 299–303

Sigband D J, Bridgewater B A (1994) FluoroPerm 151 extended wear: a clinical study. CLAO Journal 20(1): 37–40

Sloan D P (1965) Another chapter in continuous contact lens wearing. Contacto 9(4): 19–22

Stapleton F, Dart J, Minassian D (1992) Nonulcerative complication of contact lens wear. Archives of Ophthalmology 110: 1601

Stapleton F, Dart J K, Minassian D (1993) Risk factors with contact lens related suppurative keratitis. CLAO Journal 19(4): 204–210

Swarbrick H A (1988) A possible aetiology for RGP lens binding (adherence). International Contact/Lens Clinic 15: 13–19

Swarbrick H A, Holden B A (1987) Rigid gas-permeable lens binding: significance and contributing factors. American Journal of Optometry 64: 815–823

Swarbrick H A, Holden B A (1989) Rigid gas permeable lens adherence: a patient-dependent phenomenon. Optometry and Vision Science 66: 269–275

Swarbrick H A, Holden B A (1996) Ocular characteristics associated with rigid gas-permeable lens adherence. Optometry and Vision Science 73: 473–481

Swarbrick H A, Holden B A (1997) Extended wear lenses. In: Phillips A J, Speedwell L (eds) Contact lenses. Oxford, Butterworth-Heinemann, pp 494–539

Swarbrick H A, Wong G, O'Leary D J (1998) Corneal response to orthokeratology. Optometry and Vision Science 75(11): 791–799

Sweeney D F, Holden B A (1991) The relative contributions of hypoxia, osmolarity, temperature and humidity to corneal oedema with eye closure. Investigations in Ophthalmology and Visual Science 32: 739

Thakur A, Willcox M D P (2000) Contact lens wear alters the production of certain inflammatory mediators in tears. Experiments in Eye Research 70(3): 255–260

Theodore F H, Jakobiec F A, Juechter K B et al (1985) Diagnostic value of a ring infiltrate in *Acanthamoeba* keratitis. Ophthalmology 92: 1471–1479

Vannas A, Holden B A, Makitie J (1984) The ultrastructure of contact lens induced changes in the human corneal endothelium. Acta Ophthalmologica 62: 320

Vinding T, Eriksen J S, Nielsen N V (1987) The concentration of lysozyme and secretory IgA in tears from healthy persons with and without contact lens use. Acta Ophthalmologica 65: 23

Wilson G, O'Leary D J, Holden B A (1989) Cell content of tears following overnight wear of a contact lens. Current Eye Research 8: 329–335

Woods R (1989) Quantitative slit-lamp observations in contact lens practice. Journal of the British Contact Lens Association (Scientific Meetings) 12: 42–45

Yee R W, Matsuda M, Schultz R O (1985) Changes in normal corneal endothelial cellular pattern as a function of age. Current Eye Research 4: 671

Zantos S G (1984) Management of corneal infiltrates in extended-wear contact lens patients. ICLC 11: 604–610

Zantos S G, Holden B A (1977) Transient endothelial changes soon after wearing soft contact lenses. American Journal of Optometry and Physiological Optics 54: 856–858

Zantos S G, Holden B A (1978) Ocular changes associated with continuous wear of contact lenses. Australian Journal of Optometry 61: 418–426

Zantos S G, Zantos P O (1985) Extended wear feasibility of gas permeable hard lenses for myopia. International Eyecare 1: 66–75

Chapter **4**

Design variables and fitting philosophies of reverse geometry lenses

John Mountford

CHAPTER CONTENTS

Introduction   69
Basic lens fitting principles   70
Sag philosophy   70
Formulae used in lens construction   72
Peripheral curve design   74
Reverse geometry lenses   75
Design and construction of alignment peripheral
   curves   88
Accuracy of sag fitting   103
References   105

INTRODUCTION

The major difference between traditional and current orthokeratology techniques is the use of radically different lens designs and the application of videokeratoscopy in order not only to design the correct lens, but also to monitor the corneal changes that follow wear. All reverse geometry lenses have a first back peripheral radius (BPR_1) (secondary curve) that is steeper than the back optic zone radius (BOZR) (base curve), and, as a result, require a different fitting approach than that traditionally used to fit standard multicurve lenses.

The development of the fitting philosophy and lens designs has followed an evolutionary path and therefore the outline of this chapter will follow the same approach. The process began with the application of a sag-based fitting philosophy to relatively simple tricurve reverse geometry lenses and progressed to the addition of different peripheral curve constructions to maximize centration. This was followed by the analysis of the tear layer profiles produced by the lens and their effects on lens performance, which increased the complexity not only of the lens designs, but also the computer programs used as an aid to lens fitting. Additionally, there are not only different reverse geometry lens designs to consider, but different fitting philosophies that are applied to the design variations.

The purpose of this chapter is to explain in detail not only *how* reverse geometry lenses differ in design and construction from both standard lens designs and one another, but also *why* the results can differ depending on the design used. A complete understanding of all these factors is required in order to produce effective outcomes with orthokeratology.

BASIC LENS FITTING PRINCIPLES

The traditional approach to the fitting and design of rigid contact lenses is to choose the BOZR based on its desired relationship to the flattest corneal meridian (K). This led to the terminology of "flat," "on-K," and "steep" as a means of describing the actual fitting, and eventually became the commonly accepted description of the fitting philosophy.

However, standard lens designs do not have a steeper BPR_1 (commonly referred to as the reverse curve or RC), as is the case with all forms of reverse geometry lenses. The addition of the RC curve to the lens design radically alters the complexity of the fitting process, as the corneal curvature changes induced are dependent not only on the *accuracy* of the lens fit, but also on the BOZR/RC combinations used. The RC forms the tear reservoir (TR) which radically alters the efficacy of the procedure, as will be described later.

Therefore, the simple "flatter-than-K" philosophy used when fitting standard contour lenses has severe limitations when applied to reverse geometry lenses, and a more accurate approach is required.

SAG PHILOSOPHY

Any description of lens design and fitting must first start with a definition of the shape of the cornea that the lens is expected to fit. As described in Chapter 2, the corneal shape is most commonly described in terms of a prolate ellipse in that the apical radius (R_0) flattens in curvature at a relatively constant rate from the center to the periphery of the cornea (Fig. 4.1). The rate of flattening is termed the eccentricity value (e), with the mean e-value being 0.50. Population-based studies (Kieley et al 1982, Guillon et al 1986) have shown that approximately 95% of corneas have e-values in the range of 0.30–0.70.

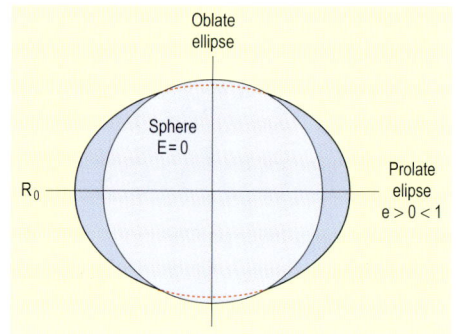

Figure 4.1 Schematic showing differences between spheroidal, prolate, and oblate ellipsoidal surfaces. The apical radius (R_0) is the radius of curvature at the center of the surface. For prolate surfaces, the radius of curvature increases (flattens) from the center to the periphery, whereas the radius decreases (steepens) in the case of an oblate. The radius remains constant for spherical surfaces.

The same studies also showed that over 90% of eyes exhibited a prolate asphericity, with the remaining eyes being either spherical ($e = 0$) or oblate, in that the corneal radius steepens as the peripheral cornea is approached.

However, the use of eccentricity as a descriptor of corneal shape is limited by an inability properly to describe oblate surfaces (Lindsay et al 1997). The other descriptors used are shape factor (p) or asphericity (Q), which are related to e by the following formulae:

$$p = (1 - e^2)$$

where p is shape factor and

$$Q = -e^2$$

where Q is asphericity.

The main attraction for using Q as a definition is that it can describe either prolate (positive Q-value) or oblate (negative Q-value) corneal shapes. Most of the currently available video-keratoscopes give both e and Q-values, with the former being quite acceptable when used to calculate corneal sag and lens design. Q, however, is preferred when describing corneal shape for scientific analysis. The common values for normal prolate corneal shapes are:

$e = 0$ (spherical) or $e > 0$ and < 1 (prolate)
$p = 1$ (spherical) or $p < 1$ and > 0 (prolate)

$Q = 0$ (spherical) or $Q <$ and > 0 (positive values are prolate, and negative values oblate).

Keratometry measures the axial radius of the cornea at a distance of approximately 1.50 mm from the apex. The flat-K reading is the mean value of the two radii along that meridian, with the same average radius value for the steeper meridian, usually set at 90° to the flattest meridian. The cornea is assumed to be spherical ($e = 0$) for the derivation of keratometry values. K readings, therefore, do not supply information as to the actual shape and asphericity of the cornea. Methods for deriving R_0 and e-values from keratometry have been developed by Wilms & Rabbetts (1977), Douthwaite (1991), and Lam & Douthwaite (1994). These techniques require the use of either a two-position keratometer (Rodenstock C-BES; Wilms & Rabbetts 1977) or a modified one-position keratometer (Lam & Douthwaite 1994). The keratometry readings, both central and peripheral, are fed into a specific computer program in order to convert the K readings into R_0 and e-values that are then used to calculate the desired lens BOZR.

As stated above, the common traditional fitting philosophies are based on describing the BOZR as a function of its relationship to the flat keratometry (K_f). This method works quite well for small total diameter (TD) lenses (9.00 mm and less) and relatively normal eye shapes. However, the accuracy of the lens fit decreases as the TD increases or if the cornea exhibits a steep or flat R_0 associated with either a high or low eccentricity. If the cornea is steep centrally with a high eccentricity, then the lens designed purely on keratometry will result in a BOZR that is usually too steep. Similarly, if the cornea is relatively flat centrally with a low eccentricity, the indicated BOZR from keratometry is usually too flat (see later).

The problems associated with these fitting inconsistencies were investigated by Bibby (1979), Atkinson (1984, 1985), and Guillon et al (1983) and the concepts of tear layer thickness and cornea and lens sags evolved. Put simply, sag-based fitting philosophy describes a situation where the sagittal height of the contact lens is equal to the sag of the cornea plus an allowance for tear layer thickness (TLT) at the apex of the

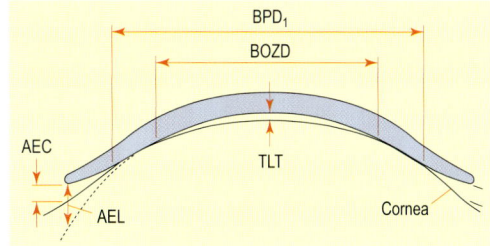

Figure 4.2   The concept of sag fitting is that the lens and cornea come into contact at the inner edge of the first back peripheral diameter (BPD_1). The lens sag is therefore the corneal sag at BPD_1 plus the apical tear layer thickness (TLT). BOZD, back optic zone diameter; AEC, axial edge clearance; AEL, axial edge lift. From Phillips (1997) with permission.

cornea over the common chord at the point of contact between the two (Fig. 4.2). The lens is fitted to the flattest corneal meridian. This gives the optimal BOZR when the corneal asphericity is taken into account, especially in the presence of astigmatism (Young 1998).

The lens is assumed to touch the cornea at the junction of the BOZR and BPR_1. An alternative is that BPR_1 is in alignment with the corneal surface, thereby creating a better distribution of pressure at the point of contact (see later). The thickness of the TLT is deepest at the corneal apex and reduces to zero at the $BOZD/BPD_1$ interface (junction of the optic zone and first peripheral curve).

The existence of a tear layer between the corneal surface and the posterior surface of the lens is essential for three reasons: firstly, for the purpose of promoting effective tear exchange for the maintenance of corneal physiology and secondly, the variations in the positive and negative fluid forces help control lens movement and centration. Finally, a tear layer between the lens and cornea is essential for preventing damage to the epithelium. The ideal TLT for contour-designed lenses is assumed to be approximately 15–25 μm.

Guillon & Sammons (1994) also point out that the alignment of the lens to the peripheral area of the cornea is of prime importance in maintaining the correct balance of tear exchange, lens movement, centration, and fluid dynamics. For this reason, the design of lenses fitted according to the sag philosophy should be primarily based on calculations derived from corneal shape, with the central parameters of the lens constructed from a correct alignment or area of touch with the peripheral cornea. The addition of the final peripheral curve has little bearing on the fitting behavior of the lens, but is essential for providing the Venturi effects that promote proper tear circulation around the edge of the lens.

The normal method of evaluating the fit of a rigid contact lens is by assessing the thickness of the postlens tear film thickness by the use of sodium fluorescein. Depending on both the concentration of fluorescein used and the degree of tear mixing present, the generally agreed *minimum* thickness of the postlens tear layer required to render fluorescein visible is in the order of 15–20 μm (Young 1988). This is of major importance when interpreting fluorescein patterns of lenses with central TLTs of 20 μm or less, and particularly reverse geometry lenses.

FORMULAE USED IN LENS CONSTRUCTION

The formula described above states:

Lens sag = Corneal sag + TLT (μm) over the chord of common contact between the two surfaces.

The sagittal height of the cornea is given by:

$$z = R_0 - \sqrt{R_0^2 - y^2\, p/p}$$

where z = corneal sag, R_0 = apical radius, y = half-chord and p = shape factor or $1 - e^2$ or $1 - Q$.

The sag of the cornea is therefore dependent not only on the apical radius and eccentricity values, but also the chord over which the sag is measured.

The calculation for spherical multicurve lenses is more complex, with the sag of all component curves needing to be added to the sag of the BOZR over the back optic zone diameter (BOZD). The basic formula for a tricurve lens is:

$$p = x_0 + x_1 + x_2$$

where x_0 = primary sag of the BOZR at the BOZD, x_1 = sag of BPR$_1$ at the BPD$_1$ – sag of BPR$_1$ at the BOZD and x_2 = sag of BPR2 at the TD – sag BPR$_2$ at the BPD$_1$.

The same general principles also apply to lenses of greater than three curves. The final formula is:

$$\begin{aligned}\text{Sag} = {} & R_1 + \sqrt{[R_1^2 - (D_1/2)^2]} + \{(R_2) - \\ & \sqrt{[R_2^2 - (D_2/2)^2]} - R_2 - \sqrt{R_2^2 - (D_1/2)^2}\} + \\ & \{R_3 - \sqrt{R_3^2 - (D_3/2)^2}\} - \{R_3 - \\ & \sqrt{R_3^2 - (D_2/2)^2}\}\end{aligned}$$

where R_1 = BOZR, D_1 = BOZD, R_2 = BPR$_1$, D_2 = BPD$_2$, R_3 = BPR$_3$, and D_3 = BPD$_3$.

A useful extension to this form of mathematical construction is to calculate the sags of the lens and cornea over small (0.10 mm) chord increments and subtract the corneal sag from the lens sag. These values are then represented on the y-axis of a graph. The x-axis represents the half-chord lengths from the center of the cornea to the edge of the lens. Such a graph then represents the tear layer profile of the lens, or, put more simply, the shape of the tear layer under the lens. Figure 4.3A represents the tear layer profile of a

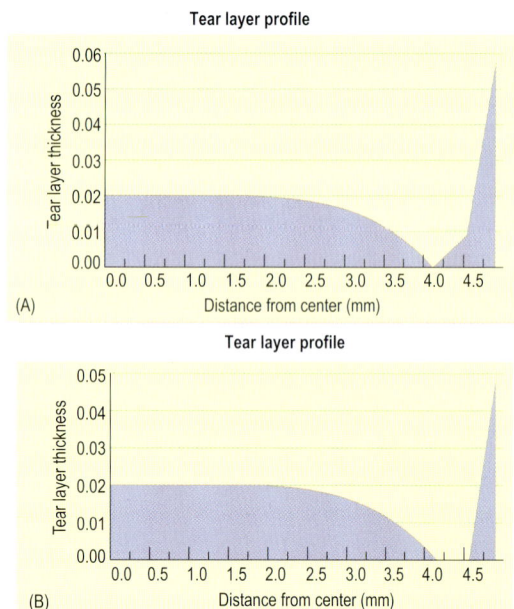

Figure 4.3   (A) The tear layer profile of a contour lens showing 20 μm of apical clearance and corneal contact at the junction of back optic zone diameter and first back peripheral radius. Note that there is a relatively sharp point of contact between the two surfaces. (B) The same lens as shown in Figure 4.3 (A), but with a change in the radius of curvature of first back peripheral radius such that the lens makes contact with the corneal surface in alignment with BPR$_1$.

contour lens with the point of contact between the lens and the corneal surface at the edge of the BOZD. Figure 4.3B, on the other hand, represents a modification of the parameters of the previous lens to allow for the common point of contact to lie along the BPR_1 at the first back peripheral diameter (BPD_1).

These lenses exhibit a central TLT of 20 μm, tapering to corneal contact at the desired point. For general lens designs, the TLT graph is assumed to show the profile along the flattest corneal meridian (Young 1998).

Manipulation of the lens design and fit can then be made by altering the lens parameters either to increase or decrease the central TLT or change the axial edge clearance to the desired amount. Decreasing the central TLT effectively involves flattening the BOZR or decreasing the BOZD, leading to a flatter-fitting lens. Conversely, increasing the central TLT involves steepening the BOZR or increasing the BOZD, leading to a tighter fit. As a general rule, changes of 0.05 mm to the BOZR lead to an alteration of 10 μm to the central TLT if the BOZD is kept constant. Similarly, changes of 0.5 mm to the BOZD will result in a change of approximately 5 μm in the TLT if the BOZR is kept constant.

By the use of lens design programs it is theoretically possible to design lenses of any appropriate combination of BOZR/BOZD to give the ideal tear layer profile at any lens diameter specified. This model of designing lenses based on the concept of an ideal tear layer profile forms the basis of most of the contact lens fitting modules in the currently available videokeratoscopes. The relative accuracy of the method can be shown by the following example.

Assuming a cornea has an apical radius of 7.80 mm, and the lens diameter is 9.60 mm with a BOZD of 8.30 mm, the indicated BOZR using keratometric values and the accepted rule of thumb of K_f + 0.05 mm would be approximately 7.85 mm. However, if the same BOZD value is kept constant, and the eccentricity of the cornea is varied, then the calculated BOZR assuming a central TLT of 20 μm would be as shown in Table 4.1.

Therefore, if the eccentricity is taken into account, a more accurate indication of the correct

Table 4.1

Eccentricity	BOZR (mm)
0.70	7.95
0.60	7.90
0.50	7.83
0.40	7.78
0.30	7.74
0.20	7.71
0.10	7.69
0.0	7.69

BOZR, back optic zone radius.

BOZR for the actual corneal shape is achieved. If the patient had a low-eccentricity cornea, then the keratometry-based choice of a BOZR of 7.85 would have led to a flat-fitting lens. Alternatively, the use of the 7.85 mm BOZR lens (fitted 0.05 mm flatter than K_f) on a cornea with an eccentricity of 0.70 would result in the lens being relatively steep compared to the calculated BOZR of 7.95 mm (Young 1998).

Chan et al (1998) compared the accuracy of the fit of rigid gas-permeable (RGP) lenses by fluorescein analysis with two methods of determining the BOZR. In the first the BOZR was determined by using the simulated keratometric readings and in the second it was calculated from the apical radius and eccentricity values given by the videokeratoscope. The definitive method of assessment was the masked choice of the correct BOZR based purely on fluorescein fit analysis. The mean differences in BOZR between the simulated keratometry values and the correct BOZR was 0.11 ± 0.05 mm, and for the fluorescein assessment and correct BOZR −0.01 ± 0.04 mm. The authors concluded that knowledge of the eccentricity from videokeratoscopy provided a more accurate prediction of the BOZR/cornea relationship than that derived from central keratometry measurements.

As previously stated, fluorescein is rendered visible when mixed in the postlens tear film at a thickness of approximately 20 μm. By drawing a line across a tear layer profile graph at the 20 μm point on the y-axis, the probable zones of fluorescein visibility can be made evident. For example, the TLT profile of the lenses shown in Figure 4.3 would indicate a light glow of fluorescein centrally, with a large mid-peripheral band of apparent alignment with the cornea until the TLT increased above the 20 μm level in the edge lift area. This concept of analyzing the tear layer profile and TLT takes on major importance when assessing the design and fit of reverse geometry lenses.

In conclusion, the design of lenses based on the correct sagittal relationship between the lens and the actual corneal shape described in terms of apical radius and eccentricity results in a more accurate and dependable relationship between the BOZR and the corneal shape. The use of tear layer profile graphs is an excellent method of visualizing the fit of the lens on the eye and the likely appearance of the fluorescein pattern. However, as stated previously, the construction of the peripheral curves also plays a very important part in the overall design of the lens and its behavior on the eye.

PERIPHERAL CURVE DESIGN

The second curve of a tricurve lens design has two major functions. It can be used either as a "blend" between the BOZR and the point of contact with the peripheral cornea, or if the primary design criterion is to have the BOZR align with the peripheral cornea, the secondary curve becomes part of the construction of the edge lift of the lens. As can be seen in Figure 4.3A, the point of contact of the BOZR with the corneal surface appears to be just that – a *point* of contact. Such apparently sharp points apply relatively high degrees of pressure over a small area, and can result in discomfort and adverse effects on lens centration.

Alternatively, the area of contact shown in Figure 4.3B shows a more even alignment with the peripheral cornea, thus distributing the pressure of contact over a larger area. The differences between the two types of peripheral contact were described in mechanical terms by Sammons (1984), who used the terms "conformal" and "counterformal" to describe the pressure effects of the two. Conformal mid-peripheral curves meet the corneal surface such that the two curves

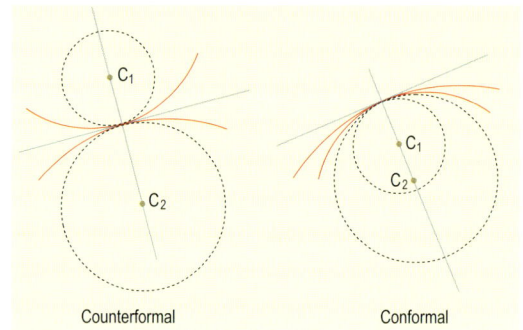

Figure 4.4 The difference between a conformal and counterformal edge design. The conformal surface has the curve oriented in the same direction as the common tangent, whereas the counterformal surface has the curve in the opposite direction. From Guillon & Sammons (1994) with permission.

(BOZR and BPR_1) are similarly oriented to their common tangent. Counterformal mid-peripheral curves arise when the two curves lie in the opposite orientation to their common tangent (Fig. 4.4). The major difference between the two lies in the degree of concentrated pressure exerted on the peripheral cornea. Conformal curves are in closer alignment with the peripheral cornea and therefore spread the pressure over a larger area. Counterformal curves result in a point of heavy pressure over a small area.

Thomas (1967) was the first to consider the pressure distribution of the peripheral area of the contact lens and introduced the concept of tangential peripheral "curves" as a means of controlling both the peripheral pressure and of maximizing lens centration. Tangent peripheries are not curves as such, but more an optical flat that meets the peripheral cornea at an approximate tangent to the surface at the point of contact (Fig. 4.5). Other conformal peripheral curves commonly used are either aspheric or parabolic (Guillon et al 1983). The major advantage of conformal peripheral curves over counterformal is enhanced centration and better pressure distribution at the lens/cornea interface. The effect that these types of alignment mid-peripheries have on the overall sag calculations must also be taken into account when constructing tear layer profiles and determining central TLT, and will be dealt with in greater detail when discussing reverse geometry lenses.

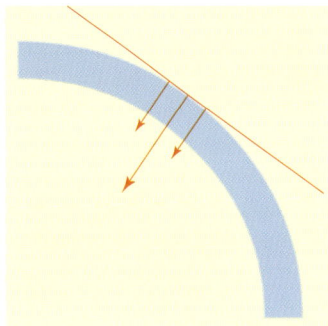

Figure 4.5 A tangent conformal periphery. Note that the "curve" is a straight line that meets the corneal surface at a tangent to the point of contact. This results in a gradient of pressure across the surface.

The accurate fitting of rigid lenses is dependent on being able to design lenses based on the shape of the individual cornea to be fitted. Furthermore, the construction of the mid-peripheral curve plays a vital role in distributing the pressure at the point of contact between the two surfaces and in centration control. The incorporation of the different lens variables into a tear layer profile graph allows for a better assessment of the lens design and also provides valuable information as to the likely fluorescein pattern. The importance of a clear understanding of these principles makes the intricate interrelationships of the variables in reverse geometry lens design easier to comprehend, and this is vital if a successful fitting is to occur.

REVERSE GEOMETRY LENSES

General background and history

Reverse geometry lenses differ from standard lens designs in that the BPR_1 is steeper than the BOZR. There are three basic designs of reverse geometry lenses, comprising three-, four- and five-zone lenses. It is the intention in this section to explain the differences in design and fitting methods using the sag philosophy. If a lens is to have an optimal fitting relationship to the cornea, the only method that is common to all designs is that the lens sag must be equal to the corneal sag over the common chord of contact between the two, plus an allowance for apical TLT. This rule applies whether there are three or 30 curves on the back surface of the lens.

All orthokeratology lenses have "proprietary curves" that are used by the manufacturer to differentiate their design from all others. However, as will be shown in the following sections, there are basic underlying principles that are inherent to all the different designs, with the major variation being the fitting philosophy or the assumptions made regarding corneal shape.

The first patent for a reverse geometry lens was granted to Nick Siviglia in 1988. The lens was designed to fit postradial keratotomy and penetrating keratoplasty cases. No reference to orthokeratology appears in the patent documents. The lens had a nominal BOZD of 6.00 mm, with the reverse curve a nominal 1.50 D steeper than the BOZR, and between 0.50 and 1.50 mm wide. The periphery of the lens was spherical. The patent has been assigned to Paragon as the basis for the CRT lens.

Wlodyga and Stoyan are credited with the original design and fitting philosophy of reverse geometry lenses for use in orthokeratology in 1986. The terminology "reverse geometry" was originally applied to the design as a means of differentiating between lenses where the second curve (BPR_1) is *steeper* than the BOZR and standard lens designs where the peripheral curves are flatter than the base curve (Winkler & Kame 1995). Fontana (1972) has been credited by some with the invention of the lens with his "bifocal" orthokeratology lens.

However, the description of the lens, which has a 6.00 mm BOZD with the BOZR 1.00 D flatter than the periphery of the lens (which is fitted "on-K"), seems to intimate that the central zone was actually a "recessed optic" which was cut into the lens after the peripheral curves were worked. It is worthwhile remembering that it has only been the introduction of computer numeric-controlled (CNC) lathes that has allowed for the manufacture of true reverse geometry lenses. This was not possible with the older single-axis lathes. The first patent for reverse geometry lenses for orthokeratology was granted to Stoyan.

Three-zone lenses (Contex OK series)

The description of three-zone fitting is based on the Contex lenses, but the same comments apply to all other three-zone lenses. The original concept of the lens was to avoid the chronic problems of induced with-the-rule astigmatism caused by the flat-fitting, poorly centering lenses that were commonplace with the traditional orthokeratology techniques. This was to be achieved by using a steeper secondary curve in order to maximize centration. However, an unforeseen effect was the apparent increase in both the degree of myopia reduction when compared to the older techniques and a reduction in the time taken to obtain the results (Wlodyga & Bryla 1989).

In general, it was stated that the lenses caused "twice the reduction in half the time" and the term "accelerated orthokeratology" was applied to the process of fitting. The original design consisted of a 6.00 mm BOZD, 3.00 D steeper secondary curve (the RC that forms the TR), an aspheric peripheral curve 0.50 mm wide and an overall TD of 9.60 mm, and was marketed under the name OK-3 (Contex, Sherman Oaks, CA). Wlodyga clinically assessed numerous lens design variations over the next few years, but the most commonly used lens remained the OK-3. By 1998, the range of lens parameters was expanded to include any combination of BOZDs from 6.00 to 8.00 mm in 0.50-mm steps and RC curves of 1.00–15.00 D steeper than the BOZR in 1.00-D increments, in both spherical and aspheric forms. The earlier OK series has been largely superseded by the four- and five-curve designs.

Traditional three-zone fitting philosophy

The original fitting philosophy was to fit the initial OK-3 1.50 D flatter than the flattest keratometry reading (K_f), and modify the fit until an area of approximately 3.00–3.50 mm central "touch" and good centration was achieved. There was no predetermined refractive change or target outcome. The practitioner simply ordered the initial lens 1.50 D flatter than K_f and an extra two sets of lenses, each 0.50 D flatter than the preceding. The course of treatment was considered over when the corneal flattening ceased.

The fitting was complicated by the introduction of an entire range of different TR curves. The use of a steeper RC meant that the BOZR needed to be flatter than that used for the 3.00 D RC lens,

and a steeper BOZR if a flatter RC lens was used. Also, if a diameter larger than the standard 9.60 mm were required, then the RC curve band would be wider, since the BOZD and BPD_2 were fixed. This led to the larger lens being relatively steeper than the 9.60-mm TD lens, so a flatter BOZR was required in order to maintain the correct fitting relationship. With over 150 different design variables available, it is no wonder that there were reports of inconsistent fitting and results reported by practitioners using the lenses. It was the inconsistency of results that led Mountford to attempt to standardize the fitting by adopting the sag philosophy to the choice of initial trial lens.

The use of a very flat BOZR leads to the presence of heavy central touch and peripheral clearance when combined with a standard contour fitting philosophy. This invariably leads to lens decentration. Guillon & Sammons (1994) defined the pressure developed by the postlens tear layer as the tear fluid squeeze pressure (TFSP), the force of which is directly proportional to the thickness of the tear film at any point on the corneal surface. The TFSP maintains lens centration by opposing the gravity and eyelid forces that cause lens decentration (Hayashi 1977). If the lens fit is flat enough, then the central TLT is zero, and the TFSP plays no role in the maintenance of lens centration. The lid force then becomes dominant, usually causing superior decentration. The lid-induced decentration causes a redistribution of the tear volume under the lens, and the final resting position of the lens is then dependent on the balance of forces developed in the postlens tear layer by the TFSP.

The inclusion of a steeper secondary curve reduces the peripheral clearance such that the lens is assumed to rest on the peripheral cornea at the junction of the TR/RC curve and the edge lift curve. The TLT therefore varies from a minimum at the corneal apex to a maximum at the BOZD/RC junction. Since the TFSP is directly proportional to the thickness of the tear layer, there will be a variation in the pressure as the TLT increases from the central to the TR area. The decentration due to the lack of a viable TFSP with a flat BOZR is then compensated by the increased TFSP induced by the deeper TLT of the reverse curve.

In this way, a flat BOZR can be combined with a steeper secondary curve and still maintain lens centration.

In sag philosophy terms, the sag of an ideally fitting reverse geometry lens is equal to the sag of the BOZR at the BOZD plus the sag of the RC curve at BPD_2. This should equal the sag of the cornea at the point of contact (BPD_2) plus an allowance for central TLT. This is the same concept described earlier for the fitting of contour lenses in that:

Sag OK lens = corneal sag + TLT over the common chord of contact

Figure 4.6 shows the relation of the lens with the various curves and the fluorescein pattern.

The apical TLT for contour lenses is assumed to be approximately 20 μm. However, this is not the case with reverse geometry lenses, where the typical TLT is assumed to be less than 10 μm or, in some cases, zero. When the initial calculations for the OK-3 lens using the sag fitting philosophy were carried out, it was found that the variation in apical TLT was extremely sensitive to alterations in BOZR. If a central TLT of zero was used,

there was no peripheral contact with the cornea at the edge of the TR curve. The minimal central TLT that provided peripheral contact was 10 μm. A central TLT of zero is possible, but only if the TR radius or diameter is varied. Furthermore, a TLT of 10 μm was felt to be more acceptable from a clinical viewpoint, as a TLT of zero would mean direct lens contact on the surface epithelium, which could result in unwanted trauma.

The advantage of fitting reverse geometry lenses according to the sag philosophy is that any combination of BOZR/BOZD and RC can be calculated to give the correct fitting relationship to the cornea. The tear layer profiles of a group of lenses with varying BOZR/RC combinations are shown in Figure 4.7. Note that, even though the shape of the tear layer profiles differ, all lenses exhibit the correct sagittal relationship to the cornea in that the central TLT is 10 μm, and the lens rests on the peripheral cornea at the junction of the RC and BPR_2. Mountford (1997a) has shown that the use of sag calculations based on corneal shape and lens sag results in a more accurate choice of initial BOZR than the traditional "1.50 D flatter than K" technique.

For a given cornea of R_0 7.80 mm and an eccentricity (e) of 0.50, the indicated BOZR using the 1.50 D rule would be 8.10 mm. However, if the

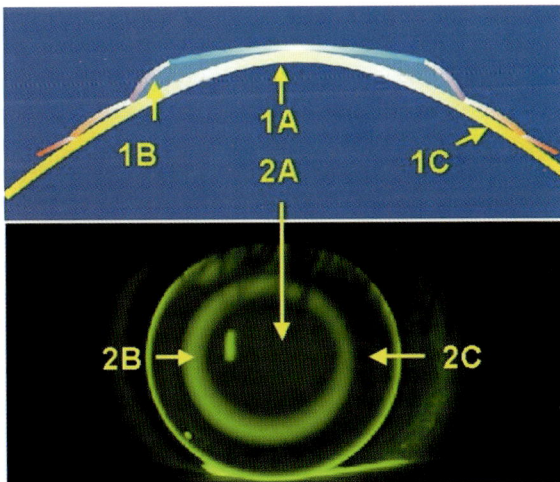

Figure 4.6   The sag philosophy applied to reverse geometry lenses. (Top) The lens and cornea come into contact at the outer edge of the alignment curve. (Bottom) The fluorescein pattern shows the common areas (1B and 2B the reverse curve, and 1C and 2C the alignment curve). Courtesy of Christina Eglund, Polymer Technology Corporation.

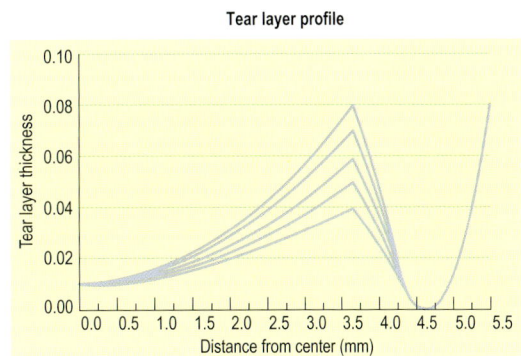

Figure 4.7   The tear layer profiles of various reverse geometry lenses having an equivalent sagittal relationship to the cornea. The variables are the back optic zone radius (BOZR) and tear reservoir (TR) curves that are 2, 3, 4, 5, and 6.00 D steeper than the BOZR. The 2.00 D TR curve has a tear layer thickness (TLT) of 40 μm at the back optic zone diameter (BOZD), whilst the 6.00 D lens has a TLT of 80 μm at the BOZD.

Table 4.2

Eccentricity	BOZR in mm (OK603)
0.80	8.45
0.70	8.40
0.60	8.35
0.50	8.30
0.40	8.25
0.30	8.20
0.20	8.15
0.10	8.10
0.00	8.10

BOZR, back optic zone radius.

eccentricity of the cornea were specified, the calculated BOZR using the sag fitting concepts for an apical radius of 7.80 mm and a lens diameter of 9.80 mm would be as shown in Table 4.2.

As can be seen from the analysis in Table 4.2, the use of the "rule of thumb" would result in a steep or tight-fitting lens unless the cornea was basically spherical ($e = 0$) in shape. Furthermore, a study involving two subject groups fitted with the same-diameter OK603, but with the BOZR chosen by the two different techniques, showed that the refractive change measured was significantly different between the groups over a 6-h period (Mountford 1997a). Group 1 (13 eyes) wore lenses fitted 1.50 D flatter than K_f and exhibited a mean refractive change of 0.91 ± 0.36 D following the trial wear period. Group 2 (10 eyes) were fitted according to the sag philosophy and showed a mean change of 1.38 ± 0.58 D. The differences were statistically significant ($F = 10.373$, $P = 0.0024$ analysis of variance), indicating that the accuracy of the fit had an effect on the efficacy of the lens with respect to the refractive change achieved.

There are over 150 different combinations of BOZD/TR available with the standard OK series lenses, so a logical approach to the determination of the most effective design is required in order to reduce the number of trial lenses necessary to carry out the fitting procedure. The ideal-fitting lens exhibits a fluorescein pattern that shows an area of approximately 3.00–3.50 mm of central "touch" surrounded by a wide and deep annulus

of tears that tapers to the peripheral contact band (Fig. 4.8). Assuming that fluorescein becomes visible at a TLT of 20 μm, then a line drawn parallel to the x-axis in Figure 4.7 will indicate the relative areas of "touch" and clearance under the lens. Areas of "touch" may be determined by drawing a line from the point of intersection of the 20 μm line and the tear layer profile to the x-axis. The diameter of the apparent touch can then be read off the x-axis.

The only lenses that satisfy the requirement of 3.00–3.50 mm of central touch are the 3.00 D and 4.00 D RC lenses. The 5.00 D RC lens shows an approximate touch diameter of 2.5 mm, and the shallow RC lenses (1.00 D and 2.00 D) show diameters larger than 3.50 mm. Bara (2000) has shown that the degree of corneal flattening is significantly greater with the steeper RC lenses than the shallow RC lenses. The main problem is that, as the relative area of central touch is reduced, the area of flattening is also reduced, which can lead to significant ghosting and haloes in dim illumination. As the pupil dilates in poor illumination, the area of corneal flattening is effectively smaller than the pupil zone, thus causing a reduction in low-contrast vision, which is made considerably worse if the lens decenters (see later).

The optimal OK design used in the author's practice was the OK704, which has an optic zone of 7.00 mm and a secondary curve 4 D steeper than the base curve. Since this RC was preset to the BOZR, the only alteration in fit possible was to flatten and steepen the BOZR. There is a significant drawback in using this type of approach, and that is that the TLT profile varies depending on the shape of the cornea being fitted. In Figure 4.7, the tear layer profiles of a group of reverse geometry lenses are shown. The variables are the BOZR and the TR curve, but, significantly, both are totally controlled by the differences in sag between the area of central clearance and the depth of the tear layer at the edge of the BOZD. Noack (personal communication) has termed this difference the "clearance factor" (CF), and for any given clearance factor, there can only be one single combination of BOZR and TR that will satisfy the requirements of the sag fitting philosophy. The CF is defined as the difference

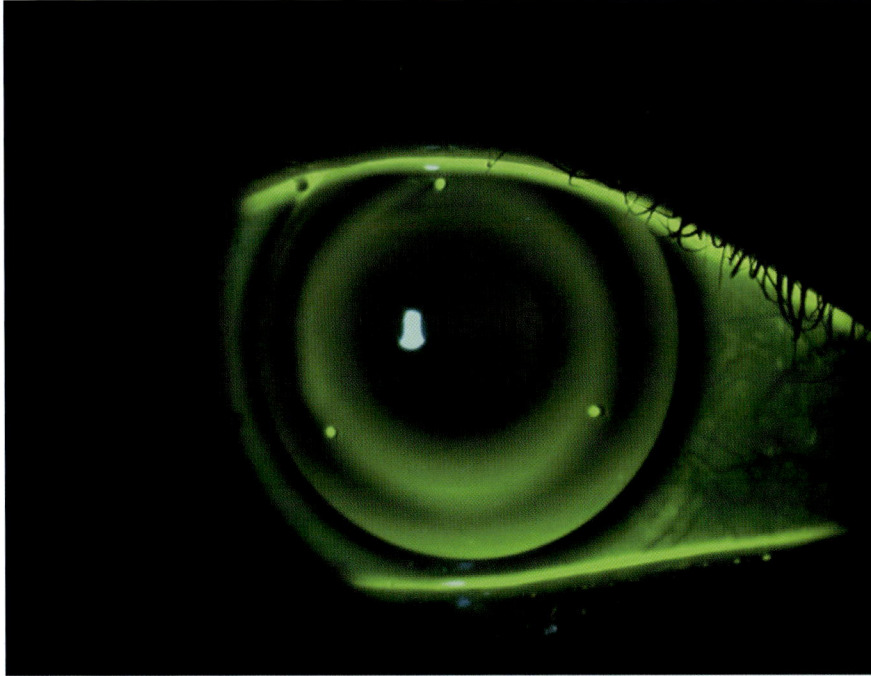

Figure 4.8 An ideal-fitting three-zone lens (Contex 704C). Note that the apical "touch" is 3.00–3.50 mm wide, and is surrounded by a wide and deep annulus of tears trapped in the reverse curve area.

between the TLT at the corneal apex and the TLT at the edge of the BOZD.

The variations in clearance factors for 10.6 mm diameter OK704T lenses over an apical radius range of 7.20–8.50 mm, and corneal eccentricities of 0.0, 0.30, 0.50, and 0.70, are shown in Figure 4.9. Note that the CFs are greatest for steep corneas with high eccentricities, and lowest for flat corneas with low eccentricities. The TLTs of two 11.2-mm diameter OK704Ts on corneas of R_0

7.20 mm and eccentricity of 0.80, and R_0 8.40 mm and 0.30 eccentricity are shown in Figure 4.10. The BOZR for the steeper cornea is 8.00 mm and the TLT at the edge of the BOZD is approximately 73 μm. The indicated area of central touch is approximately 2.60 mm in diameter. The BOZR for the flatter cornea is 8.86 mm and the TLT at the BOZD is 49 μm, with an indicated central touch diameter is 3.50 mm. These differences between tear layer profiles for different corneal

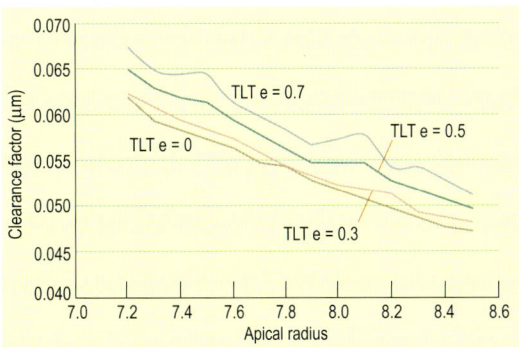

Figure 4.9 Variation in clearance factor with varying apical radii and eccentricities.

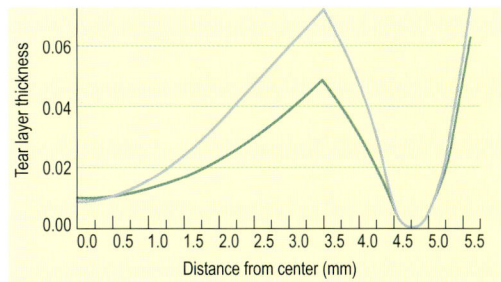

Figure 4.10 The tear layer thicknesses of two 11.2-mm diameter OK704Ts on corneas of apical radii 7.20 mm and eccentricity 0.80 (top line), and apical radius 8.40 mm and 0.30 eccentricity (bottom line).

Tear layer profile

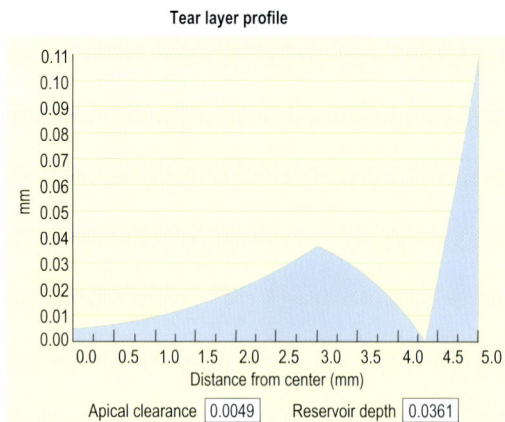

Apical clearance [0.0049]   Reservoir depth [0.0361]

Figure 4.11 Tear layer profile of a Contex reverse geometry lens.

shapes are responsible for some of the marked variations in corneal response to the lens (see Ch. 10), and are a major limitation of fixed reverse curve designs.

The major problem with the early three-zone lenses was decentration. Variations in lens diameter still led to the common problem of lens decentration, often superiorly, with the accompanying off-center corneal flattening and induced astigmatism. Since modifications of both the TLT and lens diameter were generally unsuccessful at controlling centration, the only other logical approach was to modify the peripheral curve design.

Contex reverse geometry lenses have a standard aspheric peripheral curve that is, in effect, a counterformal curve that bears a constant relationship to the BOZR (Fig. 4.11). If the BOZR is steepened in an attempt to improve centration, the RC and the peripheral curve are also steepened proportionally. This leads to marked peripheral compression at the TR/peripheral curve interface and an increase in the central TLT, resulting in a tight lens fit that can limit or reduce the corneal shape change (Mountford 1997a). The logical alternative is to modify the peripheral curve design so that it becomes conformal.

Three-zone lenses were limited by the direct relationship between the BOZR and RCs. This led to a minimum variation in apical TLT of 10 μm, and some restrictions in the efficacy of the lens with respect to refractive change. However, the

major problem continued to be decentration, and this led to the development of four-zone lenses.

Four- and five-zone lenses

There are numerous variations on the theme of four-zone lenses. The common structure of the lenses is a central optic zone, an RC, an alignment curve, and an edge lift. The five-zone lenses divide the alignment curve into two separate curves in order to produce a conformal periphery. A brief description of the main designs is outlined below.

The El Hage "aspheric mold" concept

In 1997, El Hage applied for and was granted a patent describing continuous aspheric molds for reshaping the surface of the cornea having an inner concave surface matched to the topography of the cornea (El Hage 1997a). The underlying concept was to modify a lens curve adapted from topographical data that would "include a flattened pressure zone applying relative pressure and thereby displacing underlying corneal tissue, a steepened relief zone raised away from the surface of the cornea to receive displaced corneal tissue, and a flattened anchor zone to control and direct movement of displaced corneal tissue into the relief zones." In effect, the lens consisted of a central optic zone, a second curve that was flatter than the BOZR, an RC, and an alignment curve. The central, second, and third curves were described in terms of a polynomial (Fig. 4.12). The peripheral curve is then designed to give an axial edge lift of between 80 and 100 μm.

The lens construction is designed such that the central optic zone (pressure zone) can vary with the degree of refractive error correction required, with the BOZR based on Jessen's concept of 0.20 mm flattening of the BOZR for each 1.00 D of refractive change required (the Jessen factor). A

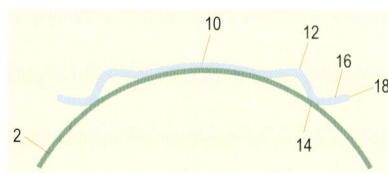

Figure 4.12
The controlled keratoreformation (CKR) lens (from El Hage 1997a).

Table 4.3 Design variables of El Hage lenses

Refraction (D)	Pressure zone diameter (mm)	d (mm)
5.50–6.00	4.00–5.00	1.20
4.00–5.00	5.00–5.50	0.80–1.00
3.00–4.00	5.50–6.00	0.60–0.80
1.00–3.00	6.00–6.50	0.20–0.60

cornea with a central radius of 7.80 mm and a refractive error of 3.00 D would therefore require a BOZR of 8.40 mm (7.80 mm + [0.20 × 3.00 D]). Also, the pressure zone is varied with the correction required. High corrections (3.50–6.00 D) have a pressure zone of 4.00–5.00 mm, and low corrections (1.00–3.00 D) a zone of 6.00–6.50 mm (Table 4.3).

The proposed mode of action is that the pressure zone, which is separated from the corneal surface by the tear film, provides a force that moves corneal tissue towards the relief curve zone. The anchor zone then limits the movement of tissue any further, and has a secondary function of maximizing lens centration. The induced redistribution of corneal tissue is then responsible for the corneal curvature and refractive change.

Corneal topography data supply the central radius (R_0), which is the mean corneal curvature over the central 2.00 mm chord. Note that this definition of R_0 differs from that of the usual definition, where R_0 represents a singularity at the corneal apex. The shape factor of the cornea is calculated as a mean of the eccentricity values of up to 360 meridians at the pressure zone diameter of choice, which is predetermined by the initial refractive error. The sagittal height of the cornea over this chord is then calculated using the derived R_0 and shape factor values. The sag of the indicated BOZR in millimeters (R_0 + 0.20 Rx) is also calculated over the same chord. The difference between the two is then assumed to be the sag change induced in the cornea by the effect of the lens. For a cornea of R_0 8.00 and BOZR of 8.60, assuming a 3.00 D refractive change, the difference in sag is 29 μm over the 5.00-mm chord of the pressure zone. This is roughly equated to 10 μm per diopter of refractive change.

The movement of the centrally displaced corneal tissue is towards the relief zone, which is "preferably raised above the reformed corneal surface by about 12 μm per diopter of correction." In the above example, this equals a sag difference of 36 μm. This is then added to the 29 μm of central sag change, resulting in a TLT of 65 μm at the edge of the relief curve. It is unclear why a sag change of 10 μm per diopter of refractive change is used for the central calculations and 12 μm per diopter in the relief zone.

El Hage obviously studied the final postorthokeratology corneal topography in detail, as the lens parameters are actually based on the *altered or final* corneal shape. The controlled keratoreformation (CKR) lens was the first orthokeratology lens design and fitting philosophy based on topography data.

The Dreimlens

The other major development or modification of reverse geometry lenses is the Dreimlens, designed by Thomas Reim. The impetus for the lens design was a requirement for enhanced control of lens centration and the corneal response to the lens. Reim (personal communication) describes the lens in terms of it being a "dual TR" design, in that there are two reverse curves on the lens back surface. The basic design consists of a 10.00 mm TD with a 6.00 mm BOZD. The first peripheral curve forms a TR that is 0.60 mm wide, surrounded by the second peripheral curve that forms a TR that is 1.00 mm wide. The final peripheral curve is 0.40 mm wide and is designed to give an adequate axial edge lift. The real difference, however, is in the relative steepness of the two RCs. The depth and width of the TR are intrinsically tied to the BOZR and BOZD and their fitting relationship to the cornea, and this is where the Dreimlens bears a major difference to the Contex designs.

The second TR (as described by Reim) is in effect an alignment zone designed primarily as an aid to centration. The first RC, being 0.60 mm wide, is therefore necessarily much steeper than the BOZR in order to maintain sagittal equivalency with the cornea. Reim applied for, and was granted, a patent (1999) for the lens due to the construction of the peripheral alignment curve to control centration. The design was altered by splitting the alignment curves in two, resulting in a five-curve lens. In those cases where lens centration could not be adequately controlled, the diameter was increased to 10.6 mm, with the alignment curves being made wider.

The fitting philosophy is a variant of the Jessen factor, where the BOZR is defined initially by the refractive change required. To this, Reim adds a further 0.75 D flattening as a "compression factor," so that, for an initial central K of 44.00 D and refractive error of 3.00 D, the indicated BOZR would be 44.00 − 3.00 − 0.75 or 40.25 D (8.38 mm). Once the BOZR has been chosen, the corneal elevation (sag) data at the point of contact of the alignment curve are read from the corneal topographer. The other lens parameters can then be calculated from the standard formulas discussed previously. The alignment curve is designed such that it meets the corneal surface at a chord of 9.20 mm for the 10.00 mm lens, with a nominal TLT of 10 μm at the junction of the alignment curve and the reverse curve. The apical clearance is set at zero.

The lens fitting is usually based on the flat-K value and an assumed corneal eccentricity of 0.50. The exact specifications of the Dreimlens are unknown, but an approximation of the TLT can be constructed using the formulas described previously. Reim intimates that there are blend zones between TR_1 and the alignment curve that are not shown in the following model. However, such small variations would have a minimal effect on the sag relationship of the lens and the cornea, and the model can therefore still be considered a useful example. The approximate TLT of a 10.00 mm Dreimlens for a patient with an apical radius of 7.65 mm (44.00 D), an eccentricity of 0.50 and a refractive error of 3.00 D, is shown in Figure 4.13.

If the 20 μm line is drawn across the TLT graph in Figure 4.13, the apparent central touch diameter is approximately 4.00 mm, surrounded by a thin, deep annulus of fluorescein. The peripheral alignment curve is approximately 1.00 mm wide. The resemblance between the calculated TLT profile analysis interpretation of the probable fluorescein pattern and the actual pattern appearance (Fig. 4.14) is obvious.

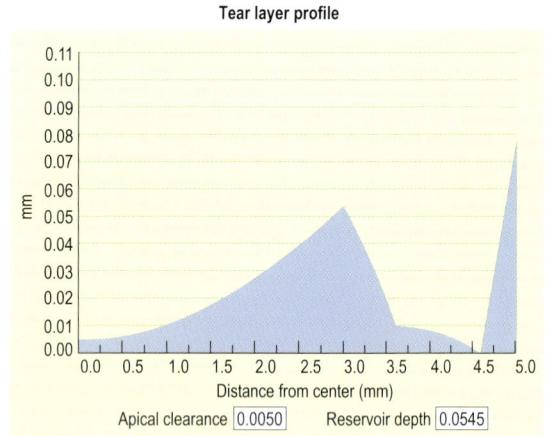

Figure 4.13   The approximate tear layer thickness of a 10.00-mm Dreimlens for a patient with an apical radius of 7.65 mm (44.00 D), an eccentricity of 0.50, and a refractive error of 3.00 D.

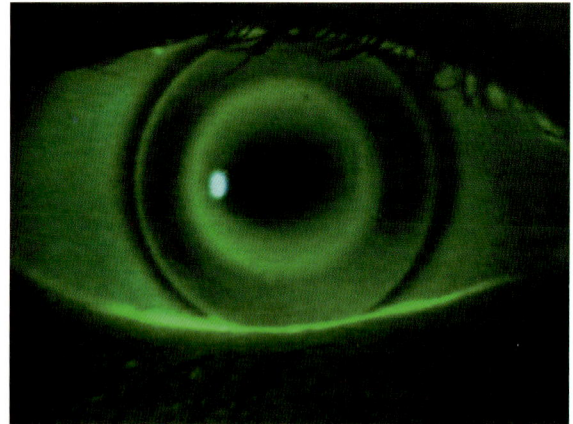

Figure 4.14   An ideal-fitting Dreimlens. Note the wide area of central "touch" and the narrow and deep tear annulus at the back optic zone diameter/reverse curve area. There is a wide alignment zone. The area of "touch" and clearance line up with the areas below and above the 20 μm line in Figure 4.13.

The tear layer profiles of the Dreimlens for 3.00 D refractive change on three different corneal shapes are shown in Figure 4.15. Note that, in contrast to the Contex three-zone design, where the reverse curve was fixed with respect to the BOZR, the differences in CF between the three lens fits is minimal. In the case of the cornea having an apical radius of 7.80 and an eccentricity

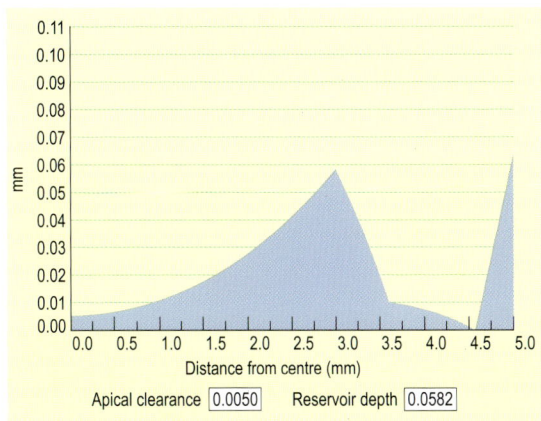

Apical clearance 0.0050   Reservoir depth 0.0582

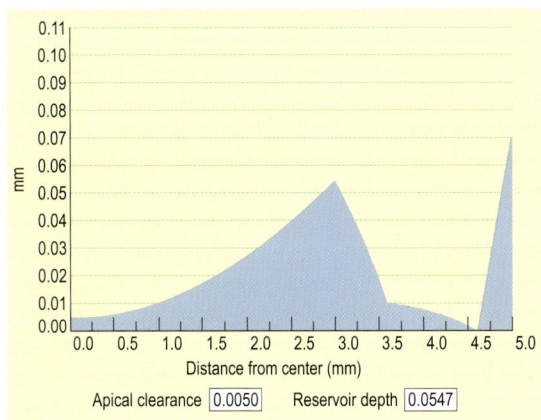

Apical clearance 0.0050   Reservoir depth 0.0547

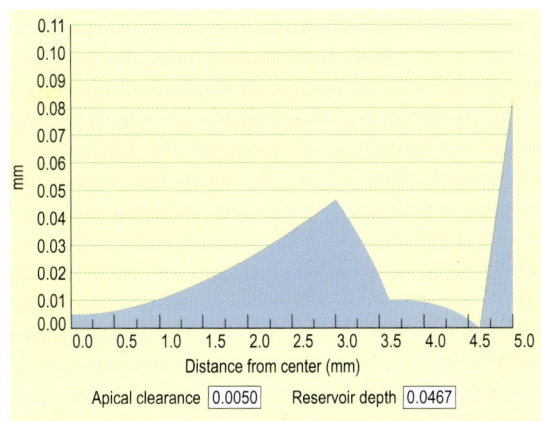

Apical clearance 0.0050   Reservoir depth 0.0467

Figure 4.15 The tear layer profiles of the Dreimlens for 3.00 D refractive change on three different corneal shapes. (A) Cornea with an apical radius of 8.20 and an eccentricity of 0.3; (B) cornea with an apical radius of 7.80 and eccentricity 0.50; and (C) apical radius 7.30, eccentricity 0.70.

of 0.50 (a 7.80/0.50 cornea), the CF is 49.7 μm, followed by 41.7 μm for the steep (7.20/0.70) cornea and 53.2 μm for the flat (8.20/0.30) cornea. When the Dreimlens was first released, it created a lot of interest, as the results achieved were more predictable than those of the Contex lenses. The reason for this was probably the enhanced centration, but the fact that the variation in CF was much better controlled also plays a part (see Ch. 10).

The alignment curve is thought to cause a second compression zone (the first being the BOZR and area of central touch) that limits the movement of tissue away from the center, and also provides a peripheral "push" in towards the center.

Reim states that the BOZR is usually limited to 4.75 D flatter than *K*, or a maximum refractive change of 4.00 D, due to early problems with corneal staining. However, he also states that this could have been caused by edema, as the incidence of staining appears to have resolved with the use of a higher-*Dk* material. The lens is currently made from Boston XO (*Dk* = 100 International Standards Organization (ISO).

Practitioners interested in fitting the Dreimlens can either supply the manufacturer with topographical or keratometric and refractive data and allow the laboratory to design the lens, or use a trial lens set to determine the optimal fit. The prime factors when assessing the lens are centration and active tear exchange. Modifications to centration are usually effected by altering the alignment curve, or by small changes in BOZR.

Other four- and five-curve designs

There are marked similarities between the Dreimlens and all other four- and five-curve designs. The Fargo lens (Jim Day) has the same basic construction, except the BOZD and RC widths are variable. Also the hyperbolic alignment curve is calculated from topography data. A compression factor of 1.00 D is used. The Nightmove lens (Tabb) has a basically aspheric alignment curve. The Orthofocus, R&R, Euclid Jade and Emerald, ABBA Optical, Contex E and Correctech designs, apart from minor differences in fitting philosophy and curve band width, are very similar to the Dreimlens.

The Scioptic EZM (Gelflex VMC) lens

This lens was designed by Mountford, who combined the BOZD/TR construction of the original three-zone Contex lens with the Thomas concept of a tangential peripheral curve in an attempt to maximize lens centration. The initial design was based on the original Conoid 9.00 mm TD and 6.50 mm BOZD lens increased to a total diameter of 10.5 mm. The standard 10.5 mm Conoid has a BOZD of 8.30 mm, so the 7.00 mm BOZD of the Contex 704 was combined with a 4.00 D reverse curve such that the combined BOZD/TR diameter became 8.40 mm. The addition of the standard 1.10 mm tangential periphery gives a TD of 10.6 mm. Based on simple sag equivalent calculations, the tangent cone angle for the lens was determined by using the cone angle of the standard Conoid based on a BOZR that was 2.50 D steeper than the BOZR of the OK704, as the calculated BOZR for the OK lens was 2.50 D flatter than the sagittal equivalent Conoid. The computer program for calculating the initial trial lens based on corneal data supplied from videokeratoscopy was written by Michael Vincent.

The trial lens is worn overnight, and the results of the trial were used to refine the final lens parameters. The main limitation is that the sag variation with this design is restricted to 10 μm (0.05 mm) steps. It was the first fenestrated orthokeratology lens, having three 0.25 mm fenestrations placed at the BOZD/TR junction at 120° intervals. The practice of fenestrating reverse geometry lenses is also done by Contex and is standard for BE lenses.

The WAVE design

Jim Edwards based the design of the WAVE lens on Keratron topography data. The lens has a 6.50 mm BOZD and a reverse zone width of 0.80 mm. The BOZR is based on the refractive change required. The alignment zone is approximately 1.00 mm wide, and the TD is 1.67 times the BOZD, resulting in a common diameter of 11.00 mm. The topography data are downloaded into the WAVE software, and the tear layer profile of the lens is generated. The design utilizes some very sophisticated computing to match the tear layer profile of the lens to the corneal shape. The

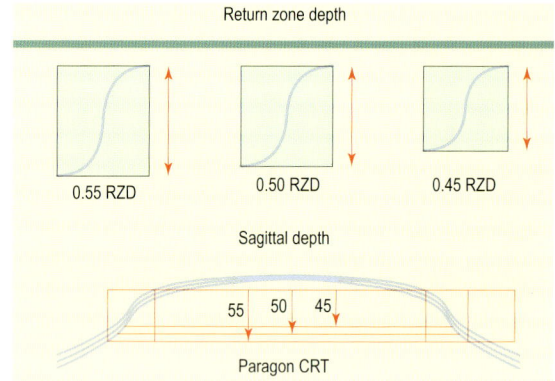

Figure 4.16 The construction of the Corneal Refractive Therapy (CRT) sigmoid proximity curve. The sag differences between the three preset curves are 0.10 mm or approximately 25 μm over the length of the curve. The sigmoid curve "blends" the back optic zone radius to the reverse curve (RC), and the RC to the tangent. RZD, return zone depth.

alignment zone and RCs include aspheric curves that are designed to control surface tension forces at the periphery of the lens in order to enhance centration. A more detailed description of the WAVE design is included in Chapter 8, covering computer-aided lens design.

Paragon CRT

The CRT lens could be considered as a three-curve lens, consisting of a spherical BOZR, a "sigmoid proximity" RC and a tangential periphery. The BOZD is 6.00 mm, with the reverse zone being 1.00 mm wide. However, the "sigmoid proximity curve" is a polynomial curve that in effect "blends" the BOZR to the RC, and the RC to the tangent (Fig. 4.16). The BOZR is based on the Jessen formula, with an added 0.50 D as a compression factor. There are five tangent angles available (see section on construction and design of tangential peripheries, below). The TD of the lens is set at 90% of horizontal visible iris diameter (HVID), or commonly 10.50 mm. A 100 lens inventory is used to determine the correct lens based on fluorescein pattern analysis, with the first trial lens being selected by recourse to a slide rule that uses the flattest keratometry reading in dioptres and the refractive change required to suggest an initial lens. A computer program is also available that can

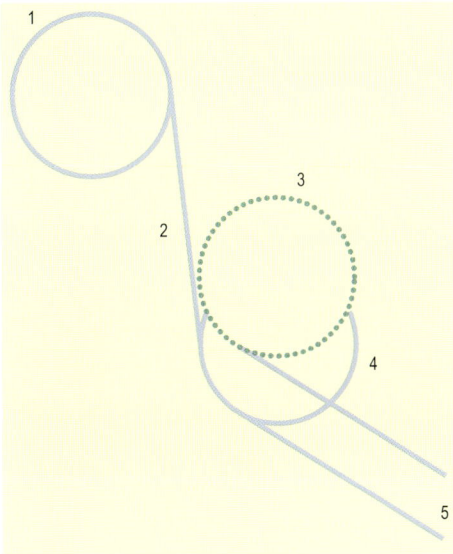

Figure 4.17   Construction of a sigmoid proximity curve. The curve (1) is the blend between the back optic zone radius and the reverse curve (2). Curve 3 represents the limit of the sigmoid curve for a given sag depth. If the sag of the reverse zone is increased (4), the sigmoid curve is lengthened. In both cases, the tangent (5) remains unaltered. In all cases, the distance in the x-axis between the two sigmoid curves is constant, and only the distance in the y-axis is altered in order to control overall lens sag.

import data from the Zeiss Humphrey Topographer and select the initial lens.

The utilization of a sigmoid proximity curve to blend the central and mid-peripheral zones of the lens is a unique design concept, but the major contribution it makes to the lens is that it is used to control variations in elevation. As shown previously with three-zone lenses, the RC is the major determinant of overall lens sag. Since the BOZR is determined by the refractive change required, and the tangents are limited to five angles, the only other means of varying the lens sag is to vary the RC. The concept of the sigmoid curve is shown in Figure 4.17. Note that, as the reverse zone is constant, changes to sag are made by altering the vertical depth of the curve. This therefore gives a far greater control of the sag variations than is usually possible with fixed reverse zone designs. The three most commonly used return or reverse zone depths are 0.525, 0.550 and 0.575mm. Variations of 0.10 mm in

BOZR lead to a change of 7 μm in lens sag, whilst a 1° change in cone angle effects a further 12.5 μm variation in sag. The depth of the reverse zone is rounded off to the closest 25 μm.

What differentiates the fitting philosophy is the assumptions made concerning the movement of epithelial tissue and how the lens design is derived based on those assumptions. CRT uses a variation of the Munnerlyn formula for refractive surgery as a basis for the assumptions regarding epithelial movement. The hypothesis is that, as positive pressure is applied by the BOZR of the lens to the corneal apex, epithelial tissue will be redistributed towards the mid-periphery, near the tangent area of the lens. The central corneal epithelium is assumed to thin down by 6 μm per diopter of refractive change required, and that the peripheral epithelium will increase by approximately the same amount. The "landing zone" or tangent is therefore initially designed with a TLT of 6 μm /D, or a degree of clearance determined by the refractive change.

As the cornea changes shape, the peripheral epithelial thickening increases to the extent that the TLT in this area is reduced to zero. In effect, this means that the lens is initially fitted with less than zero apical clearance, and up to 24 μm of clearance in the peripheral alignment zone. The published studies of Lui & Edwards (2000) and Mountford (1997b) show that the peripheral cornea is not affected by orthokeratology lens wear. Swarbrick et al (1998) have also shown that the increase in corneal thickness occurs at the edge of the BOZD, and not in the alignment curve area. It therefore appears, at least from the information to hand, that the underlying fitting philosophy is not in accordance with the published findings made about the redistribution of epithelium.

The most commonly used tangent angle is 35° (55° ISO). A cornea of R_0 7.80, eccentricity 0.50 will change to a final shape of R_0 8.176, eccentricity zero following treatment. The cone angle prefitting is 54.96°, and 55.14° postwear. The 55° cone angle is the closest match to the pre- and postwear corneal shapes.

The Paragon CRT was the first reverse geometry lens to receive Food and Drug Administration (FDA) approval for overnight orthokeratology.

BE lens (Mountford and Noack)

The BE lens is a five-zone lens comprising a variable BOZD varying between 6.00 and 7.00 mm. The first RC is 0.50 mm wide; the second RC varies between 0.45 and 0.7 mm in width. The final two sections are the tangent and a reverse perioptic edge lift. The BOZD is variable in order to create a wider treatment zone diameter for patients with large pupils. The first RC is designed to maintain the squeeze film force generated at the edge of the BOZD and hold it constant. The second RC is steeper than the first, and simply returns the lens back surface to meet the tangent. The tangent is designed according to the axial radius of the cornea at the point of contact with the tangent. The reverse perioptic curve has its radius of curvature in the opposite direction to the optic axis of the lens, and simply imparts the required degree of axial edge lift based on the cone angle.

The BOZR is not based on the Jessen factor, as control of the refractive change required is based on manipulation of the modeled squeeze film forces in the postlens tear film.

The fitting procedure is totally based on topographical data, trial lens fitting and refinement of the final lens parameters based on the evaluation of postwear topography. The lens has three fenestrations at the midpoint of the first RC at 120° intervals. The fenestrations do not prevent lens binding, but are present as an aid to tear exchange and "freeing up" of bound lenses in the morning. The preferred material for the lens is Boston XO. A more detailed description of BE fitting is included in the computer-aided design and fitting section later (Ch. 8).

Alignment curve variations for reverse geometry lenses

The major difference between three- and four-/five-zone lenses is the alignment curve or curves. Instead of a simple counterformal curve, the modern four- and five-curve lenses use conformal and tangent designs to control centration. The EZM, Paragon CRT, and BE designs all use tangents as the alignment curve. Tangents are not curves and do not have a radius of curvature, but are, in effect, "flats." The following section deals with the construction of tangents.

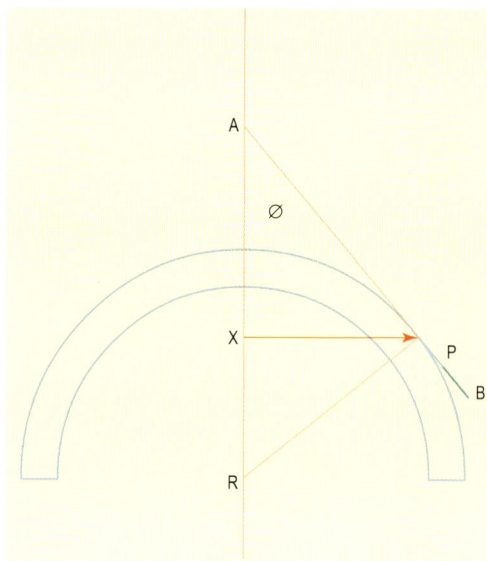

Figure 4.18   Construction of a tangent. See text for details.

Construction and design of tangential peripheries

The basic concept of a tangential peripheral curve is that it meets the corneal surface at a tangent to the surface at the point of contact. This then fulfills the requirements of a conformal curve, and theoretically distributes the pressure effects over a wider area. Thomas (1967) also postulated that there was a gradual increase in the applied pressure, being maximal at the center of the tangent (the point of contact) and decreasing as the edge of the tangent curve was reached.

A true tangent is not a curve, but a straight line that represents a cross-section of a conic section. The concept is shown in Figure 4.18. A point P on the peripheral cornea is met at its tangent by a line ($A–B$). The intersection between the line $A–B$ and the optic axis is designated the cone angle (Ø degrees), and is used as the common form of specification in writing the lens prescription. The point of contact on the corneal surface is the tangent to the axial radius of the cornea at that point, and is specified in terms of R_a and y, the half-chord from the optic axis to the corneal surface. In Figure 4.18, R_a is represented by the line $P–R$ and the half-chord y by the line $P–X$.

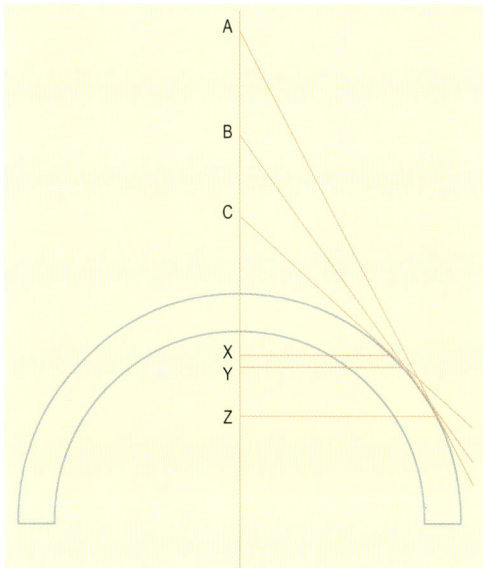

Figure 4.19   The variations in cone angle for different lens diameters.

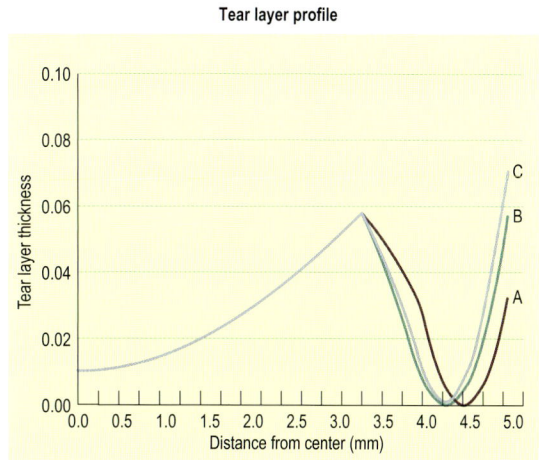

Figure 4.20   The tear layer profile of a tangential periphery reverse geometry lens with the point of surface contact set at varying points along the width of the curve. (A) $\frac{1}{4}$ tangent, (B) $\frac{1}{3}$ tangent, (C) $\frac{1}{2}$ tangent.

The axial radius is calculated using the formula:

$$R_a = \sqrt{R_0{}^2 + y^2 - y^2 p}$$

The cone angle can then be calculated by the formula;

Cone angle $(\varnothing) = 90 - \text{arcsine } y / R_a$

In order to specify the cone angle and R_a correctly, the half-chord y must be specified. In general, the chord is equal to;

$(\text{BOZD} + \text{BPD}_1 + \frac{1}{2} \text{BPD}_2)/2$ or, more simply: $\text{TD} - 2(\frac{1}{2} \text{BPD}_2)$, where BPD_2 is the width of the tangent curve, commonly 1.10 mm.

Therefore, for a lens with a TD of 11.20 mm, the chord of contact will be 10.10 mm, yielding a half-chord (y) of 5.05 mm. The cone angle is dependent on the individual R_a of the cornea, and also the diameter of the lens to be used.

Figure 4.19 shows the variation in cone angle for variations in lens diameter. As the diameter of the lens is increased, the cone angle decreases in numeric value, in that the angle actually steepens with increased diameters. However, there are two further factors that must be taken into consideration when calculating tangential peripheries for contact lenses. Firstly, the elliptical model of

corneal shape decreases in accuracy as the chord is increased. Mandell et al (1998) have shown that the peripheral cornea is in effect flatter than that described by the aspheric algorithm used in the elliptical corneal model. In practice, this means that the R_a value calculated from the above formula is in effect steeper than the actual corneal value and will result in a steeper cone angle than that actually required. Secondly, the axial edge clearance of the lens is determined by the cone angle.

Figure 4.20 shows the tear layer profile of a tangential periphery reverse geometry lens with the point of surface contact set at varying points along the width of the curve. The axial edge clearance (AEC) of the lens with the contact point midway along the width of the tangent is approximately 38 μm, with a cone angle of 51.98°. Most practitioners would consider this to be an insufficient edge lift.

Alteration of the edge clearance is achieved by manipulation of the point of contact of the tangent with the peripheral cornea. The same figure shows the lens with the contact varied to $\frac{1}{3}$ and $\frac{1}{4}$ the width of the tangent band. With the tangent set at a $\frac{1}{3}$ point of contact, the cone angle becomes 53.47° and the AEC approximately 62 μm, and at $\frac{1}{4}$ tangent the cone angle flattens to 54.17° with an AEC of 78 μm.

Tear layer profile

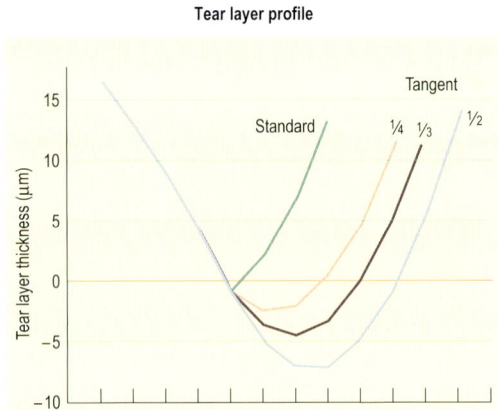

Figure 4.21   The standard Contex counterformal aspheric edge and three tangents, with 1/4, 1/3, and 1/2 points of contact.

Table 4.4 Cone angles of BE and EZM lenses over the back optic zone radius (BOZR) range

BOZR	Cone angle BE	Cone angle EZM
7.85	53.16	55.62
7.90	53.26	55.89
7.95	53.36	56.15
8.00	53.49	56.40
8.05	53.63	56.66
8.10	53.76	56.90
8.15	53.87	57.15
8.20	54.01	57.39
8.25	54.16	57.62
8.30	54.27	57.86
8.35	54.42	58.08
8.40	54.57	58.31
8.45	54.69	58.53
8.50	54.84	58.75
8.55	54.96	58.97
8.60	55.12	59.18
8.65	55.24	59.39
8.70	55.40	59.60
8.75	55.52	59.80
8.80	55.68	60.00
8.85	55.81	60.20
8.90	55.97	60.39
8.95	56.10	60.59
9.00	56.26	60.78

As a general rule, the use of the $^1/_2$ tangent on lenses with a TD of 11.00 mm or greater leads to a tight-fitting lens, due primarily to the greater corneal flattening than that assumed by the elliptical formula. The $^1/_4$ tangent gives a greater degree of freedom when trying to compensate for this effect and is preferred for the larger TD lenses. If the TD is 10.60 mm or less, however, the $^1/_2$ tangent is preferred, as the R_a and cone angle are theoretically more accurate, and the centration effect of the $^1/_2$ tangent is maximized.

Finally, the point of contact of the tangent has a direct bearing on the sag calculations for the lens/cornea fitting relationship. Figure 4.21 shows the standard Contex counterformal aspheric edge and three tangents, with $^1/_4$, $^1/_3$ and $^1/_2$ points of contact. Note how the sag difference between the lens and the cornea is affected by the edge design used. This will cause a change in the apical clearance of the lens. If the standard edge represents the ideal fit, with 10 μm of apical clearance, then the clearance will be increased by 7.5 μm if the $^1/_2$ tangent is used, resulting in a steep or tight lens fit, which will adversely affect the corneal response to the lens (see Ch. 5). As a result, the accurate fitting of the lens is dependent on calculating the initial lens, rather than using a different design and simply adding a tangent to the prescription. As a general rule, each change in cone angle of 1° causes a change in sag of 9 μm.

The BE lens uses the tangent design as outlined above. The EZM, on the other hand, uses cone angles based on a relationship to the BOZR of the lens. The point of contact with the cornea occurs at approximately $^1/_4$ the width of the tangent, which, like the BE, is 1.10 mm wide. The cone angles for the EZM and BE trial lenses are shown in Table 4.4.

The Paragon CRT lens also utilizes a tangential periphery. However, unlike the BE and EZM, the angle given as the tangent is not the angle that the tangent makes with the optic axis, but its opposite. CRT lenses have preset cone angles of 29 (61), 30 (60), 31 (59), 32 (58), 33 (57), 34 (56), 35 (55), 36 (54) and 37 (53). The values in brackets are the ISO standard cone angles for comparison with the other lenses. The cone angle is 35 (55), is the tangent for the mean corneal shape of R0 7.80 and eccentricity 0.5. A 2° difference in cone angles for the CRT equates to a difference of 25 μm in sag between lenses of identical curves except for the tangent. Each change of 2° is also related to a change of eccentricity of approximately 0.30. The range of cone angles is therefore designed to cover a wide variation in corneal shapes. The CRT system does not depend on the tangent to control the sag of the lens, but instead alters the sigmoid proximity curve to control the TLT at the BOZD.

The difference in sag change per degree of cone angle change between the BE and the CRT lens is due to the placement of the point of contact with the corneal surface.

DESIGN AND CONSTRUCTION OF ALIGNMENT PERIPHERAL CURVES

The most common form of alignment curve is either spherical or aspheric. The splitting of the four-zone lens alignment curve into two results in a five-zone lens. As with tangents, the accuracy of the alignment curve is essential if the rest of the lens construction is to be correct. There are currently two methods of calculating alignment curves for four-zone lenses. The first bases the alignment curve radius on the flat-K reading, whilst the other uses topography data to calculate the curve at the point of contact with the cornea.

Table 4.5 Comparison of alignment curves (AC) based on rule-of-thumb approach and calculation assuming a tear layer thickness of 10 μm at the junction of the reverse curve and the alignment curve

K_f (D)	Eccentricity	General rule AC (D)	Calculated AC (D)	Error (D)
43.5	0.0	43.50	43.24227	−0.25773
43.5	0.1	43.50	43.20004	−0.29996
43.5	0.2	43.50	43.0741	−0.4259
43.5	0.3	43.50	42.8666	−0.6334
43.5	0.4	43.25	42.58105	−0.66895
43.5	0.5	43.25	42.22212	−1.02788
43.5	0.6	43.00	41.79544	−1.20456
43.5	0.7	43.00	41.30739	−1.69261
43.5	0.8	43.00	40.76483	−2.23517
43.5	0.9	43.00	40.1749	−2.8251

Luk et al (2001) describe the following relationship between corneal eccentricity and the alignment curve for four-zone designs based on information supplied by various manufacturers:

1. If the eccentricity is between zero and 0.3, the alignment curve is equal to the flat-K.
2. If eccentricity is between 0.31 and 0.55, the alignment curve should be 0.05 mm (0.25 D) flatter than flat-K.
3. If eccentricity is between 0.56 and 0.70, the alignment curve should be 0.10 mm (0.50 D) flatter than flat-K.

However, this is a gross simplification of the curves required. Assuming a TLT of 10 μm at the junction of the RC and the alignment curve, the actual values for the alignment curves in order to satisfy sag fitting are shown in Table 4.5. Note that, in all cases, the rule-of-thumb alignment curves are much steeper than those calculated from the eccentricity values.

The relationship between the degree of flattening of the alignment curve with respect to the central flat-K and corneal eccentricity is as follows:

$$y = -3.465x^2 - 0.3396x + 0.26 \ (r^2 = 0.999)$$

where y is the amount flatter than flat-K for the alignment curve, and x is corneal eccentricity.

For example, if flat-K is 44.00 D, and the corneal eccentricity is 0.56, the RC needs to be $(-3.465 \times 0.56^2) - 0.3396 \times 0.56 + 0.26$ or 0.93 D flatter than flat-K or 43.07 D.

Figure 4.22 represents a four-zone lens on a cornea of flat-K 43.50 D (7.76 mm) and eccentricity of 0.50. The correct alignment curve is 7.901 mm. If the assumed alignment curve of 7.81 (K_f − 0.25 D) is fitted, the tear layer profile changes to that of Figure 4.23. Note that the lens is effectively too steep. In order to satisfy sagittal equivalency, the RC must be flattened to 7.17 mm. In general, steepening or flattening the RC by 0.15 mm (0.75 D) alters the apical clearance by 10 μm.

Some other designs assume that the corneal eccentricity is 0.50 unless advised otherwise. In general, for each variation of 0.10 in eccentricity away from 0.50, the alignment curve will alter by approximately 0.15 mm. If the eccentricity is less than 0.50, the alignment curve will require steep-

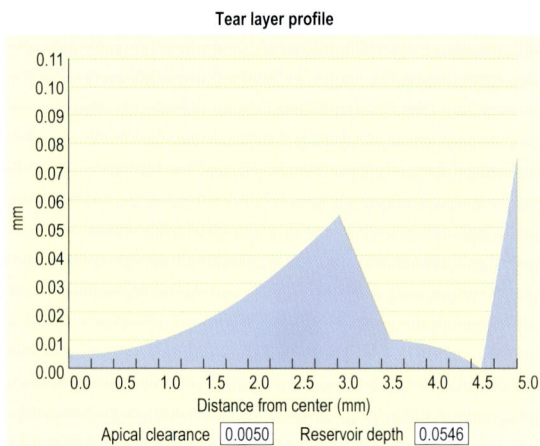

Figure 4.22   Four-zone lens on a cornea of flat-K 43.50 D (7.76 mm) and eccentricity of 0.50.

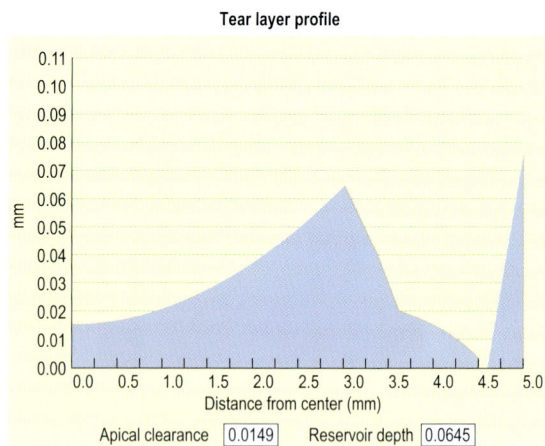

Figure 4.23   Same cornea as Figure 4.22 with the assumed alignment curve of 7.81 (K_f – 0.25 D).

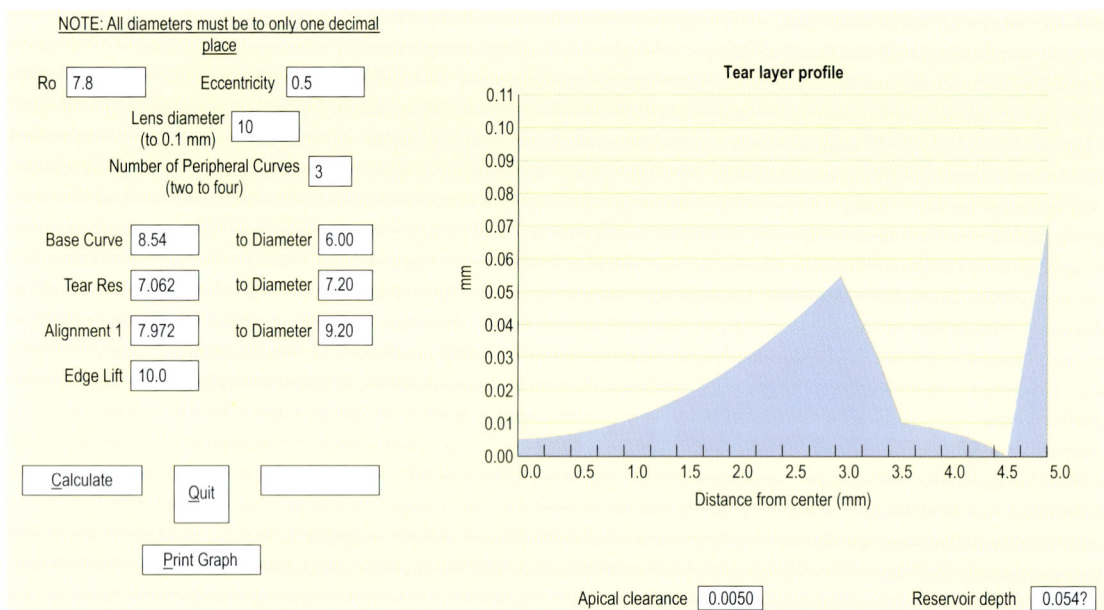

Figure 4.24   Tear layer profile of a model Dreimlens. Note that apical clearance is 5 μm, with a 10 μm clearance at the reverse curve/alignment curve junction.

ening, and conversely, flattening if the eccentricity is greater than the assumed 0.5.

Figure 4.24 shows the tear layer profile of an ideal-fitting four-zone lens. Note that in this example, the apical clearance is 5 μm, and the alignment curve meets the corneal surface at the edge of the reverse curve and the edge lift curve.

How sensitive is this curve to change, and how do those changes affect the final fit?

In Figure 4.25 the effect of steepening or flattening the alignment curve by as small an amount as 0.05 mm (0.25 D) is shown. In effect, flattening the alignment curve by 0.05 mm results in a decrease of central clearance of 5 μm, and

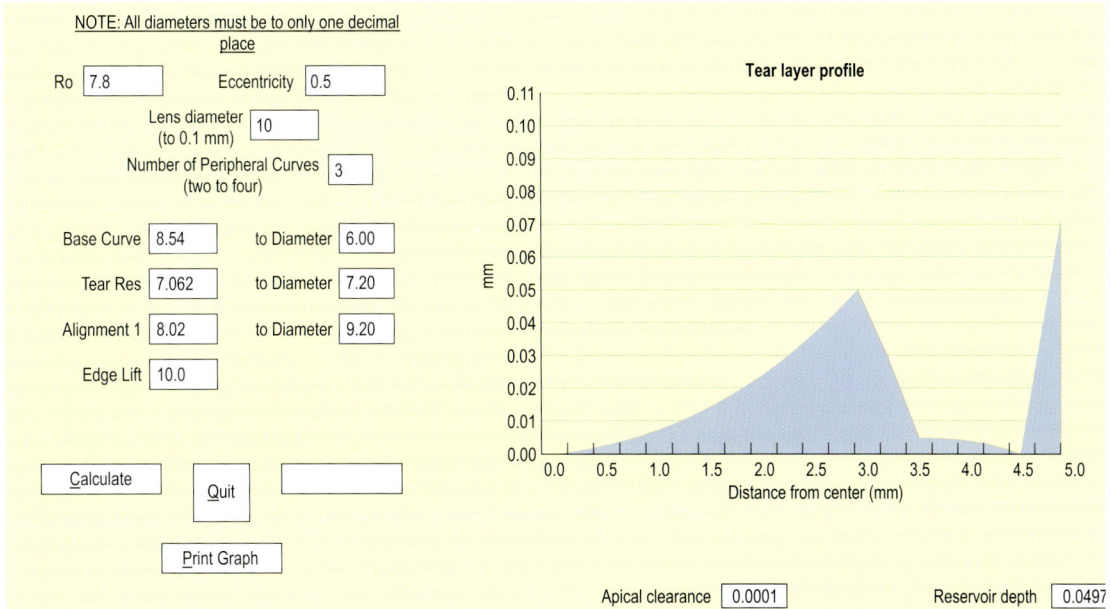

A

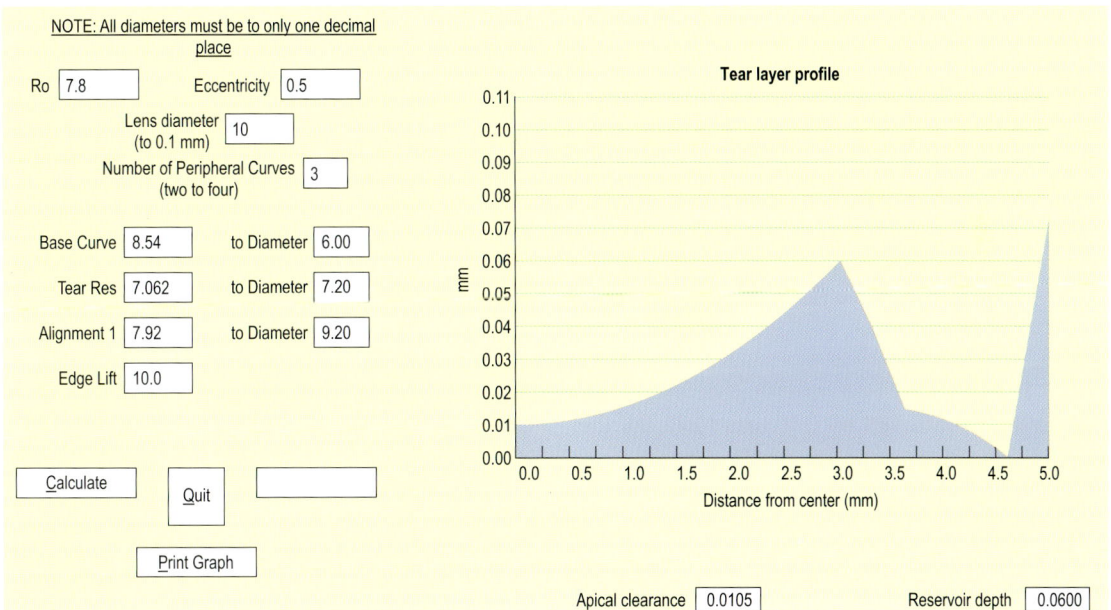

B

Figure 4.25   (A) The effect of flattening the alignment curve by 0.05 mm (0.25 D). The apical clearance is now close to zero. (B) The effect of steepening the alignment curve by 0.05 mm (0.25 D). The apical clearance is now 10 μm, and the clearance at the reverse curve/alignment curve junction 15 μm. This small change in alignment curve could cause a steep fit and associated central island, or a lack of refractive change.

steepening the curve by the same amount adds 5 μm to the apical clearance.

The above examples give some basic rules with respect to alterations to alignment curves and RC.

1. If the alignment curve is flattened by 0.05 mm (0.25 D), the apical clearance *decreases* by 5 μm.
2. If the alignment curve is steepened by 0.05 mm (0.25 D), the apical clearance *increases* by 5 μm.

Tear layer profile

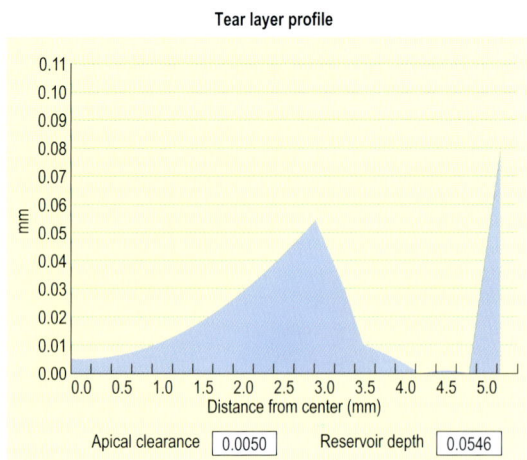

| Apical clearance | 0.0050 | Reservoir depth | 0.0546 |

A

Tear layer profile

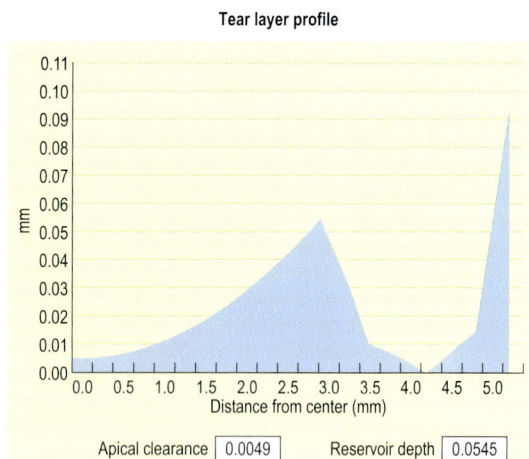

| Apical clearance | 0.0049 | Reservoir depth | 0.0545 |

B

Tear layer profile

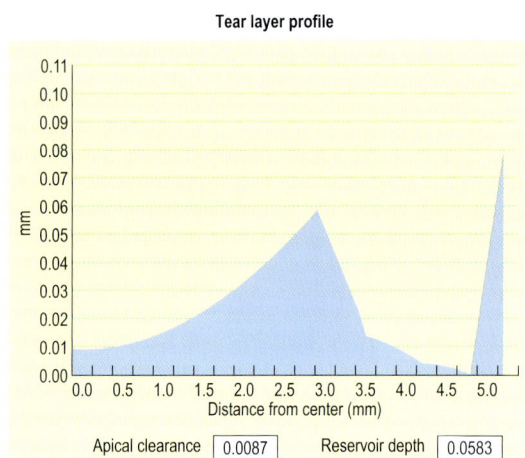

| Apical clearance | 0.0087 | Reservoir depth | 0.0583 |

C

Figure 4.26 (A) Tear layer profile of an ideal-fitting five-zone lens. (B) Effect of flattening the second alignment curve by 0.20 mm (1.00 D). Note that the apical clearance remains unaltered, but the contact point is now counterformal. (C) Effect of steepening the second alignment curve by 0.05 mm (0.25 D). The apical clearance is increased by approximately 5 μm.

3. If the RC is flattened by 0.15 mm (0.75 D), the apical clearance is *decreased* by 10 μm.
4. If the RC is steepened by 0.15 mm (0.75 D), the apical clearance is *increased* by 10 μm.

These rules only apply if one curve is changed. If both curves are changed at the same time, the results are additive.

In the case of five-zone lenses, the second alignment curve acts as a fulcrum, and is less sensitive to change than the four-zone lens. For example Figure 4.26A shows an ideal fit, whilst Figure 4.26B shows that flattening the curve by as much as 0.10 mm (1.00 D) has no effect on the apical clearance. Steepening the second alignment curve by 0.05 mm (0.25 D) increases the apical

clearance by approximately 5 μm (Figure 4.26C). If the final curve is flattened too much, a counterformal periphery results.

The major problem with counterformal periphery lenses is that the control of centration is lost, and discomfort levels increase due to the heavy point of contact between the lens and the cornea.

The most important thing to note about these apparently minor changes to the alignment curves is that they all have a major effect on the apical clearance of the lens *and are not detectable by fluorescein pattern analysis*. As stated previously, the accepted minimum TLT at which fluorescein becomes visible is in the range of 15–20 μm. All the changes used in the examples above have an effect of changing the clearance in the alignment zone by approximately 10 μm at a maximum, and as a result, these changes would not be seen in the fluorescein pattern. The same changes would occur when aspheric alignment curves are used, as the corneal eccentricity controls the eccentricity of the alignment curve. If an aspheric alignment curve is too steep or flat, the point of contact between the lens and the cornea will move, resulting in a change in the apical clearance. A flat aspheric curve would decrease apical clearance as the point of contact would move further in towards the BOZD of the lens. A tight or steep aspheric alignment curve would increase apical clearance.

The use of a simple rule to determine the curvature of the alignment curve based on a relationship to the flat-K is shown to be highly inaccurate. However, errors also occur in using topography data, as different instruments will give different eccentricity values for the same cornea, resulting in different alignment curves depending on which instrument is used. The method of analyzing these inaccuracies and their correction is covered in greater detail in Chapter 6.

Other design variables

There are three approaches that can be used to design and fit reverse geometry lenses. The first takes the Jessen (1962) concept of using the liquid lens as the correcting factor. The original "orthofocus" technique basically consisted of choosing the BOZR of the lens such that the liquid lens provided the refractive correction, resulting in all lenses having a plano power. In effect, if the patient had a refractive error of 2.00 D myopia, the BOZR was fitted 2.00 D flatter than the K_f. This invariably led to unstable fitting, especially as the degree of myopia increased.

The efficacy of this approach to fitting has not been subjected to proper analysis, as Jessen never published the results of his studies. However, the concept has been applied to the fitting of reverse geometry lenses by El Hage et al (1997), Reim (Dreimlens), Day (Fargo), Tabb (Nightmove), Stoyan (Contex BB), Breece (Correctech), Gladys (Euclid Jade and Emerald), Blackburn (Orthofocus), Legerton (CRT), and Reinhart (R&R) such

that the refractive correction required is once again the liquid lens, plus an allowance for a compression factor of between 0.00 and 1.00 D. The second curve chosen is the alignment curve, with the RC being calculated to achieve the correct sagittal fitting relationship to the cornea. This can be summarized as follows:

1. Choose a BOZR based on the initial refractive error and modify the alignment curve and TR to adjust the fit.

The second concept is to use a constant TR curve and BOZD, as in the Contex OK and EZM, and modify the BOZR until the correct sag relationship between the lens and the cornea is achieved. This approach makes no predictions as to the refractive change that will be induced by the choice of the BOZR. This can be summarized as:

2. Keep the BOZD and TR constant, and modify the BOZR.

As has been shown previously, this concept is limited by the inability to control the variations in CF for different corneal shapes, with a resultant variability in results.

The third and final method of lens design is to standardize the fitting by making the tear layer profile constant for all eye shapes. This can be summarized as follows:

3. The lens is specified in terms of TLT at the corneal apex and the edge of the BOZD. A computer program then calculates the BOZR/TR combination that will fulfill the specification.

This is the basic concept behind the BE design.

A common question is: why use a constant tear layer profile? The answer can be best described in a single word: standardization. The development of the sag fitting philosophy was based on the simple concept that different lens designs behaved differently on corneas of varying shapes, and that the "ideal" contact lens fit should have a fluorescein pattern, movement, and centration properties that could be duplicated irrespective of corneal shape.

As a result, the shape of the tear layer profile became the method of standardizing the design

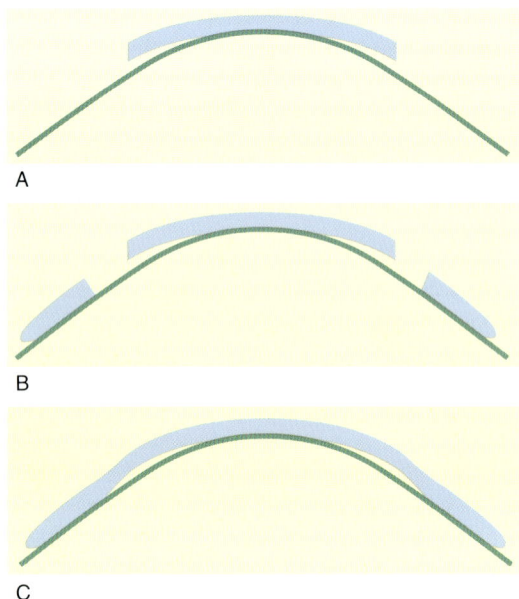

A

B

C

Figure 4.27 The construction of a four-zone lens based on the Jessen factor. The back optic zone radius (BOZR) is determined first, depending on the refractive change required. This is shown in (A). The second curve chosen is the alignment curve (AC), shown in (B). The reverse curve (C) is the final curve chosen to bring about sagittal equivalency and join the BOZR to the AC. Courtesy of Patrick Caroline.

and the fit of the lens. With the BE design, the TLT at the BOZD is *constant* irrespective of corneal shape. The refractive change is controlled by manipulating the apical clearance. The BOZR is not based on the Jessen concept, but still has an effect on the refractive change due to the change in BOZR with apical clearance.

If a lens is constructed using the first philosophy stated above, the choice of curves is as follows.

1. The BOZR is the first curve chosen due to the required refractive change (Fig. 4.27A).
2. The second curve chosen is the alignment curve, as the overall sag of the lens must equal the corneal sag at the point of contact with the alignment curve (Fig. 4.27B).
3. The final curve chosen is the RC. Note that the RC is responsible for joining the BOZR to the alignment curve in order that the requirements of sag fitting are fulfilled (Fig. 4.27C).

In the case of three-curve lenses, the BOZR can still be fitted according to the Jessen factor, but the RC will then be dependent on the corneal eccentricity. If the two are linked, as with the Contex lenses, then the sag of both curves needs to be equal to the corneal sag at the edge of the RC.

When a lens is constructed using the constant tear layer profile technique, the order of curve choice is reversed. The construction is as follows:

1. The alignment curve or tangent is derived from the axial radius of curvature of the cornea at the point of contact with the surface (Fig. 4.28A).
2. The RC is chosen to give the required TLT at the edge of the BOZD (Fig. 4.28A).
3. The BOZR is then calculated so that the curve meets the requirements of the apical clearance and the depth of the tear layer at the BOZD (Fig. 4.28B).

At first glance, these different techniques may appear to have little in common, except that they are all based on sag fitting and must obey the same rules in order for the fit to be correct.

This is the simple point that needs to be remembered. All reverse geometry lenses, irre-

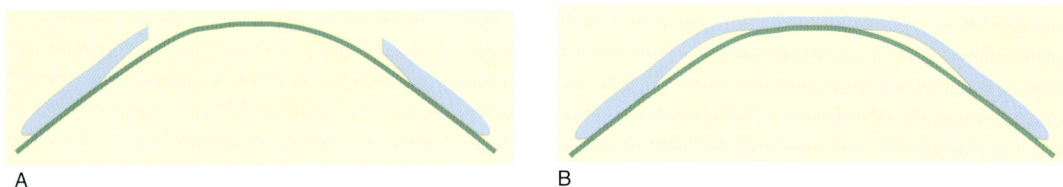

A

B

Figure 4.28 Construction of a lens based on tear layer thickness. (A) The alignment curve or tangent is chosen first, based on corneal data. The reverse curve is then calculated to give a specific tear layer thickness at the back optic zone diameter. The back optic zone radius is the final curve calculated based on the apical clearance required and is shown in (B). Courtesy of Patrick Caroline.

Relationship between BOZR and clearance factor

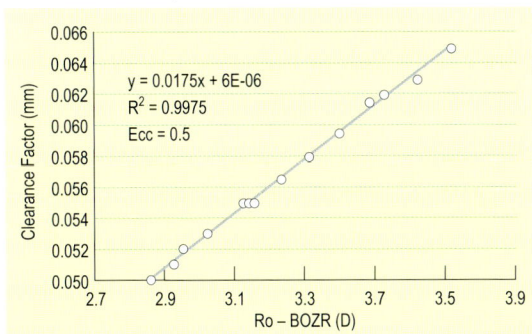

$y = 0.0175x + 6E{-}06$
$R^2 = 0.9975$
Ecc = 0.5

Figure 4.29 Relationship between flatness of fit of back optic zone radius (BOZR) to the clearance factor of OK 704T lenses. The corneal data is R_0 7.80, eccentricity 0.50.

Relationship between flatness of fit (Fo – BOZR) and TR curve

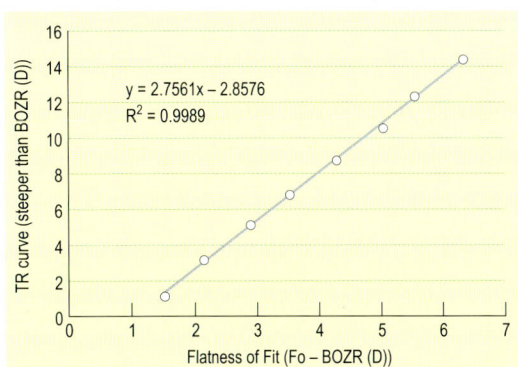

$y = 2.7561x - 2.8576$
$R^2 = 0.9989$

Figure 4.30 Relationship between flatness of fit and reverse curve steepening. TR, tear reservoir; BOZR, back optic zone radius.

spective of fitting philosophy or design variations, have the same basic construction and must be fitted according to sag philosophy if the fit of the lens is to be optimal. Where much of the variation in fitting success with the lenses occurs is in the assumptions made by various manufacturers as to the underlying corneal shape. If the lenses are empirically fitted from K readings and refraction, then the assumed corneal shape will be a prime area for inaccuracy when compared to the actual corneal shape. These variations are covered in Chapter 6.

As shown above, all reverse geometry lenses follow the same pattern of construction that is primarily based on the lens having a sagittal relationship to the cornea. The difference in TLT at the corneal apex and the edge of the BOZD (the CF) can therefore be used to examine further the similarities and differences in designs.

The definition of lens design based on the CF concept can be used to find the relationship between the fit of the lens with respect to the corneal curve and the associated steepening of the RC that is required to maintain sagittal equivalency with the cornea. In the case of the Contex lenses, if the BOZD of the lens is kept constant and the TD varied, the width of the TR curve is altered, as the peripheral curve width of all the OK series is constant depending on the design used. The Dreimlens has a constant TR width of 0.60 mm, and the El Hage TR curve varies with the TD of the lens and the BOZD

chosen. In the case of a cornea of R_0 7.80 mm and e 0.50 fitted with a 10.60 mm diameter Contex OK704T, the relationship between the CF and the difference between the BOZR and corneal curve (R_0) is shown in Figure 4.29. For the sake of simplicity, the difference between the BOZR and R_0 will be described in terms of "flatness of fit" and converted to diopters. As the CF is increased, the BOZR is flattened in a linear relationship to the clearance factor.

Figure 4.30 shows the same relationship, except the steepening of the RC with respect to the BOZR (in diopters) is used instead of the CF. Once again, there is a linear relationship between the two in that, if a specific BOZR is chosen for an individual eye, it must have a specific RC in order to maintain sagittal equivalency of fit.

However, the relationship between these two factors also varies depending on the width of the RC that forms the TR. Figure 4.31 shows the variation in steepening of the TR curve with three different RC widths, 0.30, 0.60, and 0.90 mm. If the BOZR is predetermined, then the steepening of the TR curve is also linked linearly to the width of the TR curve.

The effect of variations in CF on corneal shape and refractive change has been studied in a controlled experiment by fitting a group of six subjects with lenses of varying CFs (Bara 2000). Each of the subjects wore a lens with a specific change in CF for a period of 6 h, with a 1-week interval

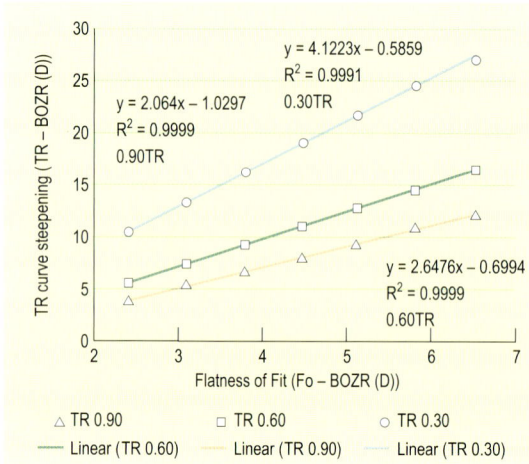

Relationship between flatness of fit (Fo – BOZR) and TR curve (TR-BOZR) for different TR curve widths

$y = 4.1223x - 0.5859$
$R^2 = 0.9991$
0.30TR

$y = 2.064x - 1.0297$
$R^2 = 0.9999$
0.90TR

$y = 2.6476x - 0.6994$
$R^2 = 0.9999$
0.60TR

TR curve steepening (TR – BOZR (D))

Flatness of Fit (Fo – BOZR (D))

△ TR 0.90   □ TR 0.60   ○ TR 0.30
— Linear (TR 0.60)   — Linear (TR 0.90)   — Linear (TR 0.30)

Figure 4.31 Relationship between back optic zone radius and reverse curve (RC) for varying RC band widths. TR, tear reservoir, BOZR, back optic zone radius.

between episodes. A control group was used for comparison. The CF variations were 30, 50, and 80 μm, with a BOZD of 7.00 mm and a tangential peripheral curve. The TD was varied during the trial wear periods to maximize centration. The changes in apical radius, eccentricity, visual acuity (log minimum angle of resolution or logMAR) and apical corneal power were measured at 1-h intervals during the 6-h wear period.

The change in apical radius for the treatment and control groups for the different CF lenses is shown in Figure 4.32A. The relationships between the lens design and change in eccentricity and visual acuity are shown in Figure 4.32B and C.

The lens with the deepest CF (6.00 D reverse curve) showed the greater and faster effect when compared to the other designs and the control group. The interesting fact to note with the results is that the refractive change appears to be related

Figure 4.32 The change in (A) apical radius R_0, (B) eccentricity, and (C) log minimum angle of resolution (logMAR) vision for a group of subjects fitted with lenses where the RC is 2.00, 4.00, and 6.00 D steeper than the BOZR. All lenses are fitted according to sag philosophy. The lens that caused the greatest change when compared to the controls is the 6.00 D lens. The 2.00 D lens changes were not statistically different to the controls. Courtesy of Christa Bara.

to the BOZR, in that greater CF values are associated with a flatter BOZR.

This is the single factor that all reverse geometry designs have in common, irrespective of the fitting philosophy used. The El Hage, Reim,

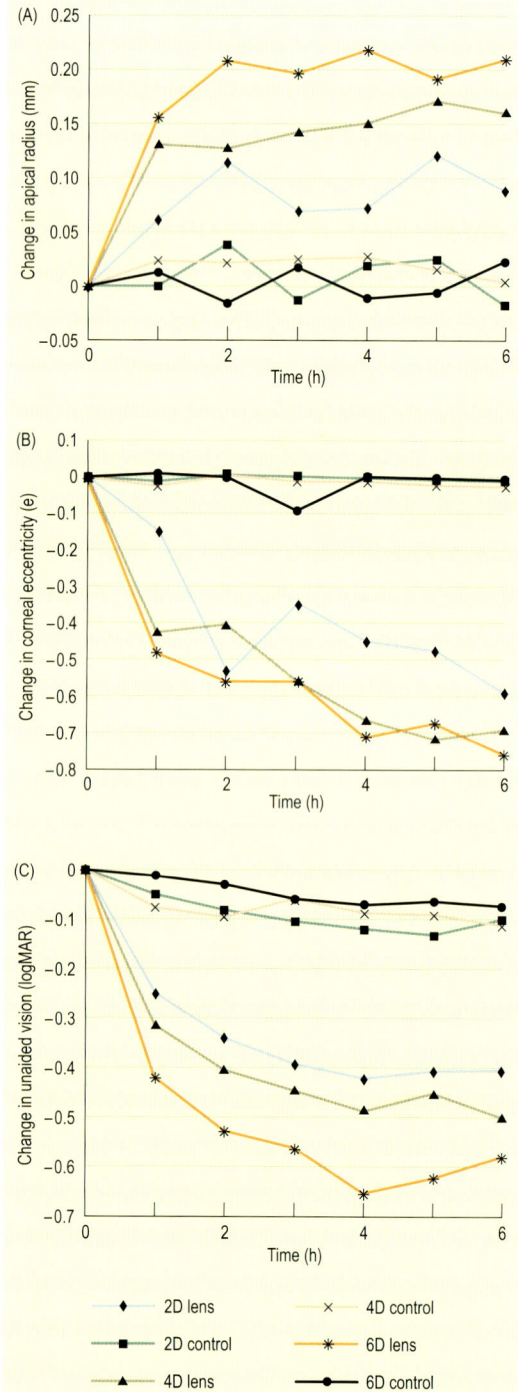

(A) Change in apical radius (mm) vs Time (h)

(B) Change in corneal eccentricity (e) vs Time (h)

(C) Change in unaided vision (logMAR) vs Time (h)

♦ 2D lens   × 4D control
■ 2D control   ∗ 6D lens
▲ 4D lens   ● 6D control

Relationship between BOZR and TR curves for 10.00 mm Dreimlens

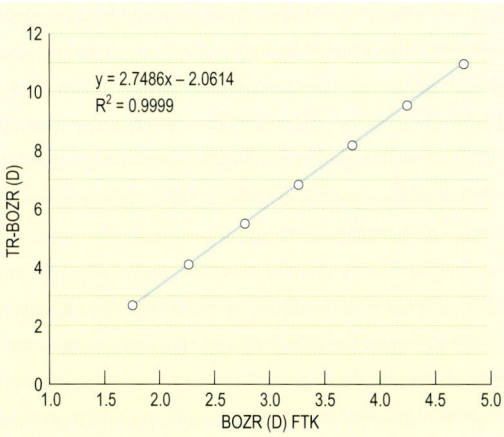

$y = 2.7486x - 2.0614$
$R^2 = 0.9999$

(x-axis: BOZR (D) FTK; y-axis: TR–BOZR (D))

Figure 4.33 Relationship between back optic zone radius (D) and reverse curve (D) for Dreimlens. The corneal data are R_0 7.80, eccentricity 0.50. TR, tear reservoir; FTK flatter than K.

Relationship between BOZR and clearance factor for 10.00 mm Dreimlens

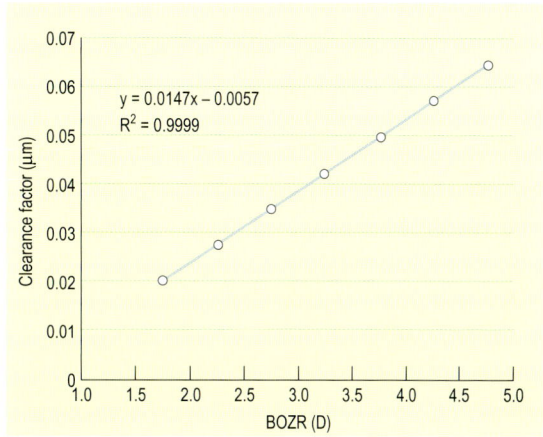

$y = 0.0147x - 0.0057$
$R^2 = 0.9999$

(x-axis: BOZR (D); y-axis: Clearance factor (μm))

Figure 4.34 Relationship between lens fit (back optic zone radius) and clearance factor.

Relationship between BOZR and clearance factor for El Hage lens (10.00 mm TD)

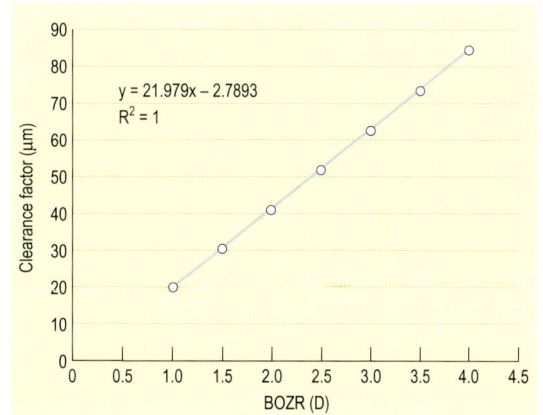

$y = 21.979x - 2.7893$
$R^2 = 1$

(x-axis: BOZR (D); y-axis: Clearance factor (μm))

Figure 4.35 Relationship between back optic zone radius (BOZR) and clearance factor for El Hage's lens.

and other philosophies are based on the selection of the BOZR as determined by the initial refractive error. The only difference between them is the amount of extra flattening used as a compression factor. However, most designs are also based on a peripheral alignment curve that contacts the peripheral cornea and are based on corneal shape, indicating constancy in the sag relationship between the lens and cornea.

In the following examples, the standard cornea of R_0 7.80 mm and e 0.50 is fitted using both philosophies. The refractive error range is from 1.00 D to 4.00 D in 0.50 D steps. Both lenses are assumed to touch the cornea centrally, with a TLT of zero.

In the case of the Dreimlens, the BOZR is equal to $(F_0 - Rx) - 0.75$ D, with a 6.00 mm BOZD, 0.60 mm TR width, and 10.00 mm TD. The relationship between the BOZR (in effect, flatness of fit in diopters) and TR curves for the different refractive error corrections is shown in Figure 4.33. Note that, once again, there is a linear relationship between the BOZR and the TR curves. Similarly, there is a linear relationship between the BOZR and the clearance factor (Fig. 4.34).

El Hage's BOZR is equal to $(R_0 - 0.2) \times Rx$, with the CF at the edge of the TR calculated by adding the difference in sag between the initial prefit corneal shape and the BOZR of the lens over the same chord. The CF is determined by adding an allow-

ance of 12 μm per diopter of refractive change at the 7.00 mm zone. Figure 4.35 shows the relationship between flatness of fit and the CF for a 10.0 mm diameter lens. As with the other reverse geometry lenses, the relationship is linear.

In effect, the main difference between the two designs is that the clearance factor per diopter of flattening is 13 μm/1.00 D for the Dreimlens, and 21 μm/1.00 D for the El Hage design. The disparity in the two is due to the difference in TR curve widths and the flatter BOZR used by Reim, but regression analysis shows a linear relationship between the two (Fig. 4.36).

Relationship between clearance factors for the
El Hage and Dreimlens

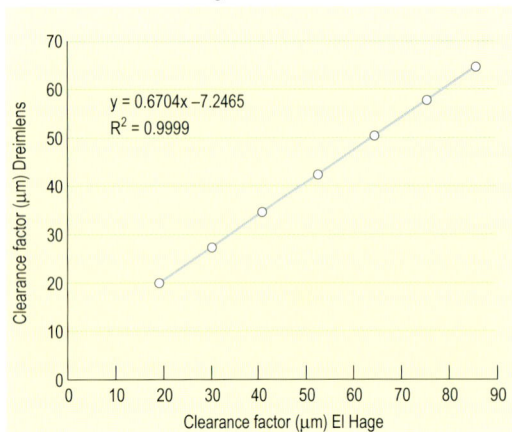

$y = 0.6704x - 7.2465$
$R^2 = 0.9999$

Figure 4.36 The relationship between the clearance factors (CFs) of the Dreimlens and El Hage lenses is linear. The difference between the two is due to the extra compression factor of 0.75 D used in the Reim design.

The above analysis shows that, irrespective of the fitting philosophy or the basic lens design, there is a direct and essential relationship between the flatness of fit of the lens and the degree of steepening of TR curve, and both factors are dependent on the CF. In effect, for *any* given BOZR, there will only be one TR curve at a specific CF that will fulfill the sag fitting requirements for an individual corneal shape. It is this constancy of the relationship between the BOZR and the RC that led to the assumption of a "dose–response" RC relationship between the refractive change and the CF at the BOZD.

In effect this is a circular argument. The reasoning is that the BOZR is directly related to the required refractive change. For any given corneal shape, a lens fitted x D flatter than the cornea will have a specific tear layer depth (CF) at a BOZD of 6.00 mm. The depth of the tear layer determines the curvature of the RC in order to maintain sagittal equivalency. This will therefore yield a linear relationship between the RC and the refractive change, but since the argument is based on the initial supposition that the BOZR controls the refractive change, the whole concept becomes a circular argument. As Bara has shown, the CF appears to control the refractive change. The CF

also determines the RC if the BOZR is preset, and the BOZR if the RC is preset.

Does the BOZR control the refractive change?

The controlled studies of the traditional orthokeratology techniques (Kerns 1976, Brand et al 1983, Coon 1984) all found no correlation between the BOZR of the lens and the refractive error correction or the final corneal shape. However, with the introduction of the four- and five-zone lens designs, the Jessen factor once again became the dominant means of programming the refractive change required. However, to date there have been no controlled studies that prove that such a relationship exists. The assumption is that the epithelium will mold itself in a 1:1 relationship to the BOZR of the lens. Therefore, if the BOZR is set at the required refractive change, the cornea will mold to it. This concept appears to have some variations in that different lens designs will use different "compression factors" added to the initial Jessen factor. The Reim design has an extra 0.75 D flattening, whereas the R&R design is 0.50 D and the Fargo 1.00 D.

If the BOZR of the lenses used had a direct "molding effect" on the cornea, there should be a good correlation between the base curve of the lens used and the change in refraction induced by the lens. To test this hypothesis, the correlation between change in apical corneal power and "flatness of fit" (F_0 – BOZR in diopters) and the calculated BOZR for four lens designs were analyzed using regression analysis. The lens used in the study was the Contex OK704T, but since it is assumed that the primary influence on refractive change is the BOZR, an assumption could be made that *any* lens that met the requirements of a correct sagittal relationship to the cornea would produce the same result. The results are shown in Figure 4.37.

There is a high correlation ($r^2 = 0.80$, $P < 0.0001$, df 59) for the relationship between the constant tear layer profile fit (IDEAL) and a poorer relationship for the 704T fit ($r^2 = 0.50$, $P < 0.0001$, df 59). However, the correlation is definitely not 1:1. If the BOZR had a direct molding effect on the epithe-

Relationship between change in apical corneal power and lens fit (El Hage)

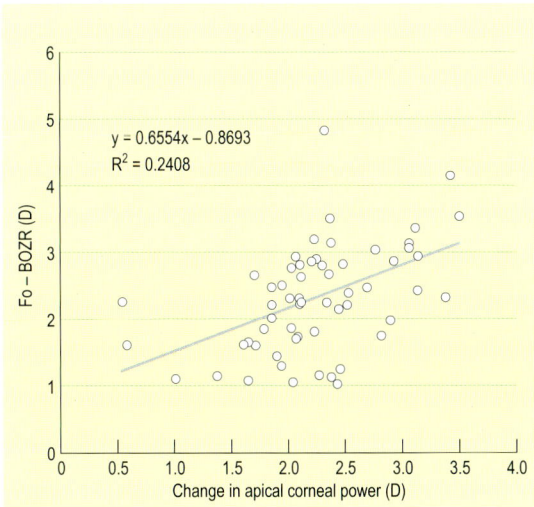

A

Relationship between change in apical corneal power and lens fit (Dreimlens)

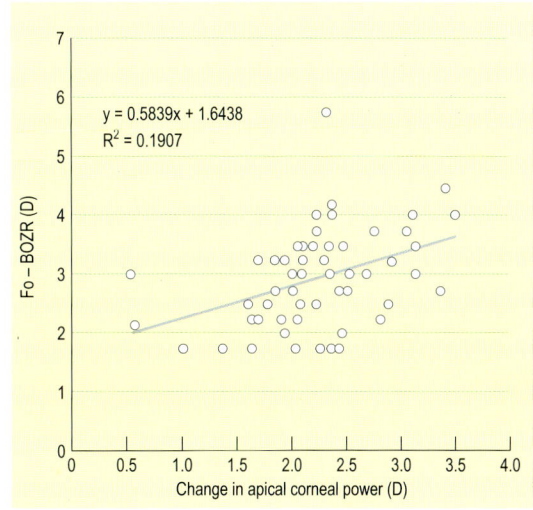

B

Relationship between change in apical corneal power and lens fit IDEAL

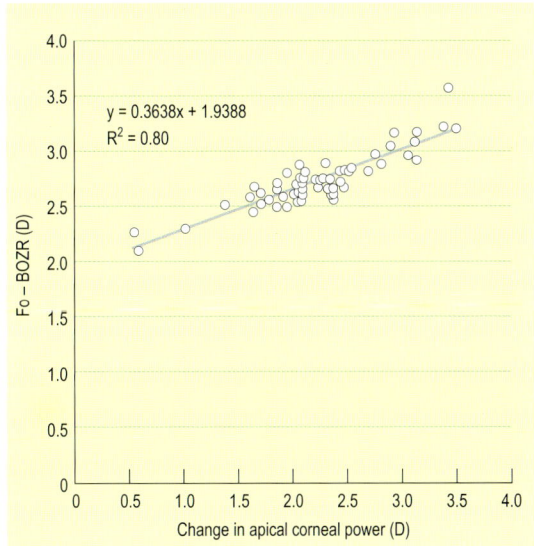

C

Relationship between change in apical corneal power and lens fit (OK704T)

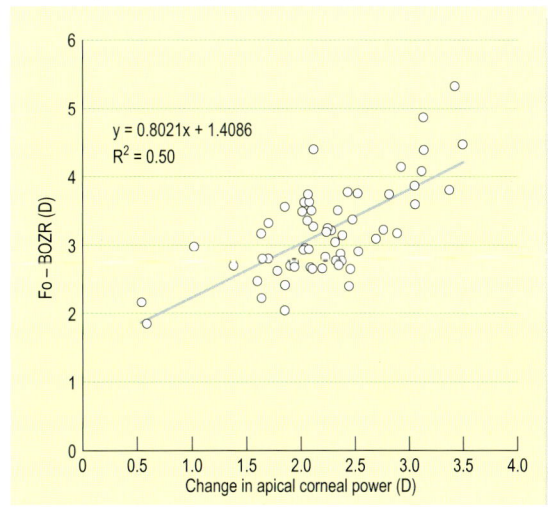

D

Figure 4.37 (A) Relationship between back optic zone radius (BOZR) and refractive change using the El Hage model. (B) Relationship between BOZR and refractive change using the Reim model. (C) Relationship between BOZR and refractive change using a constant tear layer model. (D) Relationship between BOZR and refractive change using the OK704.

lium, the regression line would be at a 45° angle between the x- and y-axes. The correlation for the fitting philosophies based on a predetermined BOZR is much poorer: Reim ($r^2 = 0.19$, $P = 0.0004$, df 59) and El Hage ($r^2 = 0.24$, $P = 0.01$, df 59). Once again, there appears to be no direct molding effect.

The results of fitting a group of subjects with the aim of a 4.00 D reduction in myopia is shown in Figure 4.38. As can be seen from the results, there is a wide variation in outcome with respect to the final refraction, indicating that there is some unpredictability in the approach.

Difference between aimed for and achieved Rx change (4.00D Aim)

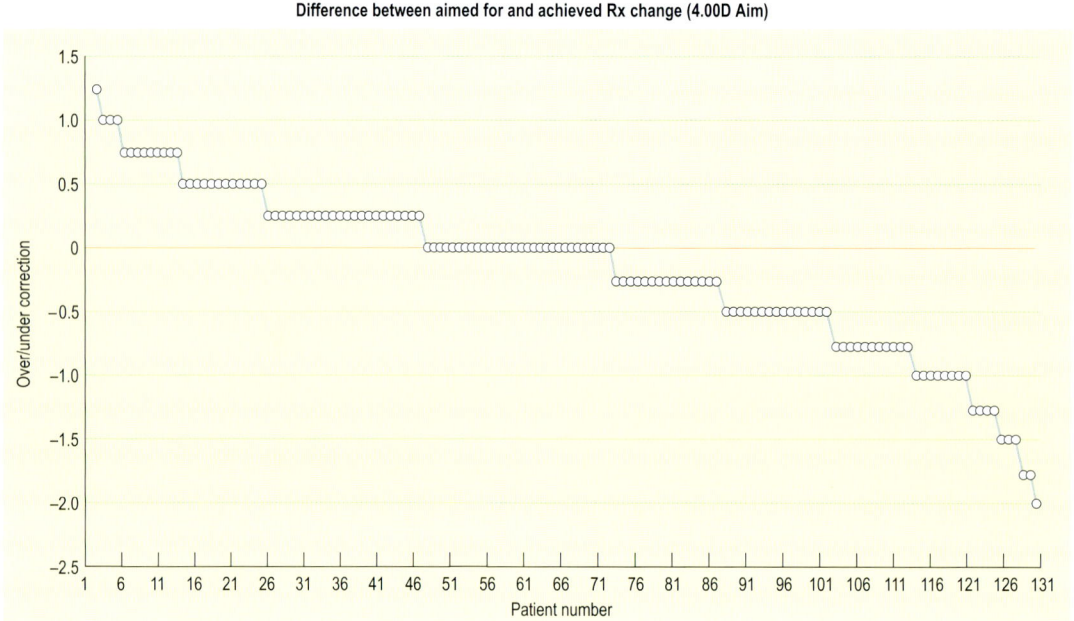

Figure 4.38   The achieved refractive changes compared to the aim of 4.00 D for a group of 131 subjects. The refractive change was based on the back optic zone radius of the lens. Courtesy of Tom Reim.

Relationship between change in apical corneal power and change in corneal sag (5.00 mm chord)

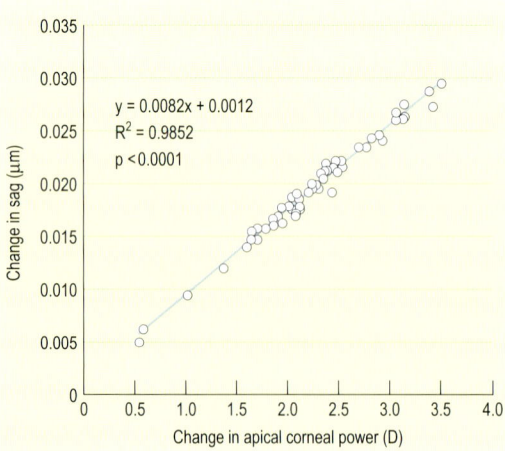

$y = 0.0082x + 0.0012$
$R^2 = 0.9852$
$p < 0.0001$

A

Relationship between change in apical corneal power and refractive change (Munnerlyns model)

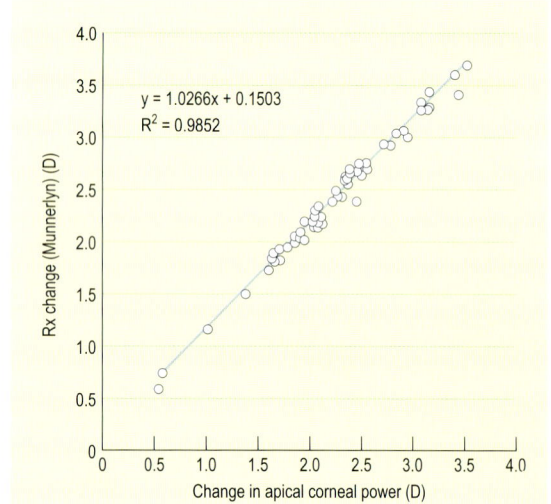

$y = 1.0266x + 0.1503$
$R^2 = 0.9852$

B

Figure 4.39   (A) Relationship between change in corneal sag (5.00 mm chord) and refractive change. (B) Relationship between refractive change and that calculated from Munnerlyn's formula over the central 5.00 mm chord.

El Hage assumes a 10 μm difference in corneal sag per diopter of refractive change. Is this correct? Essentially, the answer is "yes." In Chapter 8, the mathematical modeling of orthokeratology is approached from the viewpoint of epithelial changes researched by Swarbrick et al (1998). As part of her analysis, Swarbrick utilized a suggestion by Patrick Caroline that Munnerlyn's formula

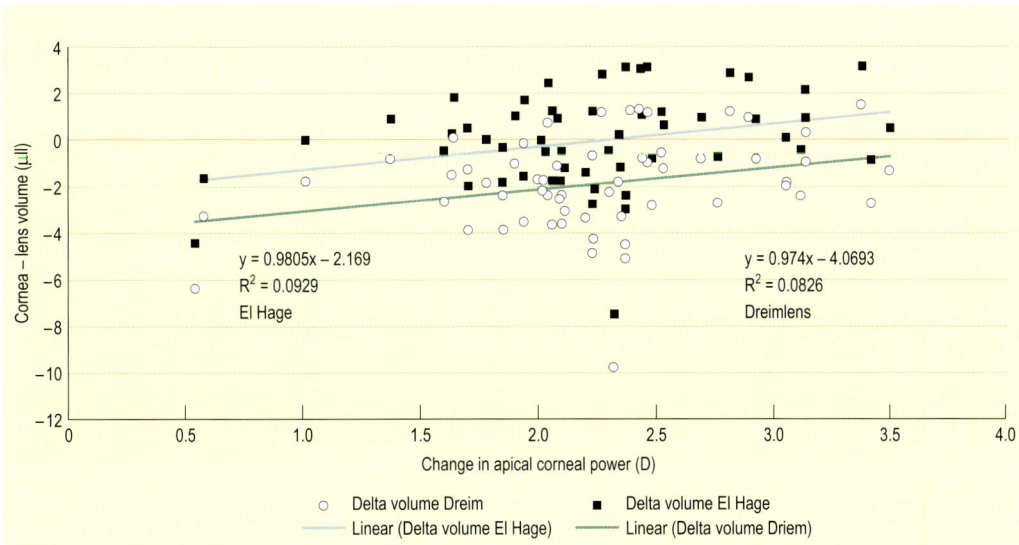

A

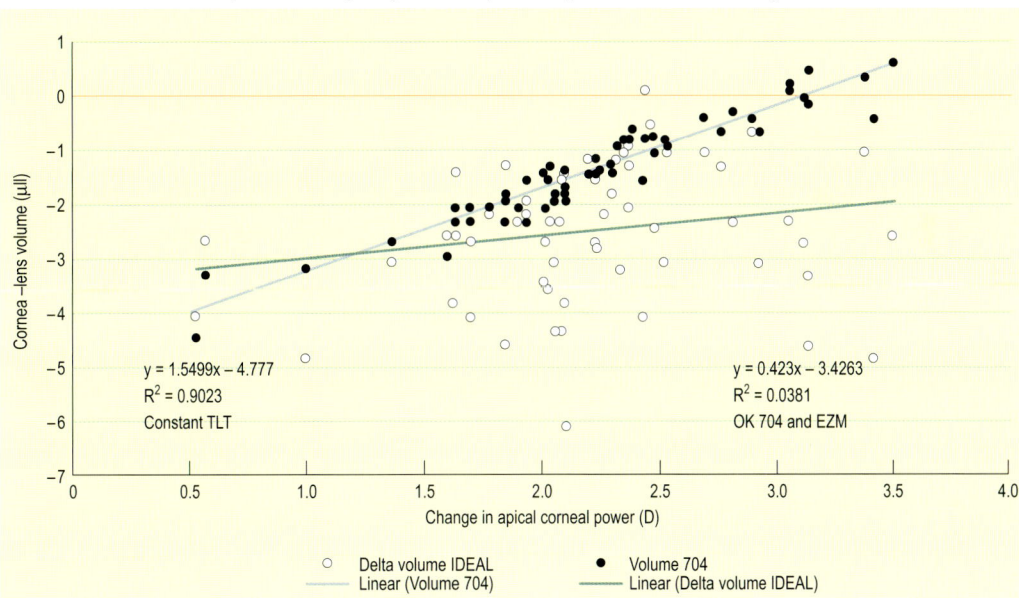

B

Figure 4.40   (A) Relationship between change in tear layer volume and refractive change using the Reim and El Hage model. (B) The relationship between refractive change and tear layer volume for the constant TLT model and the EZM and 704 models. The correlation is good for the constant TLT model.

(Munnerlyn et al 1988) for refractive surgery could be used as a means of assessing refractive changes in orthokeratology. Munnerlyn's formula states:

$$\text{Ablation depth} = (Rx\, D^2)/8\,(n-1)$$

where Rx is the refractive change required, D the diameter of the ablation zone, and n the refractive index of the cornea (1.377). From the orthokeratology context, ablation depth can be interpreted as sag change from the initial corneal shape to the final corneal shape, and D the area of corneal flattening induced by the lens.

The change in corneal sag over a 5.00 mm chord as a result of orthokeratologic treatment was calculated for a group of 60 patients. The difference in sag was calculated using the initial R_0 and e values taken from corneal topographical data and subtracting the final, posttreatment sag using the "final" R_0 value and an eccentricity of zero. The relationship between refractive change and sag change is shown in Figure 4.39a. There is a high correlation between the two ($r^2 = 0.98$, $P < 0.0001$, df 59), with the regression form indicating a sag change of 8 µm per diopter of refractive change. This is relatively close to the 10 µm assumed by El Hage. Similarly, the relationship between actual measured change in apical corneal power and the predicted change using Munnerlyn's model is highly statistically significant ($r^2 = 0.98$, $P < 0.0001$, df 59), and is shown in Figure 4.39B.

Finally, a further refinement of the model can be used to determine if there is any "molding constant" based on the different fitting philosophies. If it is assumed that the choice of BOZR in some way determines the final corneal shape induced by the lens, then there should be a correlation between the final *volume relationship* between the tear volume under the lens and the altered corneal shape, and the refractive change induced. The

change in apical corneal power represents the refractive change induced by the shape or volume change in the cornea over the 5.00 mm chord.

The regression analysis of the calculated volume differences between the cornea and the El Hage and Dreimlens postlens tear volumes and the measured change in apical corneal power is shown in Figure 4.40A. The results are quite surprising, as there is no correlation between corneal power change and the volume differences with the El Hage ($r^2 = 0.09$, $P = 0$, df 59) and Reim ($r^2 = 0.08$, $P = 0$, df 59) models, indicating that the choice of BOZR does not induce a predetermined degree of corneal power change. However, the correlations between the change in apical corneal power and the postwear tear volume difference for the constant TLT lens and the OK704 are shown in Figure 4.40B. The correlation is surprisingly good ($r^2 = 0.90$, $P < 0.0001$, df 59) for the constant TLT lens, and poor for the 704 ($r^2 = 0.03$, $P = 0$, df 59). The OK704 result is similar to the El Hage and Reim relationship, indicating a basic flaw in the concept of the lens/cornea fitting relationship. The difference between the constant TLT fitting concept and the others is the use of a constant tear layer profile irrespective of initial corneal shape. El Hage and Reim set the BOZR as the basis of lens construction, whilst the OK704 and EZM set the TR curve as the fixed basis of

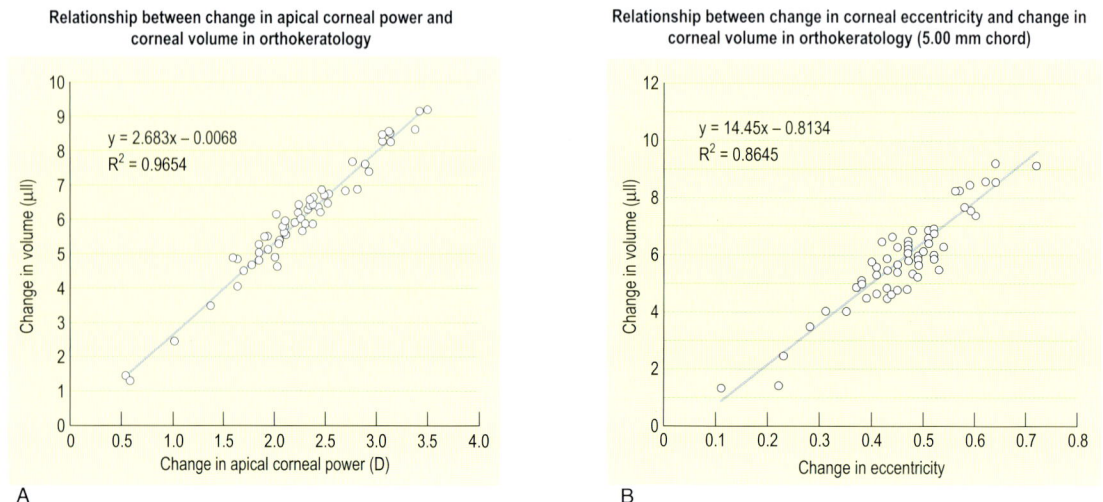

Figure 4.41   (A) The relationship between corneal volume change and eccentricity. (B) The relationship between refractive change and corneal volume.

lens design. In all of these cases, the CF will vary with the corneal shape.

The BOZR of the constant TLT lens is based on the relationship between the tear layer profile and the corneal shape remaining constant. The relationship between the final corneal shape, which causes the refractive changes, and the tear layer volume difference between the lens and the cornea is governed by the change in corneal shape, which is dependent on the change in eccentricity from a prolate ellipse to a sphere. The unifying factor between the tear layer volume pre- and postwear is the change in corneal eccentricity.

The relationship between corneal eccentricity change and corneal volume change (Fig. 4.41A) is statistically significant ($r^2 = 0.86$, $P < 0.0001$, df 59), as is the relationship between refractive change and tear volume change ($r^2 = 0.96$, $P < 0.0001$, df 59), as shown in Figure 4.41B.

The analysis shows that there is no direct relationship between the BOZR of the lens and the induced refractive change, meaning that the fitting concepts of El Hage, Reim, Mountford, and others of either a predetermined BOZR or TR curve are flawed. There is, however, a good correlation between the BOZR based on the constant tear layer profile concept and the refractive changes seen. This does not mean that lenses fitted according to the Jessen factor do not work: it simply means that the fitting concept is not validated by the analysis of the data. The reason why the choice of a BOZR based on the refractive change required actually does work as an orthokeratology lens will be discussed in greater detail in Chapter 10, but the results of the above analysis show that the margin for error of assuming a 1:1 molding relationship between the BOZR of the lens and the final corneal shape, or a modification of it, is high.

The constant–surface–area concept

Both the Fargo and Euclid lenses base the lens design on the assumption that the corneal surface area remains constant and is not altered by orthokeratology treatment. Smolek & Klyce (1998) have shown by topographical analysis that corneal surface area is in fact constant for all corneal conditions except keratoglobus. However, it appears that the constant-surface-area concept is applied to orthokeratology as a reflection of the law of the conservation of corneal power argument, as proposed by Caroline & Campbell (1991).

The Fargo and Euclid lenses derive the BOZR of the lens based on the Jessen factor, with a mild difference between compression factors. The reverse curve is then calculated such that the surface area (SA) of the pretreatment cornea is equal to the surface area of the BOZR and RCs.

Day et al (1997) use the example of a cornea with 46.00 D apical power and an eccentricity of 0.47 having a surface area of 59.00 mm² over a treatment diameter of 8.30 mm (BOZD plus BPD_1). The surface area of the BOZD of the lens used is then subtracted from the initial corneal surface area. The difference is then the surface area of the RC. The example given is that 42.50 D BOZR over a 6.00 mm BOZD has a surface area of 29.36 mm². In order for the surface area to remain *constant*, the RC must have a surface area of 29.64 mm², or a curve of 45.50 D or 3.00 D steeper than the BOZR.

Kwok (1984) gives the formula for the surface area of a rotationally symmetric aspheric surface as:

$$S = (\Pi/1 + Q)\{R^2 - (R\text{-}s\text{-}sQ)[(R\text{-}sQ)^2 + s^2Q]^{1/2} - [(R^2/(\text{-}Q\text{-}Q^2)^{1/2}][\sin^{-1} - Q^{1/2}(R\text{-}s\text{-}sQ)/R \sin^{-1} - Q^{1/2}]\}$$

where R is the apical radius, s is sag, and Q is asphericity.

The surface area of a spherical surface is:

$$SA = 2\Pi\, Rs$$

where R is the radius and s is the sag of the sphere.

If the data of Day are used ($R_0 = 7.33$ and $Q = 0.211$), the calculated corneal surface area over a chord of 8.30 mm is 59.00 mm². The total surface area of the lens follows the same mathematical rules as the sag calculations in that:

$$\text{Total SA} = SA\,R_1/D_1 + (SA\,R_2/D_2 - SA\,R_2/D_1) + (SA\,R_3/D_3 - SA\,R_3/D_2)$$

The original concept was developed for use with three-zone lenses, such that the RC came into contact with the corneal surface at a total chord of 8.30 mm. The total surface area of the lens was then

Tear layer profile

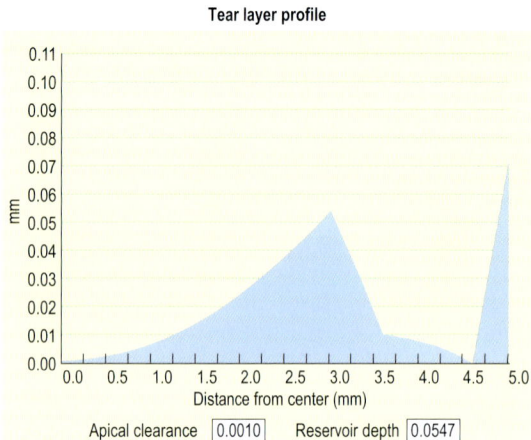

Apical clearance [0.0010]   Reservoir depth [0.0547]

Figure 4.42   The tear layer profile of a four–zone lens on a standard cornea with a back optic zone radius (BOZR) fitted 3.50 D flatter than flat-*K*.

Tear layer profile

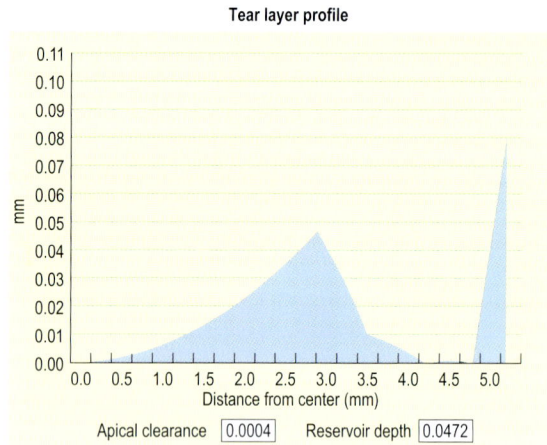

Apical clearance [0.0004]   Reservoir depth [0.0472]

Figure 4.43   A generic four-zone lens is shown fitted to the standard cornea.

29.36 mm^2 (surface area of BOZD) plus 29.63 mm^2 (surface area of the RC zone), giving a total lens surface area of 58.99 mm^2. The calculations show that the surface areas match within the limitations of the figures used (two decimal places).

Figure 4.42 shows the tear layer profile of a four-zone lens on a standard cornea with a BOZR fitted 3.50 D flatter than flat-*K*. In this case, the lens is assumed to have zero apical clearance, and the RC meets the corneal surface at the junction of the RC and alignment curve. The SA of the cornea at a chord of 7.20 mm is 42.34 mm^2, and the SA of the lens is 43.38 mm^2. Once again, given the limitations of the calculations, the results are in close agreement.

In Figure 4.43, a generic four-zone lens is shown fitted to the standard cornea. The common area of contact is now over a chord of 9.20 mm, and the SA of the cornea is 79.55 mm^2. The total SA of the lens is 80.75 mm^2 over the same chord. The technique shows close agreement for basically all correct combinations of back surface geometry if the lens is constructed using sag calculations.

However, the choice of RC and alignment curves is once again secondary to the selection of the BOZR based on variations of the Jessen factor. As has been shown previously, for any given corneal shape there is only one combination of RC and alignment curve that will satisfy the

requirements of sag fitting. SA calculations are a complex extension to the sag philosophy, and both are totally dependent on corneal shape. The fact that the SAs of the cornea and the lens match is a derivative of the sags matching, and not, as one would tend to assume, due to a 1:1 molding relationship between the lens and the cornea.

ACCURACY OF SAG FITTING

Bara (2000) noticed during the course of her study that there appeared to be a relationship between the apical radius and eccentricity value and the BOZR of the lens, in that the BOZR was approximately equal to the R_0 in millimeters and the numeric value of the eccentricity. If R_0 was 7.80 and *e* 0.50, the BOZR was approximately 8.30 mm. This led to the systematic evaluation of the sag philosophy and the traditional "flatter-than-*K*" fitting technique and the relationship to the $R_0 + e$ methods for predicting the correct BOZR. The data used for analysis had been previously published (Mountford 1997b), where a group of 60 patients who had successfully completed a course of orthokeratology were fitted with OK704T lenses. The differences in the final lens parameters used were compared to the BOZR indicated by the sag calculations, the flatter-than-*K* approach, and the $R_0 + e$ approximation.

The results showed that all the different methods *underestimated* the final BOZR by varying degrees. The average error for the sag philosophy was 0.0917 mm, 0.105 mm for $R_0 + e$ and 0.20 mm for the "1.50 D flatter than K" approach. In effect, the "1.50 D flatter than K" approach underestimated the degree of flattening of the BOZR by 1.00 D, indicating a closer rule of thumb to be "2.50 D flatter than K." If the different correction factors were added to the calculated BOZR, the relationships were:

Sag fitting   Final BOZR = Calculated BOZR + 0.10 mm

$R_0 + e$ Final BOZR = $R_0 + e + 0.10$ mm

$K_f - 1.50$ D   Final BOZR = $K_f - 2.50$ D

The relative success of the correction factors was assessed by predicting the rate of "first-fit success" for each of the methods. The use of the sag philosophy plus the extra 0.10 mm to the calculated BOZR led to a 90% success rate. The $R_0 + e + 0.10$ mm was successful in 78% of cases, whilst the $K_f - 2.50$ D was successful in only 52% of cases.

The good correlation of the $R_0 + e + 0.10$ mm ($r^2 = 0.93$, $P < 0.001$) was found to be basically a "happy coincidence," and therefore a much better approximation of the correct initial BOZR than the flatter-than-K approach. The correlation for the sag fitting plus the correction factor was also very good ($r^2 = 0.97$, $P = 0.001$). However, the rule only applies to 10.6 mm Contex OK704T lenses and no others.

What the results do show is that the fitting of reverse geometry lenses requires much greater precision than that possible with a simple flatter-than-K approach. All the current reverse geometry lens designs are based on the lens having the correct sagittal relationship to the cornea. Theoretically, if the corneal topographical data were accurate, then orthokeratology would, in effect, be a one set of lenses procedure. Bara found a constant error in that the final lens was 0.10 mm flatter than that calculated from the topography data and the lens sag formulas.

The probable cause is either in the algorithm that calculates the eccentricity value, as a difference in BOZR of 0.10 mm would equate to an eccentricity error of 0.20, or the inability of the aspheric model properly to describe the rate of corneal flattening in the periphery. If the cornea flattens at a faster rate than that assumed by the eccentricity value, then the calculated sag based on the e value would be greater than the sag of the cornea, leading to the lens being effectively too steep. The difference in calculated lens parameters based on different topography data has also been shown by McMonnies & Boneham (1997).

When EZM lens parameters were calculated using data from the EyeSys and TMS instruments, both instruments gave statistically significant differences in R_0 and eccentricity values. However, variations in R_0 were compensated by differences in eccentricity, so in the majority of their subjects, the BOZR variations between instruments was ± 0.05 mm. However, in two cases, markedly different lens parameters were calculated based on the two instruments.

Nichols et al (1998) compared the BOZR selection for OK704C lenses using the EyeSys and Humphrey Atlas instruments. Thirty-one subjects had topography measurements of R_0 and eccentricity made with both instruments, and the Bara formula of $R_0 + e + 0.1$ applied to the data to determine the BOZR. The difference in eccentricity values between the two instruments was not statistically significant, but the apical radius values were ($t = 11.14$, $P < 0.001$). The Humphrey consistently produced steeper apical radii when compared to the EyeSys, leading to a mean difference in BOZR of 0.15 ± 0.11 mm. The BOZR calculated from the Humphrey data was steeper than that of the EyeSys.

Cho et al (2002) used the data from four different topographers to design a generic four-zone lens. The lenses produced from the different instruments showed marked differences in RC and alignment curve, and none of the lenses produced from one topographer were interchangeable with those from the others (Table 4.6). These studies all show that lens selection is instrument-dependent. Corneal topographers construct a model of the corneal surface based on the algorithms used by the designers.

The accuracy of the lens fit is therefore dependent on the accuracy of the topography data used

Table 4.6 The results of a study by Cho et al (2002), who used the data from four different topographers to design a generic four-zone lens

Topographer	BOZR 6.00 mm	RC 7.20 mm	AC 9.20 mm	PC 10 mm	AC 1 μm	AC 2 μm
Medmont E300	8.57	7.56	8.20	10.00	5	5
Humphrey Atlas 991	8.52	7.00	7.90	10.00	5	28
Dicon CT200	8.59	6.98	7.88	10.00	5	28
Orbscan	8.49	6.82	7.69	10.00	5	65

BOZR, back optic zone radius; RC, reverse curve; AC, alignment curve; PC, peripheral curve; Ac1, apical clearance of the lens calculated from the topography data; Ac2, apical clearance of the lens designed from Medmont data when placed on the corneal elevation, as determined by the other three topographers.

to calculate the lens. Practitioners must appreciate that the validity of the data that are calculated by the videokeratoscope is dependent on the algorithms used by the manufacturer to determine the apical radius and eccentricity values. Also, the inability of the aspheric model to determine exactly the sag of the cornea over the chord required to calculate the lens sag means that trial lens fitting is essential in order to arrive at the correct lens parameters.

In conclusion, the differences in design of all reverse geometry lenses are basically a variation of the same theme. All lenses have a flat BOZR surrounded by a RC (s), an alignment zone (spherical, aspheric, or tangent) and a final curve giving the desired edge lift. Research to date in controlled studies shows that the results with different lens designs are almost identical. No lens design is inherently superior to the other or causes greater refractive change than the other. What differs with all the designs is the fitting philosophy. The only method of standardizing the fitting is by using sag philosophy, or alternatively, SA matching.

Both these techniques are dependent on topographical data and cannot be done accurately using keratometry data. Also, both methods require the use of sophisticated computer software that integrates the topography data with the lens design. Even though topographical fitting is not 100% accurate, it is still vastly more accurate than keratometry alone, and should be considered the gold standard for orthokeratology lens fitting. The keratometer is a redundant instrument with respect to orthokeratology as it is incapable of supplying the data required to fit and design lenses accurately.

However, the design and fitting philosophies described in this section do not explain why the lenses have the effect they have, or how the lens parameters can be manipulated to control these effects. These factors will be dealt with in much greater detail in Chapter 10.

REFERENCES

Atkinson T C O (1984) A re-appraisal of the concept of fitting rigid hard lenses by the tear layer and edge clearance technique. Journal of the British Contact Lens Association 7: 106–110

Atkinson T C O (1985) Computer assisted and clinical assessment of current trends in gas permeable design. Optician 189 (4976): 16–22

Bara C (2000) Mechanism of action of the reverse geometry gas permeable contact lens in orthokeratology. MSc thesis, University of Melbourne

Bibby M M (1979) Factors affecting peripheral curve design. Part 2. American Journal of Optometry 56: 618–627

Brand R J, Polse K A, Schwalbe J S (1983) The Berkeley orthokeratology study. Part 1. Genera conduct of the study. American Journal of Optometry and Physiological Optics 60: 175–186

Caroline P, Campbell R (1991) Between the lines. Contact Lens Spectrum 5(6): 68

Chan J S, Mandell R B, Johnson L, Reed C, Fusaro R (1998) Contact lens base curve predictions from videokeratoscopy. Optical Vision Science 75(6): 445–449

Cho P, Lam A K, Mountford J, Ng L (2002) The performance of four different corneal topographers on normal human corneas and its impact on orthokeratology lens fitting. Optometry and Vision Science 79: 175–183

Coon L J (1984) Orthokeratology part 2. Evaluating the Tabb method. Journal of the American Optometric Association 55: 409–418

Corneal refractive therapy fitting manual (2001) Paragon Vision Sciences

Day J (1998) Clinical problem solving the 4-zone series. NERF, Chicago

Day J, Reim T, Bard R D, McGonagill P, Gambino M J (1997) Advanced ortho-*k* using custom lens design. Contact Lens Spectrum 12(6): 34–40

Douthwaite W A (1991) Computerized contact lens fitting. Optometry and Vision Science 68: 770–775

El Hage S G (1997) Aspheric optical molds for continuous reshaping the cornea based on topographical analysis. US Patents Office. Patent No. 5 695 507

El Hage S G, Leach N, Colliac J-P, Dezard X (1997) Interactive software controls corneal shaping. Contact Lens Spectrum 12(8): 54–56

Fontana A (1972) Orthokeratology using the one-piece bifocal. Contacto 22(5): 9–12

Guillon M, Sammons W A (1994) Contact lens design. In: Ruben M, Guillon M (eds) Contact lens practice. Chapman and Hall Medical, London, pp. 87–103

Guillon M, Lyndon D P M, Sammons W A (1983) Designing rigid gas permeable contact lenses using the edge clearance technique. British Contact Lens Association 6(19): 22–26

Guillon M, Lyndon D P M, Wilson C (1986) Corneal topography: a clinical model. Ophthalmic and Physiological Optics 6: 47–56

Hayashi T (1977) Mechanics of contact lens motion. PhD thesis. University Of California, Berkeley

Jessen G N (1962) Orthofocus techniques. Contacto 6(7): 200 204

Keiley P M, Smith G, Carney L G (1982) The mean shape of the human cornea. Optica Acta 29: 1027–1040

Kerns R (1976) Research in orthokeratology, part 7. Journal of the American Optometric Association 48: 1541–1553

Kwok L S (1984) Calculation and application of the anterior surface area of a model human cornea. Journal of Theoretical Biology 108: 295–313

Lam A K C, Douthwaite W A (1994) Derivation of corneal flattening factor, *p*-value. Ophthalmic and Physiological Optics 14: 423–427

Lindsay R, Smith G, Atchinson D (1997) Descriptors of corneal shape. Optometry and Vision Science 75(2): 156–158

Lui W O, Edwards M H (2000) Orthokeratology in low myopia. Part 2: Corneal topographic changes and safety over 100 days. Contact Lens and Anterior Eye 23(3): 90–99

Luk B M W, Bennett E S, Barr J T (2001) Fitting orthokeratology contact lenses. Contact Lens Spectrum 16(10): 30–35

Mandell R B, Corzene J C, Klein S A (1998) Peripheral corneal topography and the limbus. ARVO Abstract no. 4789. Investigative Ophthalmology and Visual Science

McMonnies C W, Boneham G C (1997) Corneal topography validity and reliability for orthokeratology fitting. Clinical and Experimental Optometry 80(2): 69–73

Mountford J A (1997a) Orthokeratology. In: Phillips A J, Speedwell L (eds) Contact lenses: a textbook for students and practitioner, vol. 4. Butterworths, London

Mountford J A (1997b) An analysis of the changes in corneal shape and refractive error induced by accelerated orthokeratology. ICLC 24: 128–143

Munnerlyn C R, Koons S J, Marshall J (1988) Photorefractive keratectomy: a technique for laser refractive surgery. Journal of Cataract and Refractive Surgery 14: 46–51

Nichols J J, Marsich B G S, Bullimore M A (1998) A comparison of two different corneal topographers in orthokeratology base curve selection. Optometry and Vision Science 75(12s): 172

Reim T (1999) Patent no. 5 963 297. US Patent and Trademark Office

Sammons W A (1984) Lens-eye geometry. Proceedings of the European Contact Lens Society of Ophthalmology of Helsinki

Smolek M K, Klyce S D (1998) Surface area of the cornea appears to be conserved in keratoconus. Investigative Ophthalmology and Visual Science 39 (suppl.)

Swarbrick H A, Wong G, O'Leary D J (1998) Corneal response to orthokeratology. Optometry and Vision Science 75(11): 791–799

Thomas P H (1967) Conoid contact lenses. Corneal Lens Corporation, Sydney, Australia

Wilms K H, Rabbetts R B (1997) Practical concepts of corneal topography. Optician 174 (4502): 7–13

Winkler T D, Kame R T (1995) Orthokeratology handbook. Butterworth-Heinemann, Boston

Wlodyga R J, Bryla C (1989) Corneal molding; the easy way. Contact Lens Spectrum 4(58): 14–16

Young G (1988) Fluorescein fit in rigid lens evaluation. International Contact Lens Clinic 15(3): 95–110

Young G (1998) The effect of rigid lens design on fluorescein fit. Contact Lens and Anterior Eye 21 (2): 41–46

Chapter **5**

Patient selection and preliminary examination

David Ruston and John Mountford

CHAPTER CONTENTS

Introduction   109
Standards of practice and instrumentation   110
Factors affecting patient suitability for
   orthokeratology   112
Discussion of mode of wear, day or night
   therapy   130
Patient information   132
Informed consent   134
References   136

INTRODUCTION

All contact lens fitting involves a logical assessment of the physical and physiological factors with which a patient presents in order to arrive at the correct choice of lens. The aim is to achieve a successful outcome for the patient without any adverse consequences. Orthokeratology is, for many patients, an attractive alternative to the daily wear of soft or rigid gas-permeable (RGP) lenses. Careful selection of patients is just as crucial to the success of a program of orthokeratology treatment as is accurate fitting and judicious aftercare by the practitioner. The primary objective of this chapter is to give guidelines to the practitioner to enable this process to take place.

Orthokeratology is more than simply achieving an ideal fluorescein pattern: the aim is to maximize unaided visual acuity whilst maintaining epithelial integrity and corneal optics, and to do so for the long term. Figure 5.1 shows how, over a period of 4 years, a consistent change in the corneal shape was maintained. The patient selection criteria for orthokeratology are more complex than for routine lens fitting, and some are specific to the procedure. The major problem with much of the information available to the public about orthokeratology is that it is misleading. Some of the internet sites promoting orthokeratology services make no mention of the limitations or risks associated with the procedure, with the result that patients present with unrealistic expectations.

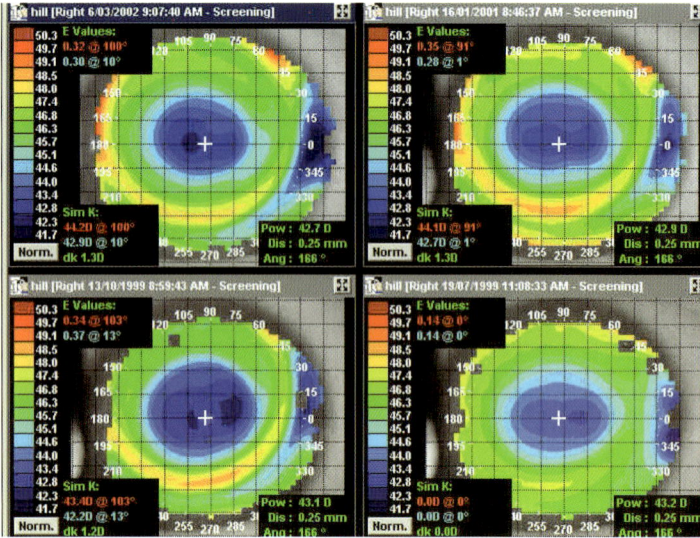

Figure 5.1 Repeated topography during 4 years of orthokeratology treatment. The plots were taken at approximately the same time following lens removal. The patient wears the lenses every second night, with vision of 6/5 (20/15). Note the consistency of the readings.

The authors have been advised by patients that they need only wear the lens for a certain period of time and their myopia will be "cured," or that 9.00 D myopia reduction is possible. The source of this misinformation is usually either friends or the websites of practitioners. It is therefore essential that those practicing orthokeratology apply the same standards of scientific objectivity to the process as that accepted as the norm for routine contact lens practice. The following section uses the data from published studies and our clinical experience in order to present a list of parameters that can be used to determine a patient's suitability for lens fitting.

However, before considering patient selection, the requirements that the practice and practitioner must satisfy will be addressed.

STANDARDS OF PRACTICE AND INSTRUMENTATION

Orthokeratology is very definitely a highly specialized form of RGP fitting. The learning curve associated with gaining expertise in the technique is longer and more challenging than in conventional RGP fitting. However, the end result in terms of patient satisfaction and quality of the refractive change make it possibly the most rewarding contact lens specialty. In view of the ease by which a poor result may be obtained and the cornea distorted, it is very important that the quality of the result in terms of topographic change and physiological compromise is closely monitored and documented. It is unlikely, therefore, that the part-time or itinerant contact lens practitioner will be able to meet its challenges.

In terms of the corneal response, it is highly desirable that topographic difference maps should show the following features:

- A zone of flattening which is centered over the pupil and which has a diameter sufficient to prevent the patient experiencing flare during normal lighting conditions. A diameter of 4–5 mm is usually adequate.
- A concentric zone of mid-peripheral steepening. The quality of lens centration and bearing can be determined by the evenness of this zone.
- A relatively unchanged periphery with minimal signs of distortion.

Such a topographic outcome is shown in Figure 5.2. To accept an inferior result to this is a disservice to the patient.

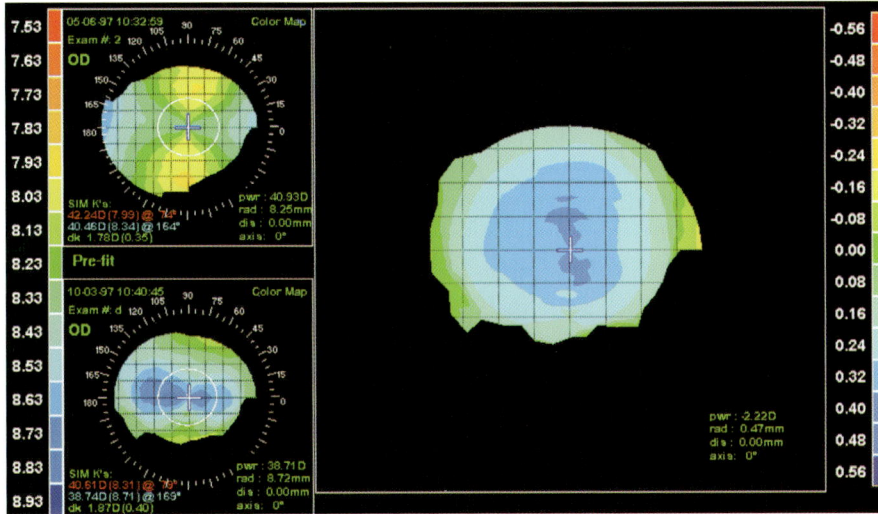

Figure 5.2 Ideal topographical change map indicating a reduction in apical corneal power of 2.22 D.

The choice of lens design and supplier is a very important one. Lens designs have been described in Chapter 4. It is important to use one design and become very familiar with it rather than pick and choose from a range of designs. As important as the design of the orthokeratology lens used is the quality of its manufacture. Inaccuracies as small as 0.02 mm make a measurable difference to the corneal response. Poor-quality surfaces may lead to reduced wetting, more rapid spoilation of the lens, tendency to parameter instability, and reduced comfort and possibly corneal staining. As well as verifying the accuracy of ordered lenses, it is recommended that the practitioner check the fitting set carefully upon receipt and then at regular intervals. If the ordered lens departs unexpectedly from the fitting set lens, then a scenario for frustration and disaster is set!

To arrive at the desired outcome, the ability of the fitter and quality of the lenses used are not the only prerequisites. Good-quality instrumentation is also required.

In terms of instrumentation, the minimum desirable list is as follows:

- Reverse geometry fitting set of lenses made in high-oxygen-permeability material. The manufacturer should be chosen with great care. As a general principle, if the practitioner does not find the conventional RGP lenses second to none, then the reverse geometry lenses will certainly be disappointing!
- Slit-lamp microscope incorporating high-quality optics, up to 40× magnification, and barrier filter to enhance fluorescence of sodium fluorescein. Extremely careful examination of the cornea is necessary before fitting commences to rule out any subtle dystrophies or corneal anomalies. The use of a yellow (Wratten 12) filter is incredibly useful to enhance the fluorescence of sodium fluorescein in blue light. The filter is placed in front of the microscope objective lens and removes the blue background light and thus enhances the contrast between the fluorescent and nonfluorescent areas. Both corneal staining and lens-fitting patterns are dramatically enhanced using this filter. All the images taken using fluorescein that appear in this book have been captured using a barrier filter.
- Computerized video keratoscope with the following features:
  - Manual editing, to remove artefacts. If this is not done the determination of the corneal eccentricity will be grossly inaccurate.
  - Accurate and repeatable determination of apical radius and eccentricity.
  - Able to give tangential topographic maps as these more closely indicate shape changes on the cornea than sagittal maps.
  - Presentation of difference maps, preferably based on both sagittal and tangential analysis.

Without a difference display it is difficult to know what the topographical change actually is and to categorize it as "bull's eye," "smiley face," or "central island."

- Test chart. This should incorporate several lines corresponding to the higher acuities (6/6 or 20/20, etc.) to prevent memorization of the chart. Ideally, log minimum angle of resolution (logMAR) charts in high and low contrast to allow data analysis and evaluate acuity at different contrasts. Illumination should be controlled during use, ideally by prior measurement using a light meter and elimination of daylight from the examination room. Alternatively, projector or computer-generated charts are very useful in that the presentation of only one line at a time helps reduce memorization.
- Focimeter. Generally, lenses for night therapy are left plano-powered. This has the advantage of minimizing thickness and therefore maximizing oxygen permeability. However, patients on day therapy will require effective refractive correction. The optical quality and accuracy of the power are obviously then as important as with any RGP lens.
- Radiuscope. It is vital for the success of any orthokeratology treatment that lenses are used that have been manufactured to a very high degree of accuracy using state-of-the-art computerized lathes. It is possible to see significant differences in treatment outcome using lenses that differ in base curve by as little as 0.02 mm. Given that the International Standards Organization (ISO) tolerance for the manufacture of RGP lenses is only 0.05 mm, then the quality standards of the laboratory itself become all-important. It is essential that the practitioner check the lens base curve before issuing the lens to the patient. In addition, trial lens parameters must be carefully evaluated and lenses may need to be verified again at aftercare visits.
- Diameter gage. Just as small errors in radius cause unexpected outcomes in orthokeratology, errors in diameter of the optic zone produce similar alterations to the expected outcome. Whilst errors of 0.03 in radius are certainly significant, larger errors, of the order of 0.20 mm, are required in total diameter or

optic zone diameter to cause alterations to treatment outcome.

- Thickness gage. As stated previously, in night therapy, the lenses used are generally plano-powered. This has the advantage of reducing the overall oxygen transmissibility by virtue of the even thickness profile. If the practitioner wishes to check the manufactured lens thickness, then a thickness gage is useful. Rigidity of the lens is important and therefore the minimum central thickness is of the order of 0.16 mm.
- Appropriate fitting software. A variety of programs are available, as set out in Chapter 8.

FACTORS AFFECTING PATIENT SUITABILITY FOR ORTHOKERATOLOGY

There are several key considerations to address when advising prospective patients as to their suitability for orthokeratology: refractive, anatomical, occupational and recreational, physiological and psychological. These are set out below. However, these considerations should be seen as augmenting the normal contact lens preliminary examination.

Refractive

Visual acuity improvement

The studies show a mean improvement in high-contrast visual acuity (VA) of approximately 5.5 lines of Snellen acuity. Thus, if a patient presents with unaided VA of 6/60 (20/200), the reduction in myopia is likely to be associated with an improvement in VA to 6/9 (20/30). The patient can then be shown the residual error and decide whether the improvement in vision is acceptable. However, it is wise to remember that the post-treatment VA is usually better than that predicted by the refractive error, and it not uncommon for patients who have a 1.00 D residual error still to see 6/6 (20/20) comfortably (Lui & Edwards 2000, Cho et al 2002). Low-contrast improvements tend to be less than those of high-contrast vision, and are more difficult to demonstrate. As far as low-contrast vision is concerned, other factors, such as pupil diameter in low illumination, treatment zone diameter, and refractive change come into the equation, and will be discussed in a later section.

Myopia

At present, single and double reverse geometry lens designs can only effectively eliminate mild to moderate amounts of myopia and are currently not effective at reducing hypermetropia. The use of high-eccentricity aspheric back surface RGP lenses fitted to give vaulting over the corneal apex may produce some hypermetropic ortho-keratology, but such designs have not been validated and are outside the scope of this book. Effective reduction is taken as being a stable reduction of refractive error, which does not compromise best-corrected VA.

Topographic sagittal change maps will indicate the quality of the refractive change in the cornea (see Ch. 2). An optimal result using current lens designs is a well-centered zone of flattening in a corneal topography difference map that is approximately 4–5 mm across (Fig. 5.2). If this is accepted as the ideal result then, at present, the mean documented refractive change is of the order of 2.25 D, with a standard deviation of approximately 0.75 D (Mountford 1997b, 1998, El Hage et al 1999, Swarbrick & Alharbi 2001, Lui & Edwards 2000, Nichols et al 2000).

However, refractive change is also determined by the initial corneal eccentricity, with the cornea changing from a prolate towards either a spherical or oblate surface (Mountford 1997a, Mountford & Noack 1998, El Hage et al 1999). The higher the initial eccentricity, the greater the refractive change possible (see Ch. 6). This finding is held in some dispute (Day et al 1997), but to date there have been no published reports to substantiate the claims.

Both the Mountford–Noack model and Day kappa function provide a means of determining the refractive change possible from prefit corneal shape data. Also, both methods are in close agreement with one another (see Ch. 8). Using the Mountford–Noack model, Swarbrick & Alharbi (2001) found a mean final refraction of +0.02 ± 0.18 D from that predicted. If the prefit corneal data are used to determine the expected refractive change for an individual, the degree of residual error can be demonstrated, and the patient given the choice to proceed. The ideal cases are those where the predicted change is greater than that required, as a small (0.50 D) degree of overcorrection can be incorporated into the treatment in order that the patient can be ultimately moved to wear every second night.

Mountford (1998) found a mean regression of 0.38 D/day, whilst Swarbrick & Alharbi (2001) and Nichols et al (2000) found approximately 0.25 D regression by day 10 of their studies. If a patient is overcorrected by 0.50 D in the morning, the regression at the end of day 1 will mean that he or she is still approximately 0.25 D overcorrected. In this situation, there is no need for the patient to wear the lens that night, as the vision and refraction are stable. This should drop to approximately 0.25 D undercorrected by the end of the second day, with some associated blur, necessitating lens wear. However, if the predicted refractive change possible is less than that required, the patient will always be undercorrected by that amount, and nightly lens wear will be required to maintain the change. The ability to limit wear to every second night has advantages in that the already low risks associated with overnight wear are probably further reduced, and the patient is more independent of the lenses.

There are patients who may feel that a reduction of 2.00 D for 3.00 D of myopia is acceptable, but others for whom the outcome may be unacceptable due to poor unaided VA. The patient should always be shown the likely improvement, leaving the final decision as to whether to proceed to the individual. For many western practitioners, the major aim of orthokeratology is a total or near-total reduction of the myopia so that the patient can experience clear unaided vision without lens wear during the day. However, in Asia, the main use of orthokeratology is to reduce the degree of myopia. By showing the patient what is possible prior to treatment, expectations can be kept realistic, and unhappy outcomes avoided.

As a simple general rule, the following formula can be used to determine the refractive change possible. This is considered in more detail below.

$$\text{Eccentricity}/0.21 = \text{Refractive change}$$

There have been anecdotal reports of much greater refractive changes occurring, but to date no studies have been published. Cho et al (2002) reviewed the results of 59 patients fitted with reverse geometry lenses (RGLs) from an ortho-keratology practice in Hong Kong. The mean prefit refractive error was –3.97 ± 2.28 D. Of the 49 patients who wore their lenses on an overnight schedule only, 44 (89%) had unaided vision of 6/6. Four subjects had less than 6/9, two having 6/36 in one eye and 6/6 in the other, one had 6/12 in both eyes, whilst the remaining subject had 6/12 in the right eye and 6/6 in the left eye. There was no statistically significant correlation between prefit refractive error and postwear unaided vision (Pearson correlation $-0.21 < r < -0.05$, $P > 0.14$).

Reim has kindly made available, prior to publication, data from a long-term study of myopia reduction with the Dreimlens. Four hundred and five subjects with refractive errors between -0.50 D and -4.00 D were fitted and wore the lenses purely on an overnight-wear schedule. The relationship between the initial refraction and the mean difference between the original and achieved change is shown in Figure 5.3. In most cases, the mean error tends towards mild overcorrection, except for the 4.00 D group, where mild undercorrection is the norm. Note

Difference between refraction and mean error n = 409

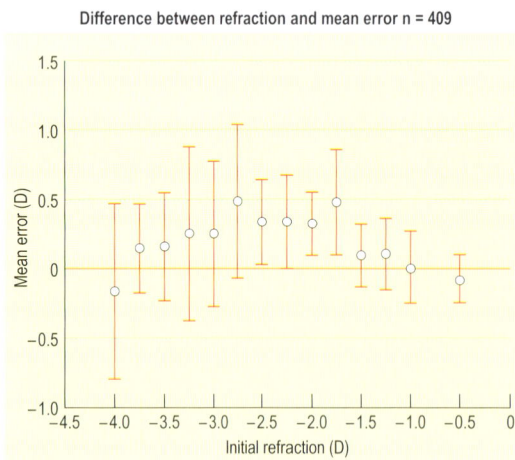

Figure 5.3 The mean error of the achieved refractive change versus the aimed-for change in a large sample group. Note that, at both extremes, the low and high myopes were undercorrected. Courtesy of Tom Reim.

also the range of results, which tend to indicate poorer predictability for the higher attempted changes. Reim states that the maximum attempted change should be 4.00 D.

The neophyte orthokeratologist is strongly advised to gain experience by correcting the lower degrees of myopia first, and then proceeding to the higher errors. Claims of consistently high refractive change should be treated with some suspicion until independent proof is forthcoming. There are practical limitations to the refractive changes possible with orthokeratology. If it were possible to correct 6.00 D of myopia, the treatment zone (TxZ) size would have to be reduced and would be less than 3.00 mm in diameter, leading to poor low-contrast vision and haloes. The aim should therefore be quality of unaided vision and corneal optics rather than large refractive changes.

Astigmatism

RGL designs do not appear to reduce against-the-rule or oblique astigmatism and may, in fact, increase it (Mountford 1997a). Therefore, a significant degree of this form of astigmatism is a relative contraindication for orthokeratology using these designs. With-the-rule astigmatism is reduced by the use of RGLs and experience to date indicates that a modest reduction will occur. Soni & Horner (1993) found a 60% reduction in the amount of astigmatism, whilst Mountford & Pesudovs (2002) found that a reduction in prefitting astigmatism of approximately 50% occurred providing the axis was with ± 30° of the horizontal. An upper limit of approximately 1.50 D for the total change has been reported (Mountford & Pesudors 2002).

Needless to say, orthokeratology can only reduce corneal astigmatism. The general principles that apply to the calculation of residual astigmatism with rigid lens fitting also apply to orthokeratology, with the added complication of a 50% reduction in corneal astigmatism. It is vital therefore to ascertain the degree of initial corneal astigmatism to the total amount in the refraction, and the influence that any lenticular astigmatism will have on the final outcome.

The following examples are used to point out the various factors that need to be considered.

1. Consider a refraction of −2.00/−1.50 × 180. The keratometry shows 1.50 D corneal astigmatism at the same axis. Therefore, all the astigmatism is corneal and the initial astigmatism will be reduced by approximately 50% to 0.75 D @ 180.

2. If the same refraction is encountered, and keratometry shows the cornea is spherical, the residual astigmatism will be a minimum of 1.50 D @ 180. In practice, the horizontal meridian is always flattened to a greater extent than the vertical, with the possibility of increased with-the-rule astigmatism to 2.00 D. This patient is a poor candidate for orthokeratology.

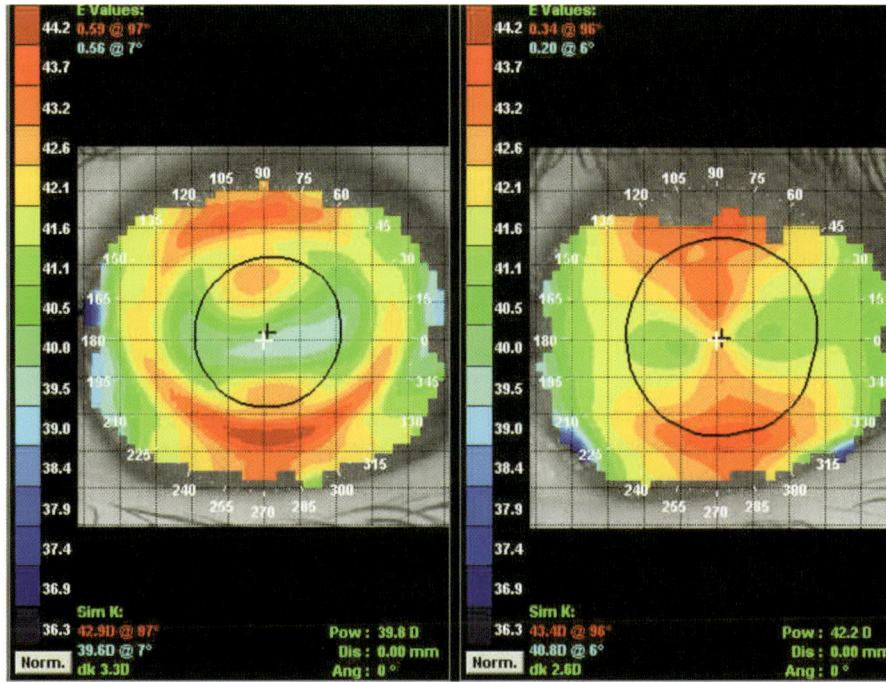

A

B

Figure 5.4   (A) The effect of orthokeratology on "wedge" or limbus-to-limbus astigmatism. Note that in the prefit plot on the right the astigmatism extends to the periphery. The postwear plot shows greater flattening of the flat meridian compared to the steep, leading to an overall increase in astigmatism. These cases are not suitable for current orthokeratology strategies. (B) Another case of limbus-to-limbus astigmatism. In this instance, the lens decentered superiorly, resulting in induced irregular astigmatism. This type of corneal topography is currently contraindicated for orthokeratology.

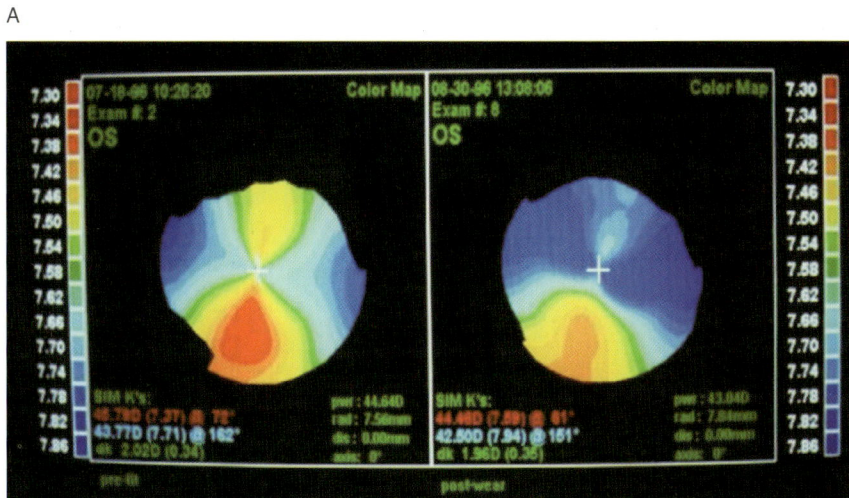

3. Assume the refraction is now −2.00/−0.50 × 180. If keratometry shows 1.50 D of corneal astigmatism at 180°, it follows that the likely outcome will be an induced against-the-rule astigmatism of approximately 1.00 D. The difference between the initial spectacle astigmatism and the corneal astigmatism is due to lenticular astigmatism, which is unaffected by orthokeratology.

4. If the refraction is −0.50/−1.50 × 180 and keratometry shows that the astigmatism is all corneal, then in theory the final Rx could be + 0.50/−0.75 × 180. This, however, is rarely the case, as the low degree of initial myopia will nearly always be overcorrected, leaving the patient unacceptably hypermetropic. In general, the astigmatic component of the refraction should never exceed the sphere if current-generation RGLs are to be fitted.

Additionally, the topographical appearance of the astigmatism is of vital importance. Clinical experience indicates that there are three distinct types of corneal topographical astigmatism: central, limbus-to-limbus, and irregular. Currently both limbus-to-limbus and irregular astigmatism are almost impossible to treat effectively with reverse geometry designs. In both of the above cases, the lenses consistently decenter superiorly, with either a smiley-face topography (and increased with-the-rule astigmatism) or, in the case of limbus-to-limbus astigmatism, greater flattening of the superior cornea than the inferior, and induced irregular astigmatism (Fig. 5.4).

Central astigmatism responds more favorably, but the 50% reduction in astigmatism occurs only over the central 2.00 mm chord (Fig. 5.5). In most cases of relatively high central astigmatism, the TxZ diameter difference between the steep and flat meridian is quite marked, and the lens does not succeed in "pushing" the astigmatism out past the pupil zone. This can result in an increase in with-the-rule astigmatism, as the flat meridian undergoes a greater change than the steep meridian, leading to a reduction in the myopic error but an increase in the astigmatism (Fig. 5.6). In general, only the classical "bowtie" type central astigmatism responds well to orthokeratology, with aberrant forms responding poorly. The current spherically based lens designs do not work well or predictably for astigmatism. In future, however, toric designs may lead to

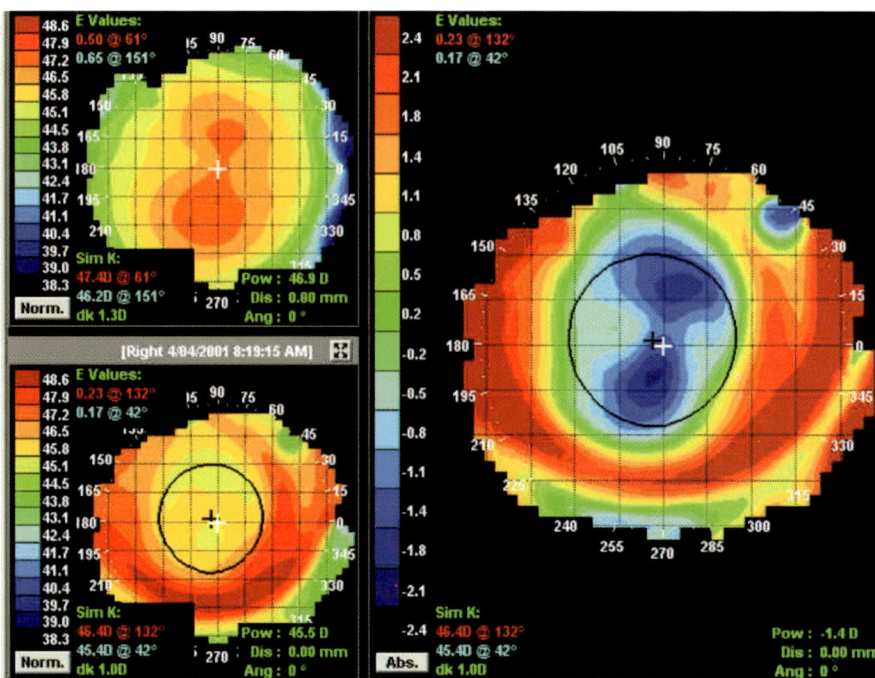

Figure 5.5   Simple central bowtie astigmatism and an ideal response to orthokeratology. Note that the steeper meridian is flattened to a greater extent than the flatter, allowing for correction of the astigmatism. Also note that the major change occurs within the central 2.00 mm chord, whilst the keratometer chord (3.00 mm) shows only a 0.70 D reduction in astigmatism.

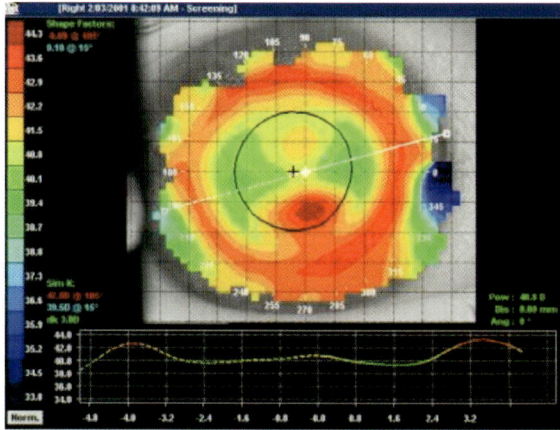

A

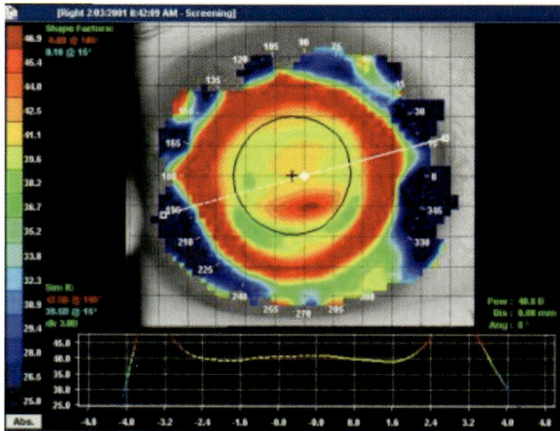

B

Figure 5.6 Axial (top) and tangential (bottom) postwear topography on a patient with high central astigmatism. Note the "island" of irregular astigmatism inferiorly. This has a detrimental effect on unaided visual acuity, and, in effect, is an increase in prefit astigmatism.

greater success. In the meantime, it is vital that not only the degree of refractive astigmatism compared to corneal astigmatism be properly assessed prior to fitting, but also the *type* of topographical astigmatism.

It therefore follows that, in general, to be considered suitable patients should have:

- low to moderate myopia (less than about 4.00 D if full correction is expected)
- mild (< 1.50 DC) with-the-rule astigmatism or no astigmatism
- no significant against-the-rule astigmatism or oblique astigmatism.

Patients with unstable refractive errors

There will be instances where the refractive error measured by the optometrist will not be representative of the true underlying error and a patient must be advised accordingly. Such instances may include:

- Long-term polymethyl methacrylate (PMMA) wearers. In many cases, such patients have either clinically significant corneal distortion or unintentional orthokeratology. Good alignment fitting of PMMA lenses results in an approximate reduction in myopia of 0.25–1.50 D on rising following daytime lens wear (Saks 1966, Rengstorff 1970a). In addition, there may be significant variation in refraction during the day, with myopia typically being lowest on rising and increasing throughout the day (Rengstroff 1970b). Furthermore, removal of PMMA lenses may result in a significant variation in the degree of myopia and astigmatism for up to approximately 3 weeks (Rengstorff 1965, Harris et al 1973), with least myopia being recorded within 2–3 days of removal (Rengstorff 1967). The average decrease is 1.32 D followed by increases for up to 3 weeks back to the level found on lens removal (Rengstorff 1967). Since there may well be corneal distortion as well as this refractive variation, it is wise to avoid performing orthokeratology on an existing PMMA wearer. If it is considered desirable to do so, then the patient should first be refitted with conventional RGP lenses and the cornea allowed to normalize for several months. Sequential topography measurements should be made until these appear stable. Since the cornea may never completely return to its prefitting state in these patients, it is probably best to avoid long-term PMMA wearers as candidates for orthokeratology.
- Existing RGP wearers. Even the best-fitted RGP lenses seem to produce some degree of sphericalization of the cornea, particularly in extended wear (Rivera & Polse 1991, Young & Port 1992). Since, as is shown below, the corneal eccentricity is a major factor to be taken into account when predicting the outcome of a period of orthokeratology treatment, it is best to allow the cornea to normalize

completely by removing the RGP lenses until sequential corneal maps show no significant change. This may take between 3 and 4 weeks. Patients wearing spherical RGP lenses on corneas with moderate astigmatism may, in addition, show a reduction in the corneal cylinder on removal of the lens. This may lead a practitioner to attempt orthokeratology when it is not really an appropriate treatment for the patient. Previous clinical records containing prefitting data, as well as removal of lenses for a period, may be helpful when advising the patient. Given the possible variability in the final refractive error and the time that it will take for the cornea to normalize, it is probably better to avoid existing RGP wearers, particularly in the early stages of one's experience with the technique.

- Existing wearers of thick, low-water soft lenses. Although evidence is sparse in the literature, clinical experience suggests that such patients can also have some degree of corneal warpage. Once again, this needs to be monitored by sequential topography, until normal corneal topography returns. Anecdotally, this appears to occur quicker than with rigid lenses. In addition, the presence of chronic edema can lead to the phenomenon of "myopic creep" where the refractive error continues to increase in adult patients, when it should have stabilized (Dumbleton et al 1999). Subsequent refitting of the patient with lenses having a higher oxygen transmissibility will lead to a reduction in myopia (Dumbleton et al 1999). Once again, it is probably wise to ensure that the cornea has completely normalized prior to embarking on a course of orthokeratology.

- Spasm of accommodation. Whilst not a particularly common clinical entity, this must always be considered when the refractive endpoint is variable and where there is not the usual close correlation between objective and subjective findings. More appropriate treatment, such as binocular vision investigation and a reading addition, should be instigated, rather than attempt orthokeratology.

Anatomical

Prefitting topographical assessment

Accurate corneal topography measurement is a vital part of the prefitting assessment. Topography has three main uses in orthokeratology:

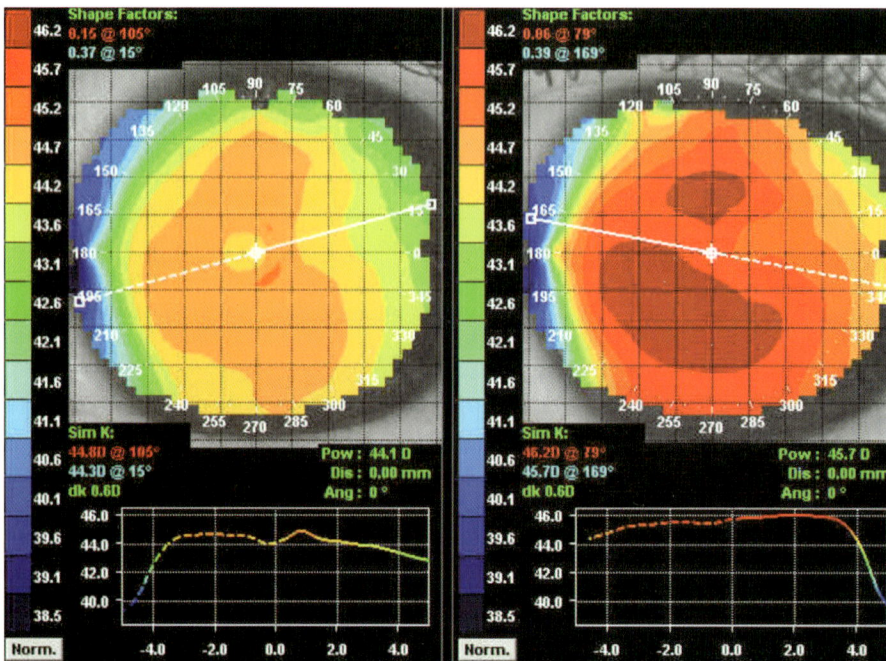

Figure 5.7 The map on the right is the initial prefitting map and is inaccurate. The map on the left was taken 2 weeks after cessation of lens wear due to an unacceptable result. The difference in apical power is 1.60 D, but the difference in sag was greater than 50 μm.

1. It provides corneal data to facilitate lens design.
2. It allows comparative analysis of the effects the lens has on corneal shape in order to optimize the lens fit and refractive outcome.
3. It acts as a permanent record of a course of treatment (Mountford et al 2002).

The single most important factor is the reliability and repeatability of the prefit topography. This not only gives the information required in order to fit the lens, but also the primary topography plot from which all postwear assessments of the lens effects will be judged. If the initial maps are inaccurate, the subsequent decisions on remedial actions will be invalid, leading to unnecessary lens reorders and more visits.

Figure 5.7 shows an invalid prefit map. The patient had three unsuccessful lens fits to the left eye, shown in the figure, compared to none for the right. Lens wear was ceased for 2 weeks and the topography repeated. The second map (left-hand side) gave totally different lens parameters to the initial lens. In the initial fitting, the lens design was based on an R_0 of 7.39 mm and a corneal sag of 1.6310 mm. The second reading gave values for R_0 and sag as 7.57 mm and

1.5794 mm respectively. The corneal response to the first trial is shown in Figure 5.8. It appears to be an ideal response, with a 2.00 D refractive change. However, the VA was 6/9 with an over-refraction of −1.00. The important thing to note is that the *whole* surface is flatter than the original cornea. However, the peripheral cornea is little affected by orthokeratology. So in this case, the *initial* map was invalid, but the postwear map was valid, giving an erroneous difference map.

The repeated reading done a few weeks later is approximately 1.50 D flatter than the original. The sag difference was 51.6 μm less than the original sag. Recalculation of the lens gave an ideal response and is shown in Figure 5.9.

Most corneal topographers derive elevation values first, and then construct the curvature values using their specific reconstruction algorithms. The crucial aspect of the whole process is the instrument's ability to determine the corneal apex. The topography plot shown in Figure 5.7 is a prime example of an inaccurate detection of the corneal apex. This can occur due to either eyelash interference or patient movement between the time taken for the instrument to detect the apex and then capture the image. The errors can be

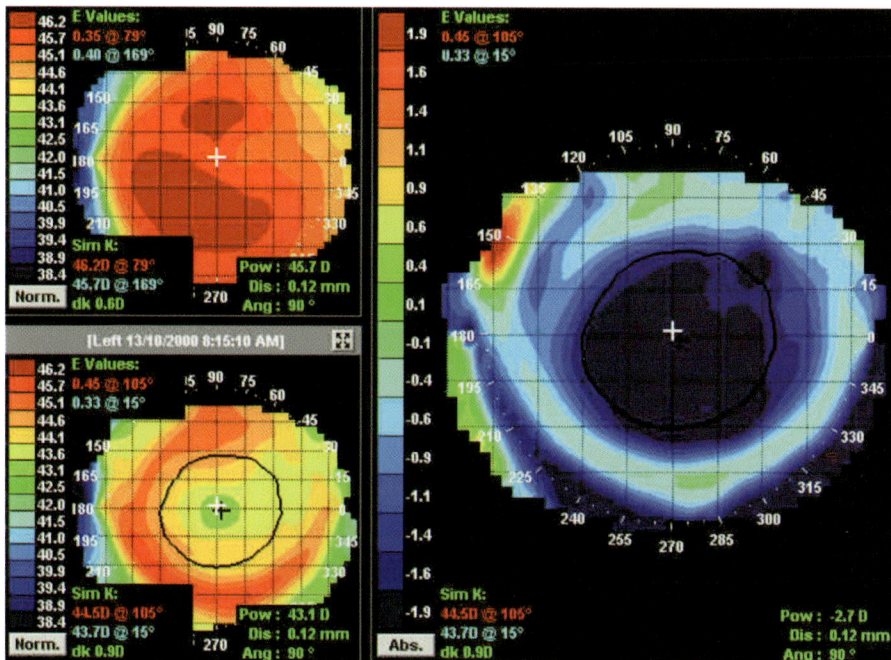

Figure 5.8 The subtractive map (right) shows the results based on the initial incorrect map. Note that the change in apical corneal power is 2.70 D, but the true refractive change was 1.50 D. Also note that the whole cornea is flatter in the subtractive plot.

quite large, as in the example shown. Indeed, once topography plots are taken, comparisons between the right- and left-eye results should be made. Both eyes in patients free of pathology should always be very similar in terms of R_0 and e-values. If the discrepancies are large (> 0.50 D), the readings should be retaken.

In order to maximize the rate of first-fit success, repeated readings in order to assess the mean values for R_0 and elevation and the standard deviation of error of the instrument are an invaluable tool, and should be considered an integral part of the prefitting assessment.

The technique used by the authors is set out in Chapter 6. Four repeated readings are taken and compared. Any clearly anomalous measurement is rejected and the remaining readings averaged. Reliance on one assessment of the corneal topography as a basis for designing the lens will lead to a low rate of first-fit success.

There are distinct corneal shapes that simply do not respond to orthokeratology. These are:

1. limbus-to-limbus or "wedge" astigmatism, as described above
2. off-center corneal apex (Fig. 5.10).

As stated previously, limbus-to-limbus astigmatism usually leads to an increase in astigmatism. In those cases where the corneal apex is decentered to a significant degree, the same problems that occur with some patients with deep-set eyes will arise: chronic smiley-face postwear plots and haloes and flare. Until better lens designs are developed for these cases, they should be considered unsuitable for orthokeratology.

The final factors to consider with the prefit topography are the quality of the tear film and the stability of the patient during the capture process. A lot of time and expense can be saved by including good topography information prior to fitting. Clearly a patient on whom one cannot obtain reliable topographic data is a poor patient to select for orthokeratology.

Eccentricity

The key anatomical consideration that arises from the prefitting topography (other than the measurement of the corneal apex) is the corneal eccentricity. Mountford (1997b) has shown that the corneal eccentricity is intimately linked to the outcome of accelerated orthokeratology using

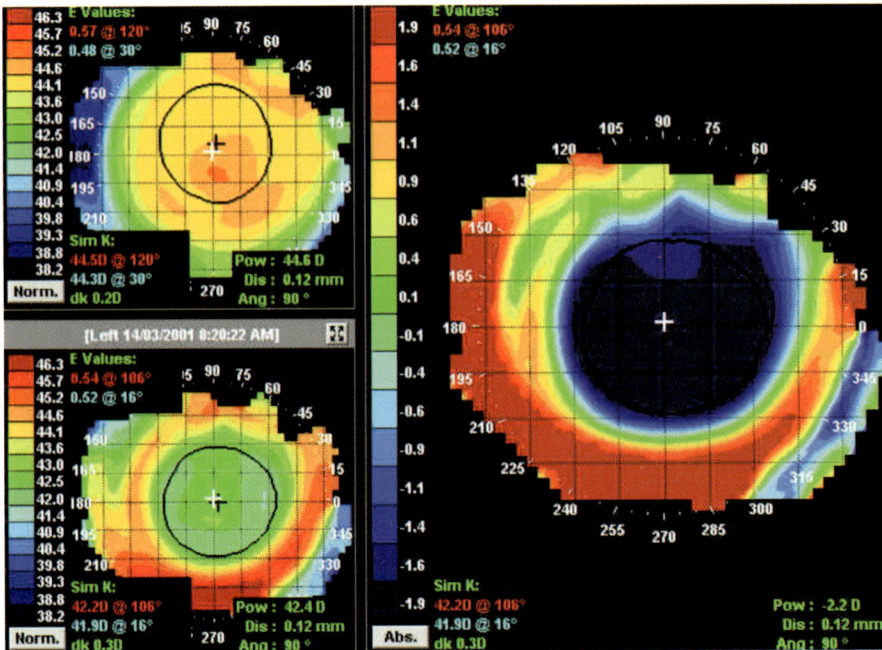

Figure 5.9   The same eye as that in Figure 5.8 following an overnight trial based on the second set of corneal data. The change in apical corneal power (2.20 D) was equal to the measured refractive change of 2.25 D. The peripheral cornea is not now flattened by the lens.

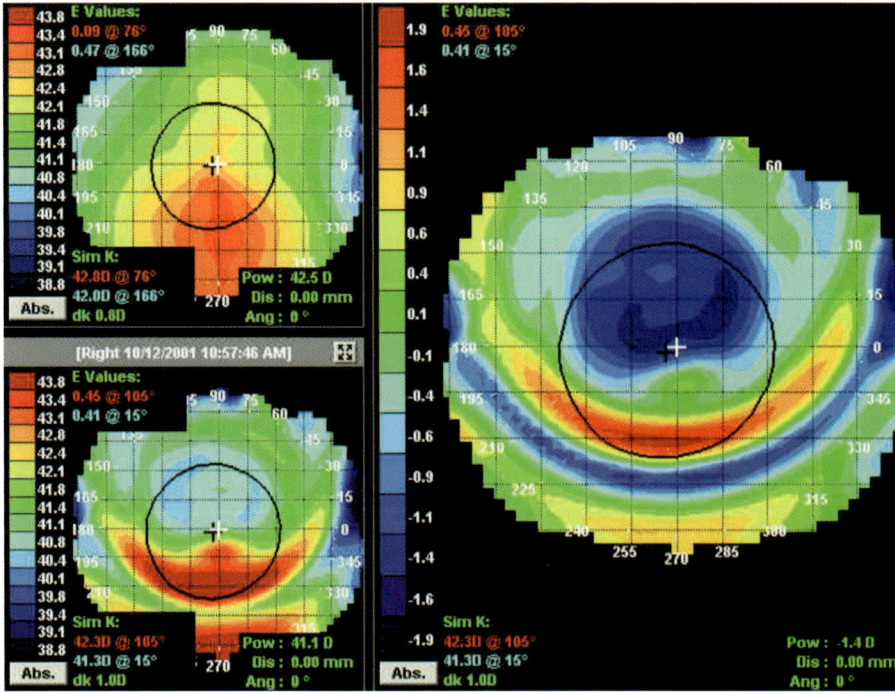

Figure 5.10 An unacceptable corneal shape with a decentered corneal apex. Four different lens trials still resulted in a smiley-face pattern due to lens decentration over the misplaced corneal apex.

one design of single RGL (Contex OK704T). He demonstrated that a reduction of approximately every 0.20 of the corneal eccentricity or *e* gives a 1.00 D reduction in myopia. The relation is not exactly linear, as shown in Figure 5.11, but this is still a useful rule of thumb.

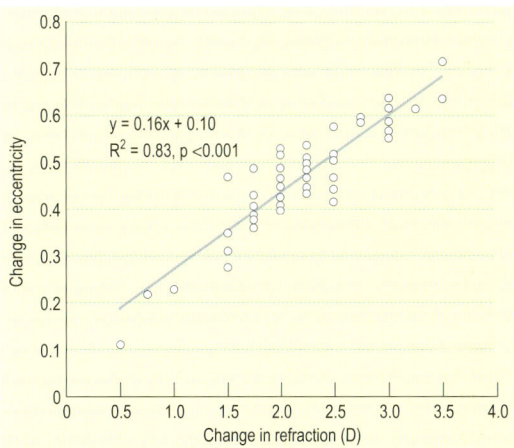

Figure 5.11 The relationship between the change in refractive error and the change in corneal eccentricity occurring after an orthokeratology treatment (from Mountford 1997b).

Therefore, if *e* is equal to the mean in the population of approximately 0.45 (Guillon et al 1986) then a likely reduction in myopia of the order of 2.25 D is possible. Mountford's analysis of the refractive changes in 60 patients showed a mean change of 2.19 D (Mountford 1997b). This must correlate reasonably well with patients' spherical refraction for them to be free of the lenses for most of the day.

If the patient has a prefitting refraction of −5.00 D, then reducing it by 2.50 D will not help greatly, unless the intention is merely to reduce the myopia, perhaps for occupational reasons. If it is −2.50 D then it is worth going ahead with a fitting if the desired outcome is emmetropia. Obviously, the higher the corneal eccentricity, the greater potential there is for reduction of myopia. The endpoint of any orthokeratology procedure has traditionally been described as a cornea with an eccentricity of zero, i.e., spherical (Kerns 1976, Binder et al 1980). Mountford (1997b) has shown that this holds true for the central 4–5 mm of the cornea. Outside this zone, there is a steepening of the cornea, so that the concept of a simple conic section breaks down.

This concept of the patient's corneal eccentricity defining the final outcome of the procedure is challenged by the latest double reverse geometry lens (DRGL) designs now available (see Ch. 4). Using the more sophisticated examples of these designs it is possible to program the required refractive change into the lens geometry to produce a unique lens for the individual topography and refractive characteristics. In these instances, the measurement of the corneal eccentricity serves to define the potential outcome using a conventional treatment zone. The extra refractive change required will reduce the size of this treatment zone. This makes measurement of the patient's pupil size important to predict the likelihood that flare will influence the quality of the visual result.

The departure from a prolate ellipse-type geometry prefitting to a more complex shape postorthokeratology means that it is not possible to use the concept of a single eccentricity value to describe the corneal shape. Whilst the new corneal shape will have an eccentricity of 0 over the central 4–5 mm, outside this, in the region of steepening, the use of the e-value becomes unworkable as there is no longer a prolate geometry. A negative e-value has no basis in mathematics. The use of a p-value can be used, but again this assumes a simple conical geometry, which may not be appropriate. Outside this zone of steepening, the cornea flattens again, in a similar way to its prefitting form.

Thus we have a three-zone surface: a central near-spherical zone of flattening, a concentric, narrow zone of steepening, surrounded by a relatively unchanged periphery. Higher-order mathematics is required to describe this changed geometry. It is for this reason that the apical radius and eccentricity values produced by the videokeratoscope do not adequately serve to establish the radius of any second lens in the same way that they can predict the initial lens.

Keratometry

The changes in corneal topography that occur in orthokeratology are not accurately detected or measured using a keratometer. Joe et al (1996) showed that the predictive expression of myopia reduction $(D) = 2(K_c - K_t) + 1.00$, derived by Wlodyga & Harris (1993), linking the relation between a temporal and central keratometry reading, is not well correlated to outcome in accelerated orthokeratology. It has been shown (Ericson & Thorn 1977, Mountford 1997b) that approximately 0.75 D of refractive change can occur before any alteration in the keratometry reading will arise. Thus there is little benefit in using a keratometer at the initial appointment. The instrument also has very little place in the aftercare of patients, as shown in Chapter 9.

However, if adapted using the method of Wilms & Rabbetts (1977) it is possible to derive a measure of the corneal eccentricity from the keratometer. Central and peripheral readings are taken from precisely defined corneal locations and a conic section fitted. Whilst this would serve adequately as a means of deriving the initial eccentricity, thereby aiding in the selection of the initial lens, it is really in follow-up of the patient that the absence of a means of determining the topography would be felt. None of the principal topographic determinants of a substandard fit is measurable using a keratometer. These are, of course, central islands, inferior and superior zones of steepening (smiley faces), and decentered treatment zones. Thus, one would be reliant on the retinoscopy reflex and subjective comments regarding visual quality as a means of defining the quality of the treatment outcome. The authors feel that this would not be commensurate with ethical practice.

Pupil diameter and treatment zone

Swarbrick et al (1998) have shown that Munnerlyn's formula can be used to account accurately for the refractive changes occurring in orthokeratology due to epithelial thinning. The maximum degree of central epithelial thinning with orthokeratology appears to be approximately 20 μm. If Munnerlyn's formula is expressed in orthokeratology terms, the relationship between refractive change and treatment zone diameter can be calculated.

The formula is:

$$\text{Epithelial thinning} = \frac{RD^2}{3}$$

where R is refractive change in diopters and D the treatment zone diameter.

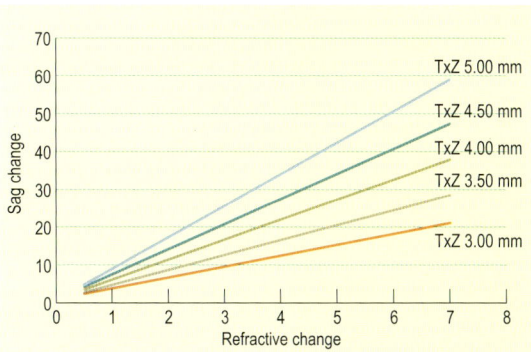

Figure 5.12   The results for a range of refractive changes plotted against change in corneal sag. Note that, as the refractive change required increases, the treatment zone (TxZ) diameter decreases.

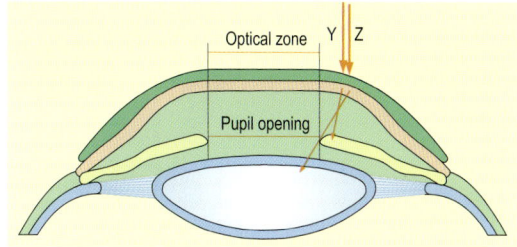

Figure 5.13   The effect of a treatment zone (TxZ) diameter being the same size as the pupil in dim illumination. The ray Y is within the TxZ and will be blocked by the pupil border. More peripheral rays (Z) will be refracted to a greater degree by the sudden change in curvature at the edge of the TxZ, and be refracted through the pupil, leading to flare and haloes.

If, as stated above, the assumed maximum thinning is 20 μm, the refractive change required can be substituted into the formula and the TxZ diameter determined. The results for a range of refractive changes are shown in Figure 5.12. Note that, as the refractive change required increases, the TxZ diameter decreases. For a nominal pupil zone of 3.00 mm diameter, a refractive change of up to 6.00 D may be feasible as the TxZ diameter and pupil diameter are the same. However, if it is assumed that the limit of the refractive change is determined by the pupil diameter in dim illumination, there is a marked reduction in effective refractive change possible. Assuming that the pupil diameter increases to 5.00 mm in dim illumination, the refractive change that gives an effective TxZ is reduced to 2.50 D. This point is of vital importance when considering low-contrast vision, as pupil dilation in dim light associated with large refractive error reductions will lead to flare and haloes, and a reduction in visual quality (Applegate & Gansel 1991).

Davidorf (1998) drew attention to this fact in regard to refractive surgery (Figure 5.13). Small treatment zones combined with large pupil diameters and deep anterior chamber depths lead to excessive flare, haloes, and decreased low-contrast vision post-Lasik. Refractive surgeons are able to compensate to an extent for these effects by manipulating both the TxZ and the method of laser ablation. This may also be possible to some

extent with different designs of RGL. The difference in TxZ for two different lens designs is shown in Figure 5.14. The refractive changes are similar, but the TxZ of one is greater than the other. Alterations to the lens back optic zone diameter (BOZD) can lead to increased TxZ diameters without compromising the refractive change but require careful calculations (see Ch. 9).

Lens design does play an important role in the TxZ diameter. Mountford fitted 14 patients with a generic 6.00 mm BOZD lens in one eye and an IDEAL lens in the other (7.30 mm BOZD). The refractive change was a mean of 1.86 ± 0.56 D for all patients. Subtractive axial power maps were used to measure the TxZ diameters following lens wear. The results are shown in Figure 5.15. Although the difference in TxZ diameter between the two designs when taken in isolation is not dramatic, it does become quite significant when compared to the percentage of pupil coverage under different conditions (Fig. 5.16). All of the currently available designs use a 6.00 or 6.50 mm BOZD, but future design improvements may allow for a greater control over the TxZ diameter.

From a clinical viewpoint, refractive changes of up to 3.00 D rarely cause symptoms of poor vision in dim illumination, but greater changes can. If a patient requires a greater refractive change, the practitioner is well advised firstly to determine the likely TxZ using Munnerlyn's formula, and then determine the patient's dilated pupil diameter. There are dedicated instruments that can be used to do this, like an infrared pupillometer, but

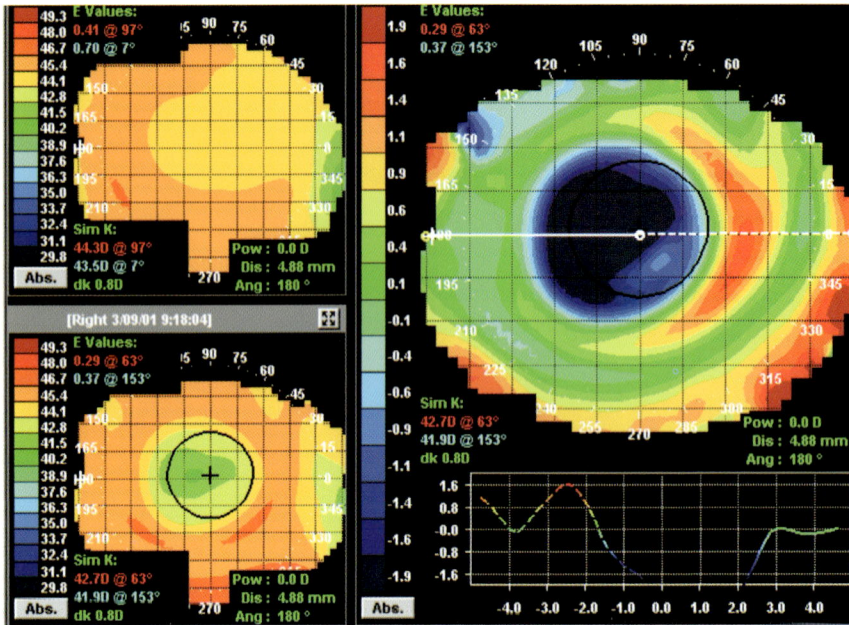

Figure 5.14 (A) A small treatment zone diameter compared with (B) a larger one for corneas of approximately equivalent shape and refractive change. The only difference lies in the lens design used.

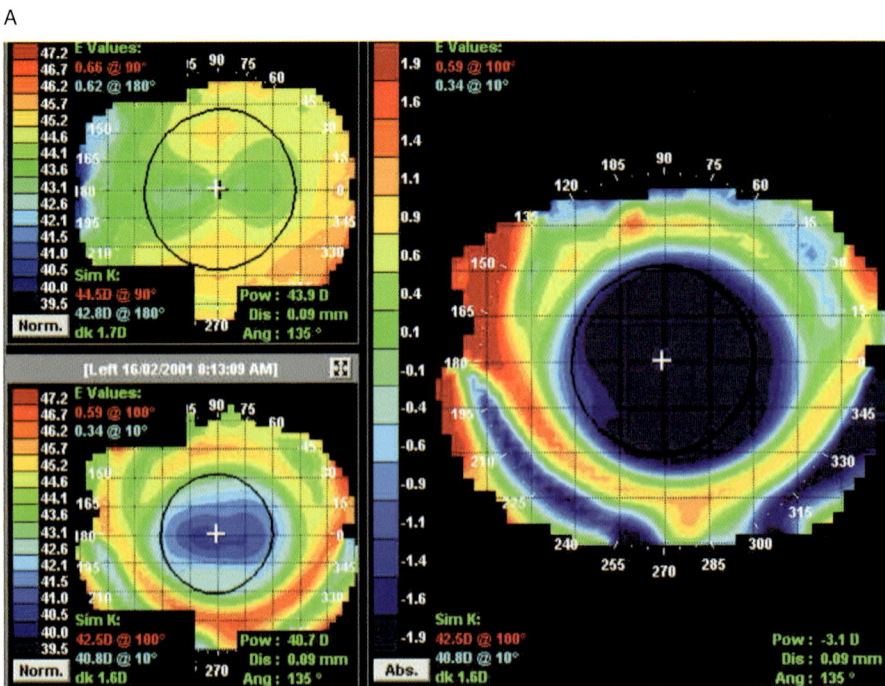

other more commonly available instruments can perform the required measurements. For example, any autorefractor or retinal camera that is infrared-driven with a television screen focusing and fixation system will work well (Fig. 5.17).

The method is to measure the horizontal visible iris diameter (HVID) on the screen and also the pupil zone when the pupil is dilated after 5 min or so in the dark. A simple fractional conversion will then give the pupil zone after dilation, e.g., if

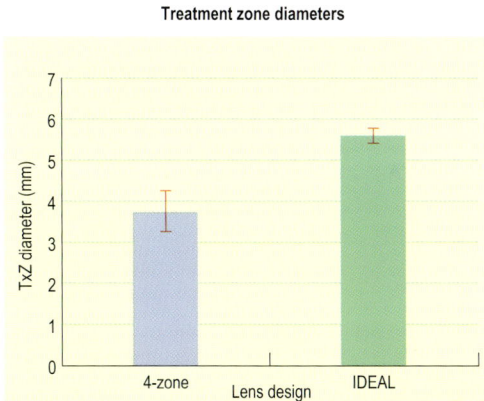

Figure 5.15 The mean treatment zone (T×Z) diameters for two different lens designs. The four-zone lens has a back optic zone diameter of 6.00 mm, and the IDEAL 7.30 mm.

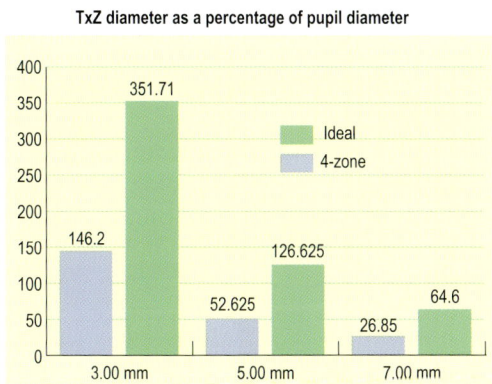

Figure 5.16 The percentage of pupil coverage of the different treatment zone (T×Z) diameters for different pupil sizes. Smaller T×Z diameters are acceptable for normal pupil sizes, but the efficacy diminishes as the pupil size increases.

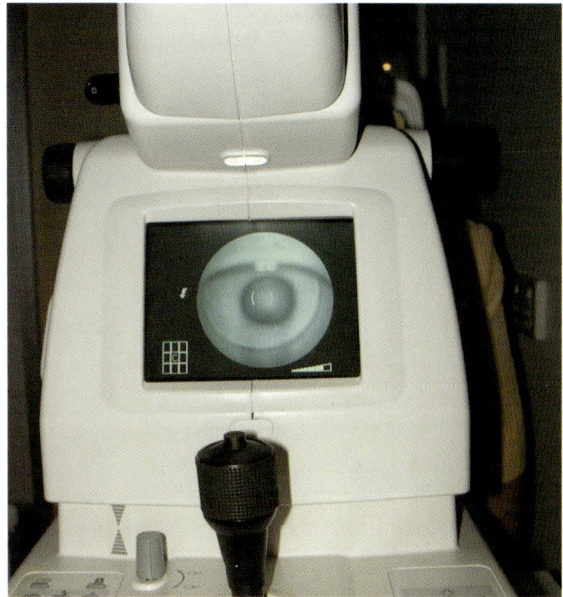

Figure 5.17 An infrared retinal camera is used to measure the pupil in dim illumination. The large circle is equal to the horizontal visible iris diameter (HVID). Simple proportional analysis of the pupil zone with respect to the HVID gives the pupil size in dim illumination.

the HVID is 12 mm, but 120 mm on screen and the pupil measures 50 mm on screen, then the "real" pupil diameter is 5 mm. If the calculated T×Z is smaller than the pupil zone in dim illumination, then it is highly probable that the patient will report symptoms of flare, haloes, and poor low-contrast vision.

If patients do present with symptoms of flare and poor vision in low illumination, the problem is easily detected with simple retinoscopy in a darkened room. Ineffective T×Z diameters will appear exactly like the retinoscopy reflex through a concentric bifocal contact lens. The approximate

increase in T×Z diameter required to resolve the problem can be determined by simply comparing the central treatment area to the pupil diameter.

Cho et al (2002) reported on the patient responses to a questionnaire about the incidence of various symptoms following overnight wear of orthokeratology lenses. Approximately 33% (21/61) reported poor vision in dim or dark conditions, so the problem does have a relatively high incidence in this patient group. The majority of the subjects (50/61) were less than 16 years of age, so the effects of the poor vision for night driving could not be gaged.

Hile & Marsden (2001) studied the effects of pupil dilation on vision and refraction in a group of eight subjects. Mean low-contrast VA decreased with increased pupil size (0.015, $P = 0.036$) and refractive error (autorefraction) increased by a mean of 1.12 D ($P = 0.01$). This is similar to the effects of small ablation zones in refractive surgery (Lohman et al 1993, Pop 1996), with a common level of complaint (30%), as found by Cho et al (2002) in a group of orthokeratology patients.

Future developments in lens design, as well as preliminary measurement of the pupil diameter, may help to reduce the incidence of the problem. The inclusion of an estimation of the pupil size in dim illumination is a valuable prefitting aid in being able to detect problem cases before they occur.

Lid position and tension

There are two main reasons for considering rejecting patients with loose lids or deep-set eyes, or those with low upper lids and narrow apertures. The first is that it can be difficult to get accurate or repeatable topography data, especially with small Placido instruments, as the cone tends to contract the orbital bones before the corneal apex can be properly located. If large Placido instruments are used, the focusing problems are not as great, but a greater surface area of the cornea is lost due to lid, nose, and brow shadow, leading to inaccuracies in the estimation of eccentricity. This will mean that potentially more trials will have to be completed until the fitting is refined.

Secondly, just as with the fitting of conventional RGP lenses, a low lower lid can result in more difficulty in attaining good centration, due to inadequate support to the lens (Carney et al 1997). This is especially the case if the low lower lid is combined with a low top lid. However, this may only be the case when daily wear is being undertaken. The authors feel that for night therapy this should not be seen as a relative contraindication and a trial should still be carried out. It is a fairly common observation that patients with lenses that sit inferiorly when the eyes are open, despite a classic fluorescein pattern, can have a perfect topographical response to overnight wear of the same lens. Presumably, with the eyes closed the centration is improved.

It may be that the lens position adopted in the consulting room, with the patient sitting upright in the examination chair and the lids and gravity exerting their customary effects on centration, is quite different from that arising when the patient is lying down with the lids closed. The effect of Bell's reflex may be significant, as the eyes may adopt a higher position relative to the primary position in which the lens is checked in the consulting room. Therefore inferior centration, but with a classic fluorescein fit, should be seen as a relative contraindication to the night treatment form of orthokeratology and an overnight trial should still be conducted to measure the quality of the corneal response. However, for daytime orthokeratology it is a definite contraindication.

In a similar way, there are instances of nasal and superior decentration, which also do not lead to decentered treatment zones following an overnight trial. The practitioner is advised to check the fluorescein pattern in a centered position. If it is thought to fulfill the attributes set out in Chapter 6 and the lens in not too small, then it is worth proceeding with an overnight trial. The position of the resultant TxZ, determined in the difference map the next morning, would serve to define the quality of the fitting. However, if the difference map indicates that decentration has occurred, it may be that fitting will have to be discontinued.

Low lid tension seems, anecdotally, to reduce the effectiveness of orthokeratology, presumably due to lowered lid forces acting on the lens. However, like abnormal lid position, it should be seen as a relative contraindication. It is still worthwhile performing a daytime or overnight trial to assess the corneal response to a well-fitted lens. The hydrostatic forces behind the lens are far stronger than the lid force and the authors have had several successful elderly patients with low lid tension achieve good outcomes with orthokeratology.

Occupational and recreational

A significant percentage of patients attending an orthokeratology practice do so in order to meet the visual standards for a particular employer or occupation. The standards vary from country to country and will not be listed here. Practitioners are advised to consult their professional body for a list of the standards that apply in their own country. In the UK the Association of Optometrists publishes these on its website at www.optometry.co.uk.

The use of visual standards in a selection process has caused many of the involved bodies significant problems in finding sufficient appropriate entrants given the rise in the incidence of myopia in the young population globally. There have been several examples where they are prepared to accept applicants who are known to use orthokeratology as a means of reducing their refractive error, whilst maintaining their corrected visual acuity.

For example, in Spain the Madrid Police Authority refers otherwise suitable applicants to an orthokeratologist for treatment with a view to allowing them to meet the vision standards (F Hidalgo personal communication). From a medicolegal perspective, the practitioner should ensure that the patient achieves excellent corrected vision after orthokeratology and realizes that it is the patient's responsibility to declare or not declare the usage of orthokeratology lenses as a device to meet the appropriate standards. Examples of patients who may seek the services of an orthokeratology practitioner are airline pilots, police officers, and firefighters. Practitioners who are concerned to be totally protected from a medicolegal point of view would be wise to write to the appropriate authority and seek clarification as to whether orthokeratology is appropriate.

There are also many patients who are active in sport who find conventional contact lenses inconvenient. The possibility of being free from optical aids whilst participating in the sport is attractive to them. Examples are swimmers who find that rigid lenses are likely to be lost from the eye and that soft lenses alter their parameters and stick to the eye whilst swimming; divers and surfers who worry about losing lenses whilst being underwater; those involved with contact sports who have had lenses displaced, and any sports people who find that lenses become uncomfortable in the environmental conditions they participate in, such as hot, dry climates or dusty, windy places.

Patients who wear lenses in night clubs can find they get dry and uncomfortable and seek an alternative. Actors and television personalities may find that having a contact lens in the eye causes them to alter their blink rate and appear less at ease than if they are free of contact lenses. Practitioners should also remember that not all patients find contact lenses convenient or comfortable in their particular situation and be receptive to the positive benefits

that orthokeratology can bring to these individuals. A particularly large group are those patients who find that they are unable to tolerate soft contact lenses all day due to dry-eye symptoms when lenses are worn (see below).

Physiological

Just as is the case for conventional RGP wear, there are physiological considerations to make when advising patients as to their suitability for orthokeratology. In essence, the contraindications to orthokeratology are either absolute, leading to immediate rejection of the patient, or relative, indicating that a cautious approach is required.

Absolute contraindications

Keratoconus   Just as with refractive surgery, this must be excluded by videokeratoscopy before attempting any fitting. The keratoconic cornea would respond quite abnormally to a RGL and there is also evidence that flatly fitted lenses cause scarring on keratoconic corneas (Korb et al 1982). Identification of keratoconus from a topography map (Fig. 5.18) can be made by consideration of five factors:

1. The apical radius. If this is less than 7.20 mm then keratoconus is more likely. However, keratoconus can occur with apical radii as flat as 7.8 mm (Woodward 1980), therefore other features must be present to confirm the diagnosis.
2. A greater eccentricity than normal. Typically, 95% of the normal population have an eccentricity in the flattest corneal meridian between 0.0 and 0.88 (Guillon et al 1986). Douthwaite's study using the EyeSys 2000 instrument (Douthwaite et al 1999) showed a narrower range of 0.0–0.71. However, in keratoconus eccentricities are typically from 0.6 to over 1.0.
3. Variation in interocular apical radius greater than 0.20 mm. Typically there is close association between both the apical radii and eccentricity between the two eyes.
4. Loss of symmetry either side of the horizontal midline. If corresponding points equidistant from the apex are considered then, in the

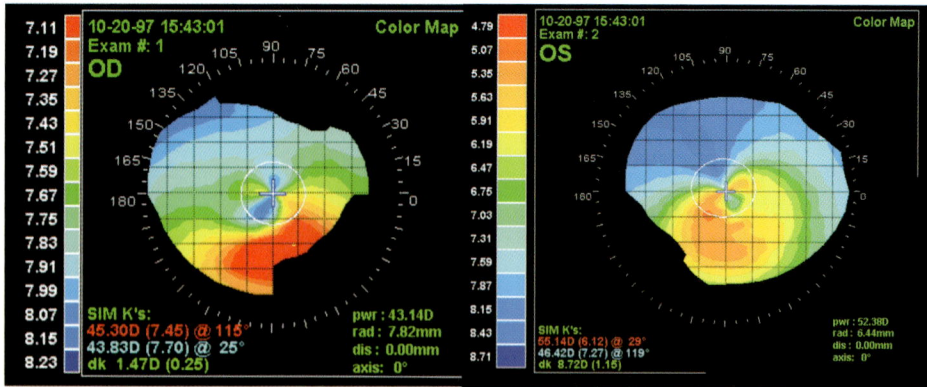

Figure 5.18   A case of moderate keratoconus exhibiting all the features described in the text. Different scales are used for the two eyes in view of the typical asymmetry.

normal eye, there are seldom variations greater than 0.20 mm (1 D). However, in the keratoconic eye there are, typically, greater than 0.60 mm (3 D) differences between these two regions on the cornea.

5. A localized area of corneal steepening, either located inferiorly (typically in 75% of cases) or centrally.

Corneal dystrophies   Nothing is known about the effect of orthokeratology on a dystrophic cornea. In the absence of such knowledge, it would be foolhardy knowingly to fit a type of lens that is thought to bring about redistribution of epithelium and possibly alter the shape of stromal tissue. Careful slit-lamp examination is essential to exclude any sign of abnormality, since many dystrophies are subtle. Direct focal, indirect, retro, and specular illumination techniques are required to exclude corneal dystrophy.

Corneal edema present without contact lenses would obviously be a contraindication to orthokeratology as even the highest-transmissibility lenses would add to the cornea's load. Signs of such metabolic stress might be centrally located, vertically oriented striae or folds in the stroma of the cornea. Other signs might be multiple epithelial microcysts or, in extreme cases, vacuoles in the epithelium.

If there is any doubt as to the presence of subclinical dystrophy, it is wise to refer the patient for ophthalmological opinion before embarking on a course of orthokeratology.

Any active anterior segment disease   The contraindications to conventional lens wear apply just as much to orthokeratology treatment. Where overnight wear is to be employed, it is more important than ever to be certain that the anterior segment is free of any active pathology which would contraindicate lens usage. It is known, for example, that blepharitis is a risk factor for infection in conventional contact lens wear (Holden et al 2000, Jalbert et al 2000, Willcox et al 2000). Therefore, all cases of significant blepharitis should be treated before a program of orthokeratology begins. Recurrent conjunctivitis is equally a contraindication until the cause is identified and treated.

Whilst it is most unlikely that a patient with active keratitis would present for fitting, careful slit-lamp examination is required to evaluate the extent and depth of any corneal staining and identify any areas of infiltrate in the asymptomatic patient. Although there is little knowledge of the potential effects, it would be unwise, for example, to fit a patient with adenoviral infiltrates until they have fully resolved. Chronic anterior uveitis may be exacerbated by lens wear, particularly if this is overnight.

Severe dry eye is equally an absolute contraindication to lens wear. The presence of gross corneal stain (grade 3 and above) or corneal filaments is indicative of pathological dry eye.

Relative contraindications

Marginal dry eye   In normal soft-lens practice, the commonest symptom reported by patients is ocular dryness, affecting 75% of wearers (Brennan & Efron 1989). This does not always correlate with the typical minor inferior desiccation stain that is commonly observed in wearers of soft contact lenses (Pritchard & Fonn 1995). This type of stain does not appear to be observed in orthokeratology patients on night therapy.

Particularly during closed-eye conditions, RGP lenses are better suited to patients with slightly reduced tear volumes than hydrogel lenses. Obviously, less evaporation occurs during closed-eye conditions, making this modality of wear more suited to marginally dry eyes. When the lipid layer is absent, the rate of evaporation from the open eye is approximately four times the normal value. Thus wearing lenses during a closed-eye situation would not be expected to lead to increased evaporation.

However, it should be remembered that truly dry eyes are a contraindication to all contact lens wear. Any patient who suffers from ocular dryness without any contact lenses and who exhibits inferior desiccation stain greater than grade 2 (mild stain) should probably be rejected as an orthokeratology patient for either modality. For other patients, it is well worth giving them an overnight or daytime trial and checking the cornea carefully using fluorescein and a barrier filter both before and after lens wear. Any increase in staining beyond grade 1 or greater than grade 2 staining (Cornea and Contact Lens Research Unit (CCLRU) grading scale) would be regarded as an adverse sign.

When there is reduced tear volume there is always the possibility of a reduced tendency for lenses spontaneously to unbind in the morning after wakening. Greater attention should be given in aftercare to identifying those patients with persistent binding. The use of artificial lubricants and the lens-loosening procedure, as detailed in Chapter 10, should be actively encouraged, as well as self-monitoring of lens adherence before removal.

Generally, those patients with substandard tears tend to show a higher level of deposition on RGP lenses with time. Given that deposits on the back surface of RGLs fitted for orthokeratology seem to cause a greater degree of corneal insult than those on conventional lenses, it is wise to ask patients demonstrating increased deposition to attend frequently for in-office inspection and cleaning. The authors find that Progent (Menicon Co. Ltd) is particularly useful at removing protein films. In addition, cleaners containing polymeric beads tend to be more effective at loosening adherent deposits and are advised for daily patient use.

Three and 9 o'clock staining with existing RGP lenses This relatively common complication of conventional RGP lens wear has not been observed by the authors in overnight RGL wear with removal of lenses on wakening. RGP lenses are remarkably comfortable with the eyes closed and this type of desiccation stain simply does not seem to occur, perhaps because there is no problem in resurfacing the tear film when the eyes are closed.

Additionally, it appears to be relatively uncommon in daytime users of the lenses, possibly because of the larger diameter than conventional lenses. Thus, it is unlikely to be a significant problem, particularly with night therapy. However, patients who are RGP lens failures on the grounds of unresolvable 3 and 9 o'clock stain should be warned that this may still be a problem if daytime wear of orthokeratology lenses is required. However, this should not preclude scheduling a trial wearing period.

Psychological

Perhaps more important than any other factor is patient motivation. It is vital that patients understand what orthokeratology is about, how it works, what their responsibility is, and that it is reversible. This last point is crucial. Time and time again one needs to reinforce the message that this is a reversible technique. This is comforting to the patient worried about the irreversible complications of refractive surgery, but is a source of discontent to some people. The authors have encountered several patients who, despite clear verbal and written advice about the complete reversibility of orthokeratology, still ask when they can stop wearing the lenses. Having written advice is important for a variety of reasons, but it is particularly useful to remind patients that they have been informed about what they may regard as a disadvantage of the technique. A patient information pamphlet and consent form are shown in Figures 5.19 and 5.20.

There are certainly patients seeking a non-existent "holy grail" treatment, who want perfect vision with minimum effort and expense. They must receive clear and detailed advice about the pros and cons of current orthokeratology techniques. Some of the extravagant claims made for orthokeratology and expounded on the internet and elsewhere make it doubly important that practitioners retain their integrity and advise the patient properly.

Patients may be motivated to undergo orthokeratology for a variety of reasons. They may have difficulties with existing contact lens modalities due to 3 and 9 o'clock staining and foreign-body problems with rigid lenses or corneal desiccation and lens awareness with hydrophilic lenses. They may wish to benefit from the considerable evidence for some degree of myopia control with rigid lenses (Stone 1976, Perrigin et al 1990). This is particularly the case for the young patient. As will be detailed later, night therapy is particularly suited to the child patient, since parents can directly supervise lens wear and there is no risk of lost lenses. There may be an occupational need for an improvement in unaided VA or a reduction in myopia below a certain level, as discussed above.

There are also a considerable number of patients who feel that, by remodeling their cornea and being free of optical aids for all or most of their waking hours, they are doing something positive about their visual defect. Providing they appreciate that orthokeratology is not a "cure," then this is a good motivating factor and should not be discouraged. Those practitioners who are not myopic may not always appreciate the degree of "disability" which myopes feel. It is this that drives their interest in refractive surgery as well as the desire to be "normal."

Additionally, patients with a history of poor compliance in previous contact lens wear are unsuitable for orthokeratology, particularly night therapy. The inability to care for lenses properly and attend for aftercare exposes the patient and practitioner to risk. At the very least, such a patient should be forced to earn the right to overnight orthokeratology by demonstrating a good response to daytime wear and showing that they will attend for follow-up and care for lenses correctly. If there is any doubt in the practitioner's mind, then it is better to err on the side of caution and not fit the patient.

Finally there are those patients who exhibit a total inability to remain still during topography. The results will always show large variations, and a high standard deviation in repeatability. This is particularly true for children when a small Placido instrument is being used. The invasion of personal space by the instrument makes them anxious and mobile, resulting in inaccurate topography data (Chui & Cho 2002). The poor-quality topographic data with low reliability mean that the procedure will be fraught with difficulties and this should be seen as a relative contraindication.

DISCUSSION OF MODE OF WEAR, DAY OR NIGHT THERAPY

For most patients, the prospect of being free of all optical aids during waking hours makes overnight wear, or night therapy, very attractive. A practitioner who has never fitted RGP lenses for extended wear may be reluctant to offer the overnight-wear modality. However, all clinical experience to date indicates that extended wear of high-Dk RGP lenses produces far less corneal compromise than current-generation hydrophilic extended lens wear. High-Dk RGP materials are sufficiently permeable to meet the criteria set by Holden et al (1984) for safe extended wear, viz. an equivalent oxygen percentage (EOP) of 10%. The incidence of microbial keratitis has been shown to be half that of extended-wear soft contact lenses (Benjamin 1992).

It should be remembered that normal overnight corneal swelling is of the order of 3–4% (Mandell & Fatt 1965, Mertz 1980). In addition, subjectively graded limbal hyperemia, an index of corneal hypoxia, is increased in soft extended wear (Holden et al 1986). The recovery from the modest levels of edema after RGP overnight wear is also more rapid than for soft lens wear. This of course has been measured with lenses in situ –

presumably it must be even more rapid when the lens has been removed on rising. Thus the practitioner unaccustomed to RGP extended wear may well be pleasantly surprised by the minimal degree of corneal physiological embarrassment induced. By the time the practitioner can first examine the patient (perhaps 1 h after waking) there should be no corneal striae or other sign of metabolic stress, nor any more than grade 1 corneal staining (CCLRU scale).

In essence, night therapy is the ideal form of orthokeratology. Lens wear occurs in a stable, regulated environment. This is particularly important where children are concerned. Parents can monitor lens usage, including insertion, removal, cleaning, and storage. Perhaps even more importantly, they can monitor the ocular response (in terms of hyperemia, discharge, etc.). There are few worries about loss or damage occurring outside the family home. Additionally, RGP lenses are remarkably comfortable when the eyes are closed. Contact with the lid margins is greatly reduced and little lens movement occurs. There are no foreign-body problems. Additionally, 3 and 9 o'clock stain is simply never observed in overnight orthokeratology. Thus the initial experience of RGP lenses can occur as an overnight trial, which will be more comfortable for the patient than a daytime trial.

The main disadvantage of night therapy is that, if patients are to be truly free of any optical aids during their waking hours, they must have the appropriate prefitting refractive error and corneal eccentricity. However, this rigid relation between eccentricity and refractive error does not hold for the DRGL designs, where more control of the corneal response can be made. In addition, a small but significant extra demand is placed on the eye's ability to cope with metabolic stress, which requires careful monitoring. The advantages and disadvantages of night therapy are summarized in Table 5.1.

There are many orthokeratologists in the world for whom daytime wear of RGLs is their only or preferred mode of treatment. They may be concerned about the reported problems with extended wear of soft contact lenses (Dart 1986, McLaughlin et al 1989, Benjamin 1992) and asso-

Table 5.1 Advantages and disadvantages of night therapy

Advantages	Disadvantages
Complete freedom from optical aids during the day	Requires appropriate refractive error and eccentricity to ensure adequate visual result
High levels of comfort	
No 3 and 9 o'clock stain	
Parental monitoring of lens usage is easy	Binding can be a problem
Less lens loss	More potential for rare but serious complications
No need for adaptation: immediate overnight trial is possible	Lens materials are more expensive
Faster results with possibly longer retention time	Quality of fitting is more crucial to ensure optimum visual result for waking hours

ciate these with RGP lenses or just feel uncomfortable with the idea of overnight wear per se. In daytime therapy, the patient has an initial 6-h trial during waking hours. Providing patients show the correct topographic response, they are allowed to increase their usage of the lens to all-day wear. The main obstacle to immediate all-day usage of the lens appears to be the lid sensitivity rather than the need for corneal adaptation to the reduced oxygen tension.

Additionally, some patients may be delighted by wearing a comfortable RGP lens which, when removed during the day, renders them substantially less myopic. It is worth considering the case of a –5.00 myope who on removal of conventional contact lenses has no functional vision, but on removal of an orthokeratology lens will have perhaps 6/12 acuity and reasonable functional vision. Once again, it is worth letting the patient decide.

The general approach in day therapy is to get the patient to wear the lens all waking hours until the unaided VA and refractive outcome have plateaued or, in other words, have reached a stable endpoint. Lens usage is then reduced to the minimum that will maintain this outcome at the end of the day. This will typically mean that the patient wears the lens for at least 4–6 h per day. Obviously, the higher the initial refractive error, the less likely it is that patients will be able to tolerate the uncorrected residual refractive error. There is no evidence that any greater reduction in refractive error occurs with daytime usage of RGLs than nighttime – in fact, anecdotally the reverse seems to be true.

There is a divergence of views amongst practitioners as to whether the final pair of reverse geometry orthokeratology lenses needs to be ultimately replaced by "retainer" lenses, or whether they form the retainer lenses themselves. In general, the advocates of the special retainer lens viewpoint maintain that long-term wear of large-diameter reverse geometry is not ideal. They feel that the lack of movement and possible potential for binding mean that it is preferable to refit the altered corneal profile with a small total diameter, but with a bigger optic zone to reduce flare. On the other hand, advocates of the opposite view, which is held by the authors, maintain that if an RGL is producing a good topographical outcome, the patient is comfortable and the corneal health maintained, why change to another lens?

There is an absolute paucity of studies concerning this area in the literature. In the circumstances, the authors feel that providing the topographic outcome is as desired and the cornea is in no way compromised, there is no logical reason for changing the lens fit. Indeed, to alter a successful RGL design by changing to a conventional design, increasing the optic zone diameter and retaining the same base curve, as suggested by Winkler & Kame (1995), must surely compromise the fitting. Theoretically, this will result in a much steeper central fit. It is difficult to believe that the new corneal profile will be maintained if such a dramatic change in the overlying lens is made.

To summarize, the classification of good orthokeratology candidates is as follows:

1. a refractive error change prediction that is within acceptable limits
2. those patients who experience dryness or discomfort with conventional contact lenses
3. those engaged in sport who find existing contact lenses inconvenient or uncomfortable

4. patients who need to meet specific occupational vision standards
5. those wishing to be free from optical aids during the day
6. low "bowtie" with-the-rule astigmats where the sphere exceeds the cylinder (maximum cylinder of 1.50 D)
7. predicted TxZ diameter is greater than the pupil diameter in dim illumination
8. normal corneal topography
9. no other contraindication to lens wear, be it refractive, anatomical, physiological, or psychological.

Additionally, prospective patients must exhibit a favorable outcome to an overnight wear trial. Such trials are crucial in ensuring that only patients who show the appropriate topographical and physiological responses enter into a treatment program. The matter of trials and trial lens fitting is addressed in the next chapter.

PATIENT INFORMATION

Most orthokeratology practitioners like to provide prospective patients with unbiased information, in written form, which sets out the basis of orthokeratology therapy. The pamphlet will typically include information on:

- what types of refractive error are amenable to treatment
- how orthokeratology seems to work
- what the typical visit schedule might be
- what takes place at each visit
- why an overnight or daytime trial is recommended
- what the costs of orthokeratology are and how payments are phased
- why orthokeratology is more expensive than conventional contact lenses (at least in the short term)
- what the advantages and disadvantages of orthokeratology are compared to refractive surgery and conventional contact lenses.

Figure 5.19 shows the information leaflet of one of the authors.

A GUIDE TO ORTHOKERATOLOGY

Mr. Expert Practitioner
BSc FCOptom DipCLP FAAO

What Is Orthokeratology?

Orthokeratology, or Orthok, involves use of specially designed rigid gas-permeable (RGP) contact lenses to alter the shape of the cornea in order to reduce or correct myopia (short-sight). It can also be effective with low degrees of certain types of astigmatism (when the front of the eye is rugby ball shaped). It has been practised in the United States for many years, but hitherto the results have been disappointing, with a variable and often minor degree of reduction in the degree of myopia. However, in the last 10 years new technology has become available to accurately scan the cornea and manufacture lenses that will achieve a controlled and precise reduction in the eye's optical imperfection. In addition new developments in lens materials have been made that enable safe overnight wear to be possible. The technique of Orthok is now a safe, viable and reversible alternative to refractive surgery. The cornea, whilst being mouldable, always returns to its original shape if lens wear is stopped. For this reason lenses are always worn nightly, alternate nights or 4-5 hours each day after the ideal corneal shape has been achieved in order to retain the effect.

Why Have Orthok Done?

The main purpose of Orthok is to be free of both contact lenses and spectacles for the majority of, or more typically, all waking hours. The freedom from any artificial aid appeals to myopic spectacle and contact lens wearers and is ideal for sportsmen, those who work in dusty or dirty environments or people who find spectacles and conventional contact lenses inconvenient. In addition, those who need to have a certain degree of uncorrected vision to satisfy their employers or a licensing body (e.g. pilots, police) can also be helped by Orthok. Most patients wear the lenses overnight and remove them on awakening, although some patients wear them solely during the day.

Possibly one of the ideal situations for using Orthok is for the child or teenager with early myopia. Not only does it have all the advantages already given above, but the procedure appears to retard the progression of the myopia (this has not yet been scientifically proven).

Is Everyone Suitable for Orthok?

No. The procedure works best up to a maximum of 4.00 dioptres of myopia and 2.00 dioptres of regular astigmatism. Errors above this may be reduced but total correction is not usually possible. In addition there are several unknown factors for each individual; the complexity of the corneal shape and the response of the cornea itself. Thus the speed of corneal moulding from one individual to the next will vary. Whilst the success rate is very high, total success cannot be guaranteed due to these factors.

What Does The Initial Visit Involve?

The initial assessment appointment includes a full eye examination and computerised corneal topographical scanning. This gives the practitioner a chance to assess both the general condition and health of the eyes and also to determine the likely effect of the procedure in that individual. Orthok contact lenses, made from highly oxygen permeable rigid material, are then fitted using the results of corneal scan to gently reshape the cornea towards less curvature and a more spherical shape. These will be worn for an initial trial and the response evaluated. This will typically take place overnight with a review the next morning. The effect should be a reduction of the myopia and astigmatism with improvement in the unaided eyesight. The corneal health will be carefully evaluated to ensure that it is not compromised. Only when the patient demonstrates an excellent response to the orthokeratology trial will the treatment programme commence.

What Does The Treatment Involve?

Once a patient has shown the appropriate response to a trial, they will start to wear lenses on a regular basis, typically overnight. For the first two to four weeks the vision may not be sufficiently good for all day-to-day activities. In these circumstances daily disposable soft lenses will be worn. After the first month, excellent vision and comfort are normally maintained whilst wearing orthok lenses. Occasionally more than one set of lenses are required to effect the desired change.

As most of the visual changes occur rapidly in the first few weeks, fairly frequent examinations and possible lens changes need to take place then. Stabilisation procedures then follow at a slower pace over the next few weeks. The programme length varies between 1 and 2 months depending upon the degree of visual error. The fees for orthokeratology treatment include all visits in the first year.

The final wearing time depends on many variables, but the treatment aim is good unaided vision all or most waking hours, with lenses being worn overnight or part of each day only. Some patients will be able to wear their lenses every second night.

Figure 5.19   Patient information leaflet.

Does Orthok Have Any Advantages Over Laser Surgery (Lasik)?

Yes
- No ethical surgeon will treat a patient until they are at least 18, or more usually 21 years old.
- It does not cause the permanent hazy vision experienced by some patients following laser surgery.
- Changes in prescription over time can be dealt with without further surgery.
- The procedure is REVERSIBLE (Lasik is not!).
- There is very significant understanding of the effects of contact lens wear on the cornea, because of the many years of lens use. Lasik's effects are not totally understood.
- There is no post-operative pain or recovery period.
- Orthok is significantly cheaper and does not preclude surgery in the future.

Cost.

The procedure is time consuming and may involve several lens changes. For this reason the initial costs are greater than conventional contact lens correction but less than refractive surgery. Once the treatment is complete, the on-going costs are significantly less than the latest options in soft contact lens wear, since the lens life may be up to two years. The current charges are £105 for the initial consultation and trial and £695 in staged payments for the rest of the treatment making £800 in all.

What Are The Advantages of Orthok?

- Good vision without spectacles or contact lenses for most of the day.
- It is not a surgical procedure.
- It is reversible.
- It is modifiable.
- It does not hurt.
- It may slow down the increase in myopia in children.
- Using well established contact lens fitting techniques mean that there are very few risks

What Are The Disadvantages of Orthok?

- You must be prepared to allow for 4-6 visits over 3-6 months.
- Continued lens wear is essential or the cornea will revert to its original shape.
- The degree of success is high but cannot always be guaranteed.
- The speed of reduction in the myopia varies from one person to the next.
- You must follow instructions implicitly for the best results.

Figure 5.19   *Contd.*

INFORMED CONSENT

It is now generally acknowledged that practitioners need to ensure that contact lens wear is an elective procedure and that all patients read and sign some form of consent prior to fitting. This is particularly important when overnight wear is being considered, since this is not a modality of lens wear generally employed in conventional contact lens practice. The statement of informed consent should include:

- the differences between orthokeratology and conventional lens fitting
- the relative risks of daily, overnight and continuous RGP lens wear
- how to recognize an adverse response
- what to do in the event of an adverse response
- an out-of-hours telephone number to contact the orthokeratology practitioner in an emergency (a pager is recommended here)
- a schedule of fees.

The informed consent form used by one of the authors is shown in Figure 5.20.

Whilst such an approach is not obligatory, it is most important that patients have a clear understanding of the costs of orthokeratology from the outset and what to do if something goes wrong. Having a statement formalizes this and helps prevent any misunderstanding later on.

London Orthokeratology Centre
12 Bloom Street
London SW1 4NL
020 7254 6789

Orthokeratology Agreement and Informed Consent

I have read the document 'All about Orthokeratology' and understand that the treatment programme requires that I wear specially designed rigid gas-permeable contact lenses either overnight or during the day to alter the shape of my corneas. The change in corneal shape should lead to a significant improvement in my unaided vision. The lenses differ from conventional rigid lenses in that they are designed to trap a specially shaped layer of tears that bring about the shape change, whereas conventional lenses have a uniform layer of tears behind them that does not change the shape of the cornea.

The likely outcome has been explained to me by my practitioner Dr _____ and if this takes place I feel that I am likely to find the outcome satisfactory. I understand that this cannot be guaranteed and that if it is not acceptable to me then the treatment can be discontinued and my cornea will return to its pre-treatment shape within 1-3 weeks and conventional means of correction such as soft lenses or spectacles can be employed once again.

I understand that orthokeratology is a totally reversible procedure and that the use of the contact lens must be continued indefinitely to retain the effect. I confirm that I will follow my practitioner's guidance on lens wear to ensure the optimum outcome and attend for follow-up examinations as advised.

Risks of the treatment

Contact lenses have been used for orthokeratology since the early 1960's and controlled scientific studies have not documented any harmful health risks to the eyes. However, with all contact lenses, whether they are worn overnight or during the day, there are potential risks of transient irritation to the eyes whether caused by allergy, reduction in oxygen access or mechanical stimulation. These effects will ease on lens removal and are not sight threatening. The only sight threatening potential complication is corneal infection and ulceration which occurs at a very low rate in rigid contact lens wearers of approximately 1-5 cases per 10 000 wearers. In the rare situation where a corneal infection does occur then providing prompt medical attention takes place any loss of vision is rare. Day-time wear and overnight wear therapies have received FDA approval in the United States.

Fee Schedule

Initial consultation:	Includes comprehensive internal and external ophthalmic examination to evaluate refractive status, state of ocular health, suitability for procedure, advice on alternatives, corneal topography measurement and determination of diagnostic lens parameters. Cost: £120 payable after examination.
Diagnostic lens trial:	An evaluation of the refractive changes and corneal topographic changes that occur following either an overnight wearing period or wear over 4-5 hours during the day. If successful treatment lenses will be ordered. Cost: £90 payable after examination.
Treatment programme:	Several visits will be scheduled during the six month programme. These will be individually set, but will occur approximately one week after lens issue and then one month, three months and six months after lens issue. Any further visits in this time will not lead to further fees being charged. Cost: £400 half to be paid at one month visit remainder at three month visit
Materials:	A pair of hyper oxygen permeable Orthokeratology lenses will be charged for at the start of the treatment programme. If refitting for clinical reasons is required during the first six months no further charges for materials will be made. Cost £190 per pair. Payable at time of supply.
Total cost:	£800

Figure 5.20   Informed consent form.

Future costs:	Six monthly review appointments will be required during which lens condition and performance will be evaluated, corneal topography measured and full review of internal and external ocular health. Cost: £90 payable at time of appointment Lens life is variable but annual replacement is prudent. Replacement and spare lenses supplied though practice replacement plan (premium £46 per year) cost £65 each
Refund Policy:	Should the treatment be discontinued by either the patient or the practitioner for any reason on or before the one month visit then the patient will pay only the initial examination and diagnostic trial costs providing the lenses are returned to the practice. Should discontinuation occur on or before the three month visit then the patient will be asked to pay half of the treatment programme costs (£200) in addition to the initial and diagnostic trial fees, providing the lenses are returned to the practice.

I have had the opportunity to discuss the treatment and costs with my practitioner and ask any questions that I may have had. I understand the possible risks of treatment and that the outcome cannot be guaranteed. I agree to follow the treatment plan and comply with the advice given to me, including caring for the lenses correctly. I understand that my practitioner will ensure that the result I obtain is the best possible and that I should always communicate any concerns, complications or difficulties arising from the treatment to my practitioner at the earliest opportunity. In the event of any pain, redness or discharge from my eyes I agree to immediately remove the lenses and contact my practitioner immediately on 020 7254 6789. In the event that he or she is unavailable then I will ring the out of hours number 020 7254 9999.

Name:

Practitioner:

Address:

Signature:

Date:

If patient is under 18 years old, then parent or guardian should sign below:

Signature parent / guardian:

Relationship to minor:

Signature witness:

Date:

Figure 5.20 *Contd.*

REFERENCES

Applegate R A, Gansel K (1991) The importance of pupil size in optical quality measurements following radial keratotomy. Optometry and Vision Science 68: 584–590

Benjamin W (1992) Risks and incidences of ulcerative keratitis. Journal of the British Contact Lens Association 15: 143–144

Binder P S, May C H, Grant S C (1980) An evaluation of orthokeratology. Ophthalmology 87: 729–744

Carney L G, Mainstone J C, Carkeet A, Hill R M (1997) Rigid lens dynamics: lid effects. CLAO Journal 23(1): 69–77

Cho P, Cheung S W, Edwards M, Fung J (2002) Orthokeratology in Hong Kong: a practice-based report (in press).

Chui W S, Cho P (2002) A comparative study of the performance of different corneal topographers on children with respect to orthokeratology practice. Optometry and Vision Science (in press).

Dart J K G (1986) Complications of extended wear contact lenses. Contax March: 11–19

Davidorf J M (1998) Pupil size and refractive surgery. Letters. Journal of Cataract and Refractive Surgery 24: 291–292

Day J, Reim T, Bard R D, McGonagill P, Gambino M J (1997) Advanced ortho-k using custom lens designs. Contact Lens Spectrum 12(6): 34–40

Douthwaite W A, Hough T, Edwards K, Notay H (1999) The EyeSys videokeratoscope assessment of apical radius and P-value in the normal human cornea. Ophthalmic and Physiological Optics 19(6): 467–474

Dumbleton K, Chalmers R, Richter D, Fonn D (1999) Changes in myopic refractive error with nine months extended wear of hydrogel lenses with high and low oxygen permeability. Optometry and Vision Science 76(12): 845–849

El Hage S G, Leach N E, Shahin R (1999) Controlled kerato-reformation (CKR): an alternative to refractive surgery. Practical Optometry 10(6): 230–235

Ericson P, Thorn F (1977) Does refractive error change twice as fast as corneal power in orthokeratology? American Journal of Optometry and Physiological Optics 54: 581–587

Guillon M, Lydon D P M, Wilson C (1986) Corneal topography: a clinical model. Ophthalmic and Physiological Optics 6: 47–56

Harris M G, Blevins R J and Heiden S (1973) Evaluation of the procedures for the management of spectacle blur. American Journal of Optometry 50: 293–298

Hile D, Marsden H (2001) The relationship of pupil size to visual performance in orthokeratology patients. Optometry and Vision Science 78: 12s

Holden B A, Sweeney D F, Sanderson G (1984) The minimum precorneal oxygen tension to avoid corneal oedema. Investigative Ophthalmology and Visual Science 25: 476–480

Holden B A, Sweeney D F, Swarbrick H A, Vannas A, Nilsson K T, Efron N (1986) The vascular response to long-term extended contact lens wear. Clinical and Experimental Optometry 69: 112–119

Holden B, Sankaridurg P, Jalbert I (2000) Adverse events and infections: which ones and how many? In: Sweeney D (ed.) Silicone hydrogels: the rebirth of continuous wear contact lenses. Oxford, Butterworth-Heinemann, pp. 150–213

Jalbert I, Willcox M D, Sweeney D F (2000) Isolation of *Staphylococcus aureus* from a contact lens at the time of a contact lens-induced peripheral ulcer: case report. Cornea 19(1): 116–120

Joe J J, Marsden H J, Edrington T B (1996) The relationship between corneal eccentricity and improvement in visual acuity with orthokeratology. Journal of the American Optometric Association 67: 87–97

Kerns R (1976) Research in orthokeratology, part 3. Journal of the American Optometric Association 47: 1505–1515

Korb D R, Finnemore V M, Herman J P (1982) Apical changes and scarring in keratoconus as related to contact lens fitting techniques. Journal of the American Optometric Association 53: 199–205

Lohman C P, Fitzke F W, O'Bart D O et al (1993) Halos, a problem for all myopes? A comparison between spectacles, contact lenses and PRK. Journal of Cataract and Refractive Surgery 9(suppl.): 572–575

Lui W O, Edwards M H (2000) Orthokeratology in low myopia. Part 2: Corneal topographic changes and safety over 100 days. Contact Lens and Anterior Eye 23(3): 90–99

Mandell R, Fatt I (1965) Thinning of the human cornea on awakening. Nature 208: 292

McLaughlin R, Kelley C G, Mauger T F (1989) Corneal ulceration associated with disposable EW lenses. Contact Lens Spectrum 4: 57–58

McMonnies C W (1987) Contact lens after-care: a detailed analysis. Clinical and Experimental Optometry 70: 121–127.

Mertz G W (1980) Overnight swelling of the living human cornea. Journal of the American Optometric Association 51: 211–215

Mountford J A (1997a) Orthokeratology. In: Phillips A J, Speedwell L (eds) Contact lenses: a textbook for students and practitioners. London, Butterworth-Heinemann, pp. 653–692

Mountford J (1997b) An analysis of the changes in corneal shape and refractive error induced by accelerated orthokeratology. International Contact Lens Clinic 24: 128–143

Mountford J A (1998) Retention and regression of orthokeratology with time. International Contact Lens Clinic 25: 60–64

Mountford J A, Noack D B (1998) A mathematical model of the corneal shape changes associated with ortho-K. Contact Lens Spectrum 13(7): 34–40

Mountford J A, Pesudovs K (2002) An analysis of the changes in astigmatism with accelerated orthokeratology. Clinical and Experimental Optometry 85(5): 284–293

Mountford J A, Caroline P, Noack D (2002) Corneal topography and orthokeratology. Contact Lens Spectrum 17: 4

Nichols J J, Marsich M M, Nguyen M, Barr J T, Bullimore M A (2000) Overnight orthokeratology. Optometry and Vision Science 77(5): 252–259

Perrigin D, Perrigan J, Quintero S, Grosvenor T (1990) Silicone-acrylate contact lenses for myopia control: 3 year results. Optometry and Vision Science 67(10): 764–769

Pop M (1996) The complicated laser: large pupils cause a devilish problem; haloes. Eye World Nov: 46–47

Pritchard N, Fonn D (1995) Dehydration, lens movement and dryness ratings of hydrogel contact lenses. Ophthalmic Physiological Optics 15(4): 40–47

Rengstorff R H (1965) The Fort Dix report. American Journal of Optometry 42: 156–163

Rengstorff R H (1967) Variations in myopia measurements: an after effect observed with habitual wearers of contact lenses. American Journal of Optometry 44: 149–161

Rengstorff R H (1970a) Overnight decreases in myopia. South African Optometrist 27(16): 18–22

Rengstorff R H (1970b) Diurnal variations in myopia measurements after wearing contact lenses. American Journal of Optometry 47: 812–815

Rivera R K, Polse K A (1991) Corneal response to different oxygen levels during extended wear. CLAO Journal 17: 96–101

Saks S J (1966) Fluctuations in refractive state in adapting and long-term contact lens wearers. Journal of American Optometric Association 37: 229–238

Soni P S, Horner D J (1993) Orthokeratology. In: Bennett E, Wisemann B (eds) Clinical contact lens practice. Philadelphia, JP Lippincott, ch. 49

Stone J (1976) The possible influence of contact lenses on myopia. British Journal of Physiology and Optics 31: 89–114

Swarbrick H, Alharbi A (2001) Overnight orthokeratology induces central corneal epithelial thinning. Investigative Opthalmology and Visual Science 42(4): S597

Swarbrick H A, Wong G, O'Leary D J (1998) Corneal response to orthokeratology. Optometry and Vision Science 75(11): 791–799

Willcox M, Sankaridurg P, Lan J, Pearce D, Thakur A, Zhu H, Keay L, Stapleton F (2000) Inflammation and infection and the effects of the closed eye. In: Sweeney D (ed.) Silicone hydrogels. The rebirth of continuous wear contact lenses. Oxford, Butterworth-Heinemann, pp. 45–75

Wilms K H, Rabbetts R B (1977) Practical concepts of corneal topography. Optician 174(4502): 7–13

Winkler T D, Kame R T (1995) Orthokeratology handbook. Newton, MA, USA, Butterworth-Heinemann, pp. 31–32

Wlodyga R, Harris D (1993) Accelerated orthokeratology. Techniques and procedures manual. Part 1. Chicago, National Eye Research Foundation, pp. 1–7

Woodward E G (1980) Keratoconus: the disease and its progression. Doctoral thesis. City University, London

Young G, Port M (1992) Rigid gas-permeable extended wear: a comparative clinical study. American Journal of Optometry 69: 214–226

Chapter **6**

Trial lens fitting

John Mountford

CHAPTER CONTENTS

Introduction   139
Empirical fitting   140
Trial lens fitting   147
Trial lens sets   147
Care and maintenance of trial lenses   151
Fluorescein pattern analysis   152
Topography-based fitting   158
How to use the topography data   161
Assessing the post-trial topography   162
Other postwear results   168
Refining the fit using postwear topography
   data   171
References   173

INTRODUCTION

Having selected a prospective patient as being suitable for an orthokeratology trial on the basis of the tests detailed in Chapter 5, the practitioner will need to fit appropriate trial lenses and schedule the trial.

At present three approaches appear to be adopted with respect to orthokeratology lens fitting. These are based on empirical, trial lens, or corneal response data.

Empirical fitting consists of supplying the manufacturer with either the keratometry readings or topography data and the refractive change required and fitting the supplied lens. Empirically fitted lenses include the Reversible Corneal Therapy (RCT) lens from ABBA Optical, Correctech, Dreimlens, Euclid Systems Emerald and Jade designs, WAVE lenses, Contex, and others.

Trial lens fitting consists of taking corneal measurements, either *K* readings or topography, and using nomograms to choose the initial trial lens. The fit of the lens is then assessed by fluorescein pattern analysis, overrefraction is performed, and the required lens is ordered. Lenses that are designed using trial lens fitting are the Dreimlens, Fargo, Contex, Gelflex EZM, Paragon CRT, R&R design, Metro Optics Orthofocus, and the BE lens.

Corneal response fitting is based purely on accurate prefit topography data in order to determine a suitable trial lens, with the corneal response to the trial lens following overnight or a period of daytime wear used to determine the prescription lens. At present, the only lens-fitting systems based solely on this technique are the BE and EZM designs.

It is generally acknowledged that fitting orthokeratology lenses is fairly complex and requires a high degree of accuracy and skill. The assessment of the three techniques will be considered with this in mind.

EMPIRICAL FITTING

Maruna et al (1989) found that approximately 50% of all contact lens practitioners order rigid gas-permeable (RGP) lenses empirically, i.e., with no trial lens fitting. The difference in success rates between empirical and trial lens fitting was studied by Bennett et al (1989), with results that are especially relevant to orthokeratology fitting. They found a much higher first-fit success rate with trial lens fitting, with the reorder rate for empirically fitted lenses being twice that of the trial lens group. Bennett & Sorbara (2000) make the following strong recommendations to practitioners who prefer to fit empirically:

1. The use of the manufacturer's recommended fitting guide in combination with having a sound knowledge of lens design to make an educated decision is essential. Sufficient experience with spherical RGP fitting should be obtained initially before empirically ordering lenses. Specialty fits, including bifocal, toric and irregular cornea lens designs (*and orthokeratology?*) *should always be diagnostically fitted.* [Italics are author's.]

2. As the cornea is aspheric and complex in its topography and because it varies in shape from patient to patient, the use of videokeratography is important if empirical fitting is to be performed.

There are two major points in Bennett & Sorbara's list that require some expansion with respect to reverse geometry lens (RGL) fitting. Firstly, they recommend a thorough knowledge of the manufacturer's design, so that some logical decisions can be made in order to rectify the fit if it is not ideal. This is simply not possible with the majority of RGLs, as the reverse and alignment curves are considered by the manufacturer to be "pro-

prietary" information. If the practitioner doesn't know the curves, then the decisions as to what curves need to be modified in order to correct a problem are left to the manufacturer.

Secondly, if empirical fitting is to be carried out, then Bennett & Sorbara recommend that corneal topography is essential. This is valid assuming that the manufacturer knows anything about topography, and how to use the data to design a lens more accurately. In most cases, according to the author's experience with empirically fitted RGLs, the only topography data used by the manufacturer are the simulated K readings, thereby negating any value that the topography data may give with respect to the real corneal shape.

Guillon & Sammons (1994) place major emphasis on three factors that are essential to the lens design process: safety, comfort, and vision. Safety is measured in terms of the ability of the lens to supply adequate oxygen to the cornea, and also in the use of design criteria that limit areas of concentrated mechanical stress on the corneal surface. Comfort is determined by the fitting relationship of the lens curves to the corneal surface, as well as the quality of lens finish with respect to edge and transition blending. Vision is the product of the relationship between the lens design, tear lens power, and the patient's refractive error.

RGL fitting is even more complex due to the lens design and accuracy required for a successful outcome (Bara 2000). This therefore seems to indicate that the first-fit success rate with empirically prescribed lenses would be even lower than that achieved with standard lenses. Poorly fitting spherical lenses may, at worst, cause discomfort and irritation, but a poorly fitting RGL can cause either marked central corneal staining if fitted too flat, or, conversely, major binding if fitted too tight (see later). The increased risk of serious corneal infection from corneal staining, as demonstrated by the high incidence of problems in China (11 cases), should be of major concern to all those who try to fit orthokeratology lenses empirically (Lu et al 2001).

There are basically three methods used by manufacturers to design lenses empirically for orthokeratology.

1. The lens has standard curves, with the back optic zone radius (BOZR) fitted 1.50–2.50 D flatter than the flat-*K* (Contex OK series).
2. The BOZR is based on the basis of the change in refraction required with an allowance for an extra "compression factor" of between 0.50 and 1.00 D. If the laboratory is only supplied with *K* readings, the eccentricity is assumed to be 0.50 (Dreimlens, CRT, Correctech, Emerald, Contex BB, Fargo).
3. The results of one topography reading are sent to the lab, and a lens design based on the data is made (Euclid Jade). Alternatively, the practitioner uses a specific computer program linked directly to the topographer as an aid to lens design (WAVE).

Table 6.1 The variation in apical radius value with changing eccentricity assuming a flat-*K* value of 7.76 mm (43.50 D)

Eccentricity	Flat-*K* (R_a)	Apical radius (R_0)
0.0	7.76	7.76000
0.1	7.76	7.75855
0.2	7.76	7.754199
0.3	7.76	7.746941
0.4	7.76	7.736769
0.5	7.76	7.723671
0.6	7.76	7.707633
0.7	7.76	7.688634
0.8	7.76	7.666655
0.9	7.76	7.641669

The sag-based fitting approach, as outlined in Chapter 4, as well as the work of Bara (2000) shows the inaccuracies that can occur if the first method is used. Mountford et al (2002) have shown that basing a lens design on the flat-*K* and an assumed eccentricity of 0.5 also leads to inaccuracies. The two values needed to design a lens based on the sag philosophy are the apical radius (R_0) and the eccentricity (*e*) or elevation at the common chord of contact between the lens and the cornea. The flat-*K* is *not* equal to the apical radius. The apical radius is the instantaneous radius of curvature at the corneal apex, and contains elements of both the steep and flat meridian. Depending on the degree of corneal astigmatism, and the eccentricity of the cornea, R_0 can be significantly steeper than flat-*K*. Table 6.1 shows the difference between R_0 and flat-*K* with varying eccentricities, assuming a nonastigmatic cornea. If astigmatism is present, the difference is greater for increasing degrees of astigmatism.

If the flat-*K* is used, and the eccentricity is known, the apical radius for nonastigmatic surfaces is calculated from the following formula (Douthwaite 1995):

$$R_0 = \sqrt{R_a^2 + y^2 p - y^2}$$

where R_0 is apical radius, R_a axial radius at the nominated chord, *y* is the half-chord (1.5 mm for the keratometer), and *p* is $(1 - e^2)$.

The accuracy of the assumptions used to generate an empirical lens design simply based on the flat-*K* value and an assumed eccentricity will be examined in detail in the following example.

A practitioner sends the laboratory the following data and asks for a lens to be made. The manufacturer designs the lens on the following basis. The BOZR of the lens is assumed to be equal to the refractive change required plus an extra 0.50 D as a compression factor. The design is a four-curve lens, with a back optic zone diameter (BOZD) of 6.00 mm, a reverse curve width of 0.60 mm, an alignment curve that is 1.00 mm wide that meets the reverse curve with a tear layer thickness of 10 μm. The edge lift is a simple 10.00 mm curve 0.40 mm wide. The apical clearance of the lens is presumed to be 5 μm.

The data supplied to the lab are Flat-*K* 43.50 D, and the refractive change required –3.00 D.

Since the corneal eccentricity was not specified, the manufacturer automatically assumes that it is 0.50 for the sake of calculations. The lens would therefore have the following specifications:

BOZR = 43.50 D – 3.00 D – 0.50 D = 40.00 D = 8.43 mm

This equates to the flat-*K* minus the Rx change required (3.00 D) minus the compression factor of 0.50 D, leaving a final BOZR of 40.00 D or 8.43 mm. The exact lens specifications and the tear layer profile of the lens are shown in Figure 6.1, and are based on an assumption that flat-*K* is equal to R_0.

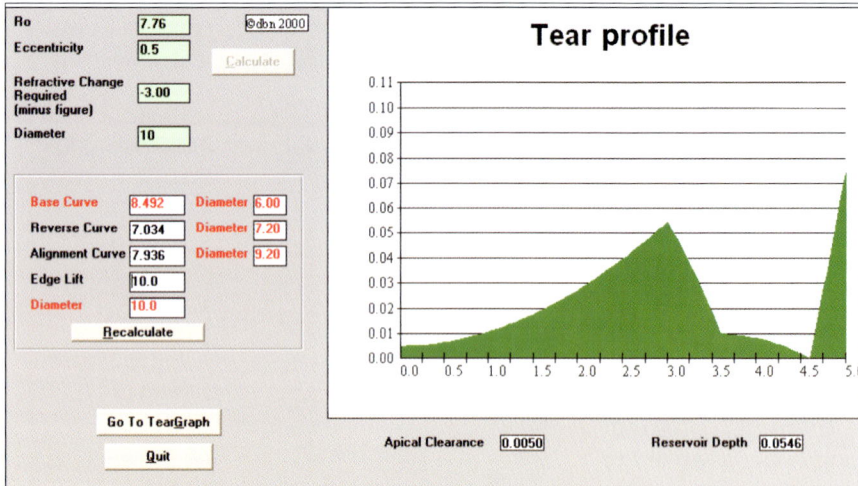

Figure 6.1   Lens parameters and tear layer profile for a lens where R_0 is assumed to be equal to flat-K.

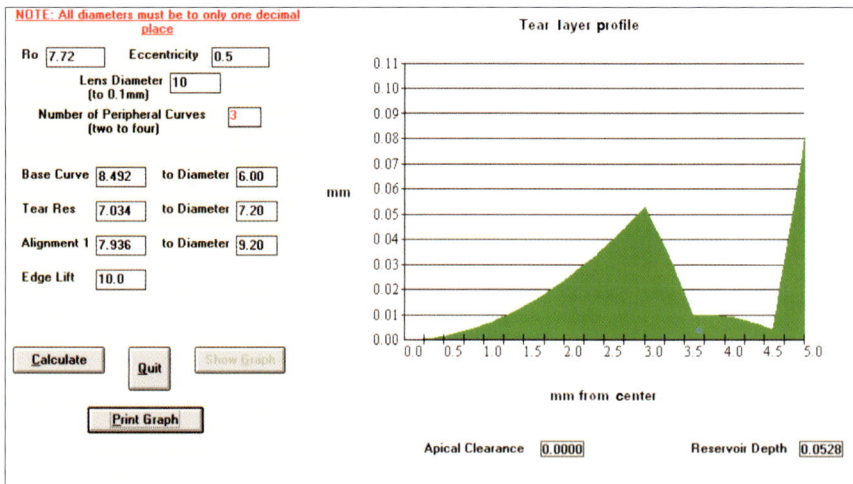

Figure 6.2   The lens calculated in the example fitted to the eye with the actual R_0 value of 7.72 mm instead of flat-K 7.76 mm. Note that the lens is too flat, with zero apical clearance, and no peripheral contact. This lens would decenter superiorly and cause a smiley-face postwear topography plot.

As can be seen from Table 6.1 R_0 is only equal to flat-K if the eccentricity is zero. The actual value for R_0 when flat-K is 7.76 mm and the eccentricity is 0.5 is 7.72 mm. If the same lens details are then fitted to the cornea with the R_0 set at 7.72 and an eccentricity of 0.5, the tear layer profile and the fit of the lens will vary. The tear layer profile of the original lens parameters on the *actual corneal shape* is shown in Figure 6.2. Note that the calculated lens parameters result in a lens that is too flat, with zero apical clearance and no peripheral touch in the alignment curve zone. This lens will commonly decenter superiorly until a tear layer under the lens is formed that causes the appropriate squeeze film and surface tension forces required for a stable fit (Hayashi 1977, Guillon & Sammons 1994).

The mean corneal eccentricity in the population is approximately 0.50, with a standard deviation of 0.15, so as a comparison in the above example, it will be assumed that the patient did not have an eccentricity of 0.5, but either 0.35 or 0.65, one standard deviation either side of the norm. The tear layer profile of the initial calculated lens on the 0.35 eccentricity cornea is shown in Figure 6.3. As with the example above, the lens design arrived at by the laboratory is too flat for the corneal shape and will decenter. In both of these cases, a smiley-face topography plot will result from wearing the lens (see later), with

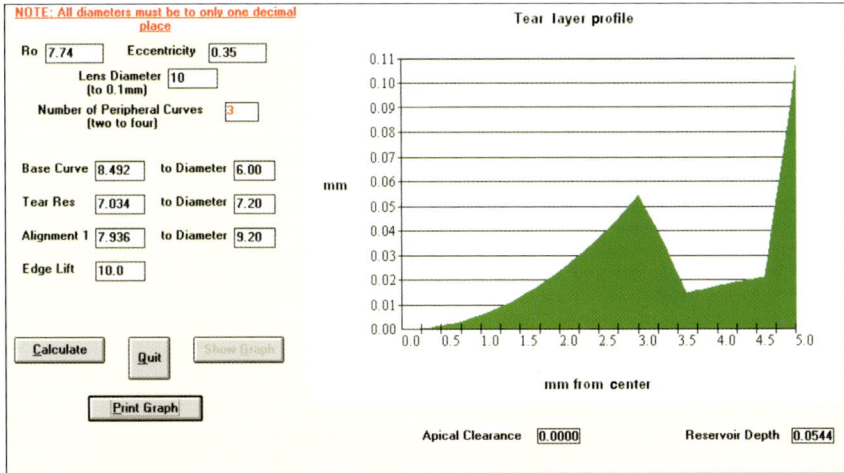

Figure 6.3   The original lens parameters fitted to a cornea with eccentricity 0.35. The R_0 of the cornea is 7.74 mm, whereas flat-K is 7.76 mm. This lens is even flatter than the last example. There is zero apical clearance, and approximately 15 µm of clearance at the alignment zone. This lens would also decenter.

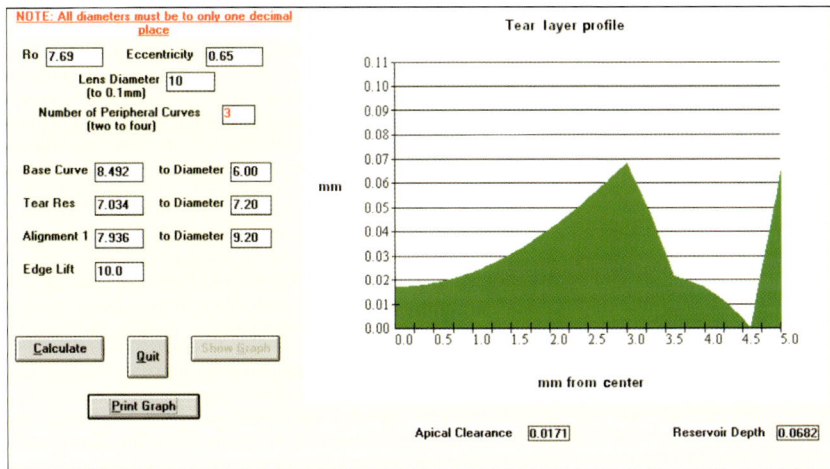

Figure 6.4   The original lens on a cornea with an eccentricity of 0.65. R_0 is now 7.69 mm. Note that the apical clearance is 17 µm, and not the required 5 µm. This lens is too steep, and will cause a "central island."

induced with-the-rule astigmatism and poor unaided acuity.

Finally, the eccentricity is assumed to be 0.65, with a resultant change of apical radius to 7.69 mm. The ordered lens on this cornea will be far too steep, with approximately 14 µm of apical clearance and a steep alignment curve (Fig. 6.4). Steep or tight lenses result in central island post-wear topography plots, with poor unaided visual acuity that is usually worse than the initial unaided visual acuity. The differences between the reverse curve and alignment curve values and those supplied by the manufacturer are shown in Table 6.2. Note that in all cases there are significant differences in the curves, and that none of the lenses are interchangeable.

If the practitioner is faced with these less than ideal responses to the lens that was sent, the only course of action is to contact the laboratory with the results and ask them to redesign the lens. The usual method of rectification with most of the empirically designed lenses is to alter the alignment curve. The alignment curve with most four-curve designs is based on the axial radius of curvature of the cornea at a chord of 4.60 mm, or the start of the alignment curve zone. The tear layer of such a lens is shown in Figure 6.5. Clinical experience showed that this curve was too flat, so the value was changed to allow for a tear layer thickness (TLT) of 10 µm at the junction of the reverse and alignment curves (Reim 2000). This, in effect, results in the alignment curve

Table 6.2 The effect of the *actual* corneal shape on the values for the reverse and alignment curves. Note that in all cases the values differ significantly from the curves used, assuming that K_f is equal to R_0 and that eccentricity is a standard 0.50

Corneal data	BOZR (6.00 mm)	Reverse curve (0.6 mm)	Alignment curve (1.0 mm)	Peripheral curve (0.4 mm)
Kf = 7.76, e = 0.5	8.492	7.034	7.936	10.00
R_0 = 7.72 e = 0.5	8.494	7.007	7.898	10.00
R_0 = 7.74 e = 0.35	8.494	6.890	7.780	10.00
R_0 = 7.69 e = 0.65	8.494	7.045	8.047	10.00

BOZR, back optic zone radius.

being approximately 0.05 mm or 0.25 D steeper than the calculated R_a. The effect this has on the tear layer profile is shown in Figure 6.6.

Luk et al (2001) cite various manufacturers' data and give the following description of the alignment curve construction. These data have already been presented in Chapter 4, but warrant repeating due to the importance in lens fitting.

- If the corneal eccentricity is between 0 and 0.3, the alignment curve should be equal to the central flat-K value.

- If the corneal eccentricity is between 0.31 and 0.55, the alignment curve should be 0.25 D flatter than the flat-K value.
- If the corneal eccentricity is between 0.56 and 0.80, the alignment curve should be 0.50 D flatter than the flat-K.

These generic values lead to gross errors, as shown in Table 6.3. Assuming a flat-K of 43.50 D, and varying eccentricities, the R_a value can be calculated at a chord of 4.60 mm. The value is then steepened by a further 0.25 D, as shown above. The resultant calculated values of the alignment curve vary dramatically with changing eccentricity.

So, what actually happens when the laboratory alters the alignment curve? In the case of the cornea with an eccentricity of 0.35 (Fig. 6.3), the advice would be that the lens was too flat, so the alignment curve would be steepened. The closest alteration is shown in Figure 6.7. This is still not an ideal situation as the depth of the tear layer at the reverse curve/alignment curve intersection is 20 μm, instead of the required 10 μm, and the alignment curve is in effect too steep. The practitioner would then try this lens, which may result in edge compression and binding, or a central island. The laboratory would be requested to alter the fit again. This time, since the alterations to the alignment curve didn't work, the reverse curve and the alignment curve would be altered. The result is shown in Figure 6.8. At this

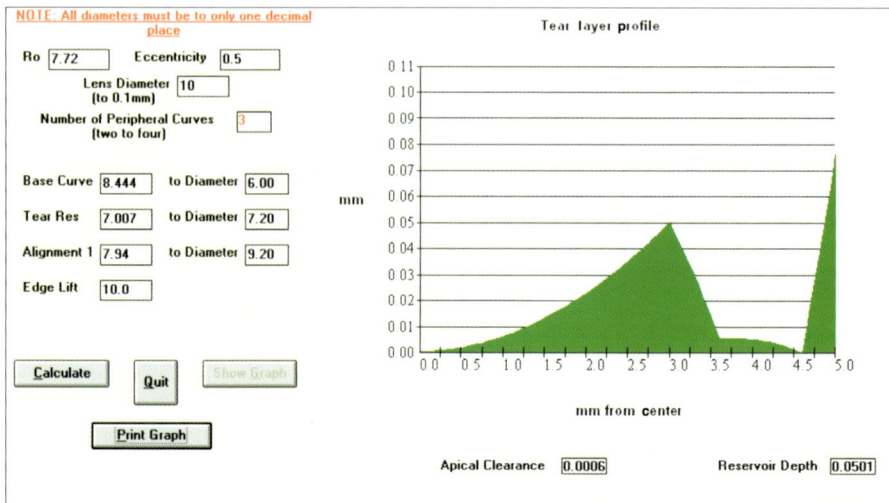

Figure 6.5 Tear layer profile of the lens when the alignment curve is equal to the apical radius at a chord of 9.20 mm. Note that the apical clearance is 0.6 μm, and that the tear layer thickness at the chord of 9.20 mm is approximately 5 μm.

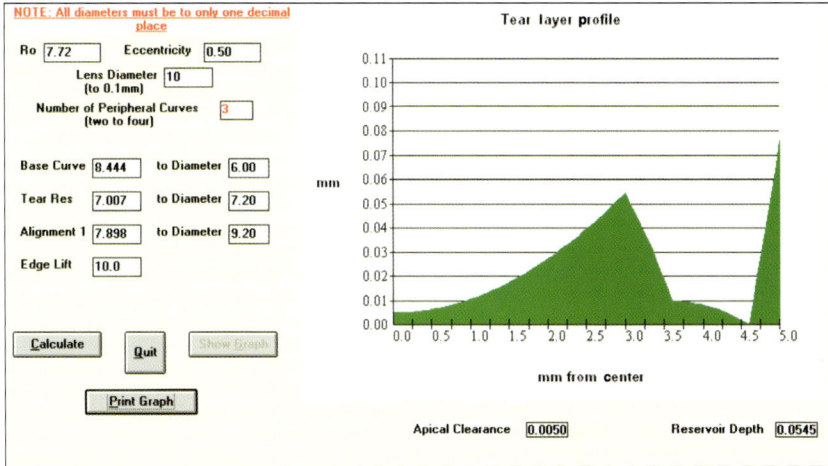

Figure 6.6   The effect of steepening the alignment curve by 0.05 mm is to increase the apical clearance to 5 μm, as well as increasing the tear layer thickness at the 7.20 mm chord to 10 μm.

Table 6.3 The flat-*K* and calculated alignment curve +0.25 D are shown. The difference between the two is shown in the third column. The values calculated from corneal data differ markedly from the generic values of the alignment curves

Flat-*K* (D)	Alignment curve (D)	Difference (D)
43.5	43.74227	0.242268
43.5	43.70004	0.200042
43.5	43.5741	0.074097
43.5	43.3666	−0.1334
43.5	43.08105	−0.41895
43.5	42.72212	−0.77788
43.5	42.29544	−1.20456
43.5	41.80739	−1.69261
43.5	41.26483	−2.23517
43.5	40.6749	−2.8251

stage, the tear layer profile is almost exactly what is required, and the final lens curves are very similar to those arrived at by calculation (Table 6.3). However, it has taken three different lenses to arrive at a lens with similar parameters to the lens based on actual corneal data.

A similar course of events would occur if the initial lens was fitted to the 0.65 eccentricity cornea. The laboratory would be advised that the lens was too tight, so the first alteration would be made by flattening the alignment curve. The result of this is shown in Figure 6.9. In this case, the alignment curve has been flattened from

7.936 mm to 8.05 mm. The usual change in alignment curve is 0.25 D at a time, so once again, three lenses would be required to arrive at the correct result that could have been achieved if the original corneal data were used. Note that in none of the cases outlined has the BOZR been altered. The entire fitting philosophy of the lens is based on a relationship between the BOZR and the refractive change required, so in effect the BOZR remains constant.

The preceding examples illustrate that empirical fitting that is based solely on keratometry data is inherently inaccurate due to the false assumptions made with respect to flat-*K* being equal to apical radius and the assumption of a mean eccentricity value of 0.50. Those practitioners who prefer empirical fitting ought to make certain that they follow the suggestions of Bennett & Sorbara (2000), in that the laboratory *must* be supplied with accurate topography data on which to base the calculations. The practitioner must also ensure that the manufacturer uses the data to design the lens, and not simply the flat-*K* values and a nominal eccentricity. Even if the lens design and fitting are based on topography (WAVE, Euclid Jade), errors are still inherent due to two main factors. Firstly, the lens fit is usually based on the data from a single topography reading, and secondly, errors due to the reconstruction algorithms used by the topographer are not taken into account. These factors will be examined in greater detail in the section on topography-based fitting (see later).

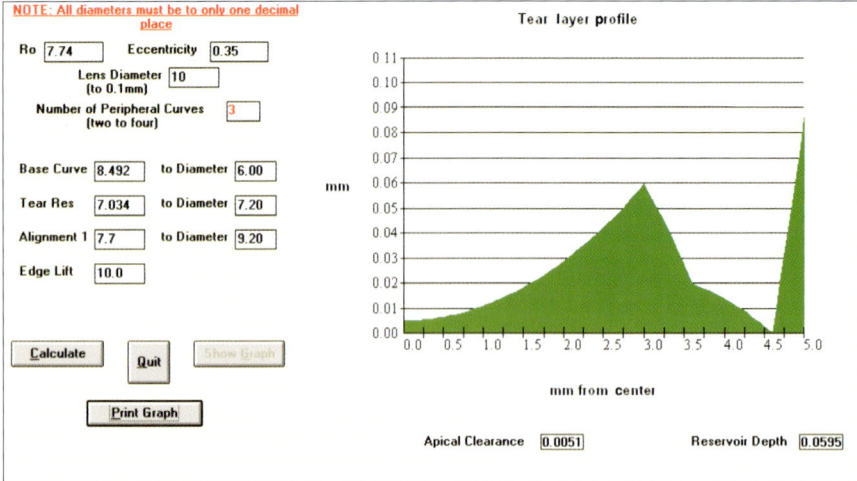

Figure 6.7 The effect of changing (steepening) the alignment curve of the lens shown in Figure 6.3 to 7.70 mm whilst keeping all the other curves constant. This is still a less than optimal fit, as the alignment curve is slightly too tight.

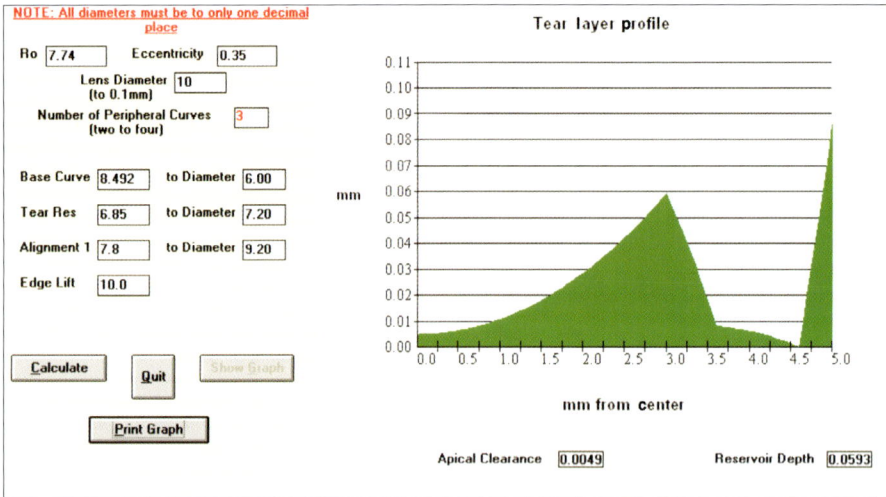

Figure 6.8 The reverse curve has now been steepened to 6.85 mm, and the alignment curve flattened to 7.80 mm. The lens is now much closer to the lens calculated from actual corneal data.

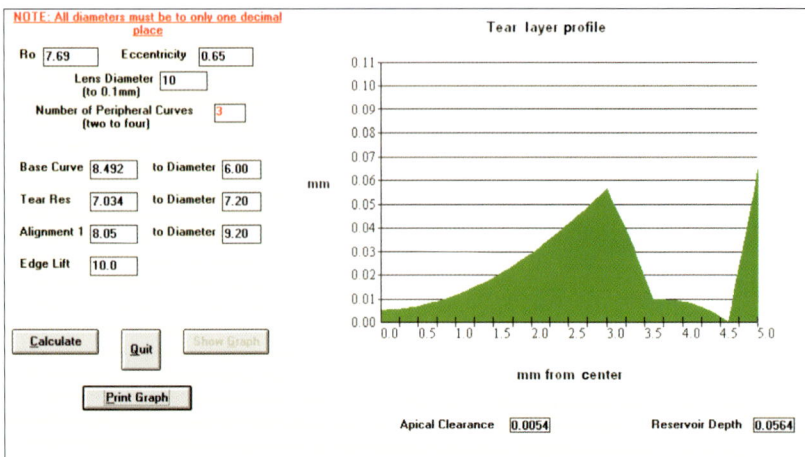

Figure 6.9 The lens shown in Figure 6.4 (eccentricity 0.50) has been altered by flattening the alignment curve from 7.936 to 8.05 mm.

To date, there has been only one report in the literature comparing the outcomes of empirical versus trial lens fitting. Fedders et al (1999) measured the changes in refraction, corneal shape, and fluorescein pattern appearance in a small group of subjects (3) following 4 h wear of OK-3 lenses. The first set of lenses were fitted by supplying the manufacturer with the K readings and the spectacle refraction. The second set were trial-lens-fitted and the fit altered until an optimal fluorescein pattern was achieved. The empirical lenses tended to be flatter in BOZR than the trial-fitted lenses, and caused less refractive change. The fluorescein patterns between the lens fits were very similar, leading to the conclusion that between fitting methods subtle differences occur that are not apparent with fluorescein pattern analysis. Further research into the differences between the first-fit success rate and corneal response to the different fitting methods is required.

Empirical fitting is potentially inefficient, time-consuming, and expensive when compared to trial lens fitting with standard spherical RGP fitting (Bennett et al 1989). It is even less efficient when applied to reverse geometry fitting.

TRIAL LENS FITTING

The basics of trial lens fitting with RGLs for orthokeratology is essentially the same as for normal lens fitting. The practitioner is given a fitting nomogram by the manufacturer in order to select the BOZR (base curve) of the initial trial lens. The nomogram is usually based on a pre-determined relationship between the BOZR of the lens and the flat-K reading. The trial lens is then inserted and the usual tests of fluorescein pattern analysis and lens movement and centration carried out. From these data, the practitioner is then able to prescribe a lens for the patient.

RGLs exhibit a totally different fluorescein pattern to that of a conventional lens. All current orthokeratology lenses show essentially the same fluorescein pattern, an area of "central touch" that is approximately 3–4 mm in diameter, a narrow and deep ring of fluorescein (the tear reservoir) approximately 0.5–1.00 mm wide, a wide alignment curve (1.00 mm), and an edge clearance. It is the appearance of the fluorescein pattern that has led to the totally false assumption of heavy central bearing with the lenses. Central bearing is always associated with epithelial insult and the formation of corneal scarring (Korb et al 1982), or lens decentration. RGLs are fitted with apical clearance. It is the limitations of fluorescein pattern analysis that give the appearance of touch.

This has been succinctly stated by UK practitioner Basil Bloom as follows:

> At no time during the orthokeratology process should a properly fitting lens come into direct contact with the corneal epithelium at the apex. Such contact will result in epithelial insult (Bloom unpublished).

TRIAL LENS SETS

There are many different designs of RGL available, but, as shown in Chapter 4, the basic mathematical relationship between all the designs means that the fluorescein patterns will all appear similar. The important factors to take into account before ordering a trial lens set are:

1. the design
2. the material from which the trial lens set is made. Is the oxygen transmissibility (Dk/t) high enough to use for a safe overnight trial?
3. the dimensional stability of the material. How often will the lenses need to be checked for warpage and steepening, necessitating replacement?
4. the cost of the lenses and replacements
5. quality and accuracy of manufacture
6. engraving of the lens or color differences so the BOZRs are not mixed up
7. Does the set come with complete fitting instructions and/or a computer program to aid in lens selection and design variables?
8. the sagittal difference between successive lenses in the set.

Various manufacturers offer different combinations of the above variables, but of prime importance are the quality and accuracy of the trial lenses, and the dimensional stability of the material. For example, trial lenses made from Boston XO have a higher Dk and appear to be more dimensionally stable than those made from Equalens 2. Mid-*Dk* materials can produce unacceptable degrees of corneal swelling on overnight trials and should be avoided for use as trial lenses.

The other important factor to consider is the logic and thought that have gone into the trial lens set design. As shown previously, the alignment curve or tangent is the major means of controlling lens centration, and varies considerably with corneal eccentricity. Since the trial lens will be required to fit a large range of different corneal shapes, the thought that has gone into varying the alignment curves or tangents in the set is of major importance. It is of little value having a trial lens set where the inaccuracies induced by too great a difference in relative sag between one lens and the next steepest or flattest lens renders the trial wear period invalid. Finally, the trial lens set should come with a complete set of instructions outlining lens design variations in order to modify the fit, and preferably a computer program that the practitioner can use to help choose the initial trial lens and then modify as necessary.

The corneal response to the lens is totally dependent on the accuracy of the lens fit, as this is what determines the tear layer squeeze film pressure and forces that initiate and control the response (see Ch. 10). If the trial lens set parameter variables limit the change in tear layer profile to a minimum of 20 μm (or 0.10 mm BOZR steps), the results can be – and will be – quite variable.

However, designing a trial lens set for RGLs is a major task. As stated previously, the common corneal shape varies in apical radius and eccentricity. Most eyes have an eccentricity in the range of 0.30–0.70, so the problem with designing a trial lens set begins with having enough lenses in the set to fit the range of eccentricities adequately, let alone the variations in apical radius. Figure 6.10 shows the total combinations of corneal sags at a chord of 9.20 mm with eccentricities ranging from 0.30 to 0.70 and a range of steep to flat apical radius values. The colored bands represent differences in sag of 10 μm. Note that for any given combination of R_0 and e there is a range of sagittal equivalent eye shapes. In order to cover this range of corneal shapes, a 49-piece trial lens set with a sagittal difference of 10 μm between lenses would be required.

However, matters are complicated by the addition of the alignment curve. If an alignment curve that is 1.00 mm wide and contacts the cornea at a chord of 9.20 mm with a TLT of 10 μm at the junction of the reverse curve is required, the range of lenses increases. The variation in alignment curve radius for the range of corneal shapes is shown in Figure 6.11. Note that there are

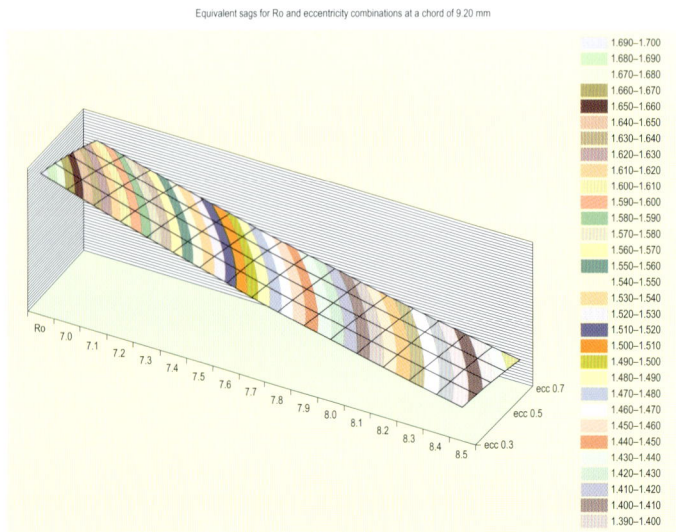

Equivalent sags for Ro and eccentricity combinations at a chord of 9.20 mm

Figure 6.10 The range of equivalent sags for combinations of R_0 and eccentricity from 7.00 to 8.50 mm. The bands of equal color are sagittal equivalents.

Relationship of alignment curve radius to apical radius for different eccentricities

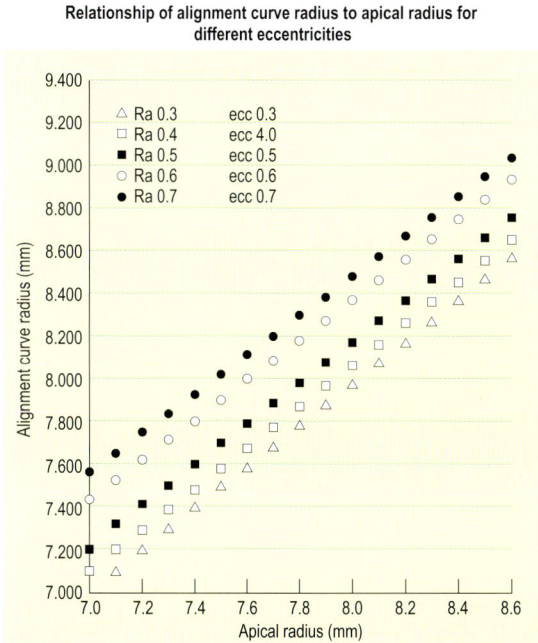

Figure 6.11   The alignment curve radius is dependent on the apical radius and eccentricity. A line drawn parallel to the x-axis at any alignment curve value shows the R_0 and eccentricity values that it will fit.

common alignment curves for various eccentricities. The design of a trial set can be simplified if the alignment curve radius is based on the mean eccentricity value of 0.5. The BOZR can be preset to a nominal 3.50 D flatter than R_0, and the reverse curves calculated for sagittal equivalency. The parameters of a trial lens set based on these assumptions are shown in Table 6.4. Note that there is an approximate sag difference of 12 μm between each lens in the series.

In order to fit the closest correct trial lens, the practitioner simply needs either to extract the corneal elevation value at a chord of 9.20 mm from the topographer, or alternatively calculate the value from the apical radius and eccentricity values. Once the corneal sag is known, the lens with the closest matching sag in the set is found. The trial lens sag should *always* be greater than the corneal sag to allow for apical clearance.

For example, assuming an apical radius of 7.43 mm and an eccentricity of 0.62, the corneal sag over the 9.20 mm chord is 1.4524 mm. The closest lens in the set is the 8.60 BOZR lens with a

Table 6.4 The parameters of a trial lens set designed on the alignment curve radius based on the mean eccentricity value of 0.5. The back optical zone radius (BOZR) can be preset to a nominal 3.50 D flatter than R_0, and the reverse curves calculated for sagittal equivalency.

R_0	Trial BOZR	Alignment curve	Reverse curve	Lens sag
7.00	7.70	7.23	6.400	1.6624
7.05	7.75	7.27	6.425	1.6499
7.10	7.80	7.32	6.450	1.6375
7.15	7.85	7.37	6.475	1.6247
7.20	7.90	7.42	6.500	1.6122
7.25	7.95	7.46	6.525	1.6011
7.30	8.00	7.51	6.550	1.5890
7.35	8.05	7.56	6.575	1.5771
7.40	8.10	7.61	6.600	1.5654
7.45	8.15	7.66	6.625	1.5539
7.50	8.20	7.70	6.650	1.5437
7.55	8.25	7.75	6.675	1.5326
7.60	8.30	7.80	6.700	1.5216
7.65	8.35	7.85	6.725	1.5109
7.70	8.40	7.90	6.750	1.5003
7.75	8.45	7.94	6.775	1.4909
7.80	8.50	7.99	6.800	1.4806
7.85	8.55	8.04	6.825	1.4705
7.90	8.60	8.09	6.850	1.4605
7.95	8.65	8.13	6.875	1.4517
8.00	8.70	8.18	6.900	1.4421
8.05	8.75	8.23	6.925	1.4325
8.10	8.80	8.28	6.950	1.4232
8.15	8.85	8.33	6.975	1.4139
8.20	8.90	8.38	7.000	1.4048
8.25	8.95	8.42	7.025	1.3967
8.30	9.00	8.47	7.050	1.3879
8.35	9.05	8.51	7.075	1.3800
8.40	9.10	8.57	7.100	1.3705
8.45	9.15	8.62	7.125	1.3620
8.50	9.20	8.67	7.150	1.3537
8.55	9.25	8.71	7.175	1.3462
8.60	9.30	8.76	7.200	1.3381

sag of 1.4605 mm that will give an apical clearance of 4.8 μm. The reverse curve is 6.85 mm and the alignment curve 8.09 mm. The tear layer profile of the trial lens is shown in Figure 6.12.

The analysis of the fit of the lens can then be refined by following the steps outlined in the section on topography-based fitting.

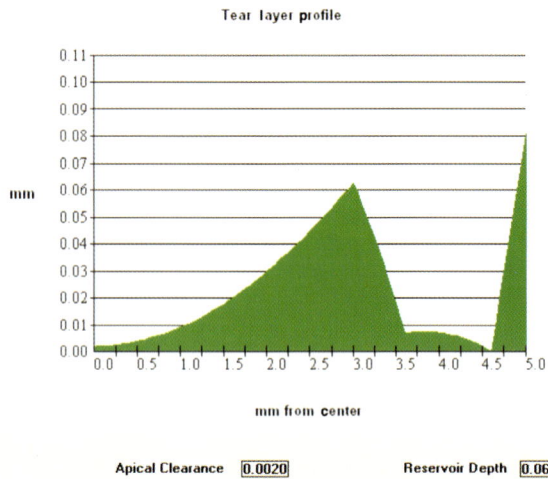

Figure 6.12 The tear layer profile for a lens designed for an apical radius of 7.43 mm and an eccentricity of 0.62, where the corneal sag over the 9.20 mm chord is 1.4524 mm. The closest lens in the set is the 8.60 back optic zone radius lens with a sag of 1.4605 mm that will give an apical clearance of 4.8 μm. The reverse curve is 6.85 mm and the alignment curve 8.09 mm.

The Dreimlens, R&R, CRT, EZM, and BE trial lens sets are designed on this type of basis, with sag differences between lenses of approximately 10 μm. Trial lens sets that have a BOZR difference of 0.10 mm (20 μm) between lenses will have a limited range of applications.

The Dreimlens trial set

The Dreimlens is not usually fitted by means of trial lenses in the USA, but this is the preferred method of fitting in Asia. The trial set was originally designed for use in Hong Kong. This is a large (56-lens) set. It is a four-zone design with a 6.00 mm BOZD, 0.60 mm wide reverse curve, 1.00 mm wide alignment curve, and a 0.40 mm wide peripheral curve. The BOZR is set at a target of 3.00 D refractive change, and the alignment curves are standard, +10 μm, –10 μm, and –20 μm.

As shown in Chapter 4, variations of 10 μm in alignment curve mean that the TLT at the reverse curve/alignment curve intersection is initially 10 μm (standard lens), and is then varied in 0.05 mm radius steps either steeper (+10 μm) or flatter (–10 and –20 μm). The BOZR of the trial lens is 3.75 D flatter than flat-K, but is labeled as the flat-K value. The initial trial lens selected is based on the flat-K value and the standard alignment curve. If the lens is too steep or flat, a lens with a looser or tighter alignment curve is used.

Alterations to the reverse curve are made by changing the BOZR. A change of 0.10 mm in BOZR alters the sag of the reverse curve by 4 μm and the alignment curve by 10 μm. The assessment of the trial lens is based on the fluorescein pattern and lens movement and centration. Lenses that decenter superiorly are considered to be too loose, and those that decenter inferiorly too tight. Lateral decentration is resolved by increasing the diameter to 10.6 mm and using a five-zone lens. Once the preferred fit is achieved, overrefraction is performed and the lens ordered. Overnight trial wear periods are not performed.

Paragon CRT trial set

This is also a large set, consisting of over 100 lenses. There are 20 base curves at 0.1 mm intervals and four return or reverse zone depths with three different tangential peripheries. Further custom lenses are available for patients with corneal topographies that fall outside the 80% of corneas that can be fitted from the inventory. The available return zone depths range from 350 to 750 microns in steps of 25 microns. These values represent the sag difference between the BOZD and the tangent. The cone angles range from 27° to 37° in 1° intervals. All trial lenses in the set have one of three preset cone angles. The BOZD is a constant 6.00 mm and the reverse zone and tangent are each

1.00 mm wide, including the sigmoid proximity blends. The common diameter is 10.50 mm. A lens with the BOZR and return zone depth and cone angle suggested by use of the slide rule lens selector is inserted and the fluorescein pattern assessed. If the centration and fitting pattern are not ideal the return zone depth is altered first to achieve the appropriate width of the central apparent contact zone and then the tangential periphery is altered to give the correct peripheral clearance and optimize centration.

The BE lens

The set consists of a minimum of 25 lenses, of either 11.00 or 10.6 mm diameter. There is a separate design and trial set for Asian eyes (A-BE).

BOZRs range from 7.85 to 9.10 mm in 0.05-mm steps. The cone angles vary with each lens, and are based on an arithmetic mean of the common ranges of eccentricities for each value of R_0. The eccentricities are weighted towards the lower end of the range for flatter corneas, and the higher range for steeper corneas. The initial corneal shape data are entered into the computer program, and the closest matching trial lens with a BOZR that gives apical clearance calculated and displayed. There is a sag difference of 8 μm between each consecutive lens in the set. The trial lens is inserted, the fluorescein pattern checked, and the patient advised to trial-wear the lens overnight. Any alterations to the final lens parameters are then made using the postwear diagnostic software.

R&R lens set

The R&R set consists of a BOZR range of 7.85–9.25 mm in 0.10-mm steps. A larger set in 0.05-mm steps is also available. The diameters are 10.00 or 10.60 mm. Assessment of fit is carried out by fluorescein pattern analysis, and the BOZR based on the Jessen factor with a compression factor of an extra 0.50 D.

The Contex E set

There is no set limit to the number of lenses in this set. It can range from as few as 10 lenses to 89 lenses. The common diameter is 10.6, and lens fit is based on the BOZR being 3.75 D flatter than K_f and fluorescein pattern analysis. At the time of writing, no further information on the set or fitting principles was available.

The Euclid Emerald set

There are 56 lenses in the set, with BOZR ranges from 40.00 D to 45.50 D based on the BOZR being 3.75 D flatter than K_f. All lenses are + 0.75 D in power, and the BOZR changes in 0.10-mm steps over a refractive range of 1.00 to 4.00 D. The alignment curves are linked to the BOZR, such that each lens in the series has an alignment curve that is 0.10 mm flatter or steeper than the next. The choice of trial lens is similar to that used for the Dreimlens, with fluorescein pattern analysis used to determine the correct fit.

Gelflex EZM lenses

The common diameters are 10.6 or 11.2 mm, with BOZRs ranging from 7.80 to 9.00 mm. As stated in Chapter 3, the cone angles vary with the BOZR. All lenses are plano-powered, with three fenestrations in at the BOZD/reverse curve junction at 120° intervals. A computer program is used to determine the correct BOZR based on inputted topography data.

Other lens designs also have trial lens sets available, but details were not available at the time of writing.

The descriptions of the various lens designs given in this section should allow the practitioner to make informed decisions as to what trial lens set is best suited to the type of fitting philosophy preferred. It is then a simple matter of approaching the manufacturer to find out what type of technical support is available for that design.

CARE AND MAINTENANCE OF TRIAL LENSES

Unlike most RGP lenses, orthokeratology lenses are preferably stored dry. This is primarily due to the possibility that dried wetting solution can bind to the lens back surface and form a rough film that is difficult to remove, but, more importantly, can cause marked central corneal staining. Following a trial lens period, the lenses should be thoroughly cleaned and then gently dried with a soft tissue and stored dry. Care must be taken to avoid dust and contaminant accumulation in the storage case, as this can cause scratching of the lens surface. If there is concern regarding the transmission of prion-related disease like variant Creutzfeldt–Jakob disease (v-CJD), then best practice dictates that the current disinfection guidelines using 2% sodium hypochlorite (Milton) are followed.

FLUORESCEIN PATTERN ANALYSIS

With spherical RGP fitting, the appearance of the fluorescein pattern is of major importance in determining the accuracy of the fit but this is not the case in contemporary reverse geometry fitting. Orthokeratology lenses are fitted with a specific outcome in mind, the controlled reformation of corneal shape, and the appearance of the fluorescein pattern of the lens gives little useful information as to the likely effect the lens has on corneal shape, other than excluding lenses with grossly inaccurate fitting patterns. Both Reim (2000) and Mountford & Noack (2001) have questioned the relative accuracy and value of fluorescein pattern analysis with RGLs. Fluorescein fitting assessment serves solely to exclude lenses showing a gross misfitting to the underlying cornea.

Fluorescein pattern analysis is a time-honored part of contact lens practice, and has been shown to be an accurate method of assessing the fit of a conventional lens (Brungardt 1961, Mandell 1974, Osborne et al 1989). Studies have shown that, with training, practitioners are capable of determining the fit of a lens to a tolerance of 0.05 mm in BOZR. Does this apply to RGLs for orthokeratology?

Figure 6.13 shows a range of "ideal" fluorescein patterns of different lens designs. The first thing to note is that a lot of the lenses have identical fluorescein patterns, irrespective of the BOZR chosen. There are commonalities in the assessment of the patterns in that the following "rules" apply to most of the designs:

1. The lens must center.
2. There should be an area of apparent "touch" over the pupil zone.

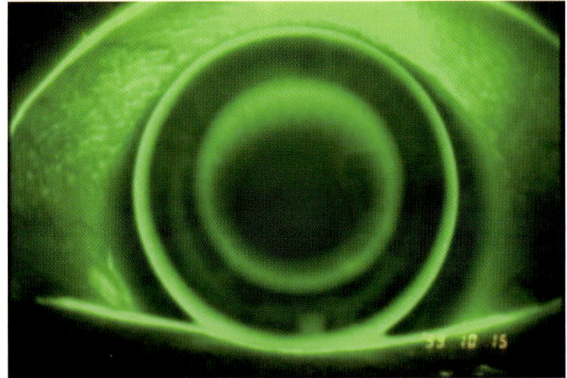

A

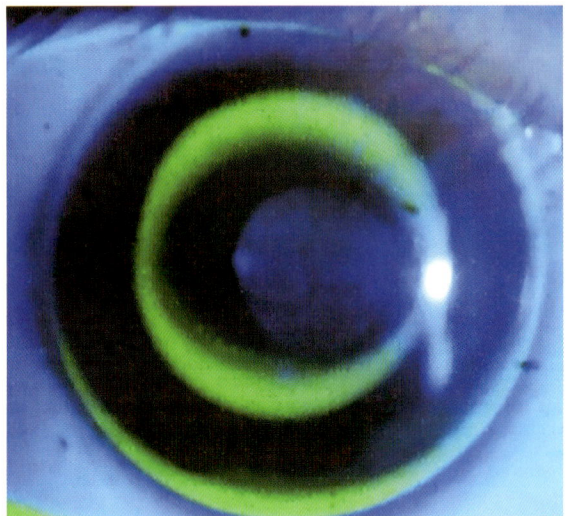

B

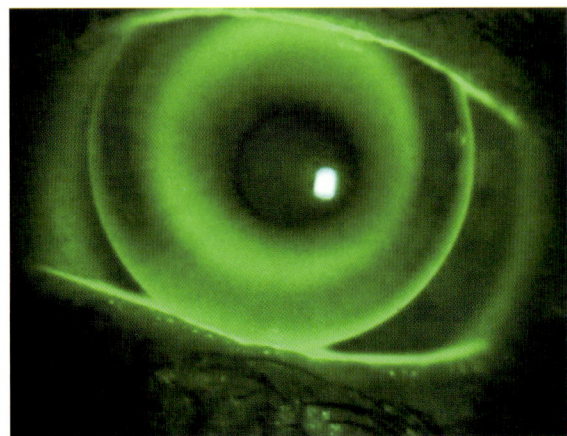

C

Figure 6.13 (A) The Context E lens; (B) the Emerald lens; (C) the CKR lens.

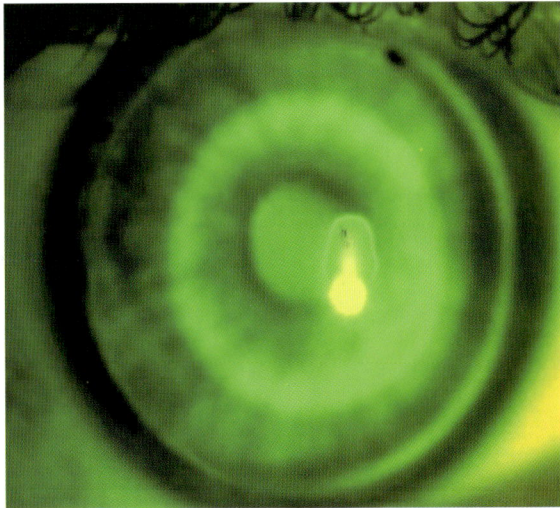

D

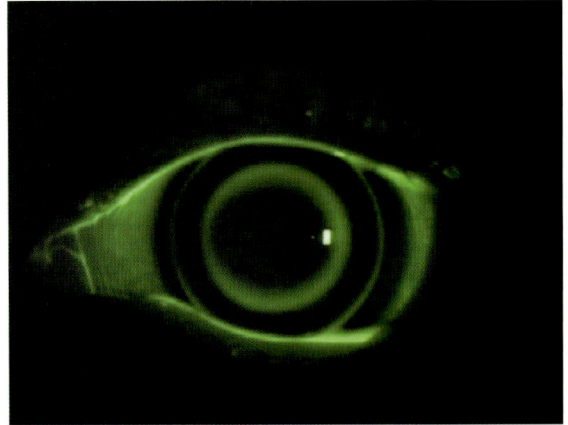

G

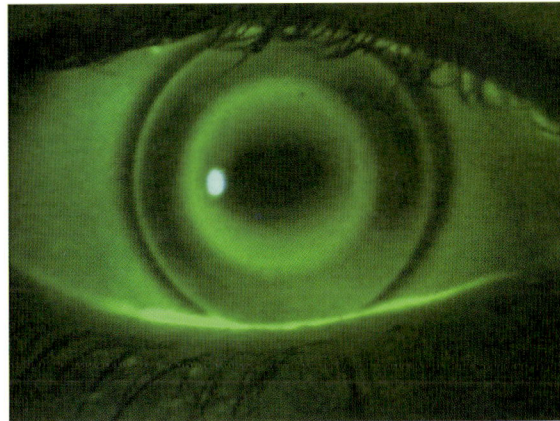

E

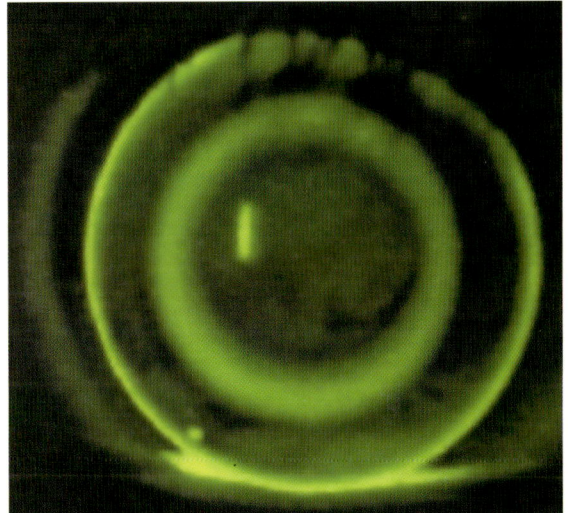

H

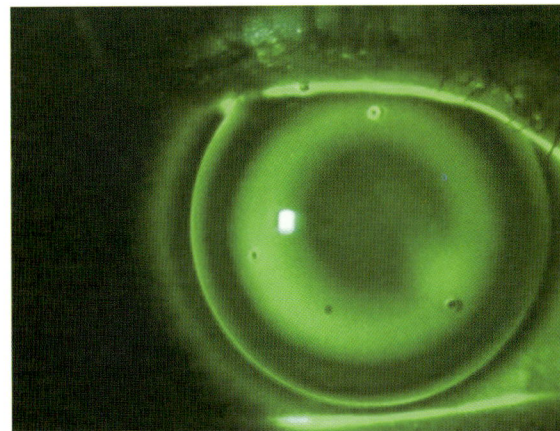

F

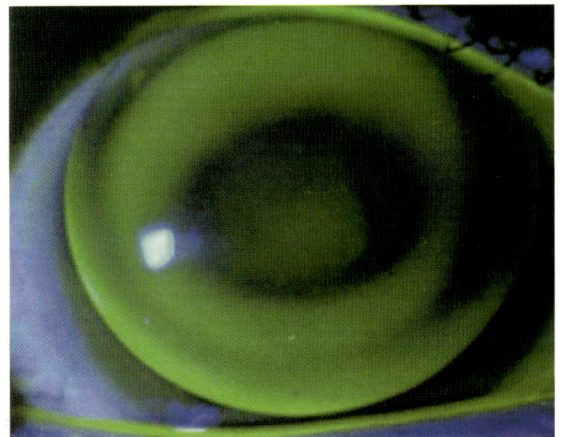

I

Figure 6.13   (D) the Reinhart Reeves lens; (E) the Dreimlens; (F) the BE lens; (G) the Nightmove lens; (H) the Fargo lens; (I) the Paragon CRT lens.

3. The alignment zone should appear as a wide band of close alignment or touch.
4. The reverse zone should be either narrow and deep (four- and five-zone) or wide and tapered (EZM and BE).

The one variant to this accepted appearance is the Contex E design, which is apparently optimally fitted with a relatively loose mid-peripheral alignment zone and some decentration acceptable. Fluorescein dissolves in the tear film, with its concentration and fluorescence dependent on the thickness of the tear film under the lens. Steep-fitting lenses exhibit greater fluorescence under the central area of the lens due to the relative concentration of fluorescein molecules present and the deeper tear layer present centrally than in the more peripheral areas. The minimum TLT required for fluorescein to become visible given the concentrations commonly used in clinical practice is in the order of 20 μm (Carney 1972, Guillon & Sammons 1994).

The tear layer profile of a four-curve lens is shown in Figure 6.14. If a line is drawn at the 20 μm point on the y-axis parallel to the x-axis, then all points above the line will appear as visible fluorescein, and all points below the line will appear as areas of touch. The fluorescein pattern of the lens is shown in Figure 6.15, with the areas of

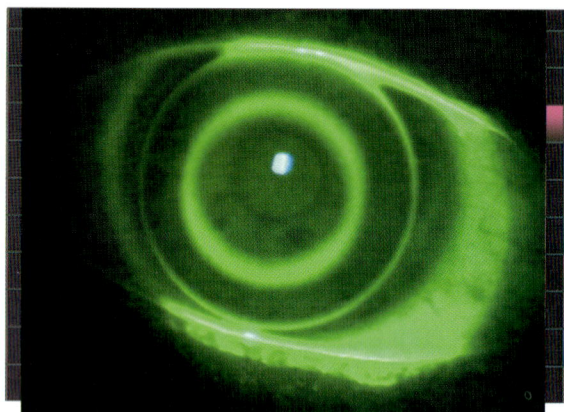

Figure 6.15 Fluorescein pattern of a four-zone lens. Note that the areas of touch and clearance are similar in area to the tear graph shown in Figure 6.14.

touch and visible fluorescein reflecting that shown in the tear layer profile graph. Theoretically, for each increase in central TLT of 10 μm, the BOZR would need to be steepened by 0.05 mm, so at best, fluorescein pattern analysis would only be sensitive to changes of ± 0.10 mm in BOZR of RGLs. This is not the case in practice, as quite large changes in BOZR often occur before distinct changes in fluorescein pattern become obvious.

Mountford et al (2003) fitted two patients, one Caucasian and one Asian, with both the Dreimlens and the BE lens, as well as standard

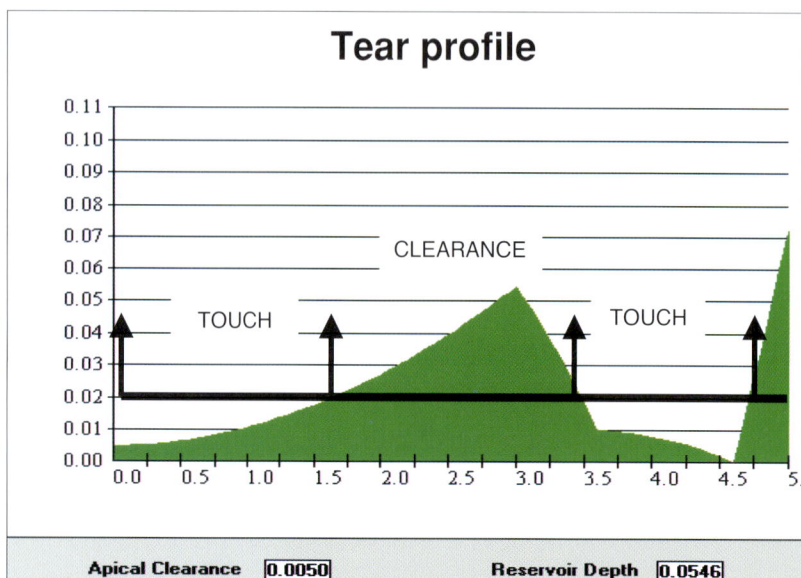

Figure 6.14 Tear layer profile of a four-curve lens. Parts of the profile above the 20 μm line will appear as clearance, or visible fluorescein, whilst those areas under the line will appear as "touch."

spherical lenses (Menicon design). The lenses were fitted according to the designer's nomograms following repeated topography readings. Each patient then had lenses fitted 0.05 mm steeper or flatter than the ideal BOZR to a maximum of 0.10 mm variation in fitting. The fluorescein patterns were photographed with a charge-coupled device (CCD) slit-lamp system until an optimal representation of each lens fit was achieved. The photos were then transferred to PowerPoint and their position on the slide randomized. A letter from A to E was then randomly applied to each photo. Two groups of practitioners, 11 experienced orthokeratologists (OK), and 21 nonorthokeratologists (NOK), were then shown the slides and asked to choose the ideal-fitting spherical and RGL and then nominate the next steepest and flattest lens in sequence. The relevant BE fluorescein patterns are shown in Figure 6.16. Forced choice was applied. Nonparametric (chi-square and Fisher's exact test) analysis was used to determine the significance of the results.

Both groups could recognize the ideal contour fit on the Caucasian eye (64% and 64%), but differed with the Asian eye, as both groups tended to choose the flatter lens as the ideal fit

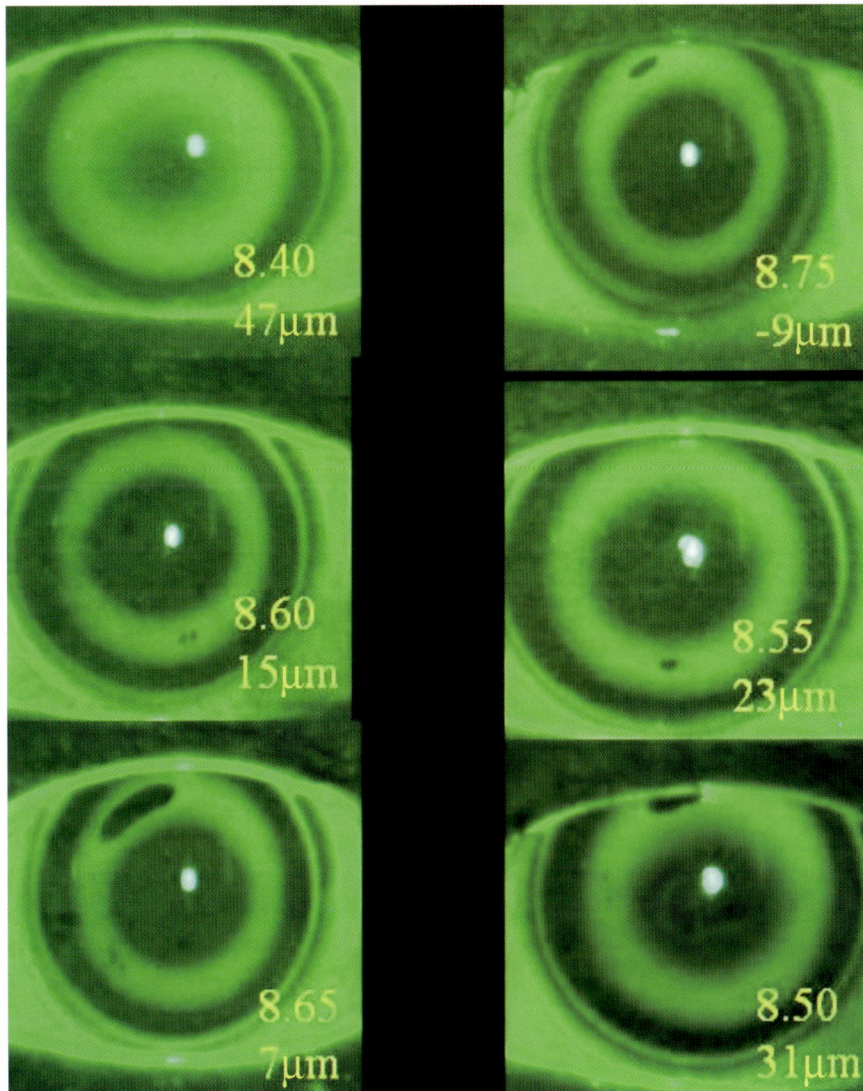

Figure 6.16 The fluorescein patterns of a range of BE lenses on the same eye are shown with calculated tear layer thickness under the apex of the lens. Even with such a wide variation in back optic zone radius (BOZR), the patterns all appear similar. The ideal fit is the 8.65 mm BOZR.

Percentage of correct choices of lens fit

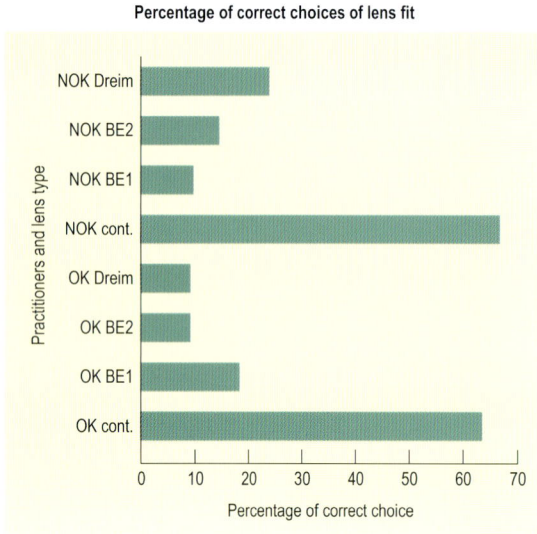

Figure 6.17 Distribution of correct lens choices for orthokeratologist (OK) practitioner and nonorthokeratologists (NOK). Both groups could accurately determine the correct alignment lens, but neither group could determine the correct reverse geometry lens. To do better than chance, the score needs to be greater than 19%; however, the NOK Dreimlens bar shown at the top of the graph was not statistically significant.

steeper RGLs. All choices were less than that expected by chance. Surprisingly, the NOKs routinely did better than the OKs in this part of the study, but the differences were not statistically significant (Fig. 6.17). Also, there was no difference in the OKs' ability to choose a lens they were familiar with (the Dreimlens) from one to which they had no previous exposure (BE).

The lenses fitted resulted in a spread of $\pm 20\,\mu m$ in apical clearance from the ideal fit. In effect, the results show that the TLT could vary from $-15\,\mu m$ to $+25\,\mu m$ at the apex of the cornea and that the difference could not be determined

(64% OK, 52% NOK). The rest of the lens choices for the alignment lenses were no better than that expected by chance. However, neither group could correctly identify the correct, flatter, or

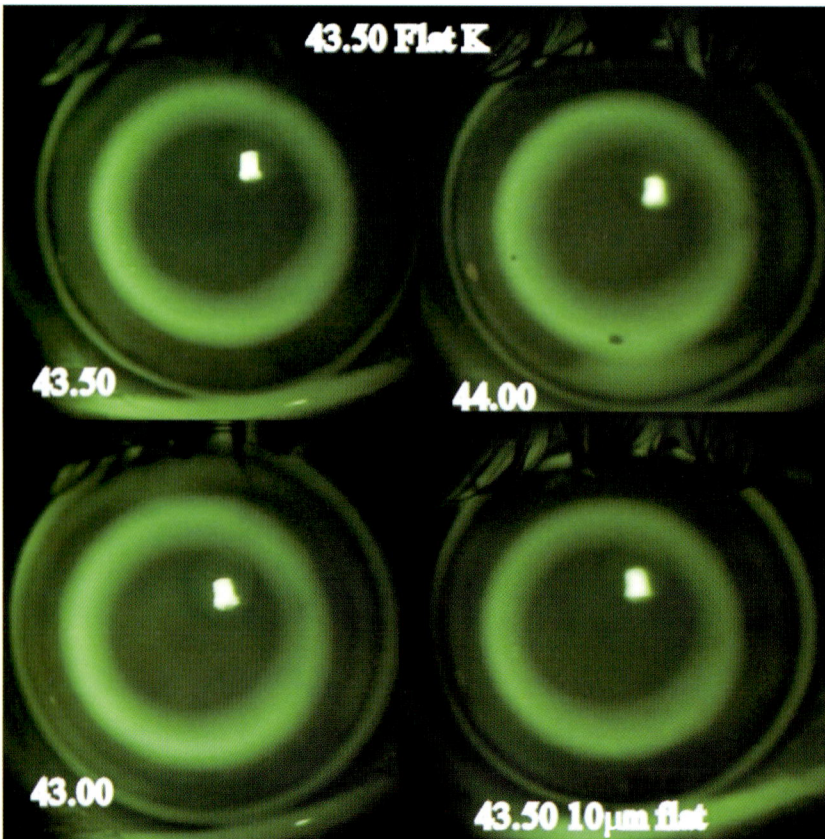

Figure 6.18 A group of Dreim lenses on the same eye. As in Figure 6.17, a lack of differentiation between successive lens fits occurs. Courtesy of Tom Reim.

by either the experienced OKs or the novices. The results of the study found that fluorescein pattern analysis of RGLs was not sufficiently accurate, and that the ability to determine the correct lens did not improve with experience.

The reason for this appears to be related to the forces acting in the postlens tear film. RGLs apply positive (compressive) force centrally and negative (tension) forces at the BOZD (see Ch. 10). This can be visualized in the old adage that flat lenses flatten the cornea and steep lenses steepen it. RGLs are the only designs that have elements of both forces acting under them. Engineers use the "surf and sand" metaphor to explain how particles move away from areas of positive force. If a wave (positive force) moves across the beach surface, the sand (particles) moves *away* from the advancing force.

Fluorescein is in solution in the tear film; however, the molecular weight of the fluorescein molecule is 346, whereas the molecular weight of the aqueous phase of the tear film is similar to that of saline (54). The difference in the molecular weights means that the heavier fluorescein molecule is the "sand" responding to the positive force under the center of the lens. The force "moves" the fluorescein molecules away from the center of the lens and into the deeper TLT at the edge of the BOZD. This will lead to an increased concentration of fluorescein in this area, with a resultant increased fluorescence. Conversely, the relative lack of fluorescein in the central area will lead to a relative hypofluorescence and the appearance of central touch. Reim makes a special point of highlighting the inability of fluorescein pattern analysis to determine the correct Dreimlens accurately (Fig. 6.18).

Also, the response appears to be time-dependent, with the visibility of the fluorescein in the reverse curve area becoming greater with time (Fig. 6.19). Experiments with BE lenses show that the first appearance of apical clearance occurs with central TLTs in the range of 45–50 μm.

Some lens designs are totally dependent on the "correct" interpretation of the trial lens fluorescein pattern in order to generate data for the correct prescription lens. From the results of the above study, it appears that reliance on the fluorescein may be misguided, unless, of course, a series of trial lens fits were photographed and the results ex-

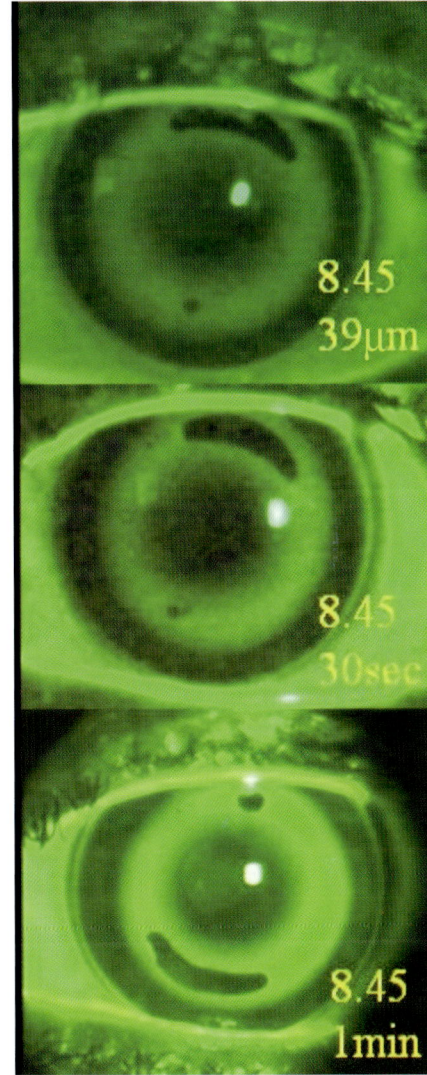

Figure 6.19 Sequence of images showing the change in fluorescein pattern over time. Note how the fluorescence appears to increase in the reverse curve area. The lens has approximately 39 μm of apical clearance.

posed to intense scrutiny in order to determine the optimal pattern. Even with such an approach, the fluorescein pattern itself will not supply any valid information as to the corneal response to the lens.

However, it is extremely worthwhile assessing the fitting using fluorescein for the following reasons:

1. Gross misfits due to poor topographical data are immediately apparent.

2. The practitioner can be certain that there is adequate peripheral clearance and therefore that the lens is not impinging on the cornea.
3. The presence of some degree of movement can be discerned.
4. The lens position can be assessed. With the lens in place, the patient is asked to close the eyes and pretend to be asleep. The eyes are left closed for approximately 20 s, and the patient is asked to open them again without consciously looking at anything. The position of the lens immediately on eye opening gives an accurate assessment of where it will center during eye closure. Lenses that are grossly off-center can be refitted immediately.

Cho et al (2002) interviewed 12 experienced orthokeratologists in Hong Kong in order to determine the type of lenses used and the general mode of practice of orthokeratology. All practitioners used trial lens fitting, with most requiring two sets of lenses to achieve the refractive goal. In general, the higher the refractive change required, the greater the number of lenses needed. The most commonly fitted lenses were the Dreimlens, Fargo 6, and Contex designs.

It is extremely important to assess the fluorescein pattern using a barrier filter. This is a yellow Wratten 14 filter held in front of the observation system of the slit-lamp microscope. Figure 6.20 shows a lens imaged with and without a barrier filter in place.

TOPOGRAPHY–BASED FITTING

As set out in Chapter 2, topographers show a very high degree of accuracy and repeatability when measuring different spherical and aspheric test surfaces (Applegate et al 1995, Hilmantel et al 1999, Tang et al 2000). The accuracy and repeatability of topographers are poorer, however, when *human eyes* are measured (Jeandervin & Barr 1998, Hough & Edwards 1999). There is one simple fact that must be understood with regard to the reported accuracy of a particular topographer on human eyes, and that is it is impossible to know what an accurate reading is, as the exact shape of the eye is unknown. Topographers determine the model of corneal shape using reconstruction algorithms to interpret the reflections of the mires from the corneal surface, so the "picture" will vary depending on the following factors:

1. the reconstruction algorithms used
2. the accuracy of the capture method (automatic or manual)
3. the stability of the patient (movement, fixation, tear layer stability)
4. the state of the instrument's calibration
5. the variation of the corneal profile from that of the model aspheric or spherical surface.

In routine clinical practice, it is common for one single topography plot to be taken of each eye, and the fit of the lens to be based on the data. However, for any given single topography plot, there are four possible outcomes with respect to the accuracy of the data, especially as regards elevation.

1. The data are accurate.
2. The topographer *overestimated* the elevation.
3. The topographer *underestimated* the elevation.
4. The data are totally inaccurate.

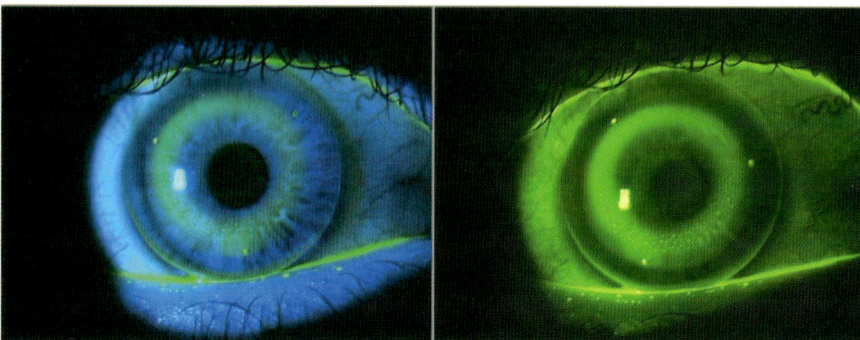

Figure 6.20 Lens imaged with (A) and without (B) a barrier filter in place.

A   B

The real problem with doing one single reading is that the practitioner does not know which of the above outcomes applies.

The ideal solution to this dilemma is to take four to six repeated readings of the eye and determine the degree of error or the repeatability of the instrument for both apical radius and eccentricity or elevation. The concept of applying statistical methods to repeated readings was introduced by Lowe (unpublished), as a means of refining the fit of the lens, and gaining greater accuracy with the final lens parameters.

Assuming that four plots are taken, the method is as follows:

1. Compare the left and right eye maps for similarities in apical radius and eccentricity. They should be similar. Marked differences between the two eyes usually indicate that one of the plots is invalid. An example is shown in Figure 6.21. Place all four maps on the screen and assess them for any gross problems like excessive brow or nose shadow, stray eyelashes, or gross discrepancies in apical radius or eccentricity values. The "rogue" readings should be discarded and a replacement plot

taken. Figure 6.22 shows repeated readings of the left eye shown in Figure 6.21. The considerable variation in apical radius values and the poor repeatability were due to a very unstable tear film. The eye was lubricated and the readings retaken.

2. Record the apical radius (in mm) and eccentricity values in different columns of a spreadsheet. If elevation data are given by the topographer, use those in preference to the eccentricity values. Make sure that the eccentricity or elevation is recorded at the chord of contact between the lens and the cornea.

3. If only R_0 and eccentricity are available, calculate the elevation or sag using the formula:

$$\text{Sag (elevation)} = (R_0 - \sqrt{R_0^2 - y^2 p}) / p$$

where R_0 is apical radius, y is half the chord of contact between the lens and the cornea, and p the shape factor or $(1 - e^2)$. Table 6.5 details the spreadsheet set-up and formulas required for the calculations.

Once the elevations are calculated, the mean and standard deviations are derived using the function wizard. This is a time-consuming task. Hough & Edwards (1999) have recommended

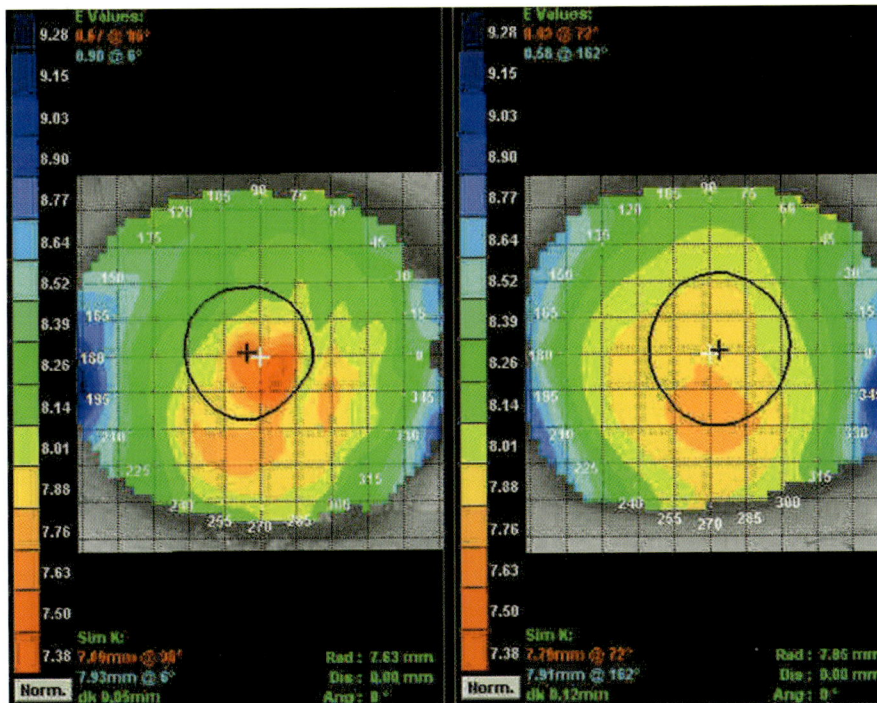

Figure 6.21 A comparison between the topography plots of two eyes. Note that the left is not similar to the right.

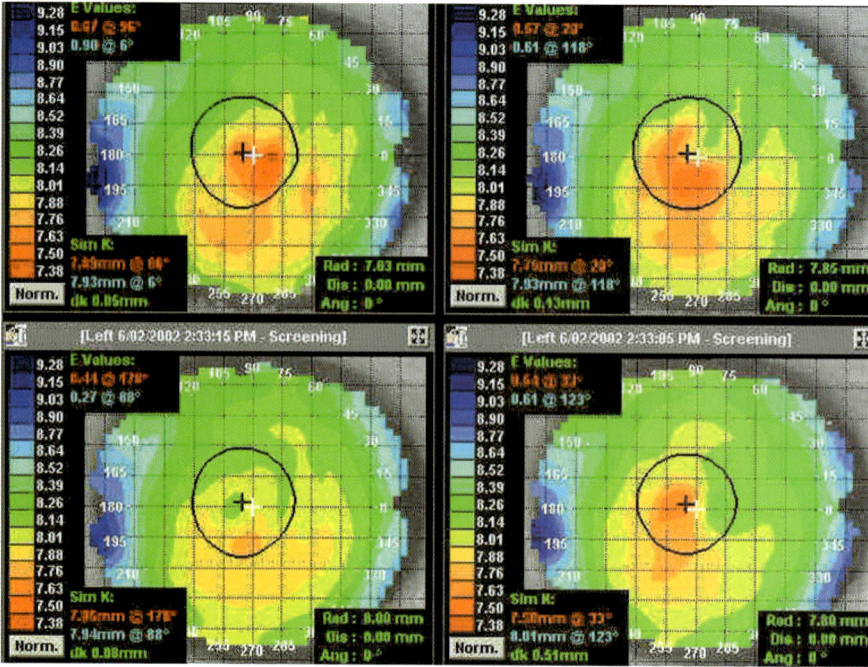

Figure 6.22   Repeated readings of the left eye shown in Figure 6.20. Note the variation in apical radius values and the poor repeatability. The patient had a very unstable tear film. The eye should be lubricated and the readings retaken.

Table 6.5   An Excel spreadsheet for determining the corneal sag. Input the relevant details and formulas so that column E contains the sag value. If a group of readings are taken, put each into column F and then use the function wizard to calculate the mean and standard deviation.

Column A1 (R_0)	Column B1 (p)	Column C1 (eccentricity)	Column D1 (1/2 chord)	Column E1 (corneal sag)
A2 = R_0	B2 = p Formula: = $(1 - C2^2)$	C2 = Eccentricity	D2 = 1/2 chord (mm) Value = 9.20 for 10.00 mm lens	E2 = corneal sag Formula = $(A2-(\sqrt{A2^2-(D2^2 \cdot B2)}))/B2$

that the different topography companies incorporate this type of statistical tool in their respective software. To date this has only been done by Medmont, who include a program that calculates the mean and standard deviation of the apical radius, eccentricity, elevation, and keratometry readings at any chord or axis chosen by the practitioner for up to four repeated readings (Fig. 6.23).

If the above seems too time-consuming, an alternative is to determine what the standard deviation of the topographer is in the measurement of the elevation data for 10 repeated measures on the same normal eye using the method set out above. Then, when measuring the corneas of the individual patient, perform two repeat measurements and only perform a third if the first two differ by more than one standard deviation. The readings that fall within one standard deviation of one another are then averaged and these data are used. This practical approach was suggested by Bloom (unpublished).

Additionally, if topography data are to be used in order to fit a contact lens to a specified accuracy, a degree of tolerance must be set that is rigorous enough to allow for proper clinical decisions. If, for example, it is required to fit the BOZR to a tolerance of 0.05 mm, then the measurement tolerance of the topographer has to be ± 0.025 mm. Similarly, if the lens needs to be fitted

Column A1 (Ro)	Column B1 (p)	Column C1 (eccentricity)	Column D1 (1/2 chord)	Column E1 (corneal sag)
A2 = Ro	B2 = p	C2 = eccentricity	D2 = 1/2 chord (mm)	E2 = corneal sag
	Formula: = (1 − C2^2)		Value = 9.20 for 10.00 mm lens	Formula = (A2 − (sqrt A2^2 − (D2^2*B2)))/B2

Figure 6.23 The mean and standard deviations of the range of corneal data values from the Medmont topographer. Note that the chord over which the measurements are taken is variable, as is the axis.

with an apical clearance tolerance of 5 μm, then the instrument measurement tolerance for elevation must not exceed ± 2.5 μm (Hough & Edwards 1999).

The stated tolerance for lens manufacture with computer numeric-controlled (CNC) lathes is in the order of ± 0.01 mm or ± 2 μm. Depending on the topographer used and the experience of the practitioner, the common range of error when measuring the elevation of human corneas can be from ± 2 μm to ± 15 μm (Cho et al 2002). The important question, then, is how many repeated readings are required in order to achieve a repeatability standard deviation of ± 2 μm?

Hough & Edwards (1999) give the following relationship that is used to determine the number of repeated readings that would fulfill the requirements set out above:

$$N = (S_r / S_e)^2$$

where N is the number of readings required, S_r is the reproducibility standard deviation, and S_e is the repeatability standard deviation.

Cho et al (2002) measured the repeatability and reproducibility of four different topographers on a group of Asian subjects, and determined the number of readings required from each instrument with the S_e limit set to 2 μm. The Medmont E300 had the best performance with only two repeat readings required. The Humphrey Atlas required 12, the Dicon 64, and the Orbscan 552.

However, this degree of accuracy in fitting is only required to determine the final lens parameters, and not the trial lens. Since the difference in trial lens sag between successive lenses is in the range of 10 μm, the tolerance for topographical elevation should be in the range of ± 5 μm.

HOW TO USE THE TOPOGRAPHY DATA

There are now two known facts that the practitioner must understand. Firstly, the *accuracy* of the topography data is unknown, but the standard deviation of error is known. Secondly, the accuracy of the sag height of the contact lens is known to a tolerance of ± 2 μm.

The concept with topography fitting is to compare that which is known (the sag of the trial lens) to that which is *not* known (the sag of the cornea) and use the corneal response to the trial lens to refine the fit.

For example, if the topographer gives a corneal elevation value of 1500 μm with a standard deviation of ± 10 μm, then the range of possible corneal elevations to the 95% confidence level is 1480–1520 μm, which is based on the 95% confidence level being equal to twice the standard deviation.

The sag philosophy states that lens sag is equal to corneal sag (elevation) plus the TLT. Taking the mean elevation value and adding 5 μm for TLT, the required sag of the trial lens is 1505 μm. In other words, the mean value is always used as the basis for determining the initial trial lens.

Once the mean and standard deviation of error of the instrument for the individual patient are recorded, the practitioner will have a good idea of the *range* of trial lenses that may be required to achieve an optimal fit. For example, in the above case where the corneal elevation range is from 1480 to 1520 μm, the number of possible trial lenses, assuming a sag difference of 10 μm between lenses, is four.

The important fact to remember is that the topographer may have a standard deviation of error of ± 10 μm, but the lens has an error of ± 2 μm.

The trial lens based on the mean value is then inserted and the fluorescein pattern assessed mainly for lens centration. If the fluorescein pattern is either grossly too steep or flat, then the initial indications are that the topography data are hopelessly inaccurate, and should be repeated. In most cases, however, the fluorescein pattern will show the typical reverse geometry appearance. The patient is then taught insertion and removal and advised to sleep in the lenses that night and return in the morning with the lenses in situ for assessment. A full description of the postwear clinical assessment is given in Chapter 9.

ASSESSING THE POST-TRIAL TOPOGRAPHY

The next step is to perform corneal topography measurements. This is probably the most valuable tool in assessing the accuracy of the corneal response to the lens, and provides invaluable information for refining the fit of the final lens design. The plot is taken and then a subtractive plot of the prefit and postwear generated.

Topographical analysis shows that there are four common outcomes from an overnight trial: a bull's-eye pattern, smiley face, smiley face with fake central island, and central islands.

Bull's eye

If the corneal data from the topographer were accurate, the trial lens will be an ideal fit, and will result in a bull's-eye postwear plot (Fig. 6.24). The diagnosis of the bull's eye is always done using the axial, tangential, and refractive power subtractive maps. The axial difference map shows the refractive change achieved at the corneal apex, and has a high correlation with the change in subjective refraction (Mountford 1997, Soni & Nguyen 2002). The refractive change achieved after the first night's wear is dependent on the number of hours the lens has been worn (Sridharan 2001) and the *actual* apical clearance of the lens (Mountford & Noack 2001). If the fit is ideal, and the apical clearance correct, the refractive change achieved in the first night of wear will be approximately 70% of the total change required (Swarbrick & Alharbi unpublished). However, the assessment of a successful overnight trial is not based on refractive change, but on the centration of the treatment zone.

The tangential power map is ideal for assessing the accuracy of centration of the treatment zone (Fig. 6.24B). Note that the "red ring" is perfectly centered around the pupil zone.

Refractive power maps also play a part in the postwear assessment of the changes. The treatment zone diameter is overestimated with the

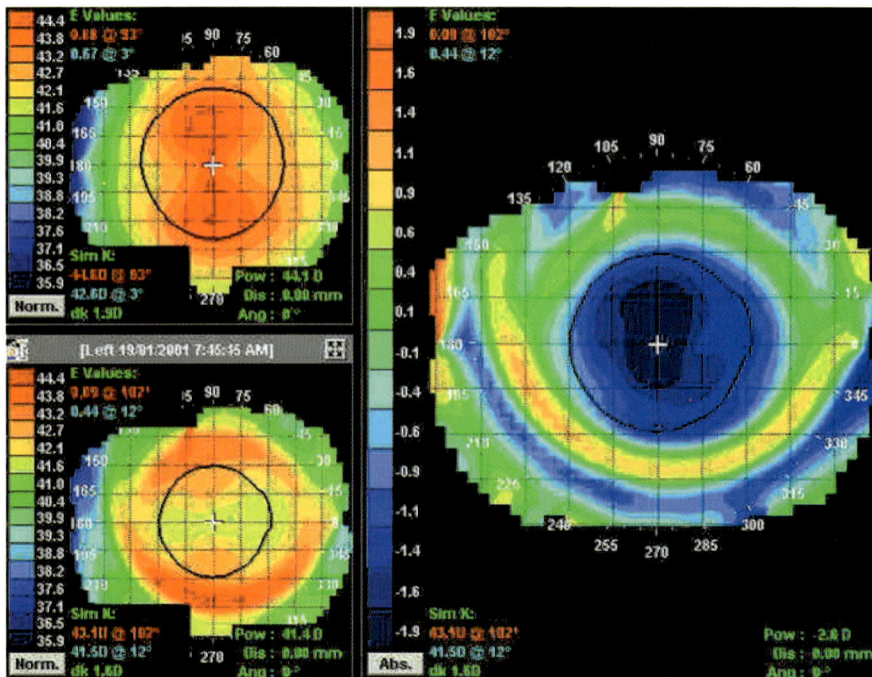

Figure 6.24 The axial (A), tangential (B), and refractive power (C) maps of a bull's-eye topography plot taken after an overnight-wear period. The axial map shows the refractive change, the tangential the centration of the effect, and the refractive map the treatment zone diameter. Note the excellent centration.

A

Figure 6.24   Cont'd.

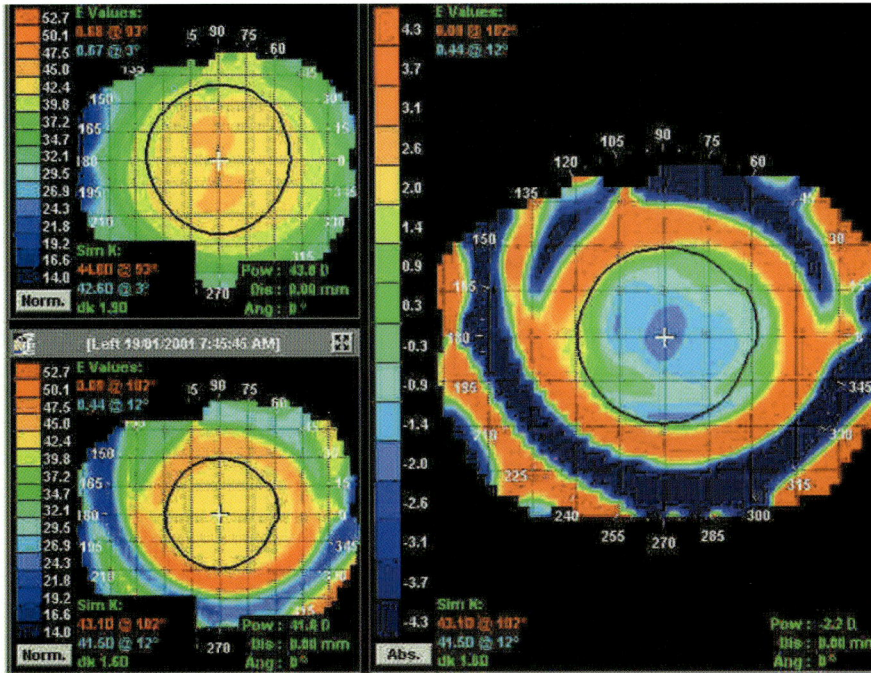

B

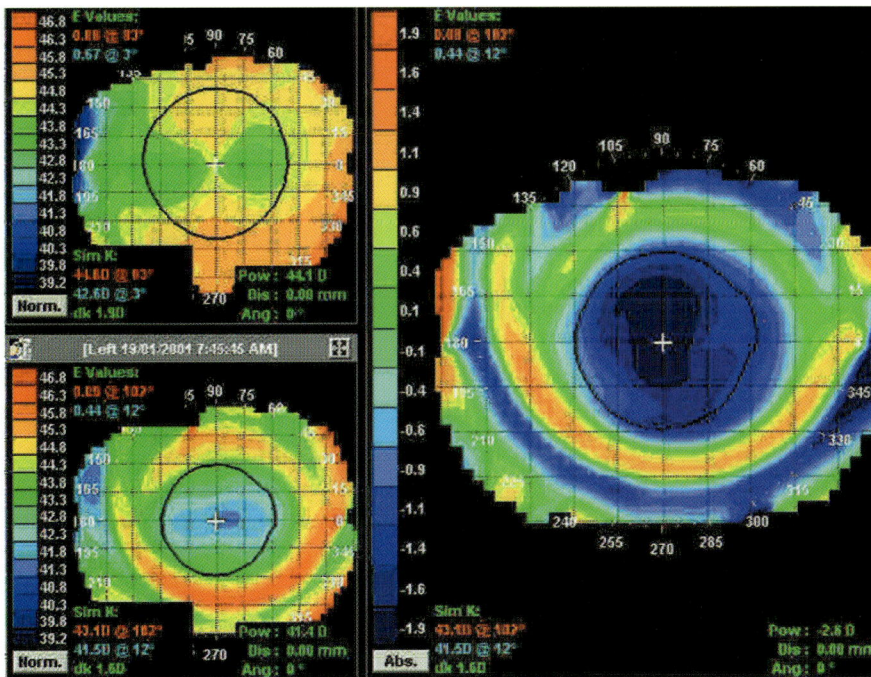

C

axial map and underestimated with the tangential map. The refractive power map gives a more accurate measure of the actual zone (Fig. 6.24C). The cursor is moved from the center of the map nasally and temporally until the point of zero change between the pre- and postwear maps is reached. The addition of the two values gives the treatment zone diameter. Also, in cases where it is difficult to make a final decision as to small degrees of decentration due to the corneal apex being decentered, the pre- and postwear refractive power maps can be used to see if the refractive change is central with respect to the initial corneal power distribution.

In cases where the initial corneal eccentricity is high, but only a low refractive change is required, the appearance of the bull's eye will not be as distinctive. Also, since the treatment zone diameter increases in diameter over the first week of wear, it is not uncommon to see incomplete bull's-eye pattern formation after the first overnight trial (Fig. 6.25). The single most important factor is the centration of the effect. Bull's-eye patterns are the only acceptable result of a trial lens fitting. The resulting corneal shape changes are well-centered and even in appearance, with little or no distortion in the central zone, resulting in good unaided visual acuity.

Smiley–face pattern

Smiley-face patterns (Fig. 6.26) are indicative of a flat-fitting lens that has decentered superiorly, typically due to instrument *underestimation* of the corneal elevation or sag. Underestimation of the elevation is equivalent to an overestimation of the eccentricity. If the eccentricity is overestimated, the alignment curve or tangent of the lens will be too flat. When the rest of the lens construction is based on this value, the result is a flat-fitting lens. Also, the apical clearance will theoretically be less than zero, and the lens back surface will come into direct contact with the corneal apex. The force of the lid, combined with a redistribution of the tear film squeeze forces behind the lens will make the lens move superior-temporally in order for equilibrium to occur.

When the lens decenters in this manner, the topography shows an area of flattening superior to the pupil, with a crescent of inferior steepening in the pupil zone. This is the classical smiley-face pattern. Figure 6.26A shows the axial power change. Refraction in theses cases usually yields a moderate decrease in myopia, but an increase in with-the-rule astigmatism. Unaided high-contrast

acuity is also usually good, but associated with symptoms of ghosting and flare. Confirmation of the decentration is best done with the tangential power map (Fig. 6.26B). Note that the "red ring" is decentered superiorly. The degree of decentration is related to the underestimation of the corneal elevation, in that the greater the decentration, the greater the underestimation of the elevation.

Smiley-face patterns are an unacceptable outcome for an overnight trial, as the resulting topography has induced corneal distortion. The patient should return for a further overnight trial with a steeper lens until a bull's-eye plot is achieved.

Smiley face with fake central island

Smiley faces with fake central islands (Fig. 6.27) represent an even greater underestimation of the corneal sag than a normal smiley face. In these cases, the lens sag is much less than the corneal sag, leading to heavy central touch that results in epithelial damage. The disruption of the surface causes distortion and linkage of the reflected mires, which the instrument then reconstructs as an area of steepening. The key diagnosis is made by the tangential power difference map (Fig. 6.27B) and the appearance of central corneal staining. Further confirmation can be made by deleting the color map from the image and inspecting the central mires for distortion (Fig. 6.28). Once again, this is a totally unacceptable outcome, and the patient must be scheduled for a further overnight trial with a steeper lens until a bull's-eye plot is achieved.

Central island pattern

Central islands (Fig. 6.29) are usually caused by a steep or tight lens as a result of instrument *overestimation* of the corneal sag or elevation. Since the development of the dual RGLs such as the Dreimlens and the BE, or lenses of larger total diameter, central islands have become the more common postwear plot, as compared to smiley faces, which are more common with the three-curve RGLs. The classic hallmarks of a central island are an area of relative steepening centrally, surrounded by an annulus of marked corneal flattening. The central island itself can be either steeper than the original cornea, or simply steeper than the surrounding annulus of corneal flattening.

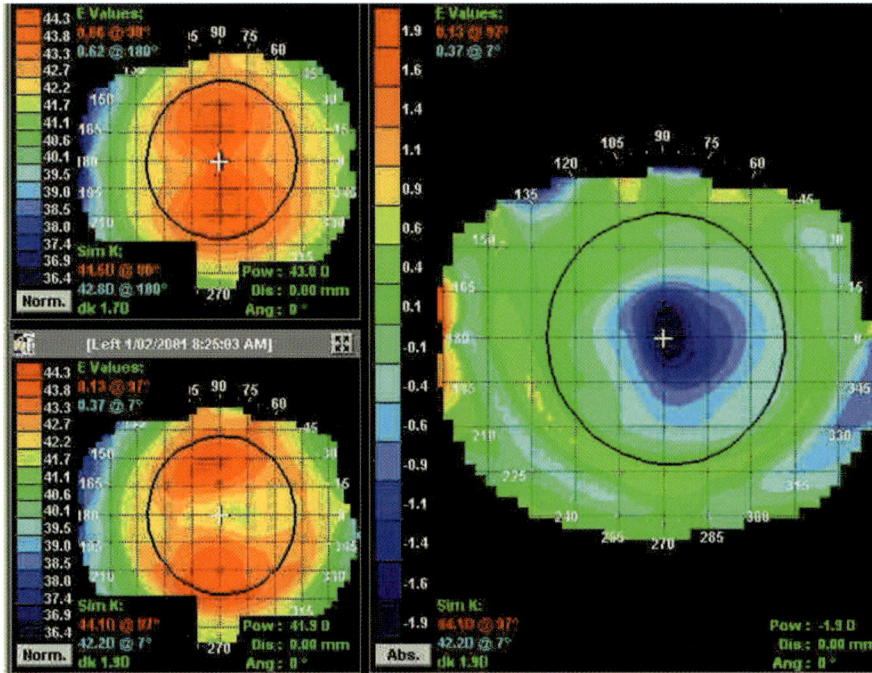

Figure 6.25 The change in bull's-eye pattern appearance between the first overnight wear (A), and that after 8 days later (B). Note the increase in treatment zone with time.

A

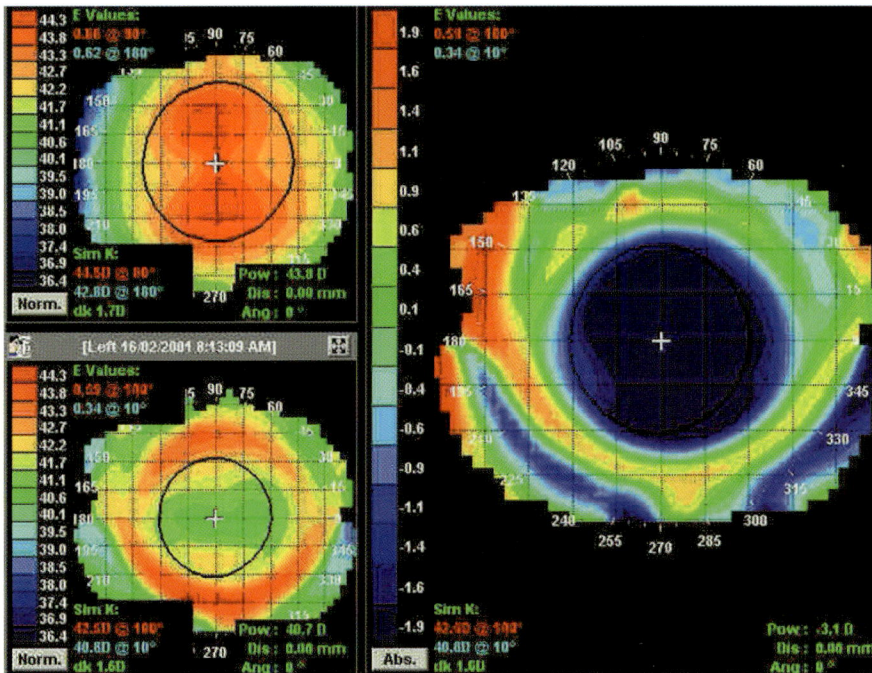

B

Clinical experience shows that small central islands (0.50 D or less) that are flatter than the original cornea, but still steeper than the surrounding area, will resolve within 1 week of lens wear. However, central islands greater than this degree, or those where the apical corneal

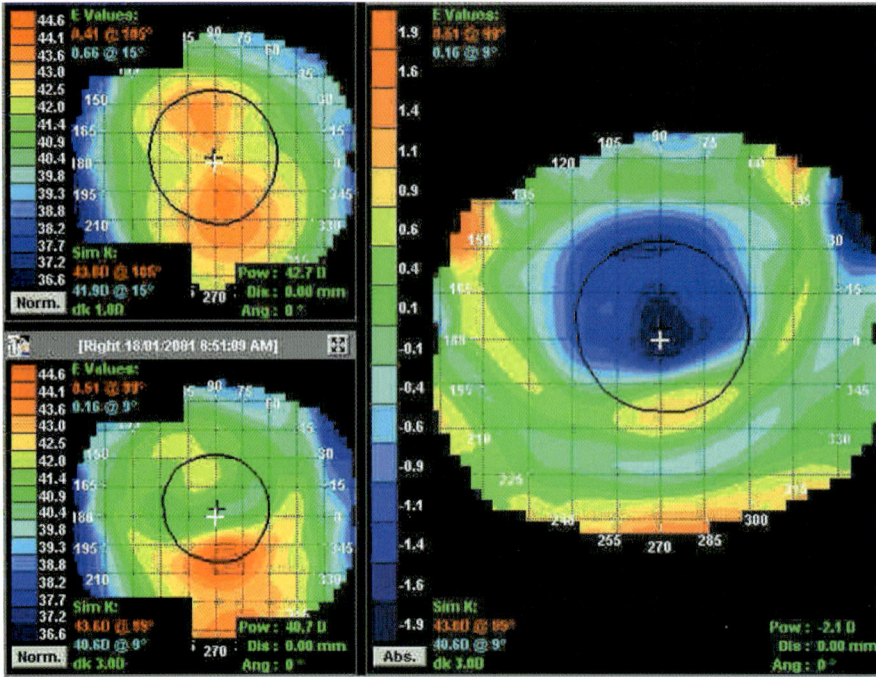

A

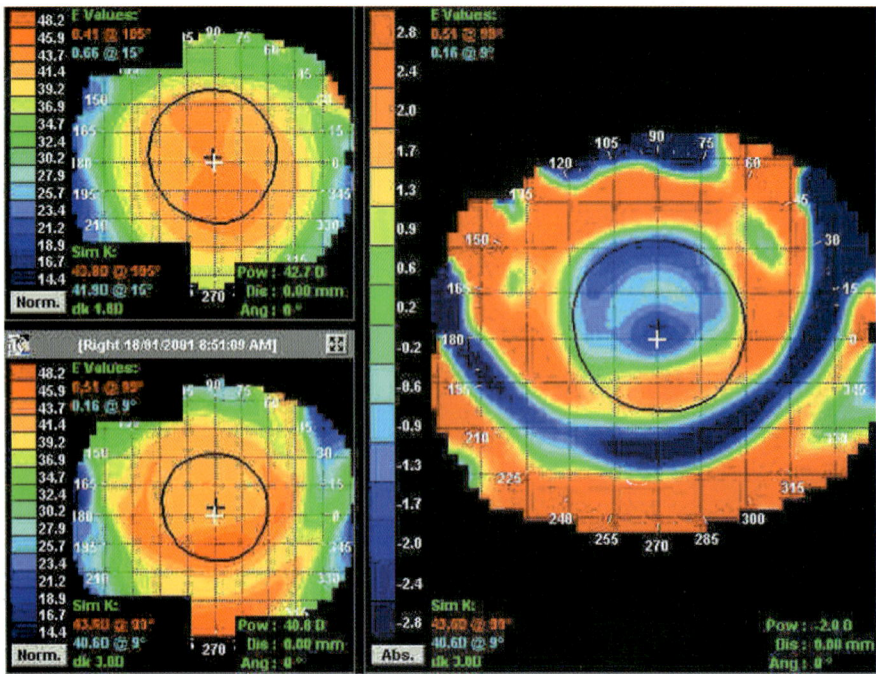

B

Figure 6.26 (A) Axial and (B) tangential maps of a smiley-face pattern. The tangential map highlights the decentration of the lens.

power is steeper than the original value, will not resolve. The difference is that a small island indicates a small degree of inaccuracy in the initial fit, whereas a steep island indicates a large degree of initial fitting error. The BOZR of the lens is usually not at fault in these cases. An

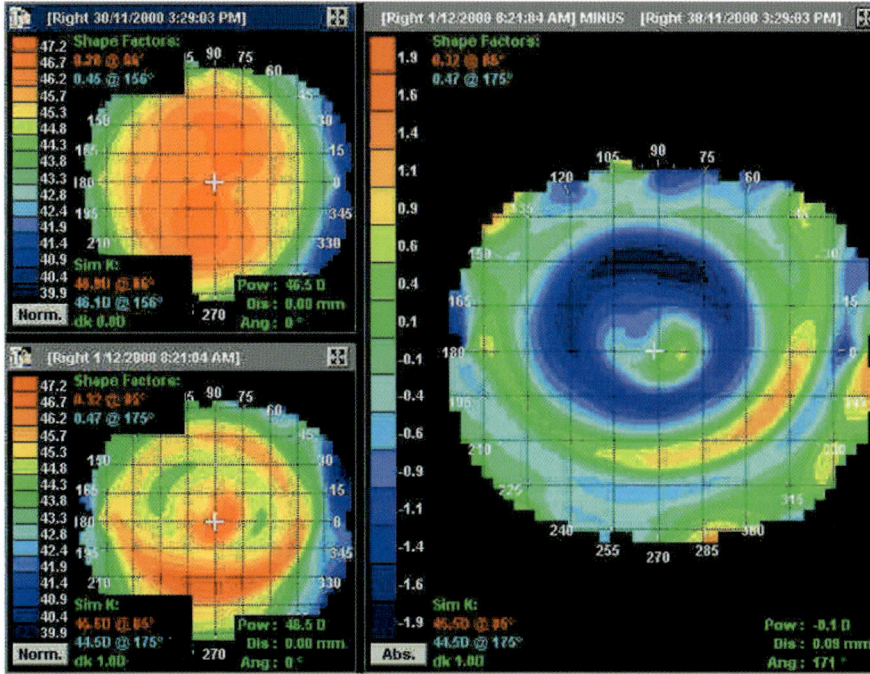

A

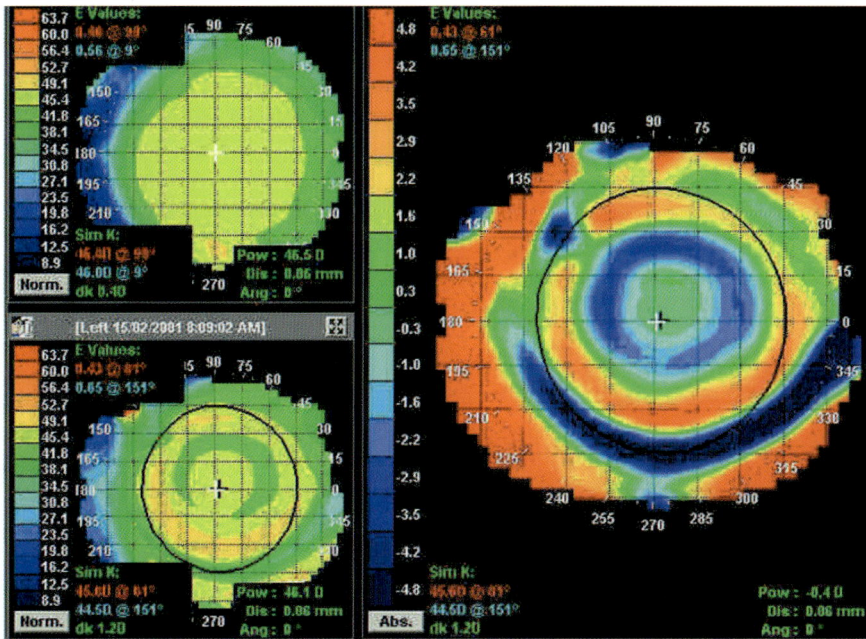

B

Figure 6.27   (A and B) A smiley face with a fake central island.

overestimation of the corneal sag will also result in a tighter cone angle or alignment curve in the periphery, and it may well be the compression caused by the tight periphery of the lens that is responsible for the formation of central islands.

The diagnosis of the central island is again the tangential power subtractive map. The centration

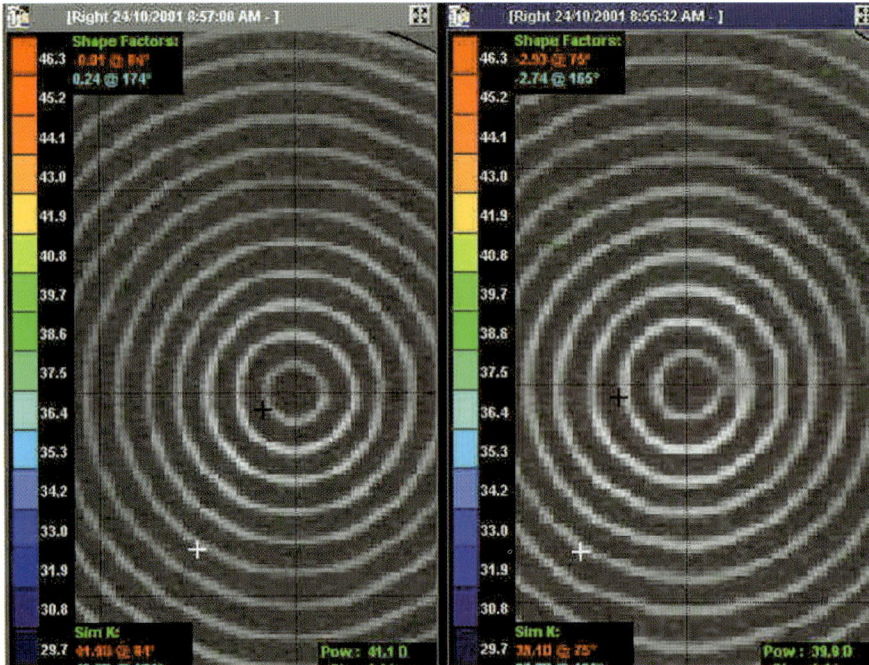

Figure 6.28 If the color map is removed, the distortion of the Placido mires becomes visible. This leads to invalid central data and the appearance of a central divot (see Figure 6.31).

with central islands is always perfect. When a central island occurs, unaided visual acuity is usually worse than the prefit values. Also, over-refraction leads to no clear endpoint, and the best corrected visual acuity is usually two lines or more less than normal. The refraction data from a central island are of no clinical importance.

It should be appreciated that some topographers, particularly the Keratron, can give false central island maps due to the reconstruction algorithm used. The Keratron does not apply smoothing to the central data, so as the arc-step method approaches the tangent normal to the optic axis, the value of the apical corneal power becomes unpredictable. Keratron users are advised to compare the refractive power maps before and after, and not subtractive, to determine if a true central island is present.

OTHER POSTWEAR RESULTS

There are two other possible outcomes from an overnight trial that occur rarely. The first is a frowny face (Fig. 6.30), where the lens appears to

be decentered either inferiorly or laterally. The cause is the same in either case: overestimation of elevation leading to a tight alignment curve, or a lens diameter that is too small. The second is termed a "central divot" (Fig. 6.31), and is caused by apical touch leading to epithelial disruption centrally. The mires of the placido become linked, and the reconstruction algorithm represents the data as a small area of gross central flattening. They can also occur if the tear layer is disrupted from a bound lens. Simply instilling a drop of lens lubricant and repeating the capture can resolve the differences. If the divot is due to tear layer instability, it will not be present on the second plot. However, if epithelial compromise did occur, the divot will still be present. Other types of abnormal topography outcomes also occur, and are discussed in greater detail in Chapter 9.

REFINING THE FIT USING POSTWEAR TOPOGRAPHY DATA

The major force responsible for the corneal shape changes seen in orthokeratology is the squeeze film

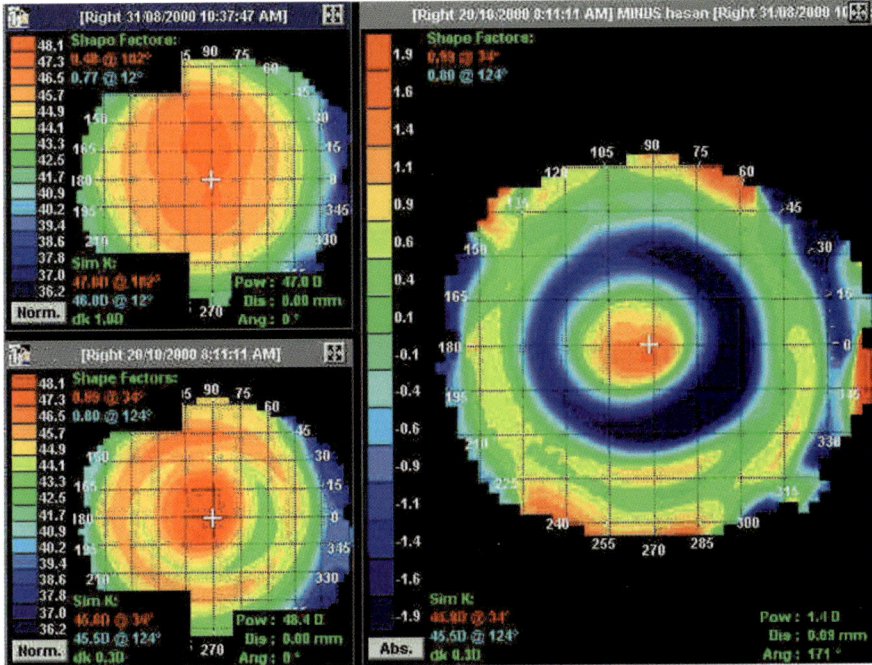

Figure 6.29   (A) Axial and (B) tangential power maps of a central island. Note the excellent centration. The steep central area is surrounded by an annulus of flattening. The unaided vision will be poor.

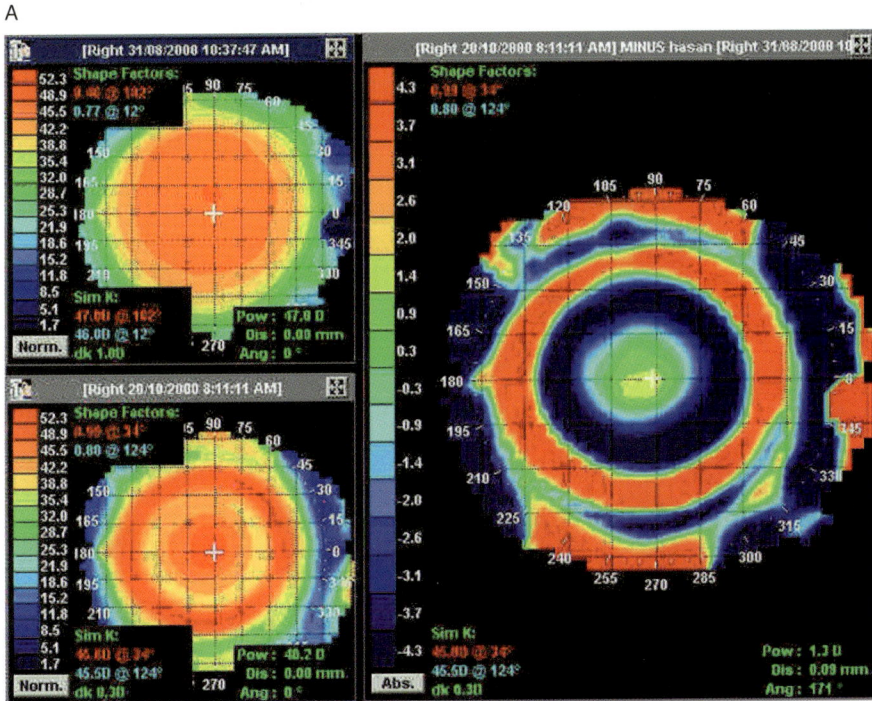

force generated by the postlens tear layer (see Ch. 10). The squeeze film force is dependent on the variation in TLT between the apex and the periph- ery of the lens. The accuracy of the lens fit is there- fore dependent on the *actual* TLT under the trial lens compared to the *calculated* TLT from the

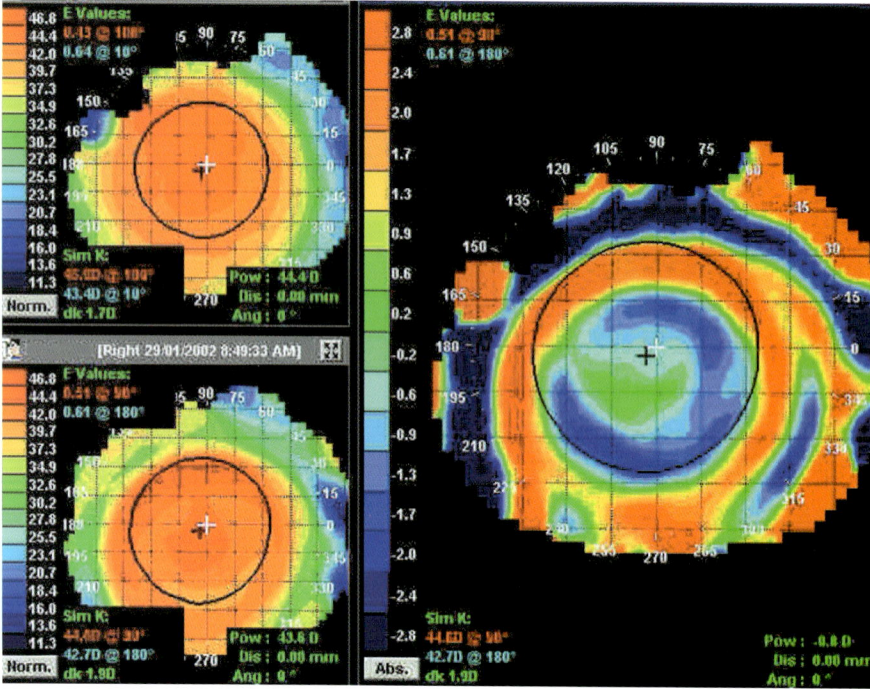

Figure 6.30 A frowny-face pattern from a tight lens. If the lens decenters laterally, this is because the total diameter is too small.

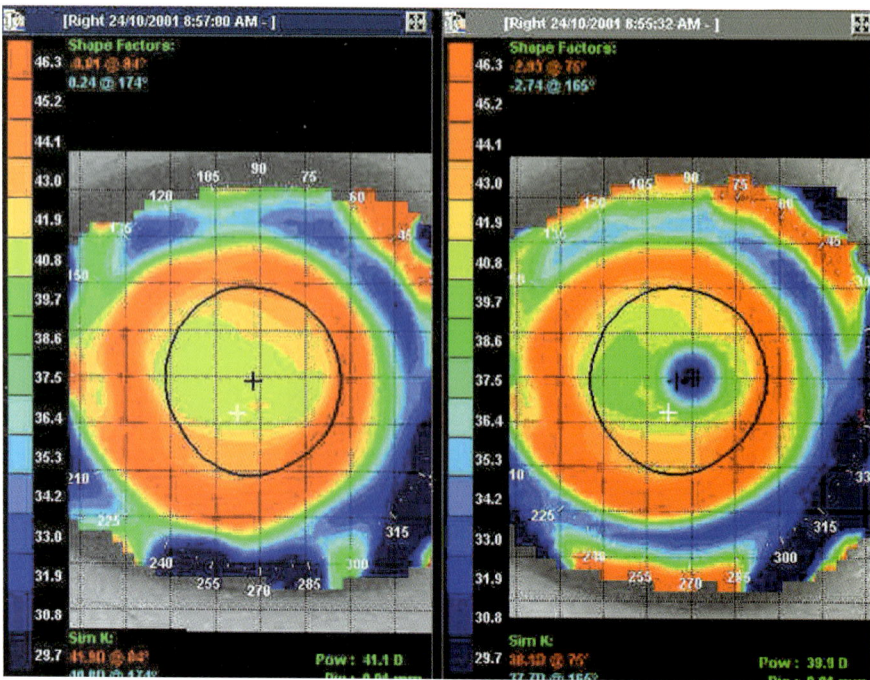

Figure 6.31 Central divot caused by tear layer disruption of the Placido mires. If lubricant is instilled and a further map is taken, the results are normal.

topography data. When the trial lens is calculated from the initial topography data, an assumption is made that the corneal sag is correct. The trial lens sag is therefore equal to the corneal sag plus the designated apical clearance, or as close to this value as possible due to the limitations in trial lens set design. Under normal circumstances, the trial lens set will need to be in 0.05 mm BOZR increments, as this will provide a sag difference of approximately 8–10 μm between each successive lens in the set. So, there are three important factors to consider:

1. The accuracy of the topography data is limited to approximately ± 10 μm over the common chord of the lens and cornea.
2. The accuracy of trial lens manufacture will result in an error of approximately ± 2.0 μm in the sag of the lens.
3. The nominal sag difference between successive trial lenses is 8–10 μm for each 0.05 mm difference in BOZR depending on the lens design.

The trial lens set or the accompanying computer program should give the sag values of the lenses in the range provided. The margin of error for the trial lens set is smaller than the error of the topographer, so it is a logical argument to compare the *known* value of the trial lens against the *assumed* value of corneal sag developed by the topography data.

The original sag formula states:

Lens sag = corneal sag + apical clearance (TLT)

The alternative perspective is:

Corneal sag = lens sag – apical clearance

So, if the subtractive plot shows a bull's-eye pattern, irrespective of the refractive change achieved, then it can be assumed that the calculated topography corneal sag value is relatively accurate. If a smiley-face pattern is evident, then the calculated corneal sag value is equal to or less than that of the indicated trial lens to a degree somewhere near the standard deviation of error of the instrument. A central island indicates that the calculated corneal sag has been overestimated by the topographer, as the sag value is greater than the difference between the lens sag and the apical clearance value.

The practitioner now has two logical choices as to which lens should next be tried if the postwear topography plots gave unacceptable results:

1. Alter the corneal sag by a value equal to the standard deviation of error of the instrument, and recalculate a new trial lens.
2. Trial fit the next flattest or steepest lens in the trial set until the best fluorescein pattern is attained. Find the difference in sag between the correct trial lens and the initial trial lens and adjust the calculated corneal sag value accordingly.

If the initial corneal sag is assumed to be 1500 μm and a trial lens of 8.45 mm BOZR and sag of 1505 μm was tried and resulted in a central island, the two choices are:

1. Reduce the corneal sag by the standard deviation of the instrument (say 10 μm), resulting in a corneal sag of 1490 μm, and a trial lens of 1495 μm assuming an apical clearance of 5 μm. The next closest trial lens has a sag of 1494 μm and a BOZR of 8.50 mm.
2. Flatten the BOZR by an amount similar to the standard deviation of error of the instrument. Assuming an 8 μm sag difference in each trial lens, the next alternate lens would be an 8.50 mm BOZR.

The same approach applies in the case of smiley faces, except that the corneal sag value must be *increased* and the sag value of the trial lens increased by steepening the BOZR.

These changes are encapsulated in the FAST rule (Bloom unpublished). The acronym stands for "flat add, steep take-away." If the corneal elevation is underestimated, the lens will be flat, so alterations are made by adding to the initial sag value. Conversely, a steep lens will require the subtraction of the standard deviation of error of the instrument or the sag difference between trial lenses.

If the above steps are taken, and the results still show a central island or a smiley face on retrial, then the error of the initial topography data must be assumed to be within the range of two standard deviations of the instrument error. If a retrial with these corrections is performed, and a poor result is still evident, then the logical assumption is that the original topography data were totally inaccurate.

The patient should then return for further corneal topography and trial lens fitting. Furthermore, if the initial indicated trial lens is obviously too steep or flat, then it has to be assumed that the topography data are highly inaccurate.

There are two approaches to this problem. The first is to repeat the topography and take the mean R_0 and e or elevation values of four or five repeated measurements and recalculate the trial lens. The second is to depend on fluorescein pattern analysis and alter the corneal sag value by the amount of difference in trial lens sags between the initial calculated trial lens and the one that gave the optimal pattern. This approach is fraught with inaccuracies, as it firstly makes the assumption that an ideal fluorescein pattern will give an ideal response, which is simply not the case. Secondly, it makes the assumption that the R_0 value of the original reading was accurate, and that the elevation or eccentricity values were at fault.

No currently available corneal topographer can measure R_0. All systems use algorithms to extrapolate from the measured area into the center to give a value for R_0. However, in order to calculate a BOZR for the trial lens, the R_0 value has to be used. If the original topography readings are within 1 SD of producing a good result, then it is acceptable to assume that the R_0 value is correct, and that the eccentricity or elevation is at fault and make corrections to improve the corneal response. However, postwear plots that produce repeated central islands or smiley faces when corrections are made indicate highly inaccurate R_0 and e values, necessitating repetition of the topography plots.

Finally, lenses that decenter laterally cause decentered treatment zones. The resolution of this problem is to recalculate for a larger total diameter. It must be emphasized that trial lens fitting in orthokeratology is primarily performed in order to validate the original topography data, especially with respect to the elevation or sag values. The corneal response to the lens is totally dependent on the accuracy of the lens fit, where the apical clearance, in particular, is of vital importance in generating the required degree of squeeze film force under the lens. The accuracy of the corneal data will determine directly the accuracy of the lens fit and the degree of apical clearance, and hence the corneal response. These factors are dealt with in greater detail in Chapter 10.

The question as to the time required between trial wear periods has been answered by Sridharan (2001), who showed that it could take up to 72 h for a cornea to return to baseline following overnight wear. If a further trial wear is initiated before the cornea returns to baseline, the results could be unduly influenced by the previous distortion still present in the cornea. It would be appropriate, therefore, to wait at least 72 h before performing a retrial, with a further prefit topography being done to ensure return to baseline.

In conclusion, it must be emphasized that the only acceptable outcome from an overnight trial is a bull's-eye pattern. Improvements in unaided acuity occur with both bull's-eye and smiley-face patterns, but the quality of the visual acuity is better with a bull's eye. Unaided visual acuity is not the standard by which an outcome is assessed, but rather the quality of the postwear topography change.

Practitioners who prefer empirical fitting should insist on knowing the design and curves on the lenses they are using, and those who judge the fitting on fluorescein pattern analysis should know the difference in sag between the lenses in the set. Orthokeratology, as stated previously, differs from standard lens fitting, as it is not the appearance of the lens that determines success, but the effect the lens has on visual acuity and the quality of the postwear corneal topography. The only fitting method that gives the practitioner total control over lens changes is the topography-based system.

At the time of writing, there have been no controlled studies into the differences in efficacy of the three different methods of fitting orthokeratology lenses. Such a study would have a direct practical benefit, in that practitioners would be better able to determine the best and most cost-effective means of fitting the lenses. As with all other types of contact lens practice, the fitting requires skill and knowledge, and should not be conducted in a hit-and-miss manner. The aim should be to get the right fit first time, all the time. This may, in practice, be unlikely due to the degree of accuracy required and the limitations of topography, but nevertheless, it should still be the aim.

REFERENCES

Applegate R A, Nunez R, Beuttener J, Howland H C (1995) How accurately can videokeratographic systems measure surface elevation? Optometry and Vision Science 72: 785–792

Bara C (2000) Mechanism of action of the reverse geometry gas permeable contact lens in orthokeratology. M Sc thesis, University of Melbourne

Bennett E S, Sorbara L (2000) Lens design, fitting and evaluation. In: Bennett ES, Henry VA (eds) Clinical manual of contact lenses, 2nd edn. Philadelphia, Lippincott Williams & Wilkins, ch. 4

Bennett E S, Henry V A, Davis L J, Kirby S (1989) Comparing empirical and diagnostic fitting of daily wear fluoro-silicone acrylate contact lenses. Contact Lens Forum 14: 38–44

Brungardt T F (1961) Fluorescein patterns; they are accurate and they can be mastered. Journal of the American Optometric Association 32: 973–974

Carney L G (1972) Luminance of fluorescein solutions. American Journal of Optometry and Archives of the American Academy of Optometry 3: 200–204

Cho P, Lam A, Mountford J, Ng L (2002a) The performance of four different corneal topographers on normal human corneas and its impact on orthokeratology lens fitting. Optometry and Vision Science (in press)

Cho P, Cheung S W, Edwards M (2002b) Practice of orthokeratology by a group of contact lens practitioners in Hong Kong. Part 2. Clinical and Experimental Optometry 86(1): 42–46

Douthwaite W A (1995) Eyesys corneal topography measurement applied to calibrated ellipsoidal convex surfaces. British Journal of Ophthalmology 79: 797–801

Fedders K, Gultranson B S, Nair B S, Horner D G, Soni S (1999) Orthokeratology: to fit empirically or use diagnostic lenses? Optometry and Vision Science 76(125): 170

Guillon M, Sammons W A (1994) Contact lens design. In: Ruben M, Guillon M (eds) Contact lens practice. London, Chapman and Hall Medical, ch. 5

Hayashi T (1977) Mechanics of contact lens motion. PhD thesis. University Of California, Berkeley

Hilmantel G, Blunt R J, Garrett B P, Howland H C, Applegate R A (1999) Accuracy of the Tomey topographic modeling system in measuring surface elevations of asymmetric objects. Optometry and Vision Science 76: 108–114

Hough T, Edwards K (1999) The reproducibility of videokeratoscope measurements as applied to the human cornea. Contact Lens and Anterior Eye 22(3): 91–99

Jeandervin M, Barr J T (1998) Comparison of repeat videokeratography: repeatability and accuracy. Optometry and Vision Science 75: 663–669

Korb D R, Finnemore V N, Herman J P (1982) Apical changes and scarring in keratoconus related to contact lens fitting techniques. Journal of the American Optometric Association 53: 199–205

Lu L, Zhou L H, Wang Z G, Zhang W H (2001) Orthokeratology induced infective corneal ulcer. Investigative Ophthalmology and Vision Science 42(4): s34

Luk B M W, Bennett E S, Barr J T (2001) Fitting orthokeratology contact lenses. Contact Lens Spectrum 16(10): 30–35

Mandell R B (1974) How valid is the fluorescein test? International Contact Lens Clinic 1: 25–27

Maruna C, Yoder M, Andrasko G J (1989) Attitudes towards RGPs among optometrists. Contact Lens Spectrum 4: 25–32

Mountford J A (1997) Orthokeratology. In: Phillips A J, Speedwell L (eds) Contact lenses: a textbook for students and practitioner, vol. 4. London, Butterworths, pp. 30–35

Mountford J A, Noack D B (2001) The BE instruction manual. Brisbane, Australia

Mountford J A, Caroline P, Noack D (2002) Corneal topography and orthokeratology – pre-fitting evaluation. Contact Lens Spectrum 17(4): 29–35

Mountford J A, Cho P, Chui W S (2003) Is fluorescein pattern analysis a valid method of assessing the accuracy of reverse geometry lenses for orthokeratology? Clinical and Experimental Optometry (in press)

Osborne G N, Zantos S G, Godio L B, Jones W F, Barr J T (1989) Aspheric rigid gas permeable contact lenses; practitioner discrimination of base curve increments using fluorescein pattern evaluation. Optometry and Vision Science 66(4): 209–213

Rah M J (2002) Patient selection and preliminary results of the lenses and overnight orthokeratology study. SECO, March 2002 (abstract)

Reim T (2000) The Dreimlens instruction manual. Dreimlens International, Alhambra, USA

Soni P, Nguyen T (2002) Which corneal parameter, anterior corneal curvature, posterior corneal curvature or corneal thickness is most sensitive to acute changes with reverse geometry orthokeratology lenses? ARVO Abstracts 3086. Investigative Ophthalmology and Visual Science

Sridharan R (2001) Response and regression of the cornea with short-term orthokeratology lens wear. Masters thesis. University of New South Wales, Sydney, Australia

Tang W, Collins M, Carney L C, Davis B (2000) The accuracy and precision performance of four videokeratoscopes in measuring test surfaces. Optometry and Vision Science 77(9): 483–491

Chapter 7

Corneal and refractive changes due to orthokeratology

John Mountford

CHAPTER CONTENTS

Introduction 175
Keratometry changes 176
The relationship between corneal topography and refractive changes 178
The nature of postorthokeratology topography 181
The effect of orthokeratology on astigmatism 185
Corneal topographical analysis in astigmatism 186
Other considerations 187
Stability and retention of induced corneal shape changes 188
Refractive changes with reverse geometry lenses 190
Visual acuity 192
Corneal thickness 194
Corneal staining 197
Short-term changes 198
Long-term changes 200
Patient satisfaction 200
Summary 201
References 202

INTRODUCTION

Although orthokeratology has been in clinical use for over 35 years, the main methods of describing the induced changes have been in terms of keratometry and improvement in unaided visual acuity (VA) (Neilson et al 1964, Grant 1981, Wlodyga & Bryla 1989, Harris & Stoyan 1992). However, since the introduction of videokeratoscopy, a better method of objective analysis has evolved.

El Hage (1995 AAO lecture) was the first to describe the use of topography in orthokeratology, not only for designing the correct lens for the eye, but also as a means of monitoring the corneal changes as they occurred. The accuracy and repeatability of the current generation of videokeratoscopes (VKCs) make them an ideal instrument for analyzing the corneal shape changes that occur with orthokeratology. For example, the repeatability of the measurement of apical corneal power (ACP) on human subjects is of the order of 0.15 D (Dave et al 1998), whereas the repeatability of postlens-wear refraction is in the order of 0.37 D (Rengstorff 1965). A correctly calibrated and automatically focusing VKC measures corneal shape changes *objectively*, whereas postwear refraction, particularly in the case of orthokeratology, where both the practitioner and patient are subject to bias, cannot be considered to be objective. However, there are limitations to the accuracy and repeatability of VKCs, particularly with respect to the measurement of human corneas (see Ch. 2).

Also, the dependence of improvement in unaided VA as a means of assessing success is also fraught with the same bias, especially if the same eye chart is used routinely. Carney (1994) points out the inherent bias and lack of objectivity of some of the earlier orthokeratology reports with respect to VA improvement, and in particular the dependence on patient-reported VA improvement by monitoring their own acuity by the supply of a "home eye chart" (Fontana 1972, Contex Fitting Manual 1997). The controlled studies (Kerns 1976, Coon 1984, Polse et al 1983b) all reported improvements in unaided VA in their orthokeratology groups that were statistically different from the control groups, but such changes in VA usually showed no correlation with the refractive change induced. The same poor relationship between improvement in VA and refraction was shown to occur in radial keratotomy (Rowsey et al 1988). Obviously, there are changes occurring in the corneal shape that have a direct bearing on the refractive changes and the VA changes, but what nature do these changes take?

Another important factor is that, although there had been many attempts to develop a predictive model for orthokeratology (Freeman 1976, Wlodyga & Bryla 1989), none could routinely be relied on to assess the likely outcome of a course of treatment accurately. This is of vital importance as one of the more commonly used examples of the nonscientific nature of the procedure was its apparent lack of predictability. The common finding of the three controlled studies of the early orthokeratology techniques was that there was a poor correlation between the lens used and the result achieved. The main problems preventing the procedure from gaining wider acceptance were the time and costs involved for what were modest clinical results, as well as the lack of predictability.

A patient presenting for routine contact lens fitting is assessed as to suitability for lens wear based on the subjective and objective data gathered by the clinician. The interpretation of the facts concerning the patient's examination is then compared to the known standards for success or failure, and an informed decision can then be made as to whether to proceed or not. To a large extent, this type of analytical approach was not in common use in orthokeratology, especially with respect to the aims and objectives of the patient. The likely outcomes were more commonly based on a "percentage success" rather than on hard evidence, which had become the norm with routine lens practice.

Orthokeratology is the deliberate alteration of corneal shape in order to effect a change in the refractive status of the eye. The concept of "corneal shape" is an interesting one. Optometrists have always known that the cornea is aspheric, but until recently have used an instrument that assumes that the cornea is a sphere for measurement. There is some controversy about what happens to corneal shape in orthokeratology: does it change from an asphere to a sphere or from a prolate to an oblate surface?

It therefore stands to reason that a process that involves the manipulation of corneal shape in order to attain a result should be primarily assessed as to the exact effects of the process on corneal shape in order to lay the foundations for a predictive model. Both Kerns (1976) and Coon (1984) suggested that the initial corneal eccentricity could be used as a predictive model, as the corneal shape following orthokeratology was basically spherical. It is the purpose of this chapter to review the changes in corneal shape and refraction, corneal thickness, and VA improvement caused by modern reverse geometry lenses. The data from both daily and overnight studies will be included together.

KERATOMETRY CHANGES

A report from Grant & May (1970) on a limited sample of cases was responsible for the adoption of the belief that the keratometric changes occurred at twice the rate of the refractive change. This belief became entrenched in the orthokeratology literature (May & Grant 1970, Nolan 1972, Patterson 1975) to the extent that it was still being reported as fact in 1994 (Wlodyga & Harris 1994).

Erickson & Thorn (1977) compiled the reported refractive and keratometric changes from 181 eyes from various authors and found that the best-fit regression between keratometric and refractive change was:

$$\Delta RE = 0.68(\Delta K) + 0.72\ D\ (r = 0.63)$$

where RE is refractive error and K is keratometry change.

Their interpretation of this finding was that there could be a change in refraction of approximately 0.75 D *before* any measurable change in keratometry occurred. The probable cause for the discrepancy was felt to be due to the inability of the keratometer to measure changes at the corneal apex, where most of the change would be expected to occur.

The authors posed three interesting questions to the orthokeratologists of the time. Firstly, why does a 0.75 D change in refractive error occur when there is no keratometric change? Secondly, why are keratometric changes, once they appear, usually accompanied by only two-thirds as much change as refractive error? The third and final question was: why does the basic 0.75 D change in refractive error and the changes in keratometry fail to account for so much of the variability in refractive error? There are two other questions that also need to be asked before initiating a course of orthokeratologic treatment and these are: what is the refractive change possible and how long will the effect last?

Wlodyga & Bryla (1989) introduced the use of "temporal" keratometry as a means of both predicting the possible degree of refractive change and also for monitoring the corneal shape changes as they occurred. Temporal-K readings are made by having the patient fixate on the nasal mire of the keratometer along the flat meridian. The measurement is then assumed to give an indication of the corneal curvature at approximately 4.00 mm from the corneal apex. The exact basis for the use of temporal keratometry is not known, but could be due in part to the relationship between the third and ninth ring of the Corneascope and the refractive change possible with earlier orthokeratology, as described by Freeman (1976). The third ring of the Corneascope corresponds to a chord of 3 mm from the corneal apex (keratometer chord) whilst the ninth ring corresponds to a chord of approximately 7.5 mm. However, as Lui & Edwards (2000) pointed out, the analysis of ring comparison methods is invalid, as the locus for the center of

curvature does not lie on the optic axis, but forms an evolute due to corneal asphericity, and cannot be used to determine peripheral curvature, as was done by Freeman.

When used as a predictive tool, the relationship between central K (K_c) and temporal K (K_t) and refractive change is:

$$\Delta Rx = 2(K_c - K_t) + 1.00$$

The extra + 1.00 D is added as an allowance for axial length change due to corneal flattening. A 2.00 D difference in K readings would therefore yield a predicted refractive change of 5.00 D. This relationship is primarily based on the assumption of May & Grant that the refractive changes occurred at twice the rate of keratometric change. The above analysis by Erickson & Thorn shows that this is not the case. Also, the predictive value of the relationship was assessed in two other studies (Soni & Horner 1993, Joe et al 1996) that found no correlation between the delta K values and the refractive changes induced. Furthermore, other authors (Coon 1984, Carkeet et al 1995) found no evidence of axial length change in orthokeratology.

The final error made by this assumption is that the temporal keratometry value is accurate. Bennett & Rabbetts (1991) have shown that the "true" value from temporal K readings is equal to half the difference between the central and temporal values. A measured 2.00 D difference is therefore closer to 1.00 D in actual value. Therefore, the "real" formula should be:

$$Rx\ change = (K_c - K_t)$$

which, in the context of the figures given previously, would result in a predicted change of 2.00 D, not 5.00 D.

When temporal K readings are taken during a course of treatment, a gradual steepening of the readings will occur, until the peripheral K readings are steeper than the central K readings. This led to the assumption of the cornea changing to an oblate surface. Figure 7.1 shows the post-orthokeratology corneal shape. The area of mid-peripheral steepening (the "red ring") coincides with the area of measurement used for temporal keratometry. The effectively steeper temporal keratometry reading when compared to the

Relationship between Rx change and eccentricity change assuming an oblate surface

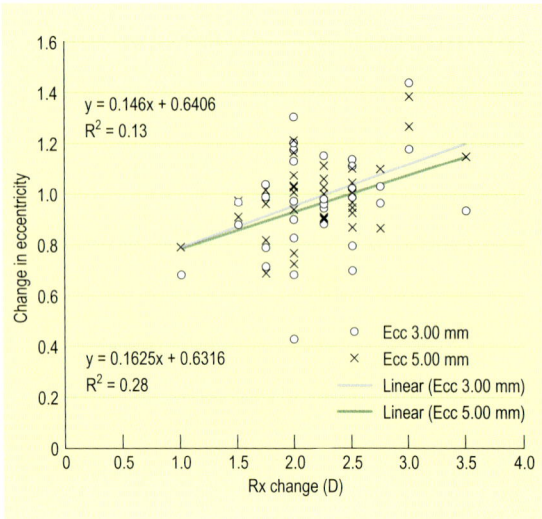

$y = 0.146x + 0.6406$
$R^2 = 0.13$

$y = 0.1625x + 0.6316$
$R^2 = 0.28$

○ Ecc 3.00 mm
× Ecc 5.00 mm
— Linear (Ecc 3.00 mm)
— Linear (Ecc 5.00 mm)

Change in eccentricity

Rx change (D)

Figure 7.1 Topographic change map (right) showing the characteristic red ring of mid-peripheral steepening centered around the blue flattened zone. This area of steepening coincides with the area of measurement used for temporal keratometry. The effectively steeper temporal keratometry reading when compared to the flatter central reading led to the assumption of an oblate surface.

flatter central reading led to the assumption of an oblate surface.

THE RELATIONSHIP BETWEEN CORNEAL TOPOGRAPHY AND REFRACTIVE CHANGES

As stated previously, El Hage et al were the first actively to use corneal topography not only to design the lens, but also as a means of monitoring the results of treatment. They reported the refrac-

Myopia reduction vs. shape factor

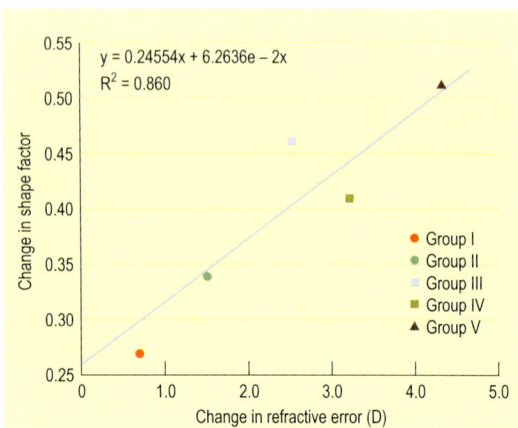

$y = 0.24554x + 6.2636e - 2x$
$R^2 = 0.860$

Change in shape factor

● Group I
● Group II
▪ Group III
▪ Group IV
▲ Group V

Change in refractive error (D)

Figure 7.2 The relationship between change in shape factor (p) and refractive change (D). Courtesy of Sammi El Hage.

tive changes occurring in 51 patients fitted with the controlled keratoreformation lens (an aspheric reverse geometry lens based on topographical fitting), and the relationship between the refractive change achieved and the change in corneal shape factor (p), as measured by the Alcon Eyemap EH-270/290.

The analysis of the data gave the following relationship between refractive change and shape factor change (Fig. 7.2):

$$y = -7.1767 + 5.929x \ (r^2 = 0.941)$$

where y = refractive change and x = change in shape factor (p).

Mountford (1997) also studied the shape and refractive changes occurring in a group of orthokeratology patients. Sixty patients were randomly selected from a large (386) group of successful orthokeratology patients, and the choice of eye randomized. Topography was performed with the EyeSys topographer (version 3.20).

All subjects underwent the same course of treatment, with regular reviews at set periods of time following the dispensing of lenses. Aftercare visits were scheduled in the morning, with the lenses in situ following overnight wear. Vision with lenses in place, slit-lamp exam, with and without lenses, postwear refraction, vision, and videokeratoscopy were routinely performed.

The postwear axial topography plot was subtracted from the original prefit plot, and the difference or change in corneal shape and power measured on repeated visits until the maximum change was recorded. This was assumed to have occurred if there was no further change over a period of 2 months. The changes in simulated keratometry (VKC), apical corneal radius, ACP, and corneal eccentricity were tabulated and used for statistical analysis.

The first thing done was to see whether the keratometric and refractive relationship was similar to that found by Erickson & Thorn. The result is:

$$\Delta Rx = 0.77\Delta K + 0.71 \ (r^2 = 0.77, P < 0.001)$$

where ΔRx is refractive change (spherical equivalent) and ΔK the change in mean K in diopters (Fig. 7.3). This is a very similar result to that found by Erickson & Thorn, in that a zero change in keratometry could be associated with a refractive change of 0.71 D.

The primary reason for the apparent discrepancy between the keratometric and refractive changes was felt to be due to the fact that the keratometer only measures the mean sagittal radius of curvature of the cornea at a point approximately 1.50 mm from center. Modern VKCs allow for a much more accurate measurement of the changes that occur closer to the corneal apex than the keratometer. A high correlation between change in ACP (the refractive power of the cornea at the absolute apex) and refractive change was also found and is shown in Figure 7.4. The relationship is:

$$\Delta Rx = 0.92\Delta ACP + 0.15 \ (r^2 = 0.91, P < 0.0001, df\ 58)$$

This can be interpreted as a 1.00 D change in ACP causing a refractive change of 1.07 D. A similar result has been found by Soni & Nguyen (2002). This must be shown in the context of the accepted accuracy of postlens wear refraction, which is approximately ± 0.37 D (Rengstorff 1965). However, there is a subtle difference, in that Rengstorff studied only polymethyl methacrylate (PMMA) lens wearers, who would therefore be expected to be suffering from some degree of corneal edema, whereas the high-Dk materials commonly used for modern orthokeratology do not cause the same problems. What the relationship also shows is that the subtractive map function of the videokeratoscope is an accurate objective method of assessing the refractive change induced by the lens.

The earlier studies on orthokeratology (Kerns 1976, Binder et al 1980) found that the endpoint of the procedure was reached when the cornea became spherical ($e = 0$). Conversely, Coon's study

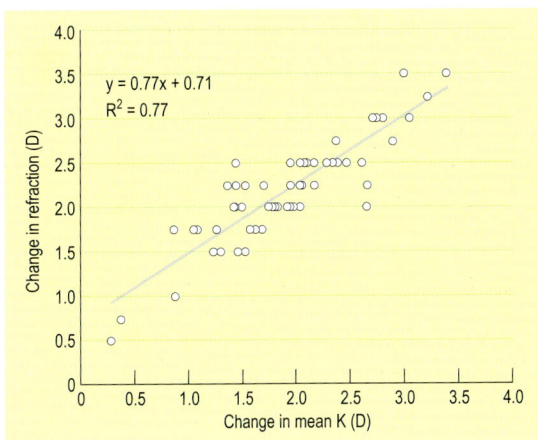

Figure 7.3 The relationship between change in mean keratometry and refractive change with orthokeratology. The relationship shows that there can be a refractive change of approximately 0.75 D before any change in K-readings occurs.

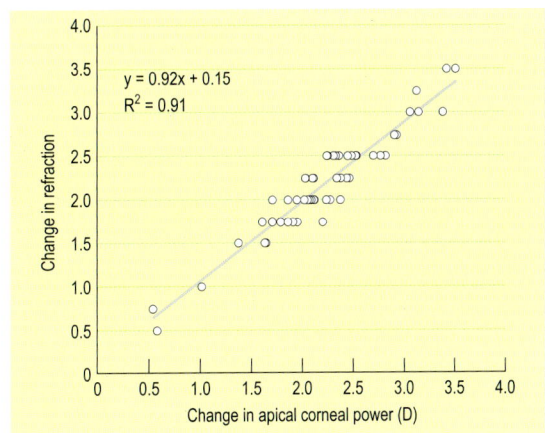

Figure 7.4 The relationship between the change in apical corneal power and refractive change. The correlation is very high, indicating that postwear changes in topography could be a good objective method of measuring spherical equivalent refractive change.

(1984), also using photokeratoscopy, found that some corneas had apparently become oblate following lens wear. If orthokeratology involves changing a prolate cornea into a spherical cornea or an oblate, there must be some correlation between the change in asphericity and the change in refraction. This relationship was assessed by comparing the change in eccentricity to both the change in ACP and the refractive change. As shown previously, the keratoscopy measurement can be considered to be an objective estimation, whilst the standard refractive technique is a subjective estimation. The relationships were found to be:

Δ Eccentricity $= 0.16\Delta$ACP $+ 0.11$ (r^2=0.84, $P < 0.0001$, df 58) and
Δ Eccentricity $= 0.16\Delta$Rx $+ 0.10$ (r^2=0.83, $P < 0.001$, df 58)

Figures 7.5 and 7.6 show the data. The results indicate that the prefitting degree of corneal asphericity can give a relatively good estimation of the refractive change likely if the cornea becomes spherical following treatment. The ratio of eccentricity to refractive change would therefore be 0.27/1.00 D, 0.42/2.00 D, 0.58/3.00 D, and 0.74/5.00 D. If the intercept of the regression was set at zero, the relationship became:

$y = 0.21x$

Where y = change in eccentricity and x = change in refraction.

If the El Hage et al regression is converted from shape factor (p) to eccentricity, the relationship becomes:

$y = 0.22x$

where y = change in eccentricity, and x is refractive change.

The results are very similar, and show that the change in corneal shape can be related to the change in refraction, and therefore used as a predictive tool for determining the refractive change possible before initiating a course of treatment.

However, the population studies on corneal shape indicate a mean corneal eccentricity of approximately 0.50, so the average change that could be expected with orthokeratology is in the range of 2.50 D using this relationship. Conversely, Joe et al (1996) found a low correlation

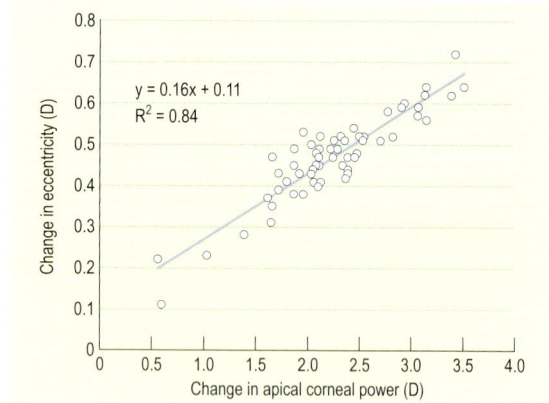

Figure 7.5   The relationship between change in eccentricity and change in apical corneal power (ACP).

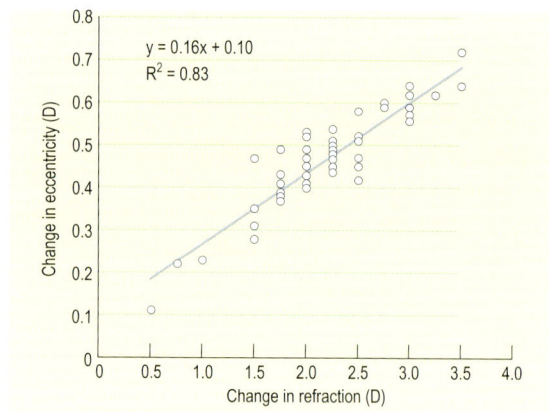

Figure 7.6   The relationship between change in eccentricity and refractive change.

between *initial* corneal eccentricity and subjective refractive change ($r = 0.526$, $P = 0.09$) and a better relationship between autorefraction and initial eccentricity ($r = 0.82$, $P = 0.002$) when reviewing the results of 15 patients fitted with the Contex OK-3.

The final factor analyzed by Mountford was the relationship between the change in eccentricity and the keratometric change (Fig. 7.7). Regression analysis gave the form:

Δ Eccentricity $= 0.132\Delta K_f + 0.22$ ($r^2 = 0.61$, $P < 0.01$, df 58)

This can be interpreted as a zero change in keratometry being associated with a change of 0.22 in eccentricity. In other words, the eccentricity could change by a value of 0.22 before

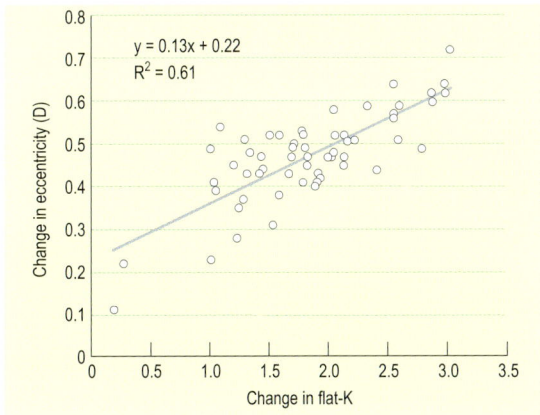

Figure 7.7   The relationship between change in flattest-K reading (K_f) and eccentricity. The eccentricity can change by 0.22 (0.75 D) prior to any changes in keratometry.

any keratometric changes became evident. If this value is inserted into the refractive change/eccentricity change relationship, then the 0.22 change in eccentricity is equivalent to a refractive change of approximately 0.75 D.

This therefore answers the first question posed by Erickson & Thorn, in that a refractive change of 0.75 D occurs prior to keratometric changes due to the initial changes occurring at the corneal apex, associated with a concurrent change in corneal eccentricity. The main reason for this effect is the inability of the keratometer to measure changes at the corneal apex. Indeed, the keratometer does not even record a change in corneal shape until the diameter of the affected zone reaches the 3.00 mm chord, where keratometric readings are made. For any given corneal shape, the keratometer assumes that the surface is spherical. If a cornea with an apical radius of 7.80 mm is assumed, but with either a high eccentricity or, conversely, a low eccentricity, then the keratometer will yield a flatter reading for the high-eccentricity cornea (as the rate of flattening is faster) than the low-eccentricity cornea.

The apparent inability of the keratometer to reflect accurately the refractive changes seen with orthokeratology is therefore due to the inherent limitations of the instrument. The assumed 2 : 1 ratio between refractive change and keratometric change is more a case of an attempt to make the readings fit the observations rather than an accurate assessment of the actual changes.

The final question as to why, when keratometric changes do occur, they only change at two-thirds of the rate of refractive change cannot be answered by the results of this study. In fact, the results appear to reach equality at approximately the 2.00 D point, and then proceed to change at the same rate. The probable reasons for the differences between Erickson & Thorn's results and those found here could be due to the fact that reverse geometry lenses cause a greater area of corneal flattening that influences the keratometry zone compared to the older orthokeratology designs.

THE NATURE OF THE POSTORTHOKERATOLOGY TOPOGRAPHY

The relationship between refractive, ACP, and eccentricity change in the previous section is based on the assumption that the "final" eccentricity value given by the instrument is correct. In the majority of cases, the final e-value was recorded as zero, indicating corneal sphericalization. However, was this really the case, or did the cornea in reality actually become oblate, and the instrument just default to an eccentricity of zero because it was not programmed to calculate oblate surfaces?

There have been reports in the literature (Coon 1984, Wlodyga & Bryla 1989, Lebow 1996, Day et al 1997) of the cornea becoming oblate following orthokeratology. The assumption is mainly based on the apparent steepening of the temporal K readings when compared to the central K readings in postorthokeratology eyes. If the cornea *does* become oblate, then the above relationship between refractive change and eccentricity change would be incorrect, as a change to an oblate surface would entail a greater change in eccentricity with respect to the refractive change.

In order to ascertain the final corneal shape properly, the axial corneal power values for 40 eyes from the group were tabulated at 0.50 mm intervals from the corneal center to the 8.00 mm chord, in the flat and steep meridians. The pre- and postorthokeratology surface powers along the horizontal meridian are shown in Figure 7.8.

In the prefit case, the typical prolate surface is evident, where the cornea appears to flatten in curvature as the periphery is approached.

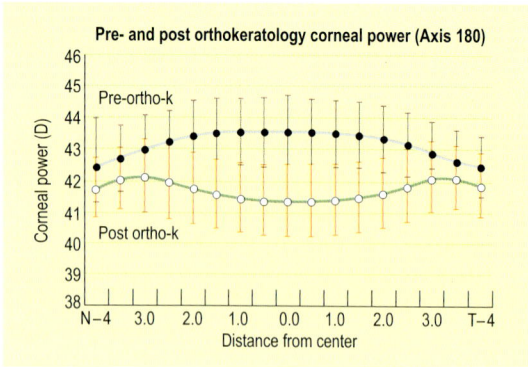

Figure 7.8   The pre- and postorthokeratology axial corneal power along the flat meridian (axis 180). Note the appearance of an "oblate" surface posttreatment.

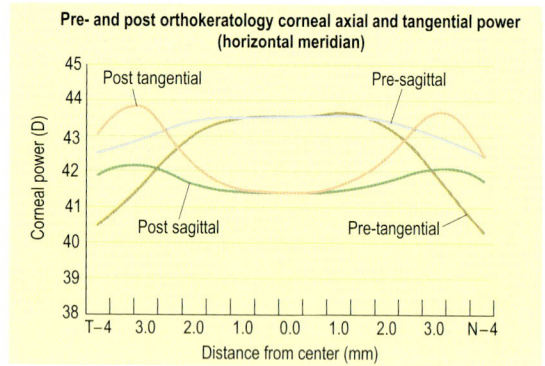

Figure 7.9   The axial and tangential corneal powers pre- and postorthokeratology. Note that the intercepts of the two sets of curves occur at different chords. The treatment zone (T×Z) diameter is the point of zero change in curvature from pre- to posttreatment. The axial power overestimates the T×Z, whilst the tangential underestimates it.

However, the postwear curve appears flatter in the center, and gradually steepens in the mid-periphery before tending to flatten again. This appears to meet the criterion of an oblate surface, especially over the central 6.00 mm chord. For each of the 40 subjects, the corneal curve in the horizontal meridian was isolated, and a "best-fit" aspheric curve fitted to the data. This led to wildly fluctuating negative asphericity values, which varied dramatically depending on the chord chosen (Fig. 7.9).

There was no correlation between the change in eccentricity from the initial prolate to the calculated "oblate" and the refractive change induced. Furthermore there was no correlation between the change in ACP and the eccentricity change if the final corneal shape was assumed to be oblate. This is unlikely to occur, due to two well-known principles. Firstly, there *must* be a relationship between shape (eccentricity) and refractive change due to the law of the conservation of corneal power, which, simply stated, means that "corneal power can never be created nor destroyed . . . just redistributed" (Caroline & Campbell 1991). Secondly, the surface area of the cornea is also a constant (except in keratoglobus) which means that the relationship between shape change and power is linked to surface area. A breakdown in both these relationships would be required for there to be a lack of correlation between corneal eccentricity and refractive surface change.

The data were then analyzed with the use of a sophisticated statistical tool (Fischer's LSD) which compared the mean and standard deviations of the curvature changes of the entire cohort at each point against each other point across the corneal surface. Over the central 4.00 mm chord there were no statistically significant differences between the points ($P > 0.05$). At the 2.50 mm half-chord, the differences did become significant ($P = 0.04$ temporal, $P = 0.01$ nasal), with the degree of significance increasing for the 6.00 mm ($P = 0.01$ temporal, $P = 0.002$ nasal), 7.00 mm ($P = 0.002$ temporal, $P = 0.002$ nasal), and 8.00 mm chords ($P = 0.04$ temporal, $P = 0.01$ nasal).

In effect, what the analysis shows is that, over the central 5.00 mm chord, the corneal surface was not statistically significantly different in shape compared to a sphere.

This result validates the use of the prefit corneal eccentricity value as a reasonably accurate predictor of the refractive change possible. The cornea starts off as an aspheric surface, but becomes spherical following orthokeratology treatment. The area of the spherical surface is dependent on complex interactions between aspheric and spherical surfaces, and will be dealt with in greater detail in Chapter 8.

The mean axial and tangential curves of pre- and postorthokeratology in 40 subjects are shown

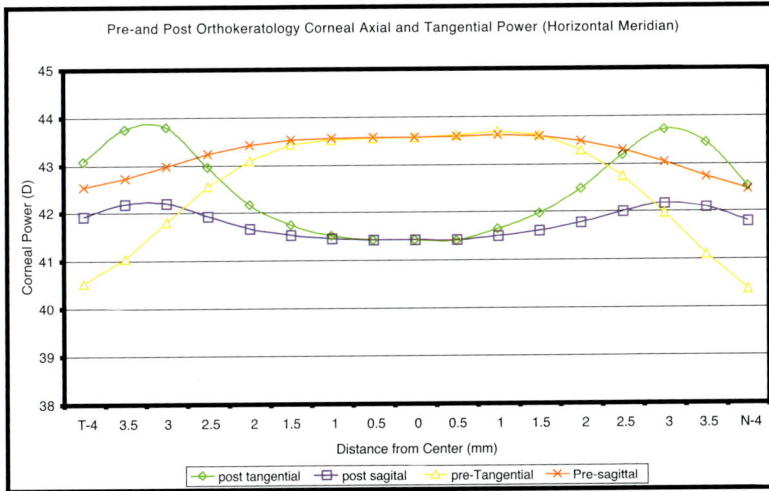

Figure 7.10 The pre- and postorthokeratology axial and tangential powers. Note that the axial power does not alter to any significant respect in the extreme periphery. The intersect of the pre and post powers shows the relative difference in sizes of treatment zones, in that axial maps tend to overestimate the treatment zone and tangentials underestimate it when compared to refractive power values.

in Figure 7.10. The axial curves in the post-treatment cornea appear to steepen in the mid-periphery and almost meet the prefit curvatures at approximately 3.50 mm from center. The tangential curves, however, intersect at approximately 2.25 mm from center. This is reflected in the topography plots as a difference in the apparent area of corneal flattening. In effect, the axial map tends to overestimate the area, whilst the tangential map underestimates the area of change. The same problem occurs when estimating the ablation zone diameter in refractive surgery (Roberts & Wu 1998). Both the axial and tangential radii give inaccurate data as to the actual area of corneal flattening due to the averaging nature of the algorithms used. The conclusion reached by Roberts & Wu was that the accurate estimate of the ablation zone following refractive surgery, and, by extension, the area of corneal flattening induced by orthokeratology (treatment zone TxZ diameter) was dependent on an analysis of the actual refractive power profiles.

Refractive power maps are based on Snell's law, and calculate the refractive power of the cornea at each point across the surface. A subtractive refractive power map is shown in Figure 7.10. The distance between the points of zero refractive change on the difference map represents the TxZ diameter as shown in Figure 7.10.

Lui & Edwards (2000) compared the effects of Contex OK704 lenses on a group of 14 orthokeratology subjects to those occurring in a control group (14 subjects) fitted with standard alignment lenses. As part of the analysis, the mean ring radius (MRR) changes from prefit to posttreatment were analyzed. Ring numbers 1 (0.6 mm diameter zone), 8 (3 mm diameter zone), 20 (7 mm diameter zone), and 26 (9.20 mm diameter zone) were used as these zone diameters related to the corneal apex (MRR1), the keratometer zone (MRR8), the maximum tear layer depth and BOZD of the lens (OK704) (MRR 20), and the contact chord in the periphery (MRR26).

Their results, over a 100-day study, showed statistically significant changes in the MRR values pre- and postwear in the orthokeratology group, particularly with MRR1 and MRR8, but not with MRR20 or MRR26. There was no statistically significant difference between MRR1 and MRR8 following orthokeratology treatment, indicating a spherical surface over this zone. Further analysis of the topography data found central corneal flattening, mid-peripheral steepening, and little or no change in the extreme periphery. They postulated that the point of zero change in the peripheral area (mean MRR23–24) should have some predictive value as far as refractive change is concerned, and found a reasonable correlation ($r^2 = 0.34$) between baseline MRR1 and mean MRR23–25.

The refractive change achieved was also correlated with the mean ring power reduction over the central five-ring area:

$$y = 1.05x + 0.09$$

where y is refractive change and x is the mean ring power change. However, there was no correlation between refractive change and change in ACP change as measured by the TMS. This was thought to be due to the fact that the majority of lenses decentered to the superotemporal direction. By using the mean of the central five-ring power change, the effects of lens decentration were minimized.

Standard OK704 lenses were used in this study whereas tangential periphery lenses were used to control centration in Mountford's study. The difference in centration between the lenses in the two groups could account for the difference in relationship between apical corneal radius and refractive change. The other factor to consider would be the difference between instruments used, and the way apical radius was determined for each.

They also found a corresponding increase in corneal shape factor (p) towards sphericalization of the corneal surface as the procedure continued. Further analysis of the p-value changes compared to the axial curvature changes using Douthwaite's method (Douthwaite 1995) showed that once orthokeratology-induced changes occur in the cornea, the ellipsoidal model breaks down, meaning that instrument-generated values of either eccentricity or shape factor become invalid. The mean change in shape factor (p) was an increase of 0.20 associated with a mean refractive change of 1.50 D. This is in agreement with the results shown in Figure 7.9, where topography-generated data were used to find the best-fit aspheric curve to the postwear shape. The lack of a correlation may be primarily due to the inability of the topographer to reconstruct nonaspheric surfaces.

Nichols et al (2000) also found variability in the postwear Q-values generated by the Humphrey Atlas, primarily due to the effects of lens decentration. However, they reported a mean change in ACP of 1.20 D associated with a mean refractive change of 1.83 D, and a mean change of 0.11 in Q-value. The studies of El Hage, Mountford, and Liu and Edwards found a relationship between change in refraction and change in corneal asphericity. The main differences between the studies is the higher correlation coefficient found by Mountford and El Hage when compared to the other two studies. The probable cause for this is the control of centration of the lenses used. Liu & Edwards used the standard OK704, which tended to center superotemporally in the majority of subjects. Nichols et al used the 704C with a wide aspheric alignment zone, but were limited by the simple algorithm used to fit the lenses, and an inability (due to the experimental design) to modify the lens fit in order to control centration.

The El Hage and Mountford studies were carried out in private practice, where lens design alterations were used to maximize centration. A lens that decenters superiorly will still give good high-contrast unaided VA, but the topography data will skew the results, resulting in a poorer correlation between the corneal asphericity changes and the refractive changes achieved. The only valid postwear topography outcome is a well-centered "bull's-eye" plot. Any lens-induced corneal distortion from lens decentration is considered to be clinically unacceptable, and the postwear refractive and shape changes basically invalid.

It is essential that the analysis of data from research into the corneal shape changes associated with orthokeratology is based on *valid* postwear information.

The conclusions that can be reached from the above analyses can be summarized as follows:

1. The predictive value of the differences in central and temporal keratometry is not valid.
2. The initial corneal eccentricity is a useful predictor of the refractive change possible.
3. There is a high correlation between refractive change and ACP change, making this a good objective method of measuring refractive change, as long as the lens centers correctly. The relationship breaks down if the lens decenters.
4. Once a reverse geometry lens starts effecting changes in corneal shape, the elliptical model of corneal shape breaks down due to the inability of the videokeratoscope's algorithms to analyze the postwear shape correctly. It is therefore not possible to fit a reverse geometry

lens using topographic data to the altered corneal shape with any accuracy.

5. Care must be taken when interpreting topography maps for the estimation of the area of central flattening. This is best performed by using the refractive power differences between the pre- and posttreatment surfaces.
6. Keratometry has severe shortcomings in monitoring the changes induced by orthokeratology when compared to corneal topography.
7. There are limitations as to the wider application of the results of these studies when using different topographers. Different topographers have different methods of calculating not only apical radius values, but also eccentricity.

However, the basic information found in the study is that there is a correlation between initial corneal asphericity and refractive change. In the case of the EyeSys topographer, the final change was found to be basically spherical, but this does not preclude the possibility of the final shape being oblate if the corneal topographer used has algorithms that can correctly calculate an oblate surface over the central 5.00–6.00 mm chord.

As will be shown in the later section on mathematical modeling of corneal shape change and refractive change (Ch. 8), there should be a correlation between these two factors even if the cornea becomes oblate.

THE EFFECT OF ORTHOKERATOLOGY ON ASTIGMATISM

One of the most problematic areas in orthokeratology is the effect of the procedure on corneal astigmatism. The earlier studies (Kerns 1976, Binder et al 1980) found an increase in unwanted with-the-rule (WTR) astigmatism, mainly due to the poor centration of the lenses used. Coon (1984) reported a decrease in WTR astigmatism using the Tabb fitting philosophy. However, the reports on the subject in the literature are mostly anecdotal, with little regard for the magnitude or direction of the astigmatic changes involved. The "accepted" limit of the correction of astigmatism is given as 3.00 D (Wlodyga & Harris 1994). However, this limit appears to be set due to the

fact that one patient had a reduction of 3.00 D in astigmatism.

The fitting philosophies also vary depending on the particular school of thought used regarding the treatment of astigmatism (Patterson 1975, Potts 1996). However, the commonly accepted method (Wlodyga & Harris 1994, Potts 1996) consists of fitting the initial lens one-third of the difference between the flat and steep meridians steeper than the flat meridian. This essentially has the effect of reducing the astigmatism prior to the active flattening of the cornea. There have been no reported studies as to the success or otherwise of this procedure, only scattered case reports. Also, the main accent is on the reduction of WTR astigmatism, as against-the-rule (ATR) astigmatism has proven almost impossible to reduce with orthokeratology. The exact reason for this is simply not known, although one study (Paige 1981) reported on the reduction of ATR astigmatism in one subject using up to 3000 transverse ocular movements per day!

There have been few reports on the effects of reverse geometry lenses and astigmatism in the literature. Soni & Horner (1993) found a 60% retention of the original astigmatism in their cohort. Liu & Edwards, on the other hand, reported no change in astigmatism in their orthokeratology subjects.

The gold standard assessment of the effect of orthokeratology on corneal astigmatism requires a vector analysis approach in order to analyze correctly the magnitude and axis changes that occur. Mountford & Pesudovs (2002) performed a retrospective analysis of 23 patients with between 0.50 and 2.00 D prefit corneal astigmatism using two different vector analysis techniques and corneal topographical analysis.

The two vector analysis techniques used in the study were the Bailey–Carney and Alpins methods. The Bailey–Carney technique (Bailey & Carney 1970) was primarily developed to measure the effects of rigid contact lens wear on corneal curvature, whereas the Alpins technique (1997) was developed in order to evaluate refractive surgery outcomes with respect to astigmatism.

Vector analysis involves the resolution of two variables so that the line joining the variables (the vector) demonstrates both magnitude and direction, which makes it an ideal method for the analysis of astigmatic changes. The results for the group of 23 subjects analyzed using the Bailey–Carney method yielded a mean reduction in astigmatism of 50.2%.

The Alpins method

Noel Alpins, a Melbourne ophthalmologist, developed this technique of vector analysis in order to assess properly the outcomes of refractive surgery, penetrating keratoplasty, and cataract surgery with respect to astigmatic changes. It is, in a lot of ways, a marked advance on the Bailey–Carney method in that the data obtained can be represented as an index of success or failure that can be subjected to statistical analysis. The subjects were divided into two subgroups for analysis: group 1 was 0.50 D or greater and group 2 0.75 D or greater.

For a total correction of 0.50 D astigmatism and greater, orthokeratology has an efficacy of 0.62 or 62%, and in order for the 100% goal to be attained, the treatment would need to be 60% more effective. Similarly, for the 0.75 D group, orthokeratology has an efficacy of 56%, and an increase in effectiveness of 80% would be required in order to correct preexisting astigmatism totally.

If a more realistic aim of a 50% reduction in preexisting astigmatism is the target, then orthokeratology is highly effective, with treatment efficacy slightly greater (7%) than that required for the 0.50 D group, and 2% less than that required for the 0.75 D group.

However, standard deviation of the angle of error values shows a markedly high degree of variability. Alpins considers a good outcome to show little deviation from the original astigmatic axis, with a small standard deviation. The comparatively large standard deviations in the angle of error caused by orthokeratology indicate a high degree of unpredictability in the axis of the post-treatment astigmatism. However, this was not reflected in the results of the 23 subjects, where the relative change in astigmatic axis from the original axis was within 10°. In fact, the deviation from sphericity locus as measured for the Bailey–Carney analysis showed a maximum deviation of 11°. The probable cause for the difference between the calculated standard deviation using the Alpins method could be partly due to the relatively small degrees of astigmatism involved. None of the cases reviewed had oblique astigmatism induced.

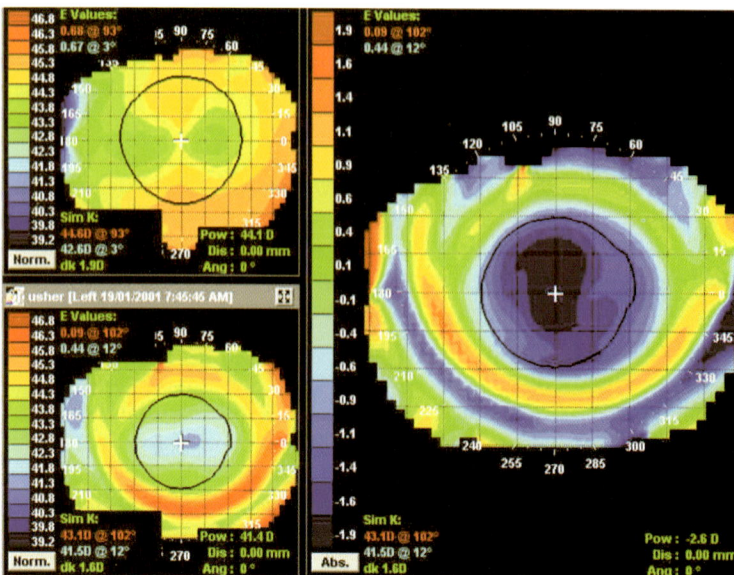

Figure 7.11 A subtractive refractive power map showing the results of an orthokeratology treatment. The white arrows show the treatment zone (T×Z) diameter.

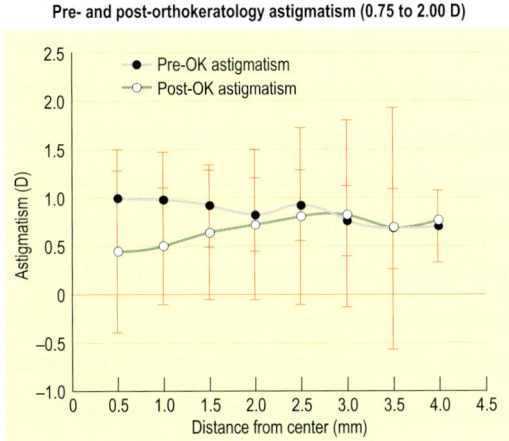

Figure 7.12   The pre- and postorthokeratology astigmatism. The major change occurs within the central 2.00 mm chord. At the keratometer zone (3.00 mm) the changes are not statistically significant.

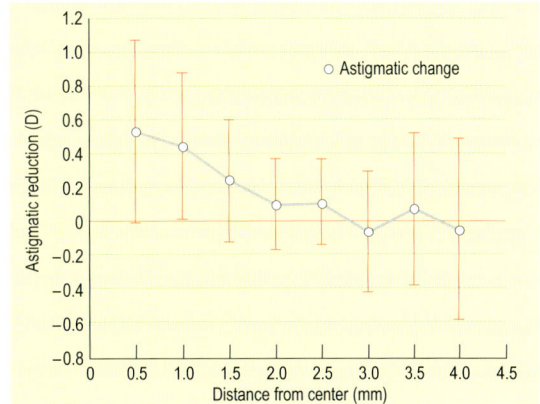

Figure 7.13   The change in astigmatism from the center to the peripheral cornea.

CORNEAL TOPOGRAPHICAL ANALYSIS IN ASTIGMATISM

Topographical analysis of the pre- and posttreatment astigmatism was performed on 16 subjects who exhibited 0.75 D or greater corneal astigmatism. The pre- and postorthokeratology astigmatism over the central 8.00 mm chord is shown in Figure 7.12.

Note that the major change in astigmatism appears to occur within the central 2.00 mm chord. This change in astigmatism is shown in Figure 7.13. Paired Student's t-tests were performed on the pre- and postwear values, with the differences over the central 3.00 mm chord being statistically significantly different. The P-values for the different half-chords were: 0.50 mm, $P = 0.004$, 1.00 mm, $P = 0.02$ and 1.50 mm, $P = 0.01$. There was no statistically significant difference for the 2.00–5.00 mm half-chords.

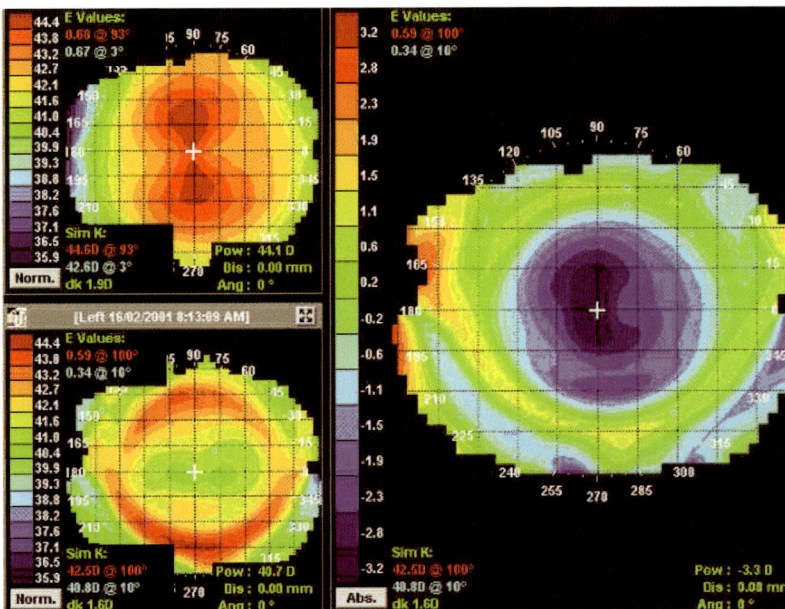

Figure 7.14   A subtractive axial power map showing the flattening of the central 2.00 mm chord with astigmatism. Note the greater change in the vertical meridian (blue bowtie).

As shown in Figure 7.11, the major change in astigmatism occurs within the central 3.00 mm chord, with the change at the 2.00 mm chord being approximately twice that occurring at the 3.00 mm (keratometer) chord. The percentage change in astigmatism for the different chords was: 1.00 mm 55.6%, 2.00 mm 49%, and 3.00 mm 29.7%. In other words, the keratometry values, if used to assess astigmatic change, would only record approximately 50% of the change occurring closer to the corneal apex.

Figure 7.14 shows a subtractive difference map of the change in astigmatism with orthokeratology. Note that the major change in the astigmatism occurs within the central 2.00 mm chord, and that the simulated keratometry values do not correspond to the reduction in astigmatism achieved. The relationship between the pre- and postcorneal astigmatism over the central 1.00 mm chord is shown in Figure 7.15. Although statistically significant, the correlation is very poor ($r^2 = 0.11$, $P = 0.04$, df 14), indicating a poor predictability between initial and final astigmatism.

All three methods of analysis point to a reduction of approximately 50% in preexisting astigmatism of up to 1.75 D if reverse geometry lenses are used. This would therefore indicate that the degree of astigmatic reduction possible with the procedure is limited to approximately 1.00 D, so

Pre- vs. post-orthokeratology astigmatism (1.00 mm chord)

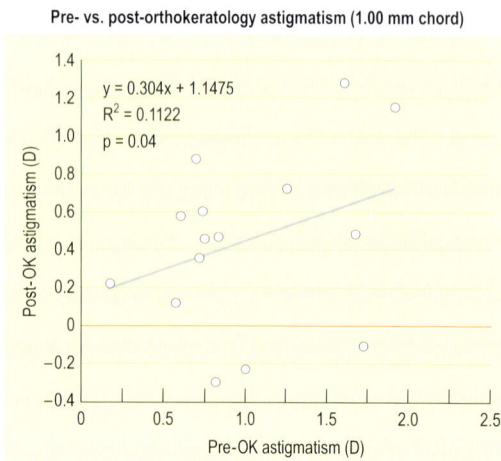

Figure 7.15   The relationship between the pre- and postorthokeratology astigmatism over the central 1.00 mm chord. Although statistically significant, the correlation is poor.

the level of preexisting astigmatism is of major importance when assessing a patient's suitability for the procedure. From a clinical viewpoint, it could be argued that a residual astigmatic error of 0.50–0.75 D would have little negative impact on unaided vision, especially if it is WTR in direction. This means that the maximum indicated error that could be treated and expected to yield acceptable results would be in the order of 1.50 D.

OTHER CONSIDERATIONS

The above analysis is based on the use of spherical reverse geometry lenses and their effect on astigmatic change, but does not take into consideration the effect, if any, of more novel lens designs and fitting philosophies. There are also some unanswered questions with respect to the treatment of astigmatism that should be addressed, namely:

1. Corneal eccentricity has been shown to be a good indicator of the refractive change possible with orthokeratology. Therefore, could a difference in eccentricity between the steep and flat meridian also play a role in determining the astigmatic change possible?
2. The shape changes induced by the lens are, in some way, related to the tear film squeeze forces developed under the lens. Could the difference in tear layer profile and thickness between the steep and flat meridian also play a role in astigmatic change?
3. Why does ATR astigmatism increase with the use of reverse geometry lenses, and what lens design variations can be used to try and control this effect?
4. Why does limbus-to-limbus astigmatism respond so poorly to orthokeratology when compared to central astigmatism?

The problem of astigmatism and orthokeratology is quite complex. Hopefully, as the sophistication of corneal topographical analysis increases, our understanding of the nature and shape of the astigmatic cornea will enable the development of specific fitting philosophies and lens designs in order to improve not only the predictability of treatment, but also the efficacy of treatment for astigmatism.

In conclusion, analysis of the data shows that orthokeratology is effective in reducing preexisting astigmatism by approximately 50%. This would therefore set the prefit level of astigmatism to an upper limit of 1.50 D with the rule.

STABILITY AND RETENTION OF INDUCED CORNEAL SHAPE CHANGES

As stated at the beginning of this chapter, one of the important factors to consider when assessing the suitability of a patient for orthokeratology is the question of the stability of the shape changes induced and how they impact on the quality of unaided vision following lens removal.

There is very little information in the literature concerning the stability of the effects of accelerated orthokeratology; however the common understanding is that those who respond faster to the treatment will lose the effect at a faster rate (Wlodyga & Harris 1994). However, some doubt was cast on this observation by Horner et al (1993), who found that the corneal response to the OK-3 lens in terms of refractive change was time-dependent, in that the longer the lens was worn, the greater the effect appeared to be. Following wearing times of 1, 2, and 4 h, the ranges of refractive change were 0.10–2.37 D (1 h), 1.01–1.81 D (2 h), and 1.43–2.56 D (4 h). The trend appears to

be increased refractive change with increased wearing time, but the other obvious factor is the variations in response, as shown by the spread of the range. Similarly, the regression of the effect to 95% of baseline levels was shown to vary with wearing time, in that the 1-h group recovered at the rate of 50.9% per hour, compared to 36.6% for the 2-h group and 30.5% for the 4-h group.

There was no correlation between the degree of induced change and the rate of recovery, in that a greater change in refraction was not related to a faster rate of recovery or regression. This was in distinct variance with the findings of Polse et al (1983a), who found that the greater the induced refractive change, the greater the "instability index" and the faster the regression.

The effect of regression and retention in a group of successful orthokeratology patients was studied by Mountford (1998). From a group of 364 subjects, 48 were isolated who fulfilled the requirements of regular reviews at 7, 30, and 90 days postfitting, with a maximum variance of ± 1 day from the required time interval. The choice of eye to be used for analysis was randomized, and the changes in apical corneal power as measured by the EyeSys topographer (version 3.20) measured at time zero (lens removal following overnight wear) and again at a mean of 8.52 ± 0.57 h postwear. Apical corneal power was chosen as the means of assessing refractive change due to the high correlation with refractive change and the objective values obtained. The end-of-day ACP values were subtracted from the immediate postwear values recorded on lens removal in the morning to yield the regression of the effect. The change in refraction from the prefit values was recorded as the change in ACP from prefit to postovernight wear. The retention of the effect was the difference between the change in ACP and the regression at the end of the day.

The mean and standard deviation values for changes in ACP, retention, and regression over the treatment period are shown in Figure 7.16. Note that there appears to be a slight increase in the change in ACP over the period, and a decrease in the overall regression with time. The ACP and retention results were analyzed with paired Student's t-tests, whilst chi-square analysis was performed on the regression data due to the non-

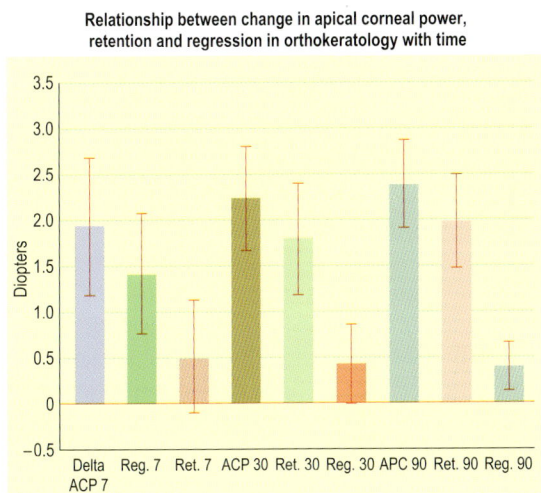

Relationship between change in apical corneal power, retention and regression in orthokeratology with time

Figure 7.16 The change in apical corneal power (ACP), retention (Ret) and regression (Reg) is shown. Note that the error bars for the regression decrease with time.

Relationship between change in ACP and regression (7 days)

$y = 0.4682x + 0.3856$
$R^2 = 0.3294$
$p = 0.06$

A

Relationship between change in ACP and regression (30 days)

$y = 0.2427x + 0.1125$
$R^2 = 0.0975$
$p = 0.6$

B

Relationship between change in ACP and regression (90 days)

$y = 0.0793x + 0.2218$
$R^2 = 0.0204$
$p = 0.26$

C

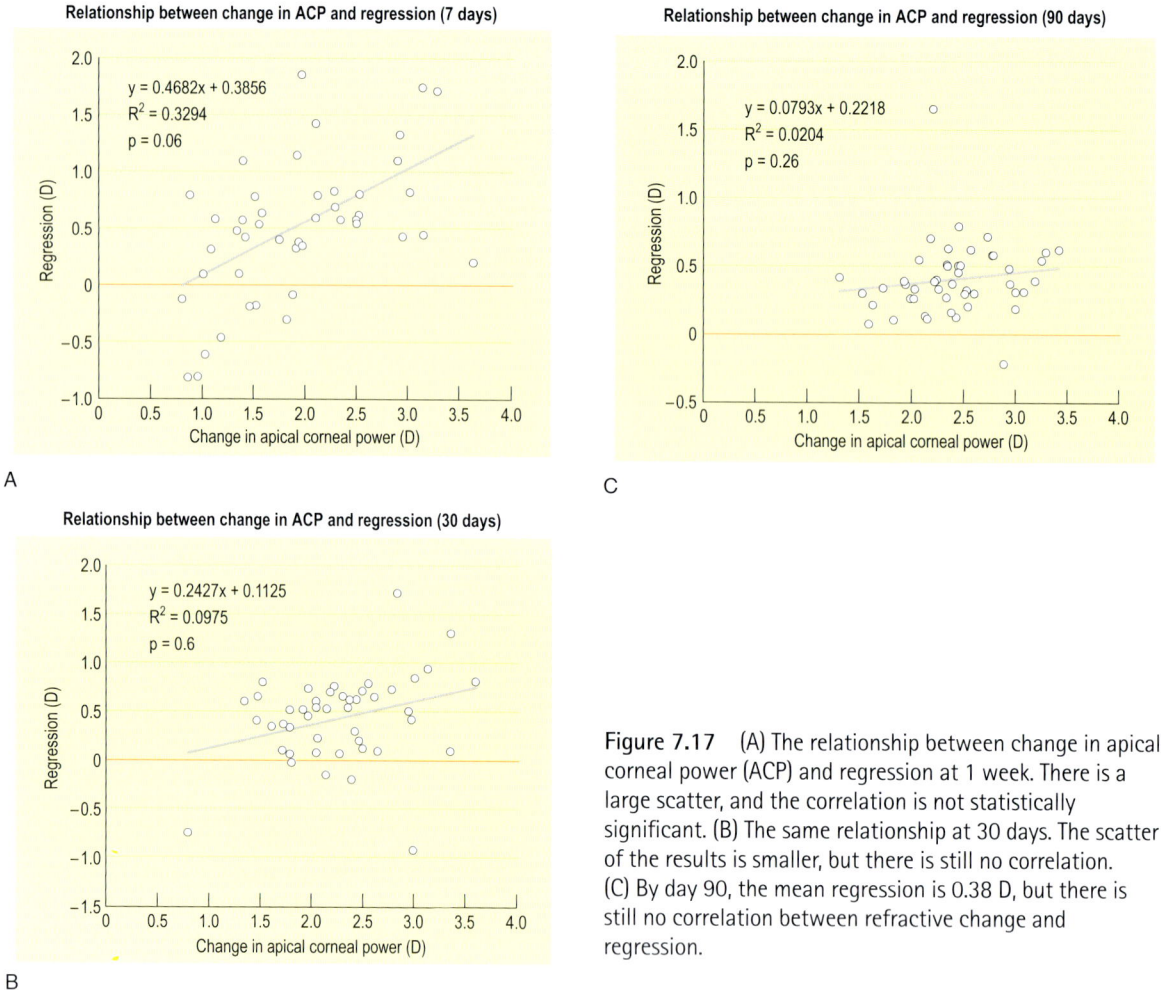

Figure 7.17 (A) The relationship between change in apical corneal power (ACP) and regression at 1 week. There is a large scatter, and the correlation is not statistically significant. (B) The same relationship at 30 days. The scatter of the results is smaller, but there is still no correlation. (C) By day 90, the mean regression is 0.38 D, but there is still no correlation between refractive change and regression.

normal distribution of the results. The change in ACP from the prefit values yielded the following results: 7 vs 30, $P = 0.014$; 7 vs 90, $P = 0.0002$; and 30 vs 90, $P = 0.06$ at the 95% confidence level. The results for the retention effects were: 7 vs 30, $P = 0.001$; 30 vs 90, $P < 0.0001$; and 30 vs 90, $P = 0.06$ at the 95% confidence level.

Two values, 0.50 D and 0.75 D, were used to determine the effects of regression using chi-square analysis. A regression of 0.50 D/day was felt to be of little clinical significance (see later) whereas a regression of 0.75 D could be considered to be more clinically significant. The results for 0.50 D regression were: 7 vs 30, $P = 0.12$; 7 vs 90, $P = 0.0012$; and 30 vs 90, $P = 0.06$. For regression of 0.75 D and less the results were: 7 vs 30, $P = 0.08$; 7 vs 90, $P = 0.003$; and 30 vs 90, $P = 0.026$.

The relationship between change in ACP and regression over the time intervals was assessed by regression analysis (Fig. 7.17).

There was a poor correlation between change in ACP and regression in all cases (7 days, $r^2 = 0.32$, $P = 0.06$; 30 days, $r^2 = 0.09$, $P = 0.6$ and 90 days, $r^2 = 0.02$, $P = 0.26$), and there was no statistical significance in the relationships. This is in agreement with the findings of Soni & Horner (1993), in that, although the degree of refractive change appears to be time-dependent, the regression is not related to the magnitude of change induced.

The major change in refraction occurred in the first 7 days, with only a small gain of approximately 0.26 D at day 30, and little if no gain up to day 90. Regression, however, appears to

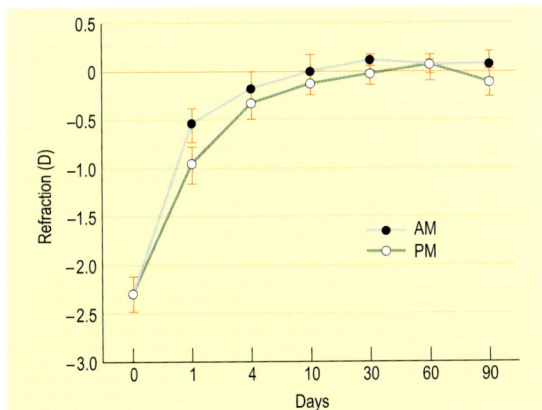

Figure 7.18   The change in refraction over time with overnight orthokeratology. Note that the major change occurs in the first night. The regression by day 10 was not statistically significant. Courtesy of Helen Swarbrick and Ahmed Alharbi.

decrease with time. The interesting point to note in Figure 7.17 is the gradual contraction of the data points over time, to the stage where the mean regression at day 90 was 0.38 D.

Lui & Edwards (2000) studied refractive change over a 100-day period of mainly daily wear of OK704 lenses. The major refractive change occurred in the first day, with approximately 80% of the total change occurring within the first 10 days. Little or no further change occurred after day 40. They did not report on the retention of the effect.

Swarbrick & Alharbi (2001) performed morning and evening reviews on a group of overnight orthokeratology subjects using BE lenses. They found a 70% reduction in refractive error on the first night, with the maximum change and stability being reached by day 10. Interestingly, they found the regression to be not statistically significant when compared to the morning results by day 10, and that the effect remained stable for the remaining 90 days of the study (Fig. 7.18).

Nichols et al (2000) found a similar result in their study using the OK704C, in that the mean regression was minimal (approximately 0.25 D) by day 60. Nguyen et al (2002) also found virtual stabilization of the refractive changes by day 10 when studying the effects of the Contex BB series. The results of both the Nguyen and Swarbrick studies differ from the Nichols and Mountford

studies in that the stability of the changes occurred at a much faster rate. Both Swarbrick & Alharbi and Nguyen et al used the newer design four-curve lenses (BE and Contex BB) whereas Mountford and Nichols et al used the older three-curve designs. There have been numerous anecdotal reports (Day et al 1997, Optcom Orthokeratology Forum) that the newer designs cause faster refractive changes than the older designs, and that the effects are better retained in a shorter period of time. The refractive and VA changes were similar for the newer designs, indicating that there really is no "superior design," irrespective of the claims made by manufacturers. However, it appears that the major difference between the original three-zone lenses and the newer four-zone designs is that the changes not only occur more rapidly, but that the regression appears to be less.

Further controlled research is required in order to determine if there are any real differences in outcome with different designs.

In general, the studies all show that, with a correctly fitted lens, the major refractive change will occur in the first night of wear, reaching a maximum change by approximately day 10. Also, by the same time period, the stability of the changes is well maintained, leading to a stable refraction and unaided VA. From a clinical viewpoint, a deliberate plan of mild overcorrection of the order of 0.50 D in order to compensate for any mild regression effects, and also as an attempt to reduce the number of nights the lenses are worn, would be a worthwhile aim for practitioners to consider.

From a purely anecdotal and clinical viewpoint, some practitioners have noted that the number of nights per week the lenses need to be worn to maintain the refractive and visual acuity gains *decreases* with the length of time the lenses are worn. If the patient is mildly overcorrected, it is not uncommon for the majority (approximately 70%) to be dropped back to every second night's wear after 3–4 weeks. By 6 months, some patients are down to as little as two nights' wear per week, and in rare cases of up to 3 years of orthokeratology lens usage, one night per week is all that is required to maintain the effect. These clinical observations raise some interesting questions as to the underlying mechanism that controls the

Difference between refraction and mean error n = 409

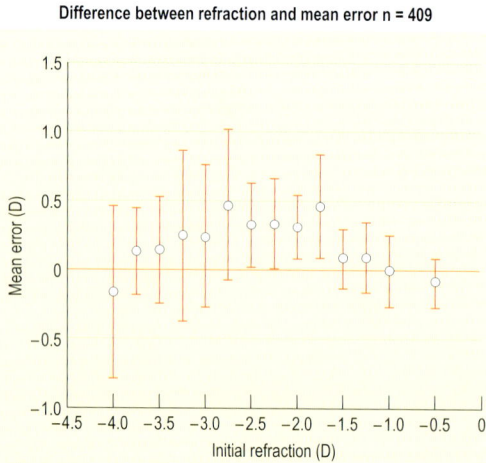

Figure 7.19 The relationship between the mean error and aimed-for refractive change in a group of 409 orthokeratology patients fitted with the Dreimlens. The x-axis represents the refractive error correction required, and the y-axis the mean error between the goal and the achieved refraction. Positive numbers indicate overcorrection, and negative numbers undercorrection. The mean error for all groups showed mild overcorrection, except for the 4.00 D group who were undercorrected. Courtesy of Tom Reim.

maintenance of the effect. If, as is currently thought, the change is purely epithelial, how can the changes be maintained for so long? Alternatively, if there is some form of stromal change occurring, then the maintenance of the effect could be viscoelastic in nature. This will be an interesting field of research for some time.

REFRACTIVE CHANGES WITH REVERSE GEOMETRY LENSES

The earlier controlled studies of Kerns (1976), Coon (1984), Brand et al (1983), and Binder et al (1980) found an overall mean reduction of myopia of approximately 1.04 D in their orthokeratology subjects compared to approximately 0.50 D in the control groups. The maximum refractive change achieved in these studies was 2.50 D. How do reverse geometry lenses compare?

The first published reports on the use of reverse geometry lenses (Wlodyga & Bryla 1989) showed an average refractive change of 2.25 D in a group of 15 subjects. This was followed by a report by Harris & Stoyan (1992) that also yielded

an average reduction of 2.00 D with the OK-3. Joe et al (1996) achieved a reduction of 2.23 ± 0.61 D in a group of 11 subjects, and Mountford (1997) a mean change of 2.19 ± 0.79 D in a group of 60 subjects.

Soni & Horner (1993) presented the results of a retrospective analysis of 120 patients as the mean change in subsets of refractive errors, with the less than 2.00 D group having a mean change of 1.12 D, the 2.00–3.00 D group 1.86 D, the 3.00–5.00 D group 2.15 D, and the high myopes (>5.00 D) a change of 2.48 D. A similar method was used by El Hage et al (1999) when reporting on the results achieved with the controlled keratoreformation (CKR) lens.

Lui & Edwards (2000) achieved a mean refractive change of 1.50 ± 0.45 D, with a maximum change of 2.62 D. In contrast, the control group had a mean refractive change of $+ 0.05 \pm 018$ D. Contex OK704 lenses were used. Swarbrick et al (1998) achieved a similar result with the same lens, with a mean change of 1.71 ± 0.59 D. The Nichols et al (2000) group results were a mean change of 1.83 ± 1.23 D over the course of the study.

Reim (personal communication) reported on the cumulative results of 409 patients fitted with the Dreimlens. The mean refractive change was 2.93 ± 1.05 D. This may at first appear to be a greater change than that achieved by other studies, but the majority of the subjects (254/409) had initial refractive errors of greater than 3.00 D. The difference between the aimed-for refractive corrections compared to that achieved is shown in Figure 7.19.

Jackson et al (2002) fitted 22 subjects with the Paragon CRT lens and achieved a mean refractive change of 2.27 ± 0.95 D (range 0.63–4.25 D).

Autorefraction was used in two studies to date to assess orthokeratology changes. Joe et al (1996) found a mean subjective refraction change of 2.23 ± 0.61 D compared to a mean autorefraction change of 1.85 ± 0.89 D. The differences between the groups were not statistically significant. However, Nichols et al (2000) found a statistically significant difference between the subjective and autorefraction results in their study. The mean subjective change was 1.83 ± 1.23 D compared to the autorefraction change of 0.64 ± 1.83 D ($t = 3.89$, $P = 0.006$). They hypothesized that the difference in the results could be due to the relatively large entrance pupil zone of the auto-refractor being adversely affected by the steep-ened zone surrounding the central treatment zone. Also, the more peripheral corneal area is less affected by the shape changes induced by the lens, leading to an underestimation of refractive change.

Orthokeratologists have noted this effect clin-ically for years, and have always preferred either subjective refraction or retinoscopy as a means of determining refractive changes. There is only one autorefractor currently available with a small entrance pupil, and that is the Nikon Retinomax. Anecdotal evidence (Mountford, Reim, Bennett) indicates that the results achieved with this instrument are in close agreement with subjective refraction. However, this needs further controlled study in order to be verified.

Taken as a whole, the refractive changes that occur as a result of reverse geometry lenses are significantly greater than those achieved by the traditional orthokeratology design lenses. In essence, the change in refraction that can be expected is in the range of 2.00–3.00 D, with higher changes being possible according to Reim's results. Also, the changes that occur appear to be stable over the course of a normal day if the lenses are worn at night.

There have been totally unsubstantiated reports and claims of up to 9.00 D myopia reduc-tion with particular designs or fitting philoso-phies. These claims have no basis in scientific fact when compared to the published literature, and should be treated with a high degree of suspicion until proven otherwise.

VISUAL ACUITY

The reports of VA change with traditional ortho-keratology suffered from a lack of standardiza-tion of measurement. Changes in vision were usually reported as lines of Snellen improvement, with the same chart used for repeated measure-ments. The mean increase in unaided VA found in the controlled studies of Kerns (1976), Coon (1984), and Polse et al (1983) was approximately 3.3 lines of Snellen acuity, from 20/100 to 20/50. As a result, studies on the effect of reverse geo-

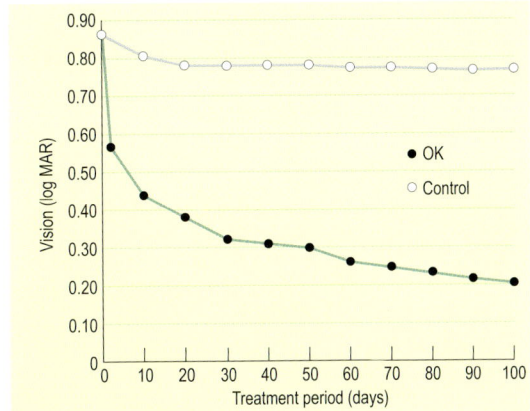

Figure 7.20   Change in log minimum angle of resolution (logMAR) visual acuity with time for the treatment and control groups for day-wear orthokeratology using three-zone lenses. Reproduced from Lui & Edwards (2000) with permission.

metry lenses on VA improvement have tended to be better standardized by the use of log minimum angle of resolution (logMAR) charts.

Joe et al (1996) found an improvement of 0.57 ± 0.25 logMAR, which equated to an equiva-lent Snellen improvement from 20/80 to 20/20. Similarly, Nichols et al (2000) found a mean change in VA of 0.55 ± 0.20 logMAR (high con-trast), equivalent to a Snellen improvement of 5.5 lines (20/66 to 20/19). The low-contrast improvement was 0.48 ± 0.26 logMAR, equating

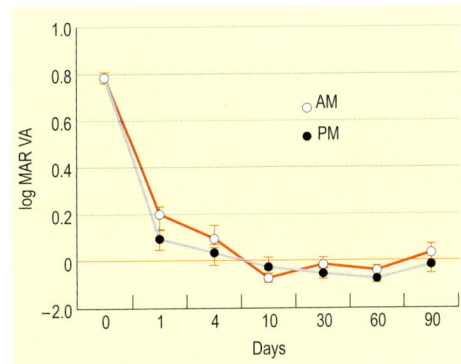

Figure 7.21   Change in log minimum angle of resolution (logMAR) visual acuity over time with night wear using four-zone lenses. The visual acuity reached stability over the course of the day by day 10. Courtesy of Helen Swarbrick and Ahmed Alharbi.

to a Snellen change from 20/100 to 20/33 over the course of the study. Lui & Edwards (2000) found a mean improvement of 0.64 ± 0.22 logMAR (or six lines Snellen equivalent), compared to a mean change of 0.09 ± 0.11 logMAR in the control group (Fig. 7.20).

The maximum change was 0.98, with the minimum 0.37 logMAR. A similar improvement was found by Swarbrick & Alharbi (unpublished), with the major improvement in VA occurring after the first night of lens wear (Fig. 7.21).

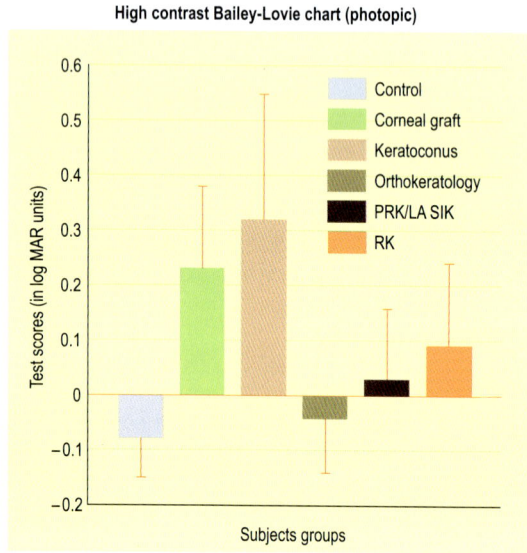

A

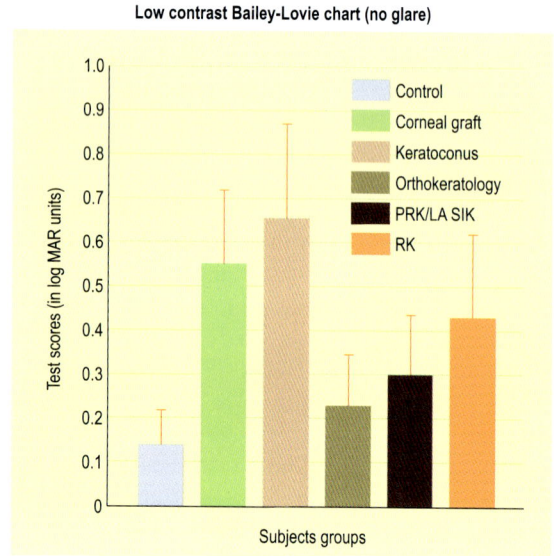

C

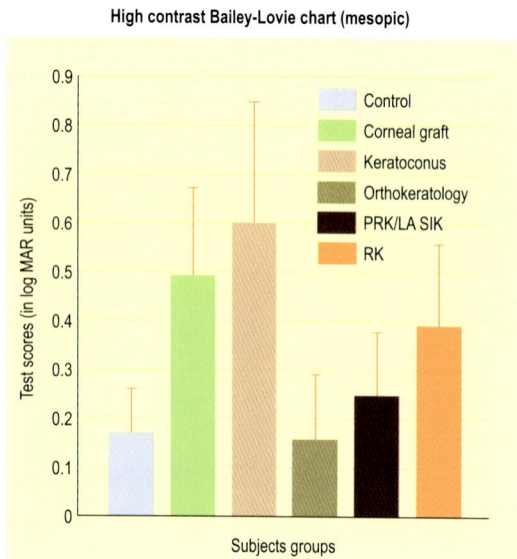

B

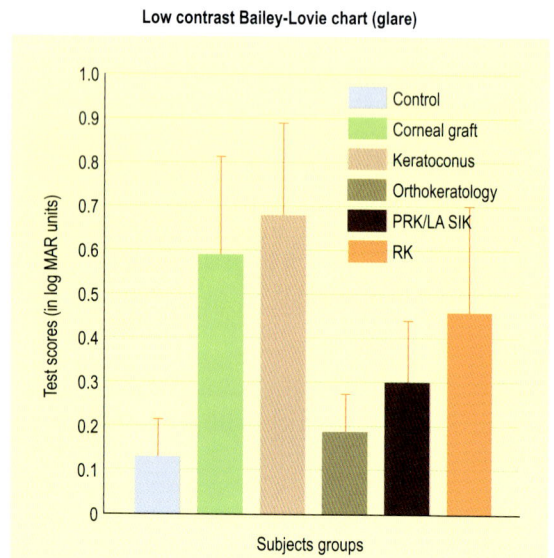

D

Figure 7.22   The differences in quality of vision for various groups of patients having altered corneal surfaces compared to normals. Orthokeratology subjects have good-quality (A) photopic and (B) mesopic vision when compared to normals. The low-contrast vision (C) without glare and (D) with glare is also reasonably good. However, the results are poorer when the Pelli–Robson chart is used (E and F). Courtesy of Wilfred Tang.

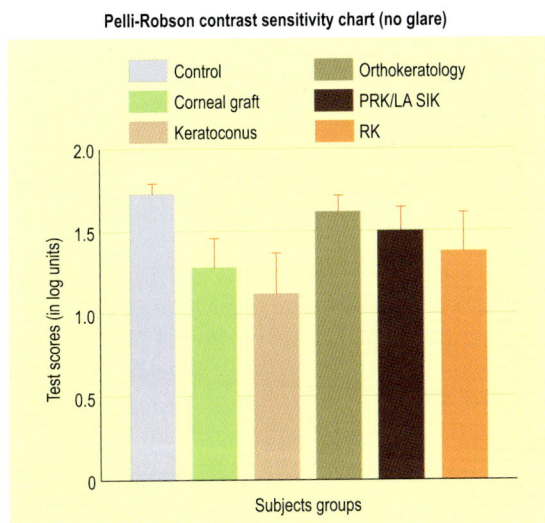

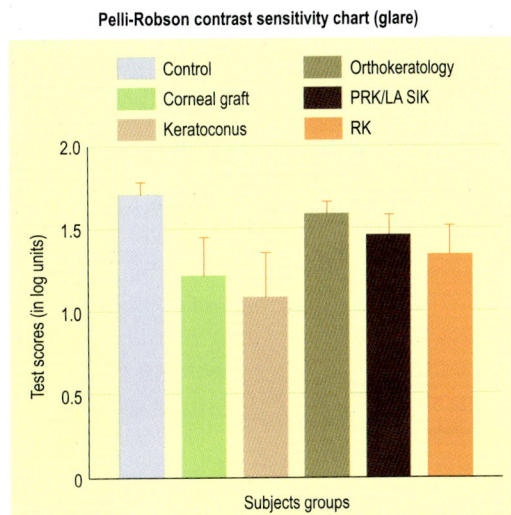

E   F

Figure 7.22   Cont'd.

The visual performance of a group of ortho-keratology subjects was assessed by Tang (2001). When compared to normals, refractive surgery patients, keratoconus, and corneal graft subjects, logMAR vision under photopic (high-contrast), mesopic (high-contrast), low contrast (with and without glare) using Bailey–Lovie charts was measured along with Pelli–Robson charts with and without glare (Fig. 7.22). The results for the orthokeratology subjects under conditions of high-contrast photopic and mesopic conditions were not statistically significantly different from normals ($P = 0.23$ photopic, $P = 0.84$ mesopic). However, the results for the orthokeratology sub-jects under low-contrast conditions with both the Bailey–Lovie and Pelli–Robson charts were poorer than for normals. This reached statistical significance for the Pelli–Robson charts at low contrast with glare. Tang postulated that the cause for this could be due to the design of the chart being set at sensitivities of three to five cycles per degree, compared to a wider range of contrast thresholds for the Bailey–Lovie charts. The results suggest that orthokeratology subjects may suffer from a loss of contrast sensitivity func-tion at intermediate spatial frequencies.

Lui & Edwards (2000) measured contrast sensitivity in both their orthokeratology and control groups at 3, 6, and 12 cycles/degree, and found an increase in both groups over all fre-quencies, with the greatest increase being in the 3 cycles/degree range, similar to that of Tang. However, their analysis showed no statistically significant differences between the treatment and control groups. This apparent change in contrast sensitivity with orthokeratology needs further investigation.

Tang also calculated the root mean square (RMS) value for total residual corneal aberration in both normal and abnormal corneal shapes under photopic and mesopic pupil diameters. Abnormal corneal shapes were due to ortho-keratology, refractive surgery (photorefractive keratectomy (PRK) and Lasik), keratoconus, postgraft and radial keratotomy. The RMS for normals under photopic conditions was 0.47 D, compared to 0.87 D (orthokeratology), 0.92 (PRK/Lasik), 1.78 D (postgraft), 3.21 D (keratoconus), and 1.98 D (radial keratotomy). The RMS for mesopic conditions increased to 0.63 D for the normals, and 1.46 D (orthokerato-logy) and 1.26 D (PRK/Lasik), indicating that the greater peripheral distortion present in these conditions leads to a statistically significant increase in corneal aberrations and their effect on visual quality.

At present, the research on the effect of accelerated orthokeratology on the quantity and quality of visual acuity change is in its infancy. The effect different lens designs may have on the TxZ diameter and the influence this may have on VA under high- and low-contrast situations is unknown. The studies all show a twofold increase in unaided VA for accelerated orthokeratology compared to conventional orthokeratology, and that the increased vision remains stable over an 8-h period.

Tang advocates the use of the Pelli–Robson low-contrast chart in preference to the Bailey–Lovie model due to its higher sensitivity to changes at the 3 cycles/degree level, and the standard Bailey–Lovie chart for high-contrast measurement. These suggestions may form the basis for standardization of VA measurement in future orthokeratology studies.

Finally, the relevance placed on improvement in unaided VA in the early orthokeratology reports is misleading. The lack of a relationship between refractive error and unaided VA has been studied in detail by Smith (1991, 1996), who demonstrated that factors such as the nonlinearity between refraction and VA, pupil size, and nonstandardization of measurement protocols meant that there could never be a single rule that would correlate VA improvement to 1.00 D of refractive change.

In conclusion, the recent controlled studies show that there is an approximate improvement of up to six lines of Snellen acuity with reverse geometry lenses, and this can therefore be used as one of the clinical indicators of the likely outcome of a course of treatment. However, VA improvement is not, of itself, a valid means of determining the success or failure of orthokeratology. What really counts is the refractive change achieved, the quality of the postwear corneal topography, and the effect this has on low-contrast vision and corneal aberration.

CORNEAL THICKNESS

Coon (1984) was the first to report central corneal thinning and increased peripheral thickening in his orthokeratology subjects, and postulated that the change in thickness could be the cause for the refractive change. This hypothesis was finally studied in detail by Swarbrick et al (1998) using

daily-wear reverse geometry lenses, and later with overnight orthokeratology (Swarbrick & Alharbi 2001). Six subjects took part in the earlier study, with pachometry carried out using the Holden–Payor optical pachometer. The daily-wear study used Contex OK–704 lenses fitted 1.50 D flatter than the flat-K reading.

Central epithelial thinning became statistically significant by day 28 (7.1 ± 7.1 μm: 9.6%) with mid-peripheral stromal thickening becoming statistically significant by day 14 (13.0 ± 11.1 μm: 2.4%). At the suggestion of Patrick Caroline, they used Munnerlyn's formula for refractive surgery to relate the thickness changes to refractive error. Munnerlyn's formula is used to determine the ablation depth required to cause a specific refractive change over a TxZ diameter, and is commonly expressed as:

$$t = -S^2 \times D/3$$

where t is ablation depth, S is ablation diameter, and D is the refractive change in diopters.

The refractive change was highly correlated to the overall sag change ($P = 0.002$), with the central epithelial thickness change also being highly significant ($P = 0.011$).

Swarbrick et al (1998) postulated that the corneal curvature change occurring in orthokeratology could be due to a redistribution of anterior corneal epithelial and stromal tissue.

Nichols et al (2000) also found central corneal thinning in their study using the Orbscan, but were unable to confirm mid-peripheral thickening. The mean change in central corneal thickness was 12 ± 11 μm. Lui & Edwards (2000) also found a decrease in central corneal thickness of 16.0 ± 8.0 μm in the orthokeratology subjects, and a mean decrease of 10.0 ± 6.0 μm in the control group. The central corneal thickness change was associated with a 1.50 D refractive change in the treatment group compared to a mean change of 0.01 D in the control group. This may, at first, appear contradictory, but as Swarbrick et al pointed out, there is a topographical difference in corneal thickness induced with orthokeratology lenses that may not occur with alignment designs.

In a more recent study, Swarbrick & Alharbi (2001) reconfirmed the presence of central epithelial thinning and mid-peripheral stromal thicken-

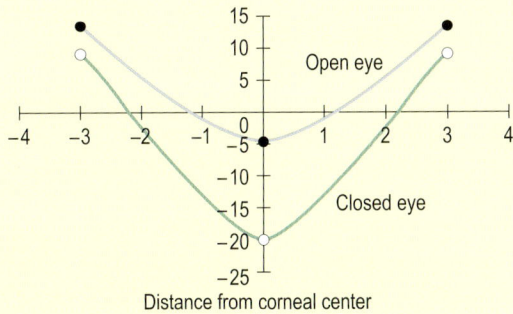

Figure 7.23   The difference in corneal thickness change (shown on the y-axis) between daily-wear and overnight-wear orthokeratology. Courtesy of Helen Swarbrick and Ahmed Alharbi.

ing in a group of subjects fitted with BE lenses on overnight wear. They found a mean change in central epithelial thickness of 17.0 μm (30%) that reached stability by day 10 over the course of an 8-h day (Fig. 7.23). The mid-peripheral corneal thickness increased by 11.0 μm (2%), and was purely stromal in origin. The refractive changes could be totally accounted for by the change in central epithelial thickness, as inclusion of the mid-peripheral stromal thickening in the calculations led to an overestimation of the refractive change achieved. Regression analysis showed a mean change of 8 μm in epithelial thickness per 1.00 D of refractive change, up to a maximum change of approximately 20 μm. This relationship is vitally important to the mathematical modeling of refractive change and orthokeratology, and will be dealt with in greater detail in Chapter 8.

The other interesting finding was that the previous hypothesis of epithelial redistribution was not supported by the data, in that, if epithelial redistribution did occur, the change in mid-peripheral thickness should have been epithelial, and not stromal. The conclusion gleaned from this study is that the refractive changes occurring in orthokeratology are mainly epithelial in origin, and not due to corneal bending.

Nguyen et al (2002) examined the changes in corneal thickness with the Orbscan. They found a 17.7 μm decrease in thickness at baseline morning review that reduced to 14.7 μm after 12 h. However, the presence of mid-peripheral stromal thickening raises some interesting questions as to the

cause of these changes. Firstly, it would appear that the stromal thickening is not due to edema, as the *Dk* of the material is theoretically high enough to avoid edema, and secondly, the stromal thickening appears to remain stable between the morning and evening readings. Also, there are inherent errors associated with off-center fixation and peripheral pachometry (Chan-Ling & Pye 1994).

The Swarbrick and Nichols studies both measured corneal thickness at approximately 3.00 mm from center, which is in the area of mid-peripheral corneal steepening, as described by Mountford and Lui & Edwards. The question that remains to be answered is this: could the stromal thickening occur as a result of stromal bending in this area, where the relative increase in thickness could be due to the effects of the slit image being somewhat magnified by the effect, if any, of the rapid change in corneal curvature?

The basis of Munnerlyn's formula is that the changes induced are purely anterior corneal, with no change in endothelial curvature. The same assumptions were made by Swarbrick et al. However, Owens (personal communication) has studied the change in endothelial curvature using Purkinje imagery, and found a change in endothelial curvature over the first 4 weeks of orthokeratology lens wear. The endothelial curvature returns to normal after 4 weeks.

The refractive changes caused by orthokeratology appear to be due to central epithelial thinning. The role that stromal changes may have could be in the retention of the effect. This is another fertile field for further research!

CORNEAL STAINING

Swarbrick et al (1998) pointed out that the measured change in central epithelial thickness, of the order of 30%, could be a cause for concern, as the loss of epithelial thickness could leave the cornea at a greater risk of infection. At present, it is not known whether the change in thickness is due to cell compression or cell loss. Greenbery & Hill (1976) demonstrated a change in epithelial thickness in the pressure zone of steeply fitted PMMA lenses on rabbit corneas. The thickness change (a decrease of 30%) was associated with flattening and widening of the basal cells, which they termed "tissue redistribution," a loss of one layer

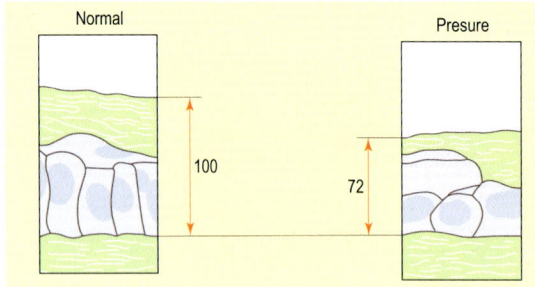

Figure 7.24 The effect on epithelial cells of pressure from a tightly fitting lens. Note that the epithelial cells are reduced in height and increased in width. The cell volume remains constant. The wing layer of cells is lost. Reproduced from Greenbery & Hill (1976) with permission from Contact Lens Spectrum.

of cells (wing layer) and an increased cell division rate in the pressure zone (Fig. 7.24).

Although this change in epithelial thickness could theoretically place the cornea at greater risk of infection, the results of clinical studies to date have failed to show a higher incidence of adverse signs than that possible with conventional lens wear. The controlled studies of conventional orthokeratology using PMMA did not show any statistically significant differences in staining between the control and orthokeratology subjects. The problem with the previous studies was a lack of standardization of grading of corneal staining, which makes true comparisons difficult.

Lui & Edwards (2000) used the Cornea and Contact Lens Research Unit (CCLRU) grading scale to record corneal staining in their treatment and control groups. Corneal staining in the ortho-keratology group was 93% (grade 1) and 7% (grade 2), compared to 92% (grade 1) and 8% (grade 2) in the control group. The difference in staining was not statistically significant. El Hage et al (1999) also used the CCLRU grading scale when reviewing the results of CKR lenses on 51 patients. Corneal staining due to foreign bodies occurred in 7.8% of patients, whilst 33.33% exhibited grade 1 staining at 12.9% of visits, and 3.92% had grade 2 staining at 2.99% of visits. Although the study also reported the incidence of 3 and 9 o'clock staining as being low (7.84% of patients at 8.73% of visits), there is no distinct delineation of the area of staining. The CCLRU grading scale also nominates distinct areas for

recording staining, and it would be beneficial if all future studies of the rate of staining included not only the degree of staining, but also the area. This would make for greater ease of comparison when assessing the effects of lens design and fitting philosophies on the incidence and severity of corneal staining.

However, in contrast to the relatively low incidence of clinically significant staining reported in the above studies, Hang et al (2000) reported a rate of 45% corneal staining in a group of 27 patients fitted with the Dynalens and Sightform designs. There was a greater incidence and sever-ity of staining in those subjects, with tear break-up times of less than 10 s and Schirmer test values of less than 10 mm. They felt that this incidence of staining was acceptable, and could be controlled by regular aftercare and treat-ment. However, this has proven to be an incor-rect assumption, as the incidence of ulcerative keratitis in both China and Hong Kong in mid-2001 reached such alarming proportions that health authorities in both areas had to step in and enforce controls on the use of orthokeratology lenses (Lu et al 2001).

The incidence of such severe complications has not occurred in other countries to date, and there are compelling reasons why this has not been the case. Firstly, anecdotal reports indicate that lenses were supplied to unqualified practitioners and that proper aftercare procedures were not followed. Secondly, the compliance of patients with regular aftercare and maintenance standards is poor (Cho et al 2002b). Thirdly, and perhaps of greater concern, is that some of the material used in the lenses supplied was totally unacceptable for overnight wear due to the lack of oxygen per-meability. The Chinese health authorities have instituted strict guidelines as to the material quality and training standards required for ortho-keratology procedures.

Although corneal staining and complication rates appear to be very low when lenses are pro-perly fitted and patients are reviewed at regular intervals, the Chinese experience shows that when these factors are compromised in any way, severe ocular complications with a resultant loss of vision *can and will occur*. As is common with all other types of contact lens practice, a strict and high standard of competency and patient after-care is mandatory for orthokeratology (see Ch. 9).

SHORT–TERM CHANGES

The effect of very short exposure times to reverse geometry lenses was initially studied by Soni & Horner (1993), who found marked changes in refraction and unaided vision following 1, 2, and 4 h wear of OK-3 lenses. Sridharan (2001) fitted 9 subjects with BE lenses in one eye and recorded the changes in refraction (ACP), unaided VA (logMAR), corneal thickness, and TxZ diameter following exposure times of 10, 30, and 60 min of open-eye wear and 8 h of overnight (closed-eye) wear. The fellow eye acted as the control. The measurement sessions were performed at 1-week intervals for each wearing time, ensuring a total return to baseline prior to the next experiment taking place.

The changes in refraction were 0.61 ± 0.35 D (10 min), 0.86 ± 0.52 D (30 min), 1.21 ± 0.52 D (1 h), and 1.63 ± 0.46 D following 8 h of eye closure (Fig. 7.25). The changes from baseline were statistically significant at all time periods. The changes in the nonlens-wearing eye were not statistically significant from baseline. The diameter of the treatment zone also increased with wearing time, being 3.86 ± 0.88 mm (10 min), 5.82 ± 1.05 mm (30 min), 5.40 ± 0.61 mm (1 h), and 5.59 ± 0.83 mm (8 h) (Fig. 7.26).

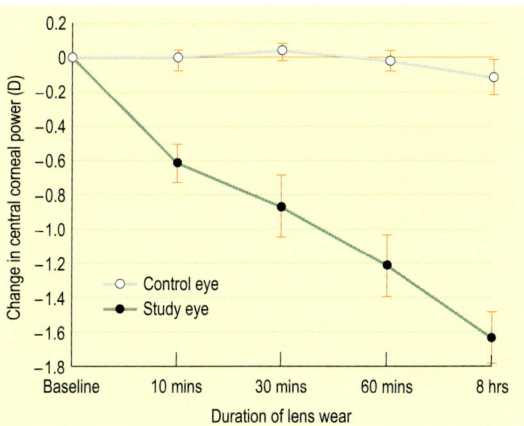

Figure 7.26 The change in treatment zone (TxZ) diameter over time. The increase is statistically significant at each interval. Courtesy of Ram Sridharan.

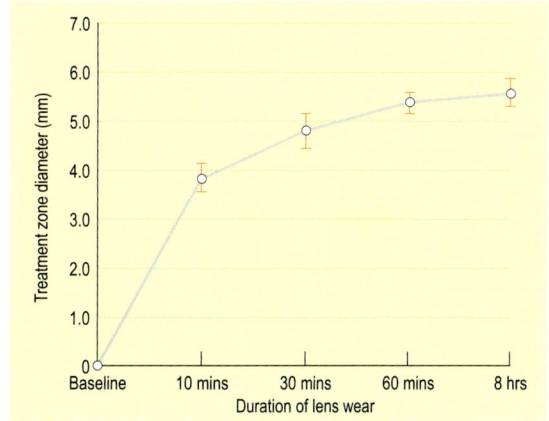

Figure 7.27 The change in corneal asphericity (Q) over time. There is a trend towards corneal sphericalization. Courtesy of Ram Sridharan.

All changes from baseline were statistically significant ($P < 0.001$). Corneal asphericity (Q) also changed towards sphericalization over the varying periods of wear. However, the change was only statistically significant after 8 h of wear (Fig. 7.27). The change in logMAR acuity was also rapid (Fig. 7.28).

Epithelial and mid-peripheral stromal thickness varied with time of wear: the central area showed increased thinning during open-eye wear, and some thickening following overnight wear. The mid-peripheral changes showed a tendency towards greater thickness, but the changes were

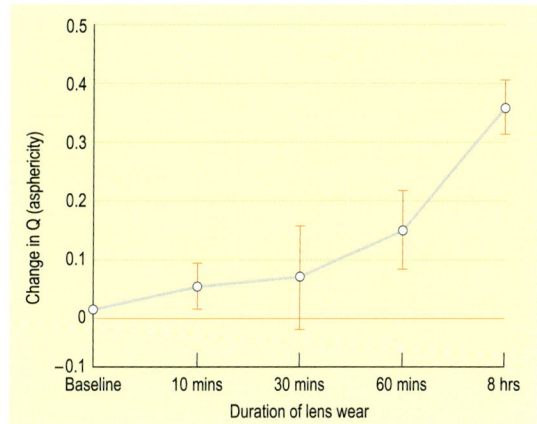

Figure 7.25 The change in anterior corneal power over short durations of exposure to BE lenses. Courtesy of Ram Sridharan.

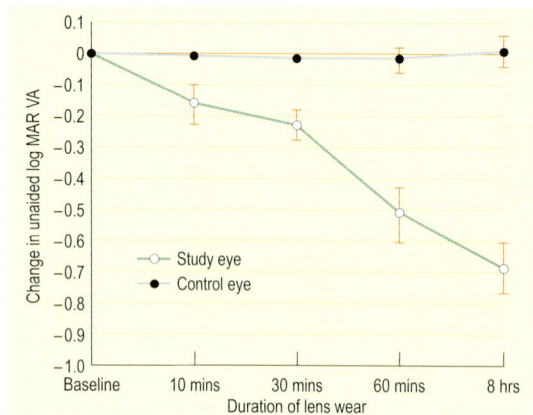

Figure 7.28 The change in log minimum angle of resolution (logMAR) vision over short-term lens wear compared to the control eye. Courtesy of Ram Sridharan.

not statistically significant. Unaided VA improved statistically from the first 10-min period and increased with longer wearing time.

The analysis also showed that the changes occurring over the short-term exposure could not accurately predict the results of the longer overnight wearing time. This then raises the question as to what period of time constitutes a "proper" trial wearing period. It appears that the results of this study indicate that an overnight wear of the lens would be the most reliable basis on which to determine the correct lens parameters.

The regression of each wearing period to baseline was also studied. The corneal parameters recovered in a nonlinear fashion, with complete recovery to baseline occurring within 24 h for all groups except the 8-h overnight trial. Recovery took 48 h for six subjects, and 72 hours for the remaining three subjects.

The results of the study seem to suggest that at least an 8-h overnight trial period is required for a predictable outcome.

LONG-TERM CHANGES

To date there have been no papers published in the literature on the long-term effects of orthokeratology lens wear. However, G Boneham (personal communication) has kindly allowed the author to present some results of a study of five long-term subjects who had worn VMC

(EZM) lenses for a period of 5 years. The mean initial refractive error was −1.66 ± 0.60 D (range 0.75–2.25 D), and mean final refractive error +0.16/− 0.23 D (range 0 ± 0.50 D). They exam-

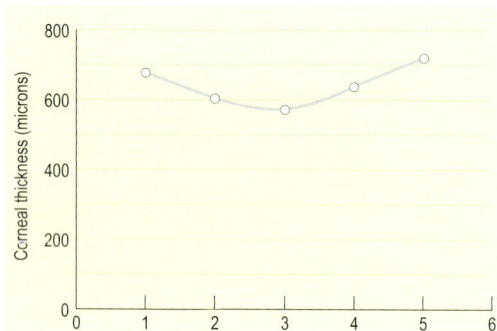

A

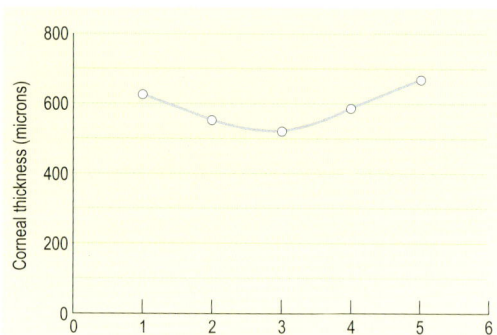

B

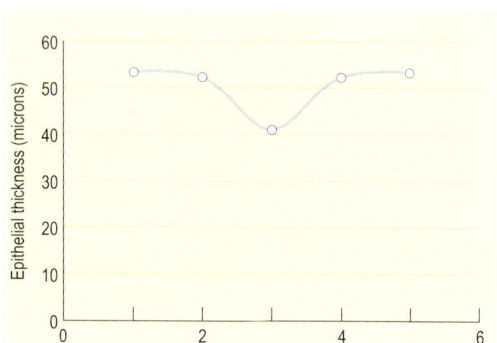

C

Figure 7.29 The change in total corneal thickness (A) over a 5-year period of orthokeratology. Points on the x-axis represent: 1 nasal periphery 4.5 mm from center; 2 nasal mid-periphery 2.5 mm from center: 3 center; 4 temporal mid-periphery; and 5 temporal periphery. (B) Change in stromal thickness; (C) Change in epithelial thickness. Courtesy of Gavin Boneham.

ined total and epithelial corneal thickness from baseline to the end of 5 years, and the changes in keratocyte populations using confocal microscopy. The changes in total corneal thickness and epithelial thickness are shown in Figure 7.29.

The central thinning of the epithelium appears to be a constant effect of the procedure, with the mean change being 12 μm.

The confocal results showed no statistically significant change in keratocyte population from baseline, indicating that there may be no long-term impact on corneal physiology.

PATIENT SATISFACTION

Perhaps the most relevant test of the efficacy of a procedure is the level of patient satisfaction following treatment. In Hong Kong, orthokeratology is seen by patient and practitioner alike as a means of myopia control, even though there is no scientific basis for the belief. Parents are keen to have their children undergo the procedure, and as a result, the majority of patients are less than 16 years of age. Cho et al (2002b) reviewed the outcomes and performed interviews on 61 randomly selected patients from a private practice.

Twelve children (24%) had been reluctant to wear the lenses overnight, but following a trial wear period only one child elected not to proceed (Fig. 7.30). The patients were also asked to rate the success of the treatment with respect to quality of unaided vision. The majority of patients (50/61) rated the outcome as either "good" or "very good," whilst one patient reported the outcome as "poor" (Fig. 7.31).

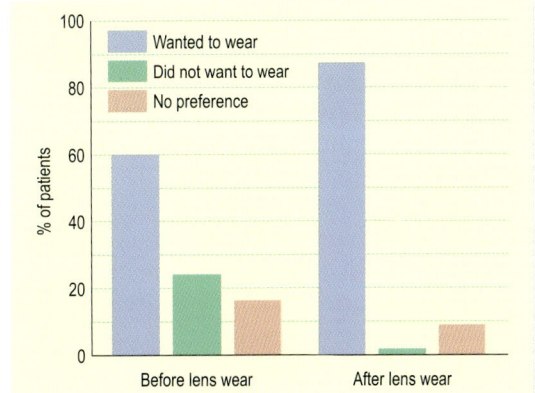

Figure 7.30   The change in perceptions or willingness to proceed with orthokeratology after a trial fitting in children. Only one child refused to proceed after the trial. Courtesy of Pauline Cho.

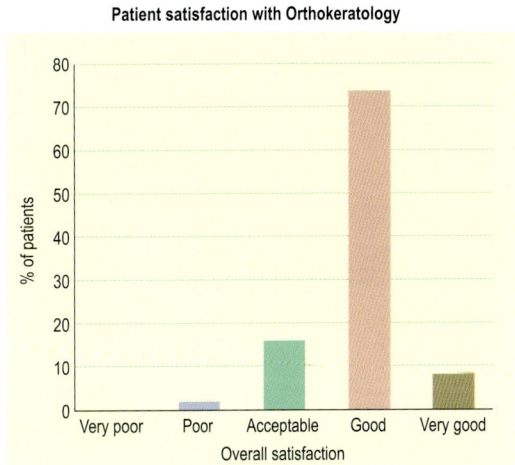

Figure 7.31   Patient satisfaction with orthokeratology. Only one patient out of 61 was dissatisfied with the treatment. Courtesy of Pauline Cho.

Table 7.1 Frequency and severity of patient reports concerning vision in the study group.

	Scores						
	0 (none)	1	2	3	4	5 (very often)	n
Poor near vision	42	13	3	2	0	0	60
Poor distance vision	22	18	16	2	3	0	61
Glare	48	6	3	2	2	0	61
Vision worse at the end of the day	25	16	14	4	1	1	61
Poor vision in dim/dark conditions	40	12	3	4	1	1	61

Courtesy of Pauline Cho.

In contrast, however, the most commonly reported problems occurred with the quality of unaided vision, in that the patients with the higher refractive errors more commonly reported poor distance or near vision, and poor-quality vision in dim illumination (Table 7.1). This is the first research into the patient satisfaction with orthokeratology, and should not be the last. It is vital that the level of satisfaction be determined, so that patients can be told the expected success rate before starting treatment.

SUMMARY

When a reverse geometry lens is applied to the cornea, things happen quickly. The central cornea flattens in curvature and the mid-periphery steepens. There is an associated reduction in refractive error and an improvement in unaided high- and low-contrast VA, although the two factors are not mutually dependent. The time for an effective reduction in myopia and improved acuity is dramatically faster than that required for traditional orthokeratology, and the changes are greater in magnitude. Also, the number of lenses required has now been theoretically lowered to one set, worn on an overnight basis, compared to an average of six sets of lenses worn on a daily-wear basis with the older techniques.

The changes in corneal shape and refraction are associated with the change in corneal asphericity, and this can be used as an accurate predictor of the refractive change possible. The refractive change, however, occurs as a direct result of central epithelial thinning.

There is a lot of scope for further research in these areas, including confocal microscopy of the epithelium and stroma, investigations on the relevance of mid-peripheral corneal stromal thickening, the optical quality of the posttreatment corneal shape and its effect on vision and, finally, the differences that lens design and fitting philosophy have on the outcomes.

References

Alpins N A (1997) A new method of targeting vectors to treat astigmatism. Journal of Cataract and Refractive Surgery 23: 65–75

Bailey I L, Carney L G (1970) Analysing contact lens induced changes of the corneal curvature. American Journal of Optometry and Archives of the American Academy of Optometry 47(10): 761–768

Bennett A G, Rabbetts R B (1991) What radius does the conventional keratometer measure? Ophthalmologic Physiological Optics 11: 239–247

Binder P S, May C M, Grant S C (1980) An evaluation of orthokeratology. Ophthalmology 87: 729–744

Brand R J, Polse K A, Schwalbe J S (1983) The Berkeley orthokeratology study. Part 1. General conduct of the study. American Journal of Optometry and Physiological Optics 60: 175–186

Carkeet N L, Mountford J A, Carney L G (1995) Predicting success with orthokeratology lens wear: a retrospective analysis of ocular characteristics. Optometry and Vision Science 72: 892–898

Carney L G (1994) Orthokeratology. Chapter 37. In: Rubin M, Guillon M (eds) Contact lens practice. London, Chapman and Hall Medical pp. 877–887

Caroline P, Campbell R (1991) Between the lines. Contact Lens Spectrum 5(6): 68

Chan-Ling T, Pye D C (1994) Pachometry: clinical and scientific applications. In: Rubin M, Guillon M (eds) Contact lens practice. London, Chapman & Hall Medical

Cho P, Cheung S W, Edwards M (2002a) Practice of orthokeratology by a group of contact lens practitioners in Hong Kong. Part 2. Clinical and Experimental Optometry 86(1): 42–46

Cho P, Cheung S W, Edwards M, Fung J (2002b) Practice of orthokeratology by a group of contact lens practitioners in Hong Kong – Part 1. Clinical and Experimental Optometry 85(6): 358–363

Coon L J (1984) Orthokeratology part 2. Evaluating the Tabb method. Journal of the American Optometric Association 55: 409–418

Dave T, Ruston D, Fowler C (1998) Evaluation of the Eyesys model 2 computerized videokeratoscope. Optometry and Vision Science 75(9): 647–654

Day J, Reim T, Bard R D, McGonagill P, Gambino M J (1997) Advanced orthokeratology using custom lens designs. Contact Lens Spectrum 12(6): 34–40

Douthwaite W A (1995) Eyesys corneal topography measurement applied to calibrated ellipsoidal convex surfaces. British Journal of Ophthalmology 79: 797–801

El Hage S G, Leach N E, Shahin R (1999) Controlled kerato-reformation (CKR): an alternative to refractive surgery. Practical Optometry 10(6): 230–235

Erickson P, Thorn F (1977) Does refractive error change twice as fast as corneal power in orthokeratology? American Journal of Optometry and Physiological Optics 54: 581–587

Fontana A (1972) Orthokeratology using the one-piece bifocal. Contacto 16(2): 45–47

Freeman R A (1976) Orthokeratology and the Corneascope computer. Optometric Weekly 67: 37–39

Grant S C, May C H (1970) Orthokeratology – a therapeutic approach to contact lens procedures. Contacto 14(4): 3–16

Greenbery M H, Hill R (1976) The pressure response to contact lenses. Contact Lens Forum July: 49–53

Hang J, Wu F, Tan T (2000) Clinical research of the effects and problems of orthokeratology. Chinese Journal of Optometry and Ophthalmology 18(1): 75–82

Harris D, Stoyan N (1992) A new approach to orthokeratology. Contact Lens Spectrum 7(4): 37–39

Horner D G, Armitage K S, Wormsely K A (1992) Corneal moulding recovery after contact lens wear. Optometry and Vision Science 69(12s): 156–157

Jackson J M, Rah M J, Jones L A, Bailey M D, Marsden H, Barr J T (2002) Analysis of refractive error changes in overnight orthokeratology using power vectors. ARVO, 2001 (abstract). Investigative Ophthalmology and Vision Science

Joe J J, Marsden H J, Edrington T B (1996) The relationship between corneal eccentricity and improvement in visual acuity with orthokeratology. Journal of the American Optometric Association 67: 87–97

Kerns R (1976) Research in orthokeratology, part 7. Journal of the American Optometric Association 48: 1541–1553

Lebow K A (1996) Using corneal topography to evaluate the efficacy of orthokeratology fitting. Contacto 39(1): 18–26

Lu L, Zhou L H, Wang Z G, Zhang W H (2001) Orthokeratology induced infective corneal ulcer. Investigative Ophthalmology and Vision Science 42(4): s34

Lui W O, Edwards M H (2000) Orthokeratology in low myopia. Part 2: Corneal topographic changes and safety over 100 days. Contact Lens and Anterior Eye 23(3): 90–99

Mountford J A (1997) An analysis of the changes in corneal shape and refractive error induced by accelerated orthokeratology. International Contact Lens Clinic 24: 128–144

Mountford J A (1998) Retention and regression of orthokeratology with time. International Contact Lens Clinic 25(1): 1–6

Mountford J A, Pesudovs K (2002) An analysis of the astigmatic changes induced by accelerated orthokeratology. Clinical and Experimental Optometry 85(5): 284–293

Munnerlyn C R, Koons S J, Marshall J (1988) Photorefractive keratectomy: a technique for laser refractive surgery. Journal of Cataract and Refractive Surgery 14: 46–51

Neilson R H, Grant S C, May C H (1964) Emmetropization through contact lenses. Contacto 8(4): 20–21

Nguyen T, Soni S, Carter D, Biehl T (2002) Corneal changes associated with overnight orthokeratology. ARVO abstract 3092. Investigative Ophthalmology and Vision Science

Nichols J J, Marsich M M, Nguyen M, Barr J T, Bullimore M A (2000) Overnight orthokeratology. Optometry and Vision Science 77(5): 252–259

Paige N (1981) The use of transverse axial oscillatory ocular movements to prevent or reduce corneal astigmatism during orthokeratological processing. Contacto 20(6): 29–30

Patterson C (1975) Orthokeratology: changes to the corneal curvature and the effect on refractive power due to the sagittal length change. Journal of the American Optometric Association 46: 714–729

Polse K A, Brand R J, Vastine D W, Schwalbe J S (1983a) Corneal change accompanying orthokeratology. Plastic or elastic? Results of a randomized controlled clinical trial. Archives of Ophthalmology 101: 1873–1878

Polse K A, Brand R J, Schwalbe J S (1983b) The Berkeley orthokeratology study, part 2: efficacy and duration. American Journal of Optometry and Physiological Optics 60(3): 187–198

Rengstorff R H (1965) Corneal curvature and astigmatic changes subsequent to contact lens wear. Journal of the American Optometric Association 36(11): 996–1000

Roberts C, Wu Y-T (1998) Topographical estimation of optical zone size after refractive surgery using axial distance radius of curvature and refractive power algorithms. Investigative Ophthalmology and Vision Science (suppl.) 39(4): S131, 111

Rowsey J J, Balyeat H D, Monlux R et al (1988) Prospective study of radial keratotomy: photokeratoscope corneal topography. Ophthalmology 95(3): 322–333

Smith G (1991) Relation between spherical refractive error and visual acuity. Optometry and Vision Science 68: 591–598

Smith G (1996) Visual acuity and refractive error. Is there a mathematical relationship? Optometry Today 36(16): 22–27

Soni P S, Horner D J (1993) Orthokeratology. In: Bennett E, Weisman B (eds) Clinical contact lens practice. Philadelphia, J B Lippincott, ch. 49

Soni P, Nguyen T (2002) Which corneal parameter, anterior corneal curvature, posterior corneal curvature or corneal thickness is most sensitive to acute changes with reverse geometry orthokeratology lenses? ARVO abstracts 3086

Sridharan R (2001) Response and regression of the cornea with short-term orthokeratology lens wear. Masters thesis. University of New South Wales, Sydney, Australia

Swarbrick H A, Wong G, O'Leary D J (1998) Corneal response to orthokeratology. Optometry and Vision Science 75(11): 791–799

Tang W (2001) The relationship between corneal topography and visual performance. PhD thesis. Centre for Eye Research, Queensland University of Technology, Brisbane, Australia

Wlodyga R J, Bryla C (1989) Corneal molding; the easy way. Contact Lens Spectrum 4(58): 14–16

Wlodyga R J, Harris D (1994) Accelerated orthokeratology techniques and procedures manual. Chicago, NERF

Chapter **8**

Computerized modeling of outcomes and lens fitting in orthokeratology

John Mountford

CHAPTER CONTENTS

Introduction 205
Surface area 205
The constant lamellar length model 207
Sphere or oblate: does it really matter? 210
Lens design and fitting software 212
Conclusions 224
Acknowledgment 225
References 225

INTRODUCTION

One of the many criticisms that have been leveled at orthokeratology is the apparent lack of a model that will accurately predict the outcome. The following section attempts to answer the criticism by using three mathematical models of corneal shape change based on the surface area and constancy of lamellar length concepts, and a modification of Munnerlyn's original formula. The second section deals with the many computer programs available to practitioners that help in the design and fitting of the lenses.

SURFACE AREA

The surface area of the cornea is considered to be constant despite localized shape changes, with the exception of keratoglobus (Smolek & Klyce 1998). The model of constant surface area as a means of predicting refractive changes in orthokeratology was developed by Day (unpublished), and is commonly referred to as the Kappa function.

In effect, the model states that the corneal surface area is a constant, and will not be changed by the effects of reverse geometry lens (RGL) wear. The cornea is assumed to change from a prolate ellipse to a sphere, with the change in apical power being equivalent to the refractive change. The surface area of the prefit cornea is calculated using the apical radius (R_0), corneal asphericity (Q), horizontal visible iris diameter

(HVID), and the resultant sag (see Ch. 4). Once the surface area is known, the equivalent spherical radius for the same surface area is found, assuming a change in sag of 9 µm/D of refractive change. Kappa function is the refractive change that occurs given an initial aspheric surface that becomes spherical following treatment.

When modeling corneal shape changes, Q (asphericity) is preferred to e (eccentricity) due to the former's ability to distinguish between prolate and oblate surfaces. For the majority of the rest of this section, the asphericity (Q) changes are related to eccentricity changes only when the cornea is assumed to change for a prolate ellipse to a sphere. If the assumption that a change towards an oblate surface occurs, only the Q value is used.

The range of refractive change for given apical radius and corneal eccentricity values assuming a HVID of 12 mm is shown in Figure 8.1. Note that the same refractive error correction exists for a number of R_0 and eccentricity values. The trend and shape of the curve are similar to

that seen for the equivalency of corneal sags, as the whole process is dependent on the initial eccentricity.

The model assumes a symmetrically rotational aspheric surface. However, in cases of with-the-rule (WTR) corneal astigmatism, the vertical curvature and eccentricity as well as the corneal diameter differ from that of the horizontal. Kwok (1984) has shown that in cases of a nonrotationally symmetrical asphere (ellipsoid), the surface area of the cornea decreases for WTR astigmatism, and increases for against-the-rule astigmatism when compared to the rotationally symmetrical model. Over the mean range of astigmatism, the error is approximately 3%, so this must be included in the kappa function in order to arrive at the correct final apical radius value. The other method of resolving the error is to use the direct integration of the variables instead of the formula (J Day, personal communication).

In the case of a model cornea of R_0 7.80, $e = 0.5$, and HVID 12 mm, the surface area is 130 mm². Assuming a sag change over the same chord of

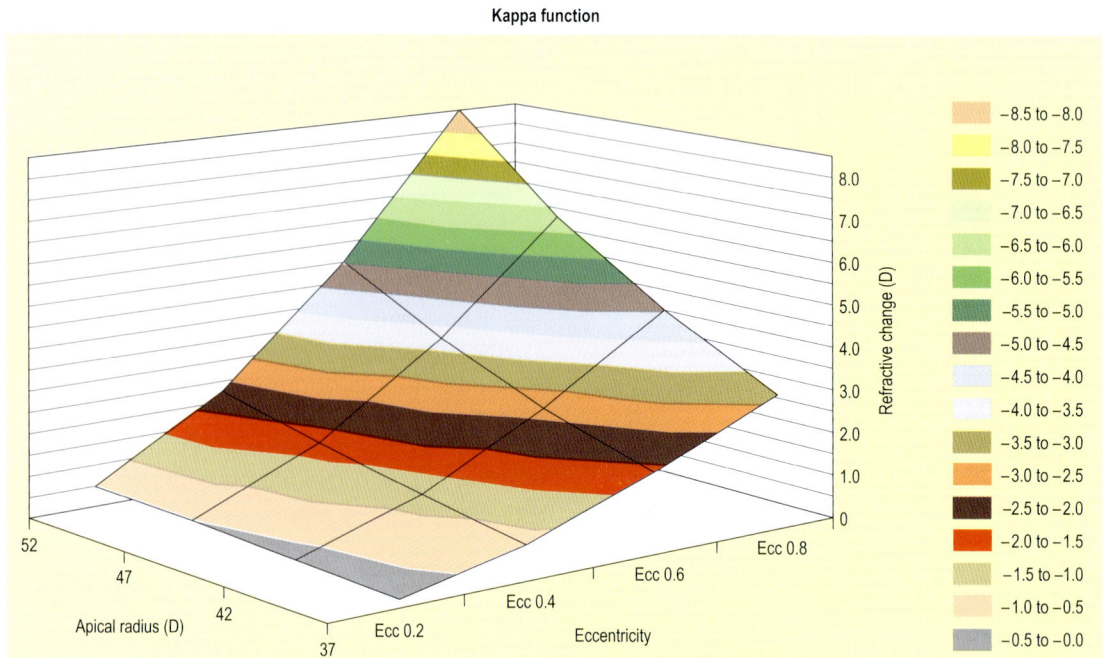

Kappa function

Figure 8.1   The kappa function showing the refractive change from a prolate ellipse to a sphere. Note the isodioptric changes in refraction for different corneal apical radius and eccentricity combinations.

20 μm, and resolving the formula to find R_0 when eccentricity is zero and the surface area 130 mm^2, the corrected final R_0 is 8.18 mm. This equates to a refractive change of 2.00 D.

The limit of astigmatic reduction can be calculated by resolving the changes for both the steep and flat meridian using the R_0, e, and HVID values in turn, and calculating surface area for both. The difference between the final apical radii gives the value for the residual astigmatism.

THE CONSTANT LAMELLAR LENGTH MODEL

This iterative model was developed by O'Leary (Mountford & Noack 1998). It is based on the fact that, under normal physiological loads, stromal lamellae can be neither stretched nor compressed. In other words, it doesn't matter what happens to the shape of the cornea, the lamellar length will remain constant. The other constant in this argument is that the corneal diameter is fixed, and is approximately 1.25 mm greater than HVID. The question therefore becomes: if the initial R_0, asphericity (Q), and fiber length are known over a specific chord, what is the relationship between R_0 and Q as the shape changes from a prolate ellipsoidal shape to a sphere and on to an oblate ellipse? The difference between the initial and "final" R_0 is equivalent to the refractive change. The calculations are iterative, and require a custom program to complete.

For the model cornea of R_0 7.80 mm, Q 0.25, and HVID 12 mm, the lamellar length is 14.474 mm. The relationship between apical radius change and change in asphericity is shown in Figure 8.2. Note that the hypothetical relationship is virtually linear, with a high correlation ($r^2 = 1.00$). The same linear relationship exists between all combinations of R_0 and Q, with only the slope of the intercept changing.

The expected refractive change is shown in Figure 8.3. The expected refractive change that occurs for a change from a prolate ellipsoidal geometry of Q 0.25 to a sphere is 2.25 D, which is indeed similar to that predicted by the kappa function. For greater refractive change, the cornea

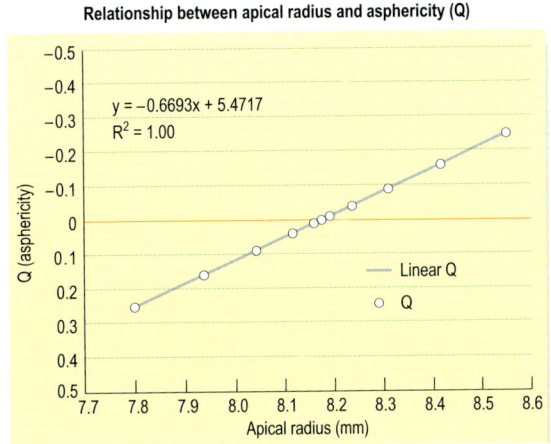

Relationship between apical radius and asphericity (Q)

$y = -0.6693x + 5.4717$
$R^2 = 1.00$

Figure 8.2 The relationship between corneal curvature change and asphericity assuming a constant lamellar length. The initial Q is 0.25 with an R_0 of 7.80 mm. As R_0 flattens to 8.176 mm, the Q value approaches zero. If the flattening of R_0 continues, the Q becomes negative or oblate.

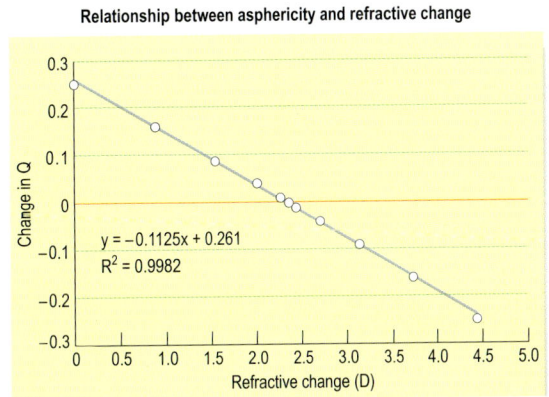

Relationship between asphericity and refractive change

$y = -0.1125x + 0.261$
$R^2 = 0.9982$

Figure 8.3 The relationship between asphericity and refractive change for a model cornea of R_0 7.80 and $Q = 0.25$. The refractive change when Q is zero is 2.25 D. If Q becomes oblate to −0.25, the maximum refractive change is approximately 4.50 D.

is assumed to become oblate, with the apical radius and asphericity changing in the same linear fashion.

Therefore, a cornea with the initial shape data as set out above has an initial limit of 2.00 D refractive change *if the "final" corneal shape is a sphere ($Q = 0$)*. If, however, the assumption is made that the cornea can become oblate with

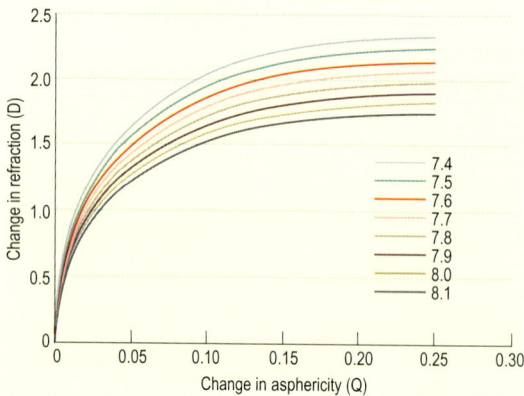

Figure 8.4 The effect that the initial apical radius has on refractive change. Starting from a Q of zero, the refractive change increases as the Q value increases. For steeper values of R_0 (given the same Q value) the refractive change is greater than that of flatter R_0 values.

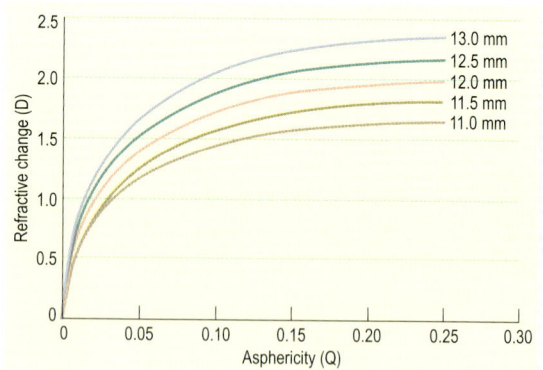

Figure 8.5 The effect that horizontal visible iris diameter (HVID) has on refractive change. Assuming an initial R_0 of 7.80 mm, the refractive change achieved as Q increases in value is greater for higher HVID values.

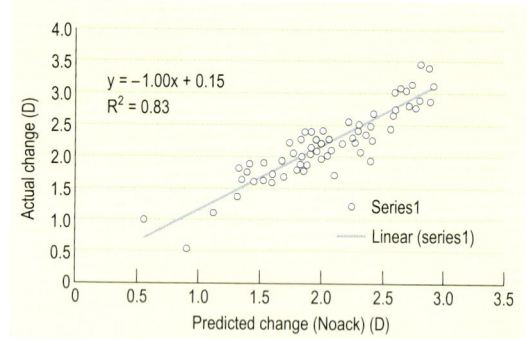

Figure 8.6 The relationship between predicted (modeled) and actual refractive change. The correlation appears to be good, with the predicted refractive change being 0.15 D greater than the measured refractive change.

orthokeratology, the maximum refractive change becomes approximately 4.00 D, when $Q = -0.2$. For smaller refractive changes, between 2.25 and 4.50 D, the cornea is assumed to "come to rest" at an oblate shape of intermediate R_0 and Q values.

The other variables analyzed were the effect of HVID and the initial R_0 value. In the past orthokeratology studies have always noted that steep corneas change to a greater extent than flat corneas, so it is interesting to note that the model supports these observations (Fig. 8.4). However, the difference, according to the model, is not that significant, with only a 0.75 D difference between the steepest and flattest R_0 values.

The model also predicts that the greater the HVID, the greater the possible refractive change, with a variance of approximately 0.75 D for an apical radius of 7.80 mm (Fig. 8.5). Unfortunately, the ideal situation of a steep cornea and a large HVID does not occur: steep corneas are generally associated with smaller HVIDs and flat corneas with larger HVIDs (Mandell 1978).

Noack extended the program to find the intercept between the prefit aspheric surface and the final spherical surface, assuming a maximal corneal thickness change of 20 μm at the apex. The result is an approximation of the treatment zone (TxZ) diameter (see later).

The accuracy of the concept was assessed by comparing the results of the predicted outcome based on the initial corneal data to the measured changes in apical corneal power using the EyeSys version 3.2 software and Contex 704T lenses on 65 randomly chosen eyes. The regression between predicted and actual changes appears quite good (Fig. 8.6), with a form of $y = 1.00x + 0.15$ ($r^2 = 0.83$). This equates to a refractive change of 1.15 D for 1.00 D predicted change, or 2.15 D for 2.00 D predicted change, and so on. This would therefore indicate that the

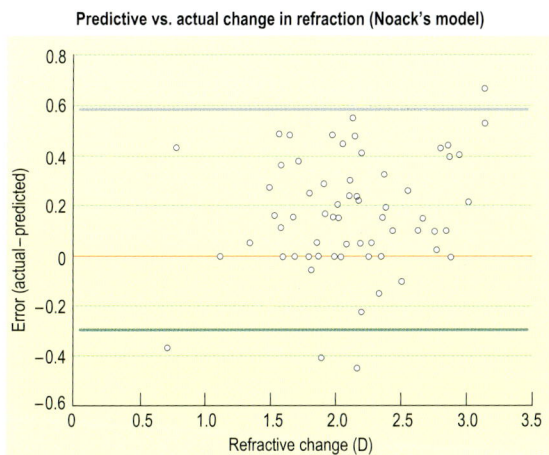

Figure 8.7 More recent analysis shows the scatter of results, indicating that the predictions are within ± 0.40 D of the actual change at the 95% confidence level.

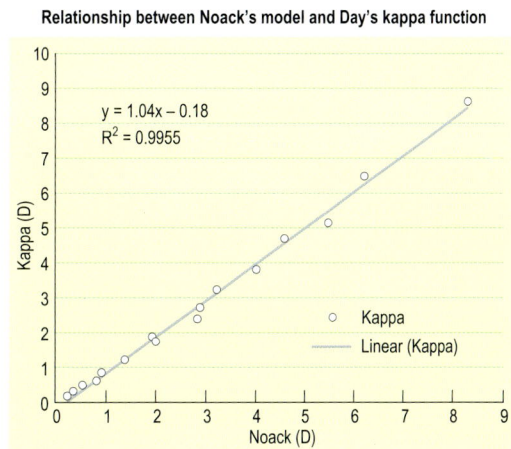

Figure 8.8 The kappa function and Noack model are highly correlated due to the fact that they both take the initial eccentricity into account. The very high refractive changes shown here are due to a combination of very steep (7.00 mm) R_0 values and high (0.90) eccentricity values. Such pre-existing corneal shapes do not occur. The "real world" changes are within 1 standard deviation of the norm, which is an R_0 of 7.80 and a Q value of 0.25. In the majority of cases, the refractive change range is approximately 2.50 ± 1.00 D.

model tends to underestimate slightly the possible refractive change.

However, more recent analysis of the data reveals a slightly different story. In order for the "true" picture to be shown, the difference between the "gold standard" (the refraction) and

Table 8.1 Calculated refractive change from initial apical radius and eccentricity for 11.50 mm horizontal visible iris diameter

Apical radius	Eccentricity									
	0.0	0.1	0.2	0.3	0.4	0.5	0.6	0.7	0.8	0.9
7.00	0	0.14	0.56	1.22	2.17	3.20	4.38	5.51	6.73	7.94
7.10	0	0.10	0.56	1.22	2.07	3.06	4.14	5.29	6.47	7.65
7.20	0	0.10	0.53	1.16	1.97	2.92	3.97	5.07	6.22	7.37
7.30	0	0.10	0.51	1.11	1.88	2.80	3.80	4.88	5.98	7.11
7.40	0	0.12	0.49	1.05	1.80	2.67	3.65	4.68	5.76	6.85
7.50	0	0.12	0.46	1.01	1.72	2.56	3.50	4.51	5.55	6.61
7.60	0	0.12	0.44	0.96	1.65	2.46	3.36	4.33	5.35	6.38
7.70	0	0.12	0.42	0.92	1.58	2.36	3.23	4.17	5.15	6.16
7.80	0	0.12	0.40	0.88	1.51	2.27	3.11	4.02	4.97	5.94
7.90	0	0.1	0.39	0.84	1.45	2.18	2.99	3.87	4.80	5.74
8.00	0	0	0.37	0.81	1.39	2.09	2.88	3.73	4.63	5.55
8.10	0	0	0.36	0.78	1.34	2.01	2.78	3.60	4.47	5.37
8.20	0	0	0.34	0.75	1.29	1.94	2.67	3.47	4.32	5.19
8.30	0	0	0.33	0.72	1.24	1.87	2.58	3.35	4.17	5.02
8.40	0	0	0.32	0.69	1.19	1.80	2.49	3.24	4.02	4.86
8.50	0	0	0.31	0.66	1.14	1.73	2.41	3.12	3.87	4.70

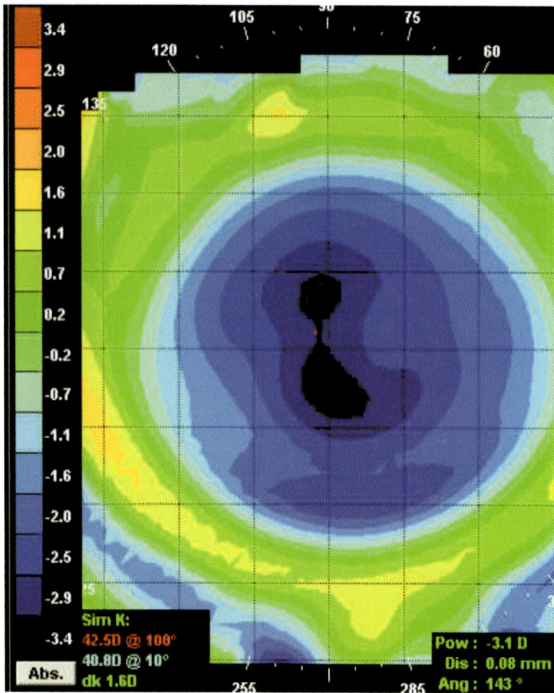

Figure 8.9   A postwear topography plot showing areas of isodioptric change. This can be viewed as representing areas of distinct spherical surfaces.

with high eccentricities will show larger changes in refractive error as the cornea is more spherical-ized by orthokeratology treatment than small, flat corneas with low eccentricity. This seems to accord with clinical experience.

SPHERE OR OBLATE: DOES IT REALLY MATTER?

A controversy exists in orthokeratology circles with respect to the final corneal shape: is it a spher-ical, or an oblate ellipse? The argument stems from the difference in refractive change possible with RGLs compared to the traditional orthokeratology techniques. The mean refractive change possible with the May–Grant or Tabb techniques is approx-imately 1.00 D, and was associated with corneal sphericalization, or a final eccentricity of zero. Since RGLs produce more than twice the refractive change associated with conventional designs, it has been proposed that the final corneal shape

the model must be calculated. This is then plotted against the mean of the two results (Bland & Altman 1986). In the above example, the mean difference is 0.18 D with a standard deviation of 0.22 D. The graphical representation is shown in Figure 8.7. This shows that, at the 95% confidence level (limits of agreement), the majority of patients will achieve an outcome that is within ± 0.50 D of that predicted by the model. The difference in outcomes could also be partly dependent on the lens design used, and this is discussed in a later section.

How well do the two theories correspond with each other? The relationship between the kappa function and Noack's model is shown in Figure 8.8. In effect, the two are identical, as both are based on the initial R_0, asphericity, and HVID, but used different methodologies to arrive at the same answer. The calculated changes for a range of corneal shapes at a HVID of 11.5 are shown in Table 8.1.

We can summarize the clinical consequences from these models as follows: large, steep corneas

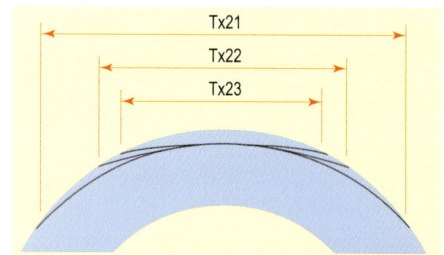

Figure 8.10   The "final" corneal shape assuming a spherical surface over different zones. Note that as the "final" spherical curve becomes flatter, the treatment zone (T×Z) diameter is decreased. The diagram shows three zones of increasing spherical curves from the center to the edge of the T×Z. Compare this with Figure 8.9.

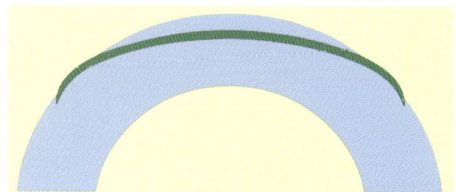

Figure 8.11   The new postorthokeratology corneal profile is shown in yellow, illustrating an oblate surface. A topographer would reconstruct this surface as zones of equal dioptric changes, as in Figure 8.9.

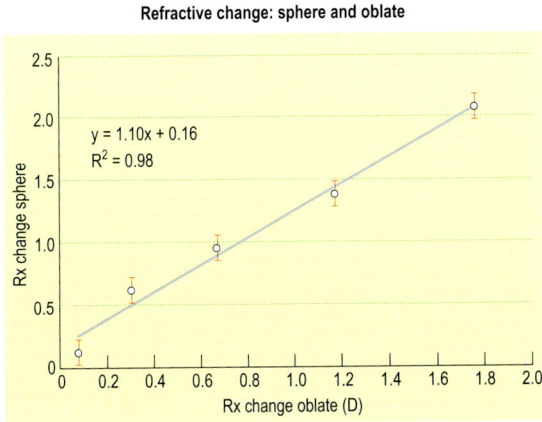

Figure 8.12 The difference in outcomes depending on whether an oblate or sphere is the model. The differences are not clinically significantly different.

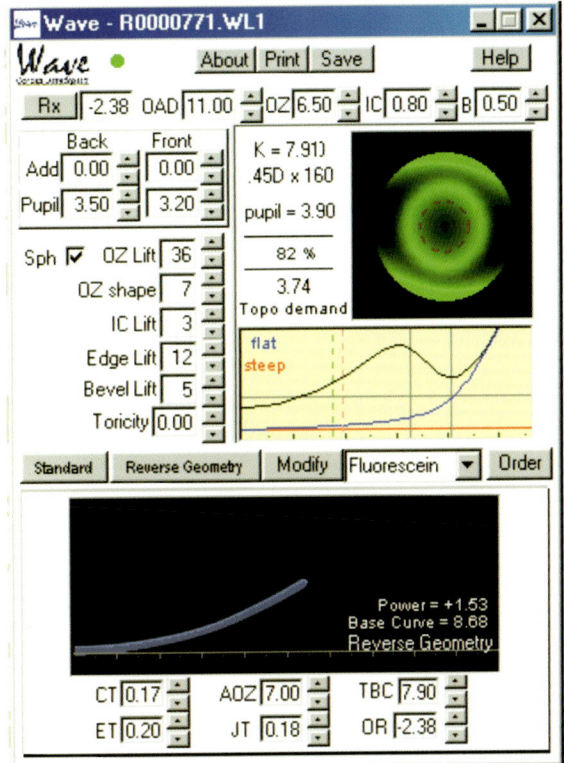

Figure 8.14 The WAVE screen output. The tear layer profile, fluorescein pattern, and allied data are shown. "Topo demand" refers to the liquid lens power of the tear layer.

becomes oblate. This would explain a greater change than that which is possible when sphericalization occurs. This is supported by the appearance of the postwear topography maps that show the central cornea to be flatter than the midperipheral cornea (Fig. 8.9).

The "spherical shape" assumption is based on the results of the earlier studies into orthokeratology. Also, statistical analysis of the postwear corneal shape shows that the radii of curvature of the central 5.00 mm chord are not statistically different from each other, indicating a spherical surface (Mountford 1997).

If a greater refractive change is required over and above that which is possible with corneal sphericalization, the following model applies. Assuming a maximum change of central epithelial thickness of 20 µm, a greater refractive change would require a flatter spherical curve over a smaller diameter, resulting in a smaller TxZ diameter (Munnerlyn et al 1988). This is shown diagrammatically in Figure 8.10.

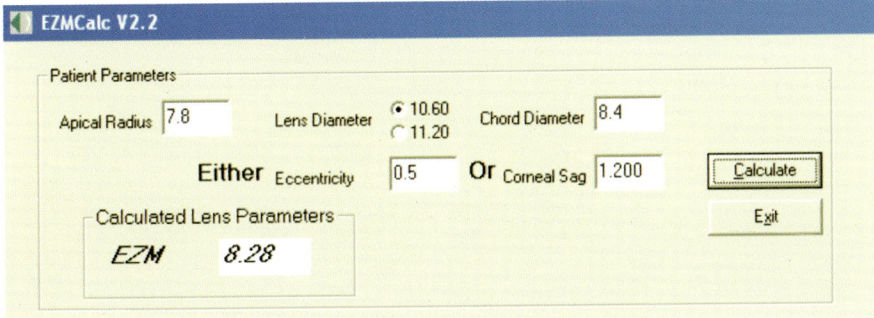

Figure 8.13 The EZM calculator, with inputs of apical radius, eccentricity, or corneal sag. The calculated back optic zone radius of the lens is shown.

The postwear corneal topography plot shown in Figure 8.9 indicates that there are differing zones of isodioptric change. This is similar to the different radius zones in Figure 8.10. However, an oblate surface, as shown in Figure 8.11, would also show the same gradations of power change over the surface. The whole question then becomes: which model best describes the refractive changes achieved?

The refractive change in excess of sphericalization for a cornea of R_0 7.80, eccentricity 0.50 when calculated using both models is shown in Figure 8.12. The oblate model underestimates the change by a mean of 0.21 ± 0.10 D when compared to the spherical model. These differences are not really clinically significant, so in effect, both models are an acceptable method of representing the final corneal shape.

LENS DESIGN AND FITTING SOFTWARE

The following section deals with the currently available computer software that can be used as a means of fitting orthokeratology lenses. It does not cover the total number of programs that are currently in development, as these were not available for inclusion at the time of writing. The most important fact that the reader has to keep in mind when reviewing these software packages is this: they are all based on the assumption that the topography data input into the program are valid and accurate. This is generally not the case, as has been shown in Chapters 2 and 9. The practitioner still needs to be able to interpret the results of the trial wear period in order to come to the correct decisions as to the remedial steps required in order to optimize the fitting.

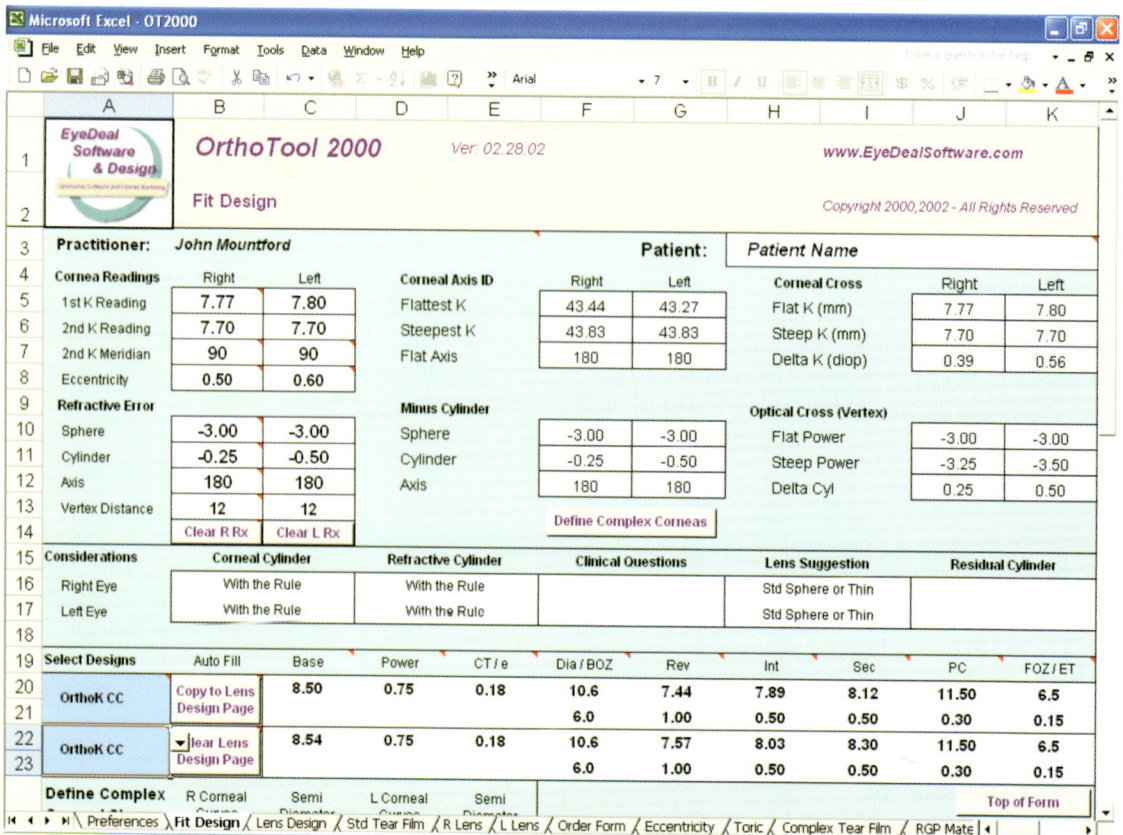

Figure 8.15   The input screen for the Ortho Tools program. The lens parameters are shown in the lower cells.

The EZM software (Gelflex)

The inputs for this program are the apical radius and eccentricity values. The choice of lens diameter is fixed to either 10.60 or 11.20 mm. The input data are then used to determine the correct base curve (back optic zone radius or BOZR) of the lens required. The lens is based on the concept of a 7.00 mm optic zone (back optic zone diameter or BOZD) with a fixed 4.00 D steeper reverse curve (see Ch. 4), with the end result of the procedure occurring when the corneal eccentricity becomes zero. The program gives no information as to the trial lens that should be fitted, but the closest BOZR in the trial lens range should suffice for a trial fit (Fig. 8.13). The chord requested is the total diameter of the lens minus 2.20 mm.

WAVE software

The software for the WAVE fitting system was developed by Jim Edwards, and is an optional extension to the Keratron topography system. The software takes the raw elevation data from the Scout or Keratron topographer and creates a lens design and tear layer profile based on the data. The system uses very sophisticated mathematics to develop a lens design. The base curve (BOZR) is based on the refractive change required, with a compression factor of 1.25 D, and the rest of the lens design follows. The diameter is variable, with the optic zone (BOZD) and reverse curve (RC) widths being automatically recalculated. The optimal optic zone diameter is 1.00 mm greater than the pupil diameter.

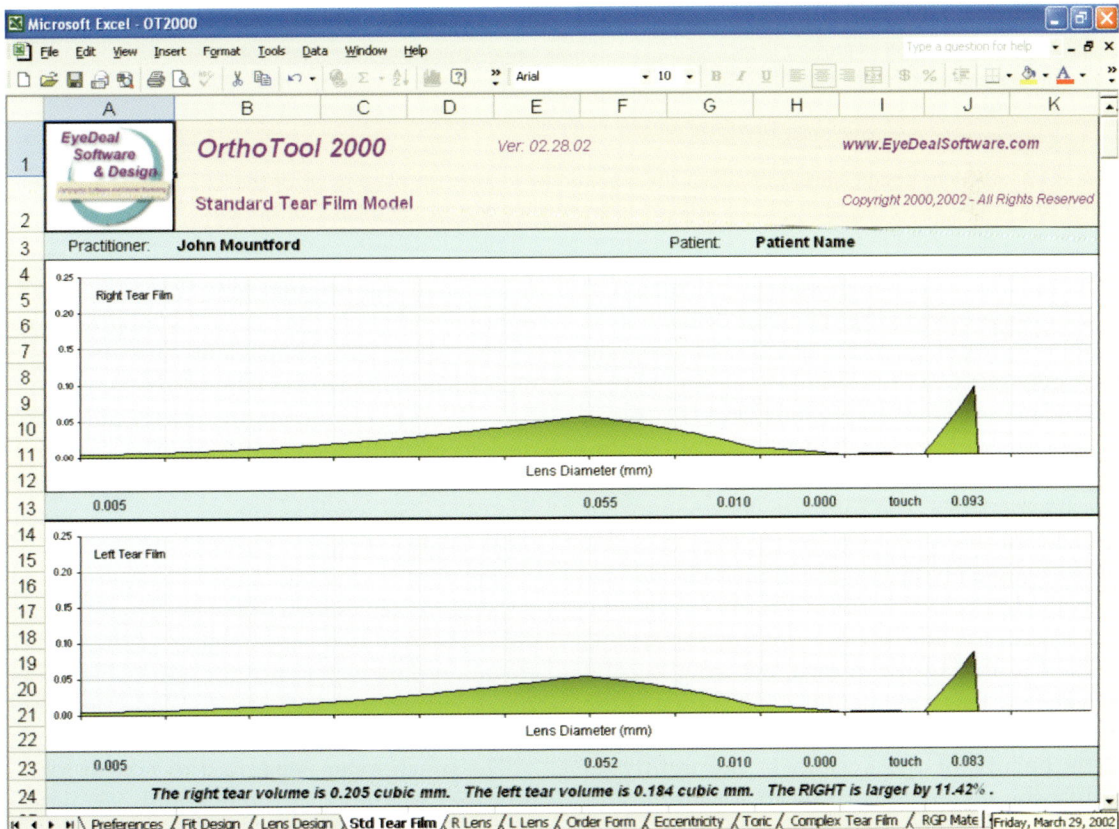

Figure 8.16   The tear layer profile of the lens on the eye. Note that the tear layer thickness is shown at each zone diameter, as well as the tear volume behind the lens.

Microsoft Excel - OT2000

File Edit View Insert Format Tools Data Window Help

EyeDeal Software & Design

OrthoTool 2000 Ver: 02.28.02 www.EyeDealSoftware.com

Lens Design Worksheet Copyright 2000,2002 – All Rights Reserved

Practitioner: John Mountford **Patient:** Patient Name

Clear Right Lens	Fill Right Lens	OrthoK CC		RIGHT	Material / Vertex	LEFT	OrthoK CC		Fill Left Lens	Clear Left Lens
BC Diopters			B	XO		XO	B			BC Diopters
39.63		Sphere	Flat	Steep		Flat	Steep	Sphere	39.50	
	touch		8.50		Base Curve / Ecc	8.54			0.005	
Front Radius (mm)			0.75		Power / Ecc	0.75			Front Radius (mm)	
8.43		Sphere	0.18	Steeper	Center Thickness	0.18	Steeper	Sphere	8.46	
	Tear Film	Alt. PCs	10.6	Flatter	Diameter	10.6	Flatter	Alt. PCs	Tear Film	
Diopters	0.056					6.0			0.052	Diopters
40.00	0.084	0.80	**Reverse Curve Width**			7.57		1.00	0.010	44.63
42.75	0.074	0.50	Range: (0.00 to 3.00 mm)			8.03		0.50	0.000	42.00
41.63	0.074	0.50	8.12		Secondary Curve	8.30		0.50	touch	40.63
29.38	0.167	0.30	11.50		Peripheral Curve	11.50		0.30	0.083	29.38
8.48		<- Flange	6.5		Front OZ	6.5		Flange ->	8.25	
0.174		<- J.T.	0.150		Edge Thickness	0.150		J.T. ->	0.189	
0.015		<- R.E.L.	0.019		Axial Edge Lift	-0.036		R.E.L. ->	-0.028	

The right tear volume is 1.341 cubic mm. The left tear volume is 0.184 cubic mm. The RIGHT is larger by 629.44%.

Effective R. E. L.		Effective OZ	Effective BC		Effective Curves	Effective BC		Effective OZ	Effective R.E.L.
0.068		10.00	8.26			8.09		10.00	0.074
Front Surface		22.7	0.06	Lentic	Angle & Lset	Lentic	22.6	-0.23	Front Surface

Preferences / Fit Design / Lens Design / Std Tear Film / R Lens / L Lens / Order Form / Eccentricity / Toric / Complex Tear Film / RGP Mate

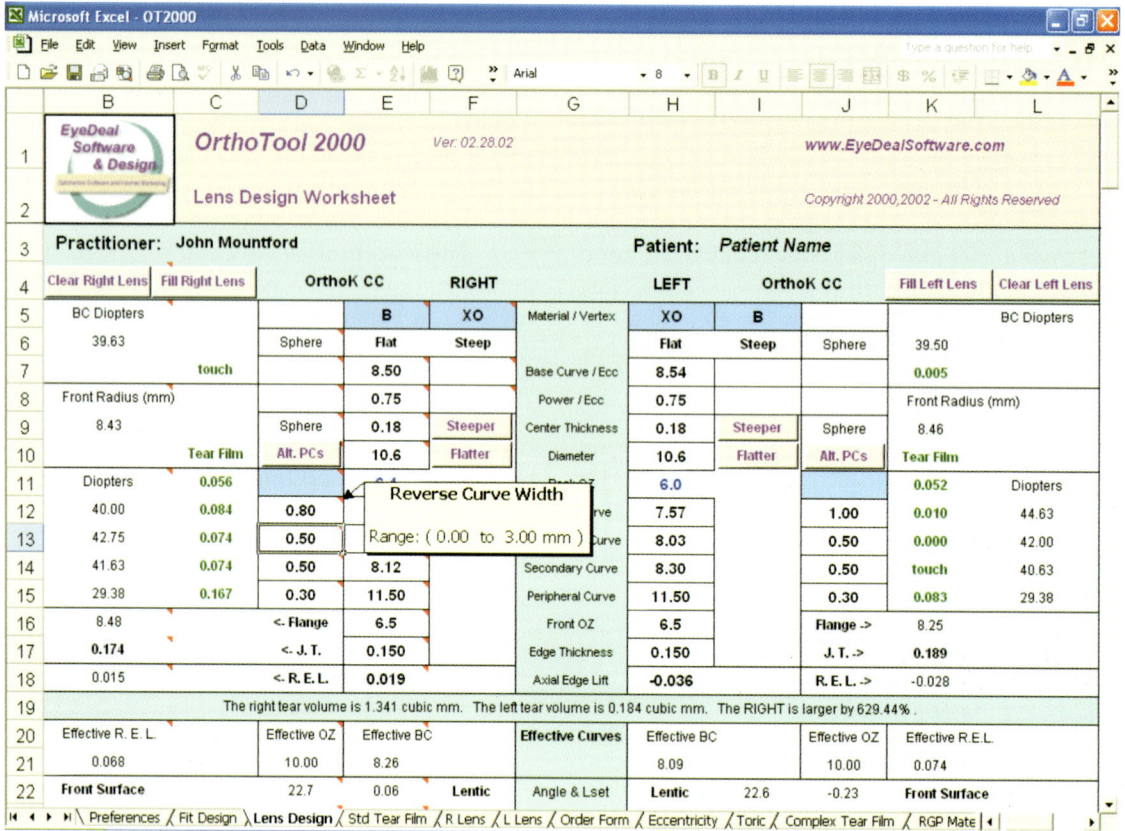

Figure 8.17 The lens design worksheet allows the practitioner to alter the parameters of the lens. In this case, the width of the reverse curve has been altered without corresponding changes to the rest of the lens.

The reverse zone is then initially calculated to be 12% of the BOZD. The diameter of the lens is 1.67 times greater then the BOZD. The program then generates a representative fluorescein pattern and tear layer graph of the lens (Fig. 8.14). The practitioner is then free to manipulate the tear layer profile to optimize the fit depending on clinical experience. The software does not output the exact curves of the lens as they are complex aspheres based on the raw elevation data and tear layer thickness. At varying points across the corneal surface, the surface area of the lens is matched to that of the cornea, assuring sagittal equivalency. This information is not shown in the outputs.

The beauty of the system is the ability to modify the tear layer profile in real time and assess the results. Also, a comprehensive problem-solving system allows the practitioner to reinstall the original lens that was less than optimal and make the necessary modifications.

The data are then sent directly to the Optoform lathe at the laboratory for manufacture. WAVE also contains programs for the design of multifocals and bitorics, as well as nonsymmetrically rotational aspheres for complex cases such as keratoconus and postsurgical fitting.

The first-fit success rate is therefore highly dependent on the accuracy of the topography data. The reported repeatability of the Scout for elevation data is ± 12 μm for adults (Berrer et al 2002) and up to ± 0.25 mm for children (Chui & Cho 2003).

The practitioner is advised to take at least six repeated readings of the eye and calculate the mean and standard deviation of error. The map closest to the mean value should then be used to

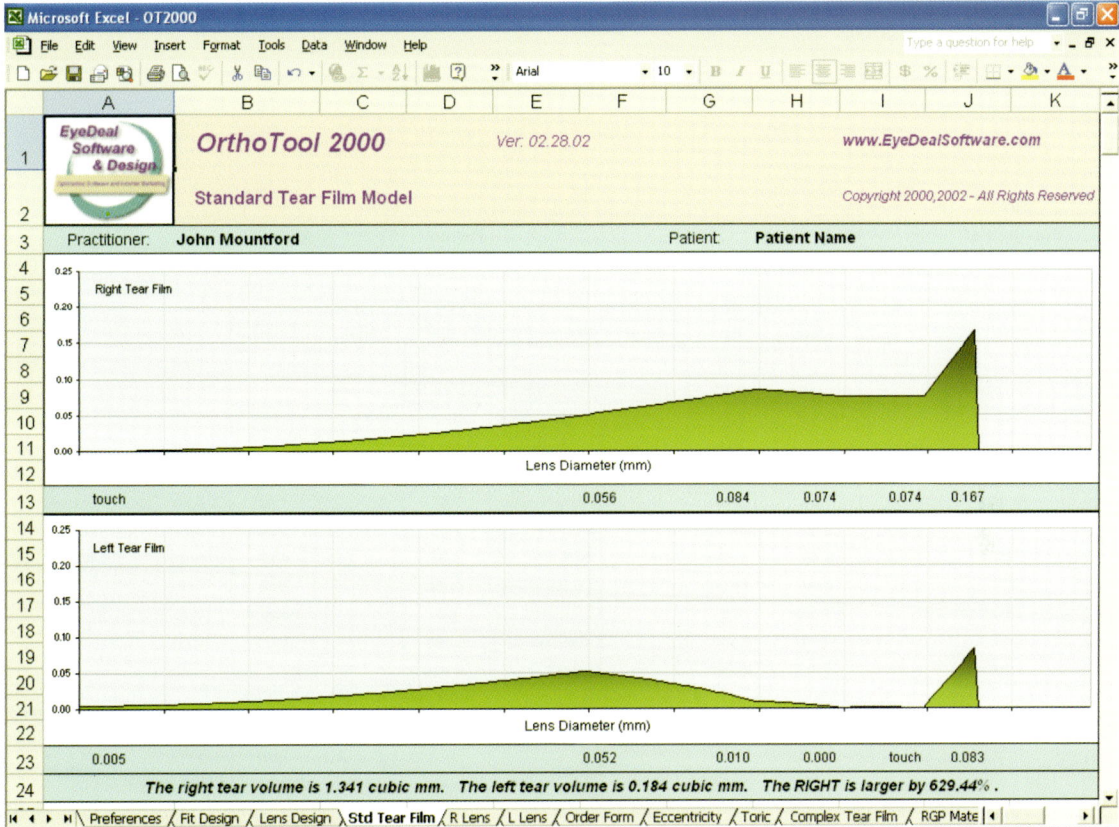

Figure 8.18   The resultant tear layer profile. Simply changing one individual curve band totally alters the lens fit. Compare the top graph of the altered right eye to the unaltered left eye.

design the lens. The error values can then be used if refinement of the fit is necessary.

Ortho Tool 2000 (EyeDeal software and design)

The Ortho Tool program was written by Tom Geimer. It is based on a Microsoft Excel platform and is very easy to use. The opening statement in the instruction manual sets the tone: "It's a simple truth, everyone hates user's guides. Software developers hate writing them. Users hate reading them." Thus begins an enjoyable read through one of the best user's guides the author has ever read. The program will design standard alignment lenses, aspherics, bitorics, and RGLs for orthokeratology. There are two options for RGL design, either a practitioner pre-

ference design (controlled clearance) or the Reinhart R&R design. The input data are the keratometry values, the corneal eccentricity, and the refractive error. The program also includes a very useful section where the central and temporal K readings can be entered and the apical radius and eccentricity calculated. Alternatively, the apical radius can be calculated from K readings and eccentricity.

The lens design and fitting are based on sag calculations, with the resultant tear layer profiles graphically presented. The practitioner is free to manipulate the clearance values and the program calculates the required curves.

In this case, a cornea of K_f 7.77 mm, eccentricity 0.50, and a refractive error of -3.00 will be used to design a controlled-clearance five-zone RGL. The input data are shown in Figure

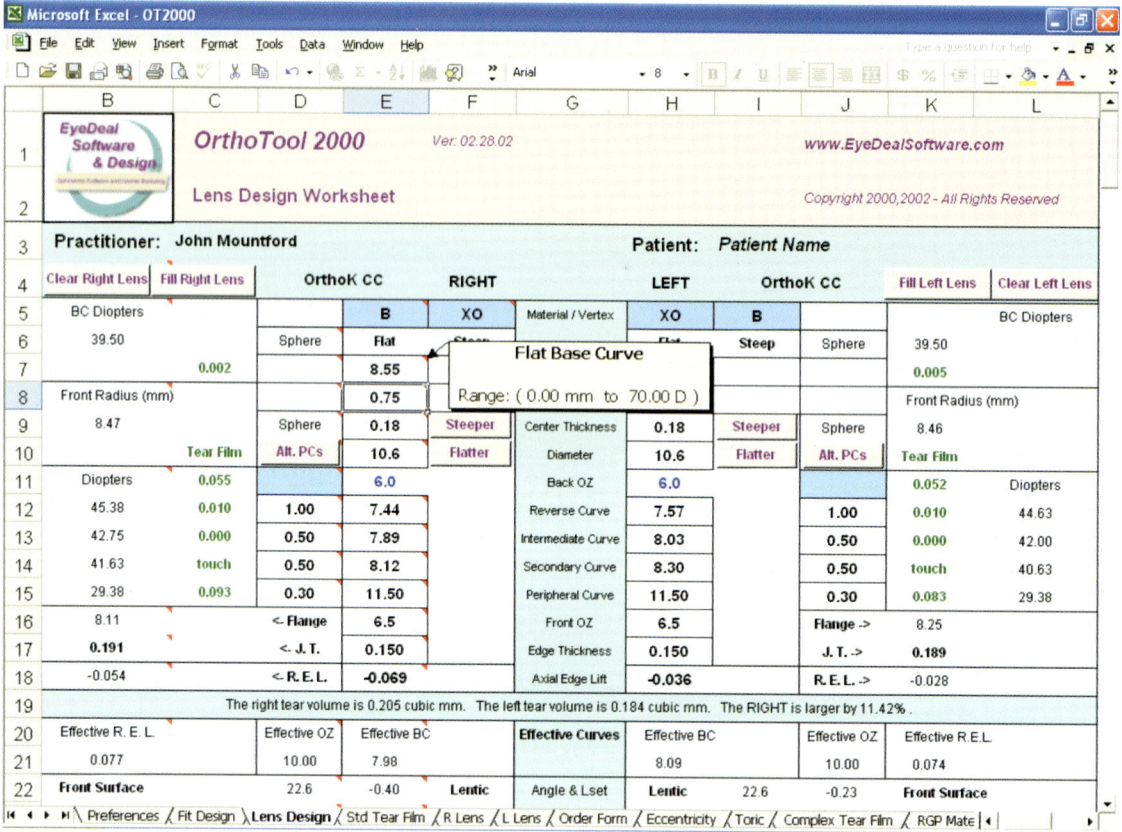

Figure 8.19   The back optic zone radius is altered from the calculated 8.50 to 8.55.

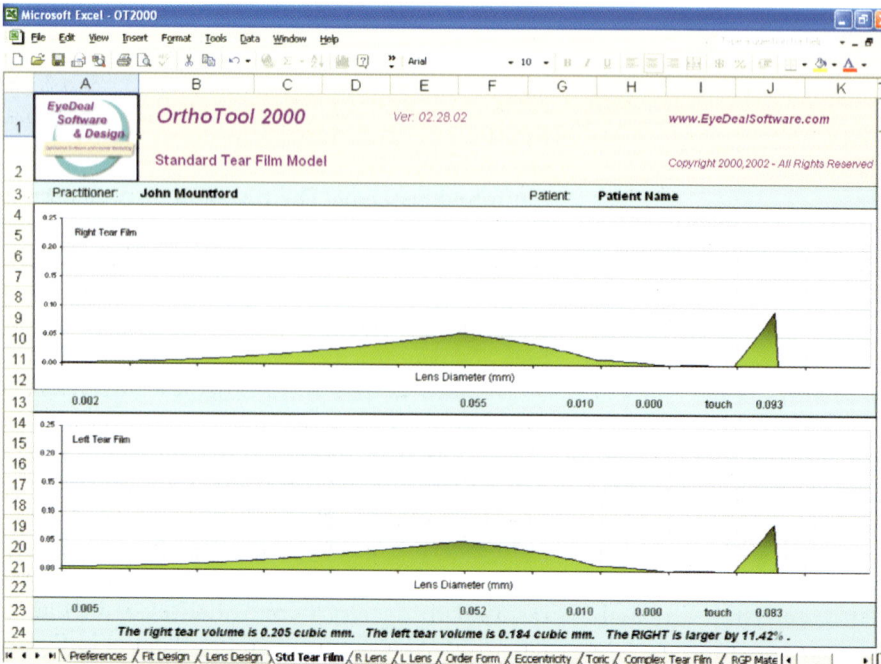

Figure 8.20   The effect of altering the back optic zone radius is shown by the decrease in apical clearance to 2 μm.

8.15. Note that the parameters of the lens are shown in the lower section of the sheet. The tear layer tab is then pushed, and the tear layer profile of the lens is shown (Fig. 8.16). The thickness of the tear layer at each zone of the lens is displayed, along with the calculated tear volume under the lens.

The lens design sheet allows the practitioner to change any of the variables like BOZD, RC width, and so on. In this case, the RC width has been changed to 0.50 mm from the original 1.00 mm (Fig. 8.17). The effect this has on the lens fit is shown in the tear layer sheet (Fig. 8.18). Note that the lens is now a poor fit, being too flat with no peripheral touch. If changes are made to the design section, all the lens parameters must be altered. The beauty of this program is that the simple act of manipulating the data is an excellent teaching tool for learning the interdependence of all the curves required for good contact lens design.

Figure 8.19 shows the effect of flattening the original BOZR from 8.50 to 8.55 mm. The change in tear layer thickness at the apex has been reduced to 2 μm (Fig. 8.20). The Ortho Tools software can be used with either topography data or keratometry values. The most important thing to remember is that sag fitting is dependent on the eccentricity of the cornea. Those practitioners who do not use topography will therefore need to calculate the eccentricity values using the program that converts temporal *K* readings over specific chords to an eccentricity value.

Free Choice OK

The Free Choice program was written by Don Noack. The RGL section is shown here, but it also contains design data for aspherics and standard lens designs. The inputs are topography-based, with apical radius and eccentricity used to calculate the lens based on sag fitting.

The first page gives the practitioner the choice of lens design for a specific refractive change, with three-, four-, and five-zone variations (Fig. 8.21). A standard compression factor of 0.50 D is used for all designs. In this case, the standard cornea of R_0 7.80 mm, eccentricity 0.50, and a 3.00 D refractive

change will be used as an example. The data are entered and the program shows the various curves and diameters for the lens assuming a 5 μm apical clearance (Fig. 8.22). In order to alter any of the lens parameters, the practitioner must choose the tear graph option. This then shows all the same data again (Fig. 8.23).

However, the program is intended to be used as a problem-solving device, so the tear graph page allows for alteration of all the curves in order to refine the fit. For example, if the original lens, designed for a corneal eccentricity of 0.50, is worn and results in a central island, then the likely tear layer profile of the lens on the cornea can be visualized by changing the eccentricity value to 0.55. This is the original 0.50 with the assumed standard deviation in determination of eccentricity of 0.05 added. Thus the lens was effectively too steep due to the eccentricity being underestimated. The standard deviation of the eccentricity measurement is added to the original value. The lens now appears too steep (Fig. 8.24).

The practitioner then applies the rules outlined in Chapter 4 for refining the fit.

1. If the alignment curve is flattened by 0.05 mm, the apical clearance decreases by 5 μm. Steepening the alignment curve by 0.05 mm increases the apical clearance by 5 μm.
2. If the RC is flattened by 0.15 mm, the apical clearance is decreased by 10 μm. Steepening the RC by the same amount increases apical clearance by 10 μm.

In the above example, the apical clearance is 16 μm, so the first step taken is to flatten the RC by 0.15 mm from 7.062 to 7.212 mm (Fig. 8.25).

The resultant tear layer profile shows a lens with tight alignment curves. The apical clearance is approximately 8 μm, so flattening the alignment curve by 0.10 would lead to a drop of 10 μm in apical clearance. Alterations to the second alignment curve do not effect as great a change in apical clearance, so in this case, both alignment curves will be flattened by 0.05 mm, which will reduce the apical clearance to approximately zero. The final alteration is then to steepen the RC by 0.05 mm, which will increase the apical clearance to the 5 μm level required. The result is

Free Choice OK

○ 1.50 Rx Shift - Three Curve

○ Over 2.00 Rx Shift - Four Curve

○ Over 2.00 Rx Shift - Five Curve

○ TearGraph

Quit

©dbn 2000

The first three listed programmes are representations of the 3, 4, and 5 curve programmes currently being used for OrthoKeratology in the USA. These programmes determine the curves required relative to the Ro and eccentricity of the eye for these lenses utilising the appropriate preset formulae relating to the particular design. It is possible to enter the final programme "TearGraph" completely independent of these programmes. "TearGraph" is a programme which gives tear profiles for lenses completely independent of any preset values. It is recommended that initially "TearGraph" be entered only indirectly in this manner, but after becoming familiar with the system, it can be entered directly from this form.

NOTE Figures in red indicate that they cannot be altered without exiting and re-entering the programme

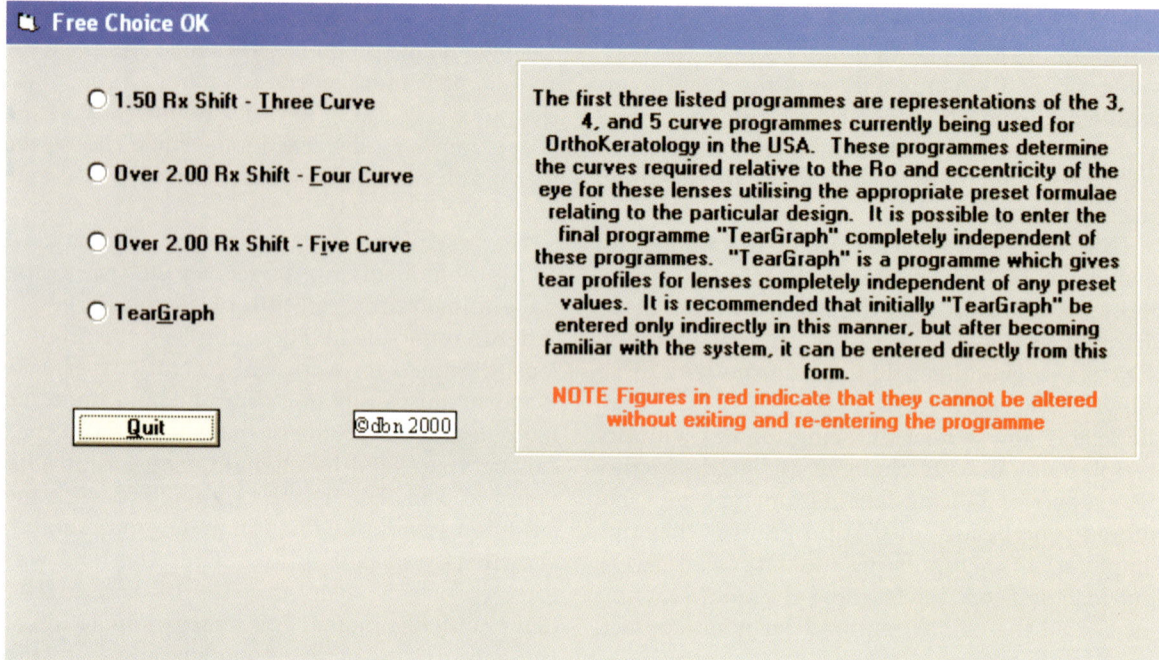

Figure 8.21 The opening page of the Free Choice OK program. The practitioner can choose between three different designs of reverse geometry lenses.

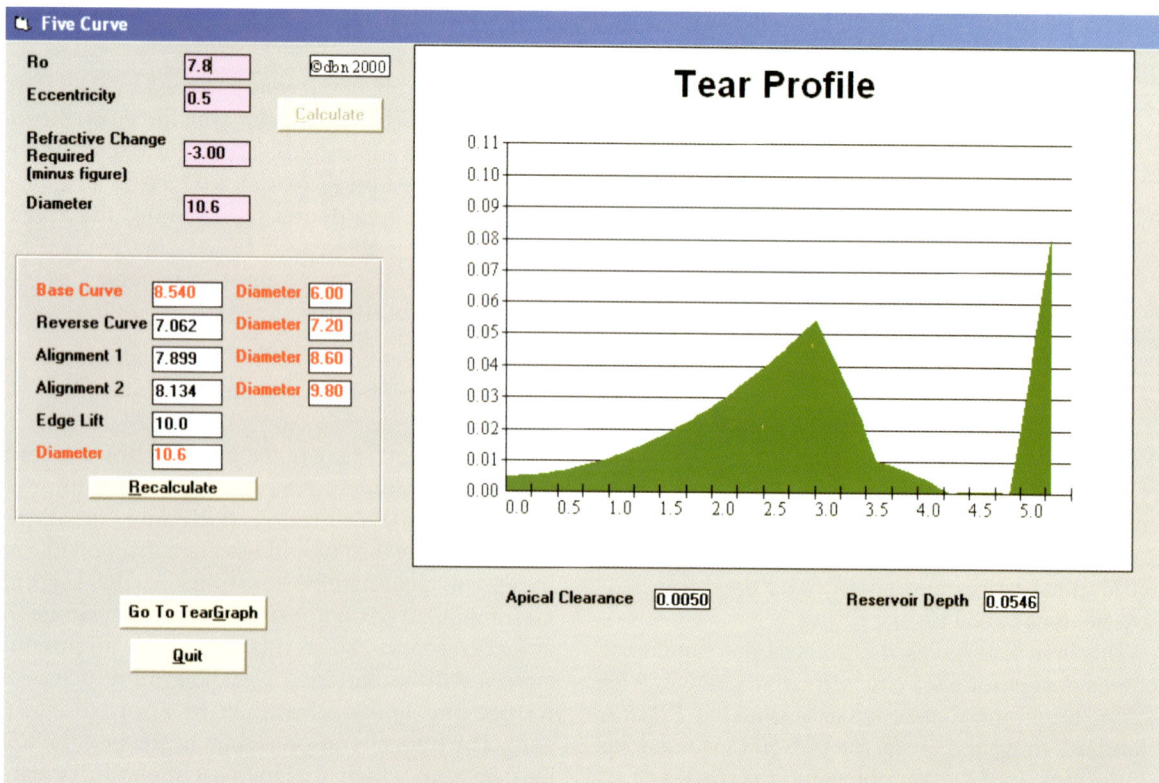

Five Curve

Ro	7.8
Eccentricity	0.5

©dbn 2000   Calculate

Refractive Change Required (minus figure)	-3.00
Diameter	10.6

Base Curve	8.540	Diameter	6.00
Reverse Curve	7.062	Diameter	7.20
Alignment 1	7.899	Diameter	8.60
Alignment 2	8.134	Diameter	9.80
Edge Lift	10.0		
Diameter	10.6		

Recalculate

Go To TearGraph

Quit

Tear Profile

Apical Clearance 0.0050   Reservoir Depth 0.0546

Figure 8.22 The entered data are displayed along with the tear layer profile of the lens. The apical clearance and the clearance at the edge of the optic zone are also shown.

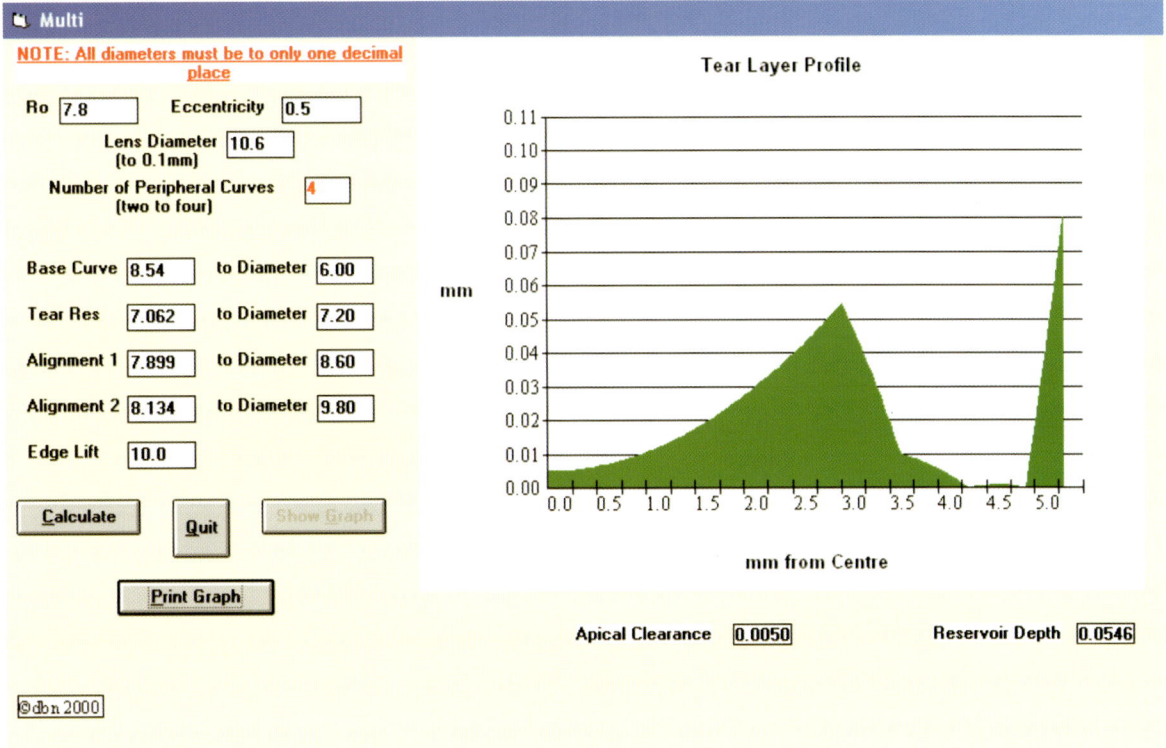

Figure 8.23   The same data transferred to the tear graph section.

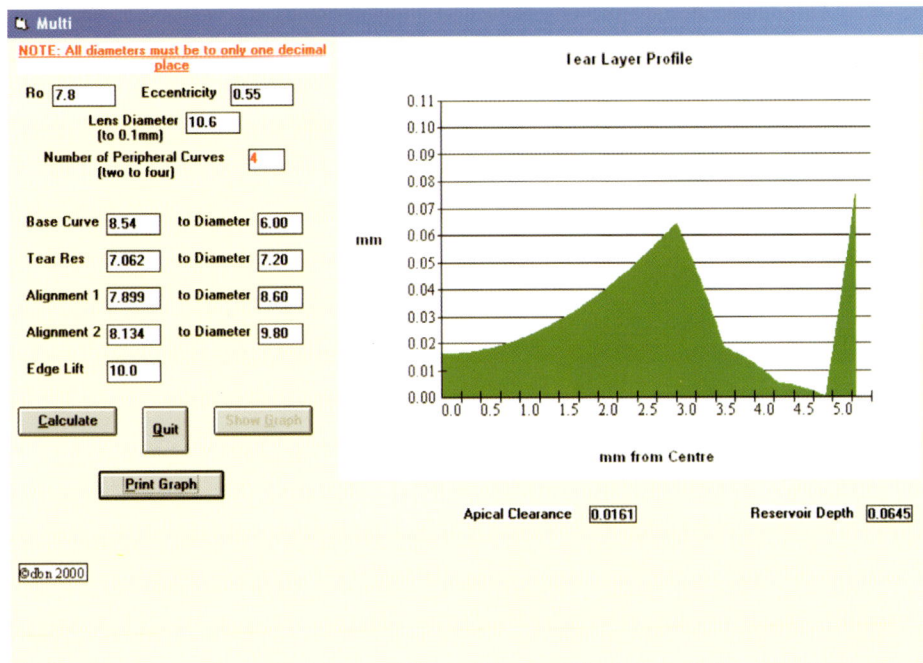

Figure 8.24   The standard deviation (SD) of eccentricity error (0.05) is input into the eccentricity value, and the tear layer profile of the original lens parameters on the altered corneal shape shown. Note that the lens now appears too steep.

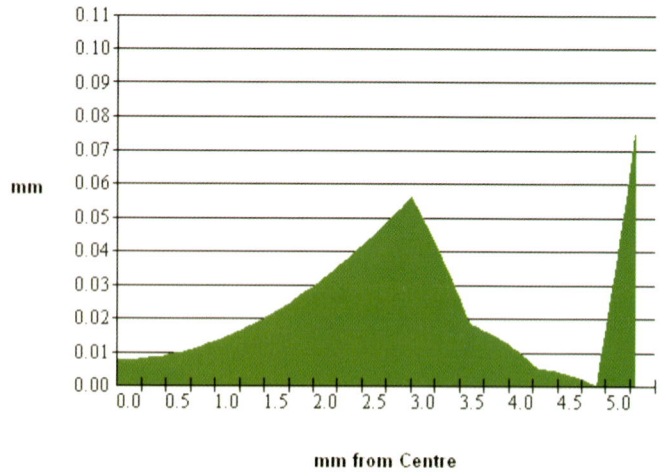

Figure 8.25   The effect of steepening the reverse curve by 0.15 mm. The alignment curves are still too steep.

shown in Figure 8.26, with the alignment curves flattened by 0.05 and the RC steepened by 0.05 from those shown in Figure 8.25.

The program also allows for alterations in the width of the curves; the practitioner is then able to alter the radii of the zones until the ideal tear layer profile is achieved. Like the Ortho Tool program, this is an excellent teaching aid for practitioners to understand the interrelationships of curves and diameters for sag fitting.

BE software

The BE lens and fitting software was developed by Don Noack and John Mountford. It is a purely topography-based system, and requires inputs of apical radius, eccentricity, or elevation in order to calculate the lens. It is used to:

1. calculate the elevation or sag values from R_0 and eccentricity for those topographers that do not give elevation data. Several repeated measurements on the same eye can then be entered into a spreadsheet and the mean and standard deviations calculated. This allows the practitioner to predict the likely variations in topographic data
2. determine the optimal trial lens based on the corneal data
3. refine the final lens prescription by using a postwear analysis system.

The first page (Fig. 8.27) gives the practitioner the choice of calculating the sag of the aspheric cornea, or the choice of tangent contact points for the prescription lens. These are preset to $1/4$, $1/3$, or $1/2$ tangents. The most commonly used tangent is the $1/4$, with the wider tangents being

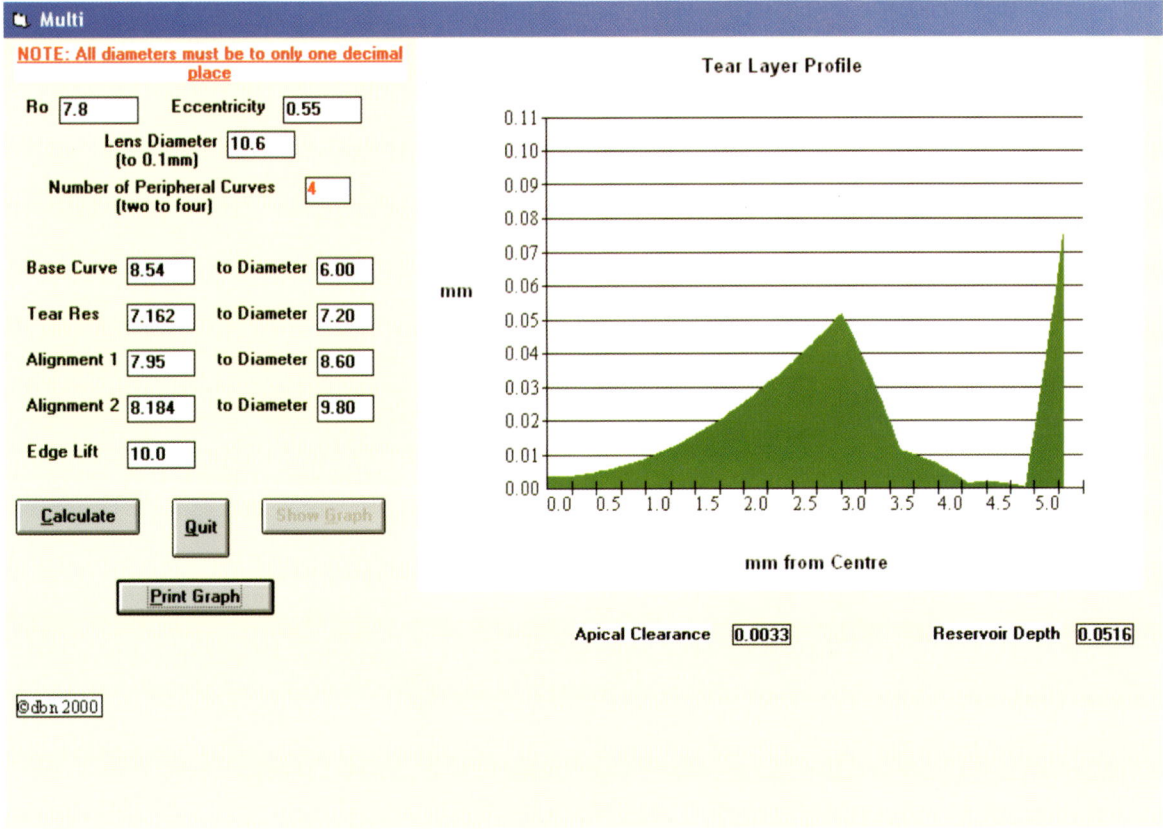

Figure 8.26 The alignment curves have been flattened by 0.05 mm each, and the reverse curve steepened by 0.05 mm, giving an ideal tear layer profile, and the parameters of the lens.

used for smaller lens diameters. Figure 8.28 shows the aspheric sag calculation page. The apical radius and eccentricity values of the repeated topography plots are calculated in turn and the mean and standard deviation calculated by transferring the results into a spreadsheet. The sag is calculated over the chord of contact between the lens and the corneal surface, which, for an 11.00 mm TD lens with a $^1/_4$ tangent, is 9.35 mm.

Once the tangent option is chosen the program moves to page 2, where the relevant apical radius, eccentricity, or elevation values are entered. The refractive change possible with corneal sphericalization as well as the final R_0 and TxZ diameter are shown (Fig. 8.29).

The "extra refractive change" box has two functions. Firstly, if the refractive change required

is less than that calculated for corneal sphericalization, the difference can be typed in and taken into account for later calculations. For example, the calculated refractive change in this case is 3.00 D. If the patient had a refraction of −1.50, the lens would cause overcorrection. Allowing for an initial overcorrection of 0.50 D, the actual required refractive change is 2.00 D, not 3.00 D. The "extra" +1.00 D would therefore be placed in the "extra refractive change" box.

Secondly, assuming that the Rx change required is 3.00 D, an extra −0.50 D is added to take regression into account. The limit of the exercise is an extra 1.00 D over that value predicted. If an extra 2.00 D were to be placed into the box, the practitioner would be warned that the TxZ diameter would be too small. Also, there are absolute limits as to the refractive change possible

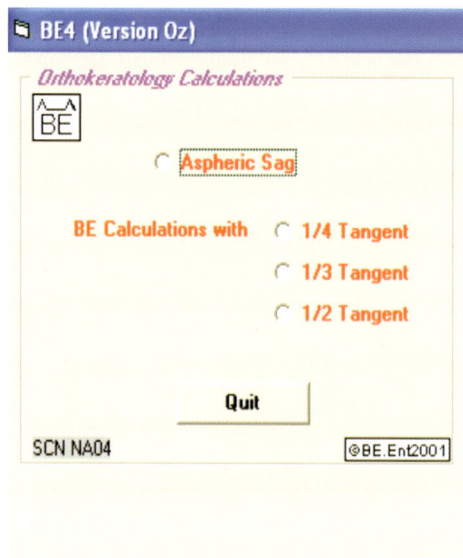

Figure 8.27 The first page of the BE software. The practitioner can choose between the aspheric sag calculator and the tangent width required for the lens.

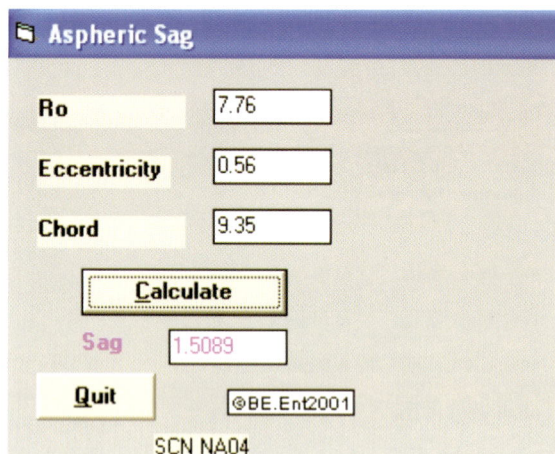

Figure 8.28 The aspheric sag calculator. The inputs are the apical radius, eccentricity, and chord. The sag is then calculated.

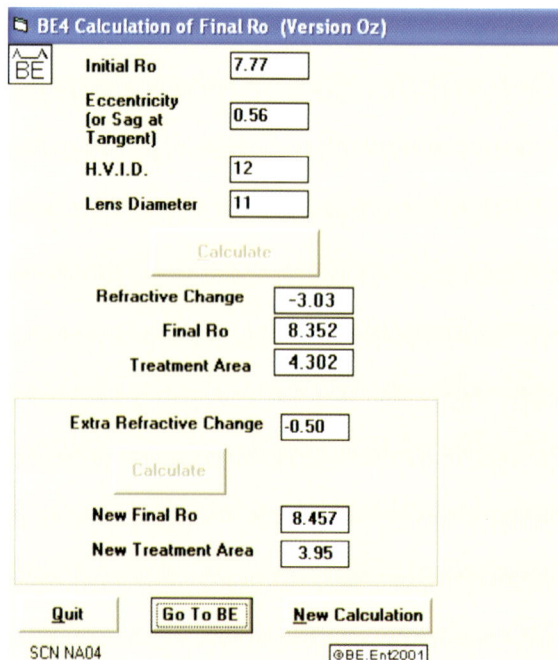

Figure 8.29 Second screen of the BE software. The corneal data are input and the refractive change calculated. Extra refractive change to a limit of an extra 1.00 D can be included.

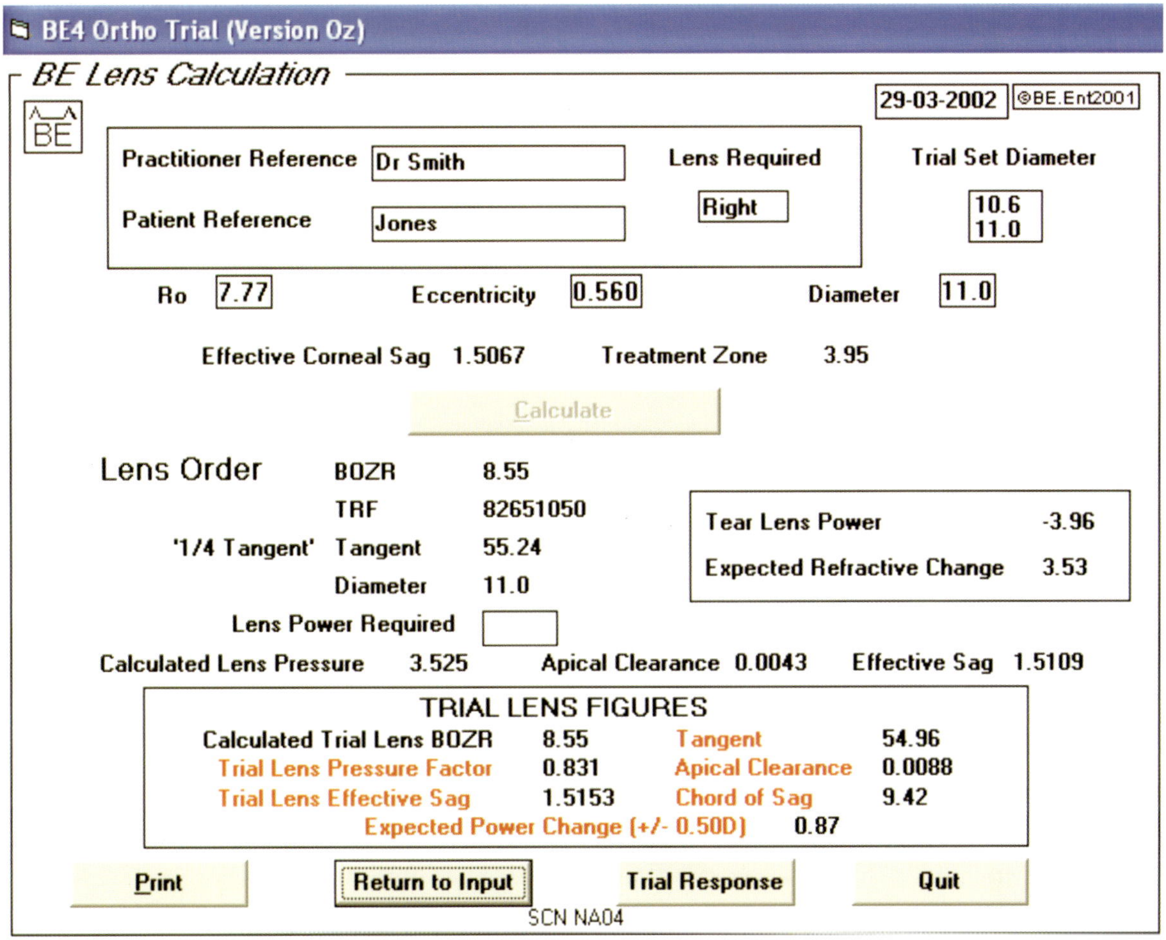

Figure 8.30   The trial lens screen showing the differences between the "calculated" lens and the trial lens. The predicted refractive change from the lens is also shown.

with RGLs so the limit of refractive change past that predicted by the initial corneal shape is approximately 1.00 D.

Once all the data are entered, the "go to BE" button is pressed. The parameters of the "calculated" and trial lenses are displayed (Fig. 8.30). Patient and practitioner references are added, and the trial lens diameter box is checked. The lens can be ordered in diameters from 10.20 to 12.00 mm, but the trial set is restricted to two common diameters of 10.6 and 11.00 mm. The results of the trial wear with the lens are then used to calculate the parameters for the different diameter, if required.

The important information is the trial lens that will be used for the overnight trial. Note that the BOZR is 8.55 mm, but the trial lens has a calculated apical clearance of 8.80 μm compared to the required apical clearance of 4.30 μm for the actual prescription lens. The trial lens will contact the cornea at a chord of 9.42 mm, and not the required 9.35 mm, and this is the cause of the increased apical clearance.

BE lenses use squeeze film force models to predict the refractive change, and this is dependent on the apical clearance. The greater the apical clearance, the less the refractive change will be, so the expected refractive change from the trial lens

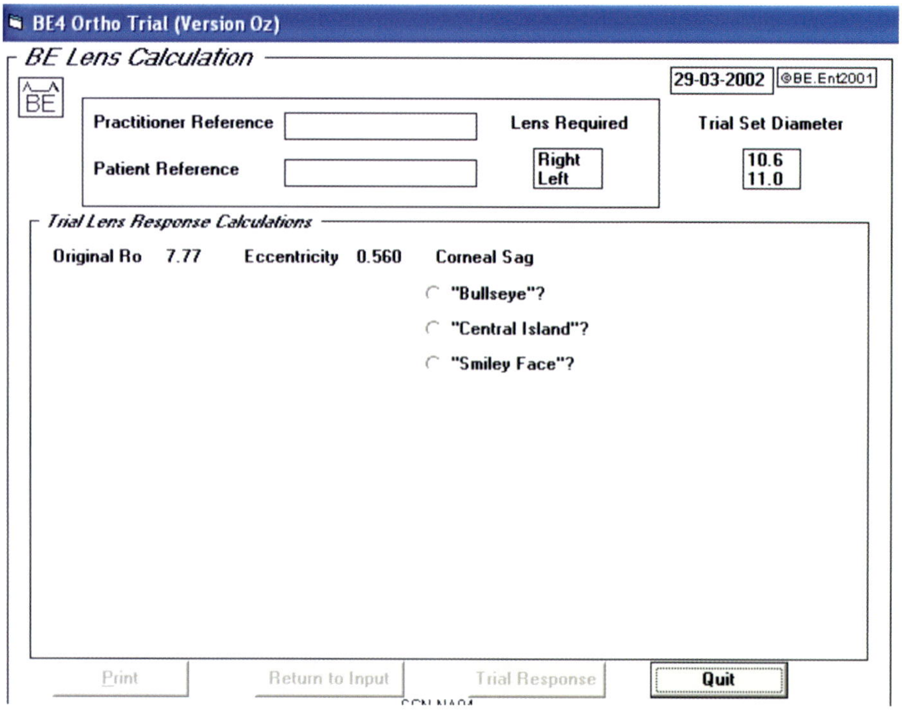

Figure 8.31 The "postwear" analysis screen. The practitioner enters data as required in order to determine the optimal outcome and final lens parameters.

is given. In this case, if the topography data are correct, the lens will cause approximately 0.87 D of change overnight. The trial lens is inserted, and the results assessed the next morning.

The original data are entered into the program, and the "trial response" button activated. The practitioner is then given three choices: did the trial result in a bull's eye, smiley face, or central island (Fig. 8.31)? In this case, a bull's eye is assumed, but the refractive change that occurred was 2.25 D, and not the predicted 0.87 D. This is entered into the program, and the screen then gives the parameters for the correct prescription lens. Since the refractive change was greater than that predicted, the apical clearance of the trial lens must have been less than the calculated 8.8 μm. Proprietary algorithms are used to link the refractive change to the estimated squeeze film force and apical clearance. The corneal elevation is then corrected, and the final lens parameters calculated.

If a smiley face or central island occurs, the program asks for the standard deviation of error of the topography readings in the determination of the elevation data. If a smiley face occurred,

the standard deviation is added to the original data and a new trial lens selected for a second trial. The opposite occurs for central islands, where the standard deviation is subtracted from the data. Trial wear periods are performed until a bull's eye is achieved, and only then will the final lens parameters be derived.

The BE program is based on the assumption that the lens sag is known, and the corneal sag is a value within the mean and standard deviation of the range of repeated values. The squeeze film force model allows for direct comparisons of calculated versus achieved outcomes based on the relationship between the force and the apical clearance. It gives the practitioner control over refinements to lens fit and corneal response.

CONCLUSIONS

The use of computer software to design and fit orthokeratology lenses is in its infancy. As the designs become more complex in order to resolve problems like astigmatism and corneal optics, the sophistication of the programs will increase. Also, as practitioners become more aware of the advantages of topography and sag-based fitting over the older and less accurate keratometer-based fitting, they will demand software to help with design and fitting.

Steps are already being taken by some designers to have their programs fully integrated into topography platforms, like the WAVE system, further simplifying the whole process. However, the final accuracy of the whole process is still dependent on the topography data, so there will always be a margin of error involved.

ACKNOWLEDGMENT

The author wishes to extend his sincere thanks to the people who so kindly gave their different software packages for inclusion in this book.

REFERENCES

Berrer R, Bende T, Jean B (2002) Assessment of topography systems for customized ablations. ARVO abstracts 158: B133. Investigative Ophthalmology and Visual Science

Bland J M, Altman D G (1986) Statistical methods for assessing agreement between two methods of clinical measurement. Lancet 1: 307–310

Chui W S, Cho P (2003) A comparative study of the performance of different corneal topographers on children with respect to orthokeratology practice. (in press).

Kwok S (1984) Calculation and application of the anterior surface area of the model human cornea. Journal of Biology 108: 295–313

Mandell R B (1978) Contact lens practice, 4th edn. Illinois, Charles C Thomas, pp. 127–128

Mountford J A (1997) An analysis of the changes in corneal shape and refractive error induced by accelerated orthokeratology. International Contact Lens Clinic 24: 128–143

Mountford J A, Noack D B (1998) A mathematical model for corneal shape changes associated with Ortho-K. Contact Lens Spectrum 13(6): 21–25.

Munnerlyn C R, Koons S J, Marshall J (1988) Photorefractive keratectomy: a technique for laser refractive surgery. Journal of Cataract and Refractive Surgery 14: 46–51

Smolek M K, Klyce S D (1998) Surface area of the cornea appears to be conserved in keratoconus. Investigative Ophthalmology and Vision Science 39 (suppl.)

Chapter **9**

Lens delivery, aftercare routine and problem-solving

David Ruston, Trusit Dave, and John Mountford

CHAPTER CONTENTS

Verification 228
What can be measured? 229
Inspection of edge profile 234
Surface quality 234
Tolerances 236
Lens delivery 236
The instruction session 238
Wearing schedules 238
Scheduling aftercare visits 240
The first aftercare 242
Symptoms and history 243
Vision with lenses in situ 245
Lens movement and position 245
Fluorescein fit assessment 246
Postremoval visual assessment 247
Decision on continuing suitability for
    orthokeratology treatment 252
Visual correction during the first week 252
Further aftercare visits 253
Emergencies 253
Problem-solving 254
Corneal staining 255
Contact lens papillary conjunctivitis 263
Epithelial iron deposition 264
Sterile peripheral ulcers 265
Microbial keratitis (MK) 265
Loss of the effect 265
References 266

The fundamental routine of aftercare employed in modern orthokeratology practice is very similar to conventional contact lens aftercare in terms of symptoms and history, examination of the anterior eye with and without lenses, and finally a management strategy to address any potential problems. However, there are a number of specific tests and questions that relate solely to the practice of orthokeratology. With a growing number of patients choosing to have their refraction managed using the principles of orthokeratology, it is important that contact lens practitioners familiarize themselves and ensure that they are able to perform a competent follow-up even if they are not practicing orthokeratologists. The main reason for this is that once treatment is complete many patients choose to return to their "regular" practitioner as many travel considerable distances for the treatment.

As detailed in Chapter 6, it is the opinion of the authors that any prospective orthokeratology patient ought to take part in a trial wearing session. This means that trial lenses will have been worn overnight or for 6 h or more during the day and the outcomes assessed by the practitioner. The outcomes that are relevant are the changes in unaided vision, refractive error, corrected vision, corneal topography, and corneal physiology. Where trial lenses are not available, the authors are of the opinion that this trial should still take place but with the lenses that have been ordered empirically.

Once a successful trial has taken place the practitioner will be in a position to order the final lenses or issue the empirically ordered lenses for further wear. It is foolhardy to commence a program of orthokeratology treatment until the practitioner can be certain that the patient shows the appropriate responses to the lenses.

Whichever method of fitting is used, whether trial-lens-based or empirical, a pair of lenses that have been ordered for the specific patient will need to be issued. This chapter covers the delivery of those lenses to the patient and how and when the patient should be reexamined.

Prior to final lens issue, lens verification is most important and this is dealt with below.

VERIFICATION

As has already been outlined in Chapter 6, orthokeratology as a clinical technique is heavily reliant on the quality of lens manufacture. If the laboratory does not supply exactly what has been requested by the lens fitter, then the favorable results of the orthokeratology trial will not be reproduced with the patient's final lenses. The tolerances typically applied to conventional rigid gas-permeable (RGP) lenses are simply not rigorous enough if applied to orthokeratology lenses. As has already been outlined, inaccuracies as small as 0.03 mm in back optic zone radius (BOZR) appear to lead to discernible differences in the visual and topographic outcomes. Ultimately, responsibility for the quality and subsequent clinical performance of contact lenses rests with the practitioner who supplies them. For all RGP fittings, it is essential that every contact lens is measured and inspected carefully to determine both its quantitative and qualitative accuracy. However, this is crucial when orthokeratology is being undertaken.

It is obvious from the above that lenses should be checked to verify their accuracy prior to supply to the patient. However, verification should also occur in the following circumstances:

- to establish the specification of the patient's existing lenses
- to confirm lenses are being worn in the correct eyes
- to confirm that current and old lenses have not been mixed up

- when lens parameters are thought to have altered, e.g., distorted
- to verify the accuracy of trial (diagnostic) lenses.

The BOZR and back vertex power (BVP) are arguably the most important dimensions in respect of any rigid contact lens. The former is crucial to the success of orthokeratology and is potentially vulnerable to change and distortion over a period of time. It therefore requires validation at each and every aftercare examination where problems with the lenses have been reported or observed.

Typically in orthokeratology, the specifications of the right and left lenses may be very similar. Patients frequently transpose lenses and may be unaware of this. To help prevent this, lenses may be supplied in different colors. Unless this is done and/or the lenses are clearly engraved to differentiate right from left, verification may be required to identify right from left.

In orthokeratology, we have historically used a sequence of two or three lenses to refine the fitting as the cornea changes. This is now typically the case when the practitioner is going through the "learning curve" of becoming an experienced orthokeratology practitioner. It is most important to be able to differentiate between lenses whose base curve may differ only very slightly so that we can be sure the patient is wearing the latest lens supplied and has not confused it with an earlier lens.

As one's experience and reputation in orthokeratology grows, one may attract patients who are already wearing orthokeratology lenses, perhaps fitted overseas. Where the details of the lens specification are not available, it is crucial to be able to establish as well as one can what is being worn. Even if details of the lens specification are available it is prudent to verify that these are the lenses being worn or indeed whether these lenses have become distorted with time.

Notwithstanding the above, it is, of course, impossible to verify completely the intricacies of the peripheral curve design and thus the practitioner will have to assume that certain aspects of the lens specification have been correctly manufactured. Ultimately the performance of the lens on the eye serves to confirm whether the lens matches the trial lens in terms of comfort and topographic changes.

WHAT CAN BE MEASURED?

The standards employed in the UK are those of the British Standards (BS) Institution and the International Standards Organization (ISO) and are summarized at the end of this section. In other parts of the world slightly different standards may apply. In almost all cases, these standards will not be rigorous enough to guarantee the ideal outcome in orthokeratology. The practitioner must, therefore, establish with the laboratory the standards that he or she will apply to orthokeratology lenses rather than conventional RGP lenses. The list of parameters that can be readily checked in the consulting room situation is as follows:

- power (BVP)
- radii (BOZR)
- diameter (total diameter or TD)
- lens sag
- center and edge thickness (t_c and t_e)
- edge form
- surface quality
- special features.

Measurement of power

The instrument used will be the focimeter. It is used to determine the prescription of the lens as follows:

- Place the instrument in a vertical position.
- For BVP measurement, place the concave surface towards the focimeter.
- The lens should be placed as close as possible to the focimeter, ideally by using a very small stop. If the standard stop is used (designed for spectacle lenses), then the reading will be more plus or less minus than the true BVP. However, the difference for the relatively flat curves on orthokeratology lenses is small.
- Note the quality of the image; distortion indicates a poor optical quality.
- A good image does not guarantee a distortion-free optic because a small aperture stop is

being used and therefore only the center of the lens is being measured. Therefore to access optical quality use a larger stop and, ignoring the power reading, examine the quality and regularity of the image itself.

Measurement of radii

Back optic zone radius

The instrument typically used is the radiuscope. A typical instrument is shown in Figure 9.1. The principle is based on Drysdale's method (Drysdale 1900), which measures the distance

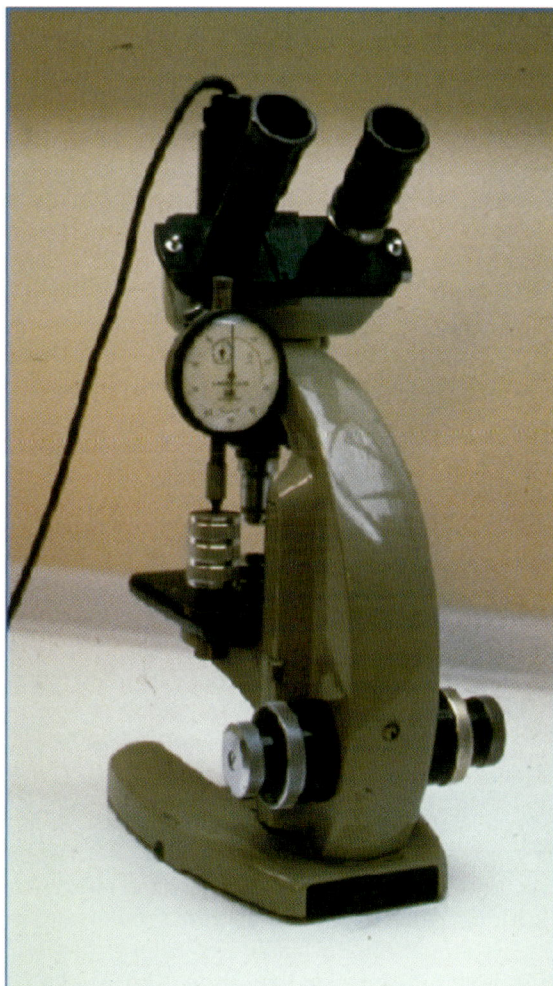

Figure 9.1 Typical radiuscope for checking lens back optic zone radius.

between the lens surface and the center of curvature. The procedure for using a radiuscope is as follows:

- A few drops of water or saline are placed in the concave recess of the lens support to reduce reflections from the front surface of the lens. Too much water on the support will allow the lens to move around whilst it is being measured. After use, the water should be removed by drying with a tissue to avoid deposits forming on the lens holder.
- The lens, which must be cleaned and dried, is placed with its front surface in contact with the water upon the support. The lens must be handled with care to avoid flexing, which may give rise to a distorted or even toric reading. In addition, the technician's hands should be clean to avoid transferring grease to the lens surface as this would produce a distorted reading.
- The microscope is focused upon the aerial image at the center of the back surface of the lens and the stage is adjusted until the image of the spoke-patterned target appears exactly centered.
- The dial gage is set to zero.
- The microscope is next focused using the fine adjustment control upon the surface of the lens. Traveling from zero to the second position, the image of the bulb filament is seen. On an old lens, particles of debris and scratches will facilitate identification of this image.
- The image at the lens surface is usually much larger and brighter than at the center of curvature and will show up any surface imperfections.
- Three readings are taken, each of which must be obtained by focusing first upon the aerial image and then upon the surface image or vice versa.

The issue of hydration and radius measurement is somewhat contentious. Many practitioners, including the authors, believe that the latest generation of fluorosilicone acrylate materials are highly dimensionally stable and do not alter their radius significantly on hydration. Thus they may be supplied and measured in the dry state and the measurement will not change once they are hydrated either by soaking prior to issue to the patient, or by hydration in the patient's tear film. However, others believe that all RGP lenses, including orthokeratology lenses, should be hydrated for 24 h before being checked, or should be supplied in the hydrated state by the manufacturer. Any practitioner in doubt may wish to perform a simple experiment on five lenses or so. Take delivery of the lenses in the dry state and take three readings of base curve on each of them. Then repeat the same measurements after 24 h of hydration in contact lens soaking solution. The difference in the mean of the two sets of readings will indicate whether the issue of hydration is important in clinical practice.

In the absence of a radiuscope, several companies produce devices that are designed to attach to the head-rest of a keratometer in order to measure the lens BOZR. The keratometer is used with a special contact lens holder that utilizes a mirror with the front surface silvered and a lens support. The lens rests on the water in a small depression on a horizontal support. The mirror is set at 45° to the optical axis of the instrument and reflects light from the instrument on to the surface being measured.

The majority of keratometers will require the practitioner to use specially modified scale or conversion tables since these instruments are primarily intended for the measurement of a convex surface (the cornea) and not a concave lens surface. Whilst the rule of thumb of adding 0.03 mm to the reading is adequate for conventional RGP lenses (Bennett 1957), it is not for orthokeratology and thus conversion tables should be used. A major problem with the keratometer is that the scale does not read generally in fine enough steps to enable readings to be taken to the nearest 0.01 mm.

Given that a radiuscope is not a particularly expensive instrument, it is worth investing in one, since the nuisance of having to check RGP lenses on the keratometer soon becomes apparent.

Peripheral radii

In some cases, it is possible to measure peripheral radii of a conventional lens with a radiuscope if the lens is tilted on the holder. However the bandwidth of the curve needs to be at least 1 mm and be fairly well demarcated. In practice, both the narrow width of the peripheral curves on orthokeratology lenses and the presence of blending render this measurement impossible.

The keratometer measures radius utilizing two points on either side of the lens axis which are separated by a distance of approximately 3 mm – hence peripheral radii cannot be measured by this means.

The issue arises as to whether the peripheral radii can be verified using a videokeratoscope. Whilst in theory this is perfectly possible, in reality the algorithms used to derive the radius from ring separation are based on convex surfaces. Thus significant errors are introduced. Certain videokeratoscopes provide a facility for changing the set of algorithms to measure a concave surface, like a RGP contact lens, but the accuracy of these on reverse geometry lenses for orthokeratology has not been established by scientific investigation. However, they may be useful to indicate the qualitative form of the back surface of the lens.

Measurement of diameters

Total diameter

There are two instruments in widespread use. These are the band magnifier and the V-gage.

The band magnifier shown in Figure 9.2 consists of an engraved graticule plus an adjustable eyepiece with a lens giving typically × 7 magnification. The contact lens is repositioned on the scale for the measurement of different zones. This is obviously easier if the transitions are sharp. Typically the transitions in orthokeratology (and modern conventional RGP) lenses are too subtle to allow any measurement other than the TD and the optic zone diameter. It is important to ensure that the lens is dry as capillary attraction can make it difficult to remove from the smooth glass surface. It is also important to avoid parallax errors by ensuring that one looks normal to the surface of the graticule when reading off the measurement.

The V-gage shown in Figure 9.3 consists of a V-shaped channel graduated between 6.0 and

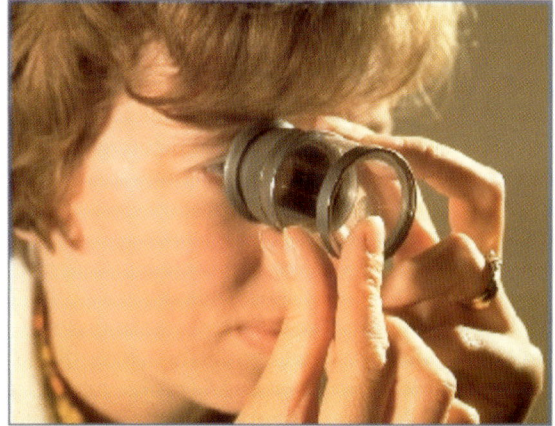

Figure 9.2   A band magnifier in use to measure the total diameter of a lens.

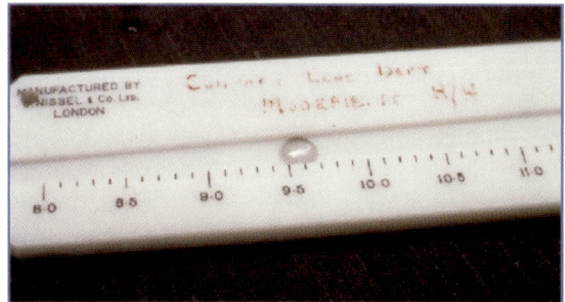

Figure 9.3   A V-gage being used to determine the lens diameter.

12.5 mm. The lens is allowed to slide down the channel until it stops due to friction against the walls. At this point the diameter is read off the scale. Due to the nature of the technique, it can only measure the TD. It is important that the lens is not forced down the scale, but that it simply falls under the influence of gravity, otherwise the lens can be distorted and a falsely low reading obtained for diameter.

Other diameters (BOZD and BPZD)

Back optic zone diameter (BOZD) and back peripheral zone diameters (BPZD) can be measured using a band magnifier in a similar manner to TD.

In practice, location of these diameters may be extremely difficult due to blending of transitions. Generally, only the edge of the BOZD will be discernible. Generally orthokeratology lenses are supplied in relatively low powers and thus there is no front optic to confuse with the back optic. Measurements should be repeated in different meridians in order to verify that the back optic zone is circular.

Measurement of lens sag

The practitioner is somewhat limited in the ability to assess accurately the parameters of a reverse geometry lens, with the exception of those outlined in this section. However, if the BOZR measurement is correct, does that provide any evidence that the reverse and alignment zones or tangents are correct? To date, there have been no published reports on the accuracy and reproducibility of reverse geometry lenses. Many practitioners have been mystified and frustrated by the simple fact that sometimes a "duplicate" lens does not perform to the same standards as the original lens, but are routinely assured by the laboratory that the lens was accurate. Laboratories cannot measure the reverse or alignment curves of the lenses, and work on the assumption that, if the lathe is correctly zeroed and programmed, then the lens will be accurate.

A simple solution to the problem has been developed by Mountford and Noack, and is based on the simple assumption that, for the lens to work correctly, it must have the correct sag.

The lens sag can be calculated using a dedicated computer program. An example of the inputs and read-outs from such a program written by Noack is shown in Figure 9.4. The BE program automatically supplies the sag of the calculated trial lens at a chord of 9.35 mm (11.00 mm TD lens) and 8.95 mm (10.6 mm lens). However, laboratories that wish to keep their lens designs proprietary need only supply the practitioner with the BOZR and the sag of the lens at a chord corresponding to the edge of the alignment curve to enable the lens to be verified.

The basis of the instrument is that the sag of the lens is equal to the total height of the lens at a fixed chord minus the center thickness of the lens. Specially machined mounts were made for the two diameters (11.00 and 10.60 mm) with a total

A   B

Figure 9.4   (A) The sag of a five-zone lens at a chord of 8.95 mm is shown. The sags of the intermediate curves are also given. Program courtesy of Don Noack. (B) The calculator for determining the sag of a BE lens is shown. The lens is then placed in the holder and the sag measured at a chord of 9.35 mm. Program courtesy of Don Noack.

aperture 0.10 mm greater than the TD of the lens. This allows for minor discrepancies in the TD of the finished lens, with the calculated decentration induced by the lens causing a maximum sag error of 0.7 μm. A shelf of exactly 9.35 or 8.95 mm is raised above the base of the mount, so that when the lens is placed back surface down into the mount, it makes contact with the mount at the exact chord length over which the theoretical sag of the lens has been calculated.

The lens is placed front surface down into the device and the center thickness measured. A Mitutoyo Absolute dial gage, which is sensitive to 1 μm, is used to take the measurements. The weight of the spring is set to the minimum amount, so that the probe does not induce lens flexure. The gage is connected to a DP-1VR Digimatic miniprocessor, which takes repeated measurements of the values, calculates the mean and standard deviation, and gives the sag of the lens with a repeatability of 1 μm and an error of ± 1 μm.

The instrument is mounted on a solid granite base that has been precision-machined to create a flat surface (Fig. 9.5). Measurements on trial lenses with known sag values show the instrument to be highly accurate and repeatable. Six repeated measurements of a lens take approximately 4 min.

The practitioner can then simply verify the sag of the lens on delivery. If the measured sag is over ± 3 μm from that ordered, the lens should be rejected and remade. Lenses that are steep are worse than lenses that are marginally flat, as the increased apical clearance of the steep lens will decrease the efficacy of the lens. The instrument, complete with the miniprocessor and mounts, is approximately one-half of the cost of a radiuscope. Don Noack's program is available to practitioners and manufacturers who wish to use this accurate and relatively straightforward method of ensuring that their lenses have the correct sag.

Measurement of thickness

Center and edge thickness (t_c and t_e)

The instrument used is the dial thickness gage. This consists of a spring-loaded, ball-ended

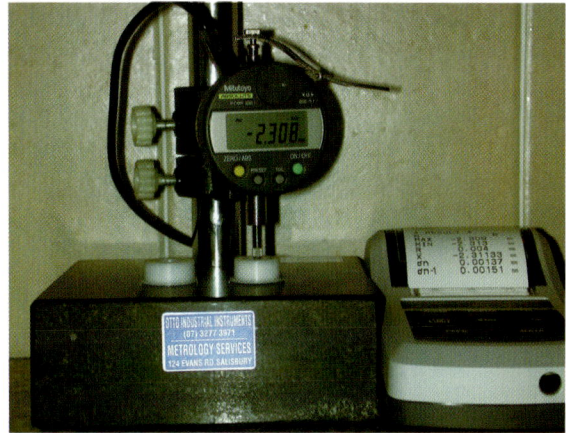

Figure 9.5   The Mountford–Noack lens sag gage. The lens is placed in the specially designed mount, and the central thickness and total sag subtracted. The statistical analysis of the repeated readings is performed by the attached miniprocessor.

probe geared to a direct reading scale. The scale will typically give a reading in 0.01 mm steps. The scale is first zeroed with no lens in place. Then the lens is introduced by pulling the probe up. The lens is placed concave side down and the probe gently lowered on to the part of the lens to be measured. Both center and edge substance should be verified and compared to that anticipated. It is worth taking several readings around the lens edge, as thickness may vary around the circumference. It is important that the reading is taken right at the edge of the lens, but care must be taken not to damage the edge.

Whilst it is possible to measure both radial and axial edge thickness, in practice we measure the radial thickness, viz. the thickness normal to the lens surface at the point of measurement. The axial thickness, which is the thickness measured along the primary axis of the lens, is the value that arises from laboratory computations based on sagitta. It is important that laboratory and practitioner know which thickness they are talking about when they refer to edge thickness. Pearson (1986) derived conversion formulae linking axial to radial thickness, but in practice it is the laboratory's responsibility to ensure that the edge substance is set according to the practitioner's wishes.

As well as understanding that the practitioner is measuring radial edge thickness, it is equally important that the laboratory should know at what distance from the edge apex the measurement is being taken. Port (1987) described a modified-thickness gage that enabled this distance to be set. In normal clinical situations, it is believed that the nearest to the edge that it is reasonably possible to measure is 0.50 mm.

INSPECTION OF EDGE PROFILE

The shape of any contact lens edge can have a significant influence upon its comfort in wear. It has been suggested that edge quality may be assessed by rubbing the lens edge on the wrist or fingers. Such tests are capable of disclosing grossly unacceptable edge forms but the profile is not determined.

A simple and relatively quick method is to inspect the lens using the magnification of a hand loupe, stereomicroscope, or slit lamp. At high magnifications it is useful to support the lens on a holder. The edge should ideally have either a centrally or posteriorly displaced apex. The apex is visible as a thin white line when the edge is well-illuminated. The use of a smooth rolled edge has been shown to be crucial for good RGP comfort (La Hood 1988). In addition, it has been shown that the anterior edge profile is more important than the posterior profile in terms of comfort (Picciano & Andrasko 1989). Careful verification of the lens edge is important to ensure the patient receives the most comfortable lens possible.

Whilst it is possible to take a plaster cast of the lens edge and then inspect this on the slit-lamp microscope, this is beyond the bounds of what most practitioners would consider reasonably achievable at every verification. However, it is a useful way of checking that the laboratory is producing consistent edges, if it is performed from time to time. A small pool of dental stone is placed on top of an elastic band that has been stretched around a plastic surface. The lens is inserted at right angles to the rubber band. When the dental stone has set, the lens is removed. This needs to be done with care if the lens is to remain in one piece! The dental stone is then snapped about the scoring imparted by the elastic band.

The form of the lens edge can then be inspected as an impression in the dental stone. Given the risks of damaging the lens whilst removing it from the dental stone, this is a "gold standard" edge inspection technique best reserved for occasional use on specially ordered lenses.

SURFACE QUALITY

The quality of the lens surface, particularly the rear surface, is vital to the clinical success of orthokeratology. Imperfections such as scratches or deposits on the back surface or poorly finished fenestrations can be a cause of corneal staining. In orthokeratology, the lens back surface may be only 3–10 μm from the underlying corneal surface in the center of the lens. There are three possible instruments that can be used to examine the surface – the slit lamp, the band magnifier, and the radiuscope. Since a magnification of 20× or more is essential to detect surface defects that have been caused by poor manufacture, the band magnifier is inadequate. The authors prefer to hold the cleaned lens gently at the slit lamp between thumb and first finger and rotate whilst looking for any pitting, scratches, lathe marks, signs of incomplete polishing, or burning and mottling. Surface burning or mottling results from excessive heat during manufacture and is likely to cause poor in vivo wetting.

There are some special features to note and record. These include:

- engravings
- laboratory codes
- fenestrations – number, position, size, and finish
- tint
- carrier design – assessed by edge measurement.

Engravings may include a dot or letter to indicate whether the lens is destined for a right or left eye. It is important that these are not too deeply sunk into the lens as they can give rise to accumulations of deposited material that cannot easily be removed. In the longer term these can cause ocular irritation. In addition deep engravings can weaken the lens, giving rise to splitting, perhaps after several months of use. Due to the ease with which lenses can be switched and the highly customized nature of modern orthokeratology lens designs, the authors do recommend some means by which the patient can differentiate the right from the left lens. This may take the form of different tints for each eye. Certain laboratories prefer to mark the lens with a black dot from an indelible pen rather than permanently mark the lens. This is less than ideal as eventually the ink wears off and the issue of toxicity from the ink also arises.

Some laboratories engrave the lens with a code indicating the type of construction that the lens has. This might be vaguely useful if the patient goes to another practitioner who is unable to access the patient's complete lens specification, but, in the main, the clinical record should contain all the information required to duplicate the lens. It therefore seems a relatively pointless exercise to mark the final lens in such a way. However, the marking is very useful on a trial or inventory lens.

Fenestrations are often incorporated into orthokeratology lenses, particularly when night therapy is being used, as it is thought they enable adherent lenses to unbind more easily. A typical order is for three fenestrations, at 120° intervals, just within the optic zone of the lens. Thus in verification, the practitioner establishes that the fenestrations are present, that there are the correct number, and that they are in the correct position. Ideally, the practitioner should specify the size of the fenestration, or at least be aware of what the laboratory usually produces. A figure of 0.2 mm is fairly typical. Even more important than the size of the fenestration is the quality of polish around it. It is most important to inspect each fenestration on the slit lamp to see that there are no sharp edges or splits around it. Generally, polishing fenestrations has to be done by hand and it is an area where laboratories with even the best-quality lathes may fall down. Some laboratories are now producing fenestrations using a laser.

Generally there are two reasons why RGP lenses are tinted. The first is to aid location once the lens is out of the eye. The second is to reduce any photophobia associated with the use of the contact lens and perhaps impart some degree of ultraviolet protection. In night therapy these latter issues are an irrelevance, but it is still worth ordering a tint as it helps the patient enormously in locating the lens and ensuring that it is in

the case after removing it in the morning. For daytime wearers the issue of reducing photophobia and offering some ultraviolet protection is no stronger than for a conventional RGP wearer. In fact, with modern lens designs and high-Dk materials, photophobia is rarely a reported symptom.

When verifying the tint of a contact lens, the important thing is to ensure that the color is as specified and that the density of tint is in line with expectations based on the thicknesses concerned. In typical orthokeratology work, the final thickness will not depart greatly from the trial lens thickness and so the trial lens will, in most cases, serve as a good reference for the tint hue and saturation.

The form of the carrier requires careful skilled interpretation. Where a negative carrier or lenticulation has been requested (normally to raise the habitual riding position of a positive lens), measuring the edge and junctional thickness is the best technique. In the case of a negative carrier, the junctional thickness should be less than the edge thickness. For an orthokeratology lens with a negative carrier and a positively powered BVP, the junctional thickness will typically be the lowest thickness recorded on the lens. This is found by carefully moving the lens in steps across the thickness gage (withdrawing the probe each time to avoid scratching) until the lowest thickness is measured. An alternative is to cast the lens in dental stone, as described above, but with the concomitant risks of breaking or scratching the lens.

Where a positive carrier or lenticulation has been specified, usually in the case of a negative lens that rides high, then the junctional thickness will be greater than the edge thickness. In fact, the junctional area in a negative lens will be the thickest point on the lens surface. Thus in a similar manner to that described above, the lens is moved over the surface of the thickness gage until the thickest point is found. This should be greater than the edge substance, demonstrating that a positive lenticulation has been made.

However, in night therapy different carrier forms have little effect in altering habitual lens resting position. In fact, it is a common observation that a lens that rides high or low with the eyes open in the primary position will produce a perfectly centered zone of flattening on the cornea overnight providing it is correctly fitted. This indicates that the centration of the lens with the eyes closed is correct.

TOLERANCES

The dimensional tolerances for rigid contact lenses are set out in Table 9.1, which quotes from British Standard BS 7208: Part 1: 1992; ISO 8321-1: 1991 (E).

Unfortunately, although all of these tolerances may be adequate for conventional RGP lenses, they are inadequate for reverse geometry orthokeratology lenses in the case of the standards for the BOZR. As has already been mentioned, this parameter needs to be specified to an accuracy of ± 0.02 mm to ensure reliable outcomes in orthokeratology. This imposes a high level of understanding between laboratory and practitioner if they are to work together in a professional manner. In addition, both parties must ensure that they have properly calibrated instrumentation to determine the lens radius. The laboratory has to be using a computer numeric-controlled (CNC) lathe with a good-quality diamond-tipped tool and a regular servicing calibration protocol. Although the standards on radius have to be tight, it is the authors' experience that a good laboratory can rise to the challenge and produce excellent, accurate reverse geometry lenses to the practitioner's and the patient's satisfaction.

Table 9.1 Dimensional tolerances for rigid gas-permeable lenses

Dimension	Tolerance
Back optic zone radius	± 0.05 mm
Back peripheral zone radius (where measurable)	± 0.10 mm
Back optic zone diameter	± 0.20 mm
Total diameter	± 0.10 mm
Front optic zone diameter	± 0.20 mm
Center thickness	± 0.02 mm
Back vertex power 0 to ± 7.00 D	± 0.12 D
Back vertex power from ± 7.25 D to ± 14.00 D	± 0.25 D
Back vertex power from over ± 14.25 D	± 0.50 D
Prescribed prism	± 0.25Δ

Reproduced from Hough (1998) with permission.

LENS DELIVERY

Assuming that a satisfactory trial of orthokeratology has taken place and the patient's lenses are verified to meet the specification, then the insertion and inspection of the final lenses should not produce any surprises. The fitting pattern should be as the trial lens and, assuming the initial overrefraction was performed carefully, the vision should be good. As has already been stated, generally in night therapy the lenses are left planopowered to give the best transmissibility profile. Thus there will often be a small, and insignificant, overrefraction. Obviously daytime wearers require full and accurate correction with the lenses in place.

The issue of anesthetic use was raised in Chapter 6. Whilst it is extremely useful to enable a rapid appraisal as to the quality of a trial lens fitting, by virtue of the reduction in reflex lacrimation, it arguably serves less purpose at the time of the final lens issue. Particularly when night therapy is being employed, comfort is not a major issue, providing the lens fit and material are appropriate. Even in daytime wear, the large diameters used in orthokeratology designs mean that the lens comfort is usually superior to any rigid lens the patient may have worn previously. Even soft lens wearers are frequently surprised, and vocal, about the high level of initial comfort with their new lenses. Furthermore, since handling instructions will usually immediately follow the issue visit with the practitioner, the cornea needs to have full sensitivity for these to be carried out safely. Therefore the use of an anesthetic is not recommended at this time.

The typical protocol to follow at the issue visit is as follows:

- practitioner to wash hands
- remove any existing lenses and check corneal integrity
- clean patient's lenses, rinse with saline, and apply wetting solution
- insert lenses and ask patient to take up fixation with head supported and gaze lowered
- after a few minutes, measure the visual acuity and check for residual overrefraction
- check quality of fit using slit lamp and barrier filter

- if all is satisfactory, patient is instructed on insertion and removal and lens care
- first aftercare visit is scheduled.

The importance of demonstrating good hygiene in all aspects of contact lens practice cannot be overstated. Whilst the risks of developing infection with all RGP lenses are low, patients need to be set a good and clear example of procedures to follow when handling their lenses on all occasions. All practice staff need to be similarly instructed.

The patient's existing lenses may be rigid or soft. In either case, they should be removed, cleaned and rinsed, and then stored. If patients do not have their case with them, then the practitioner needs to have a supply of temporary cases to hand, so that patients can leave the practice with their original lenses safely stored away in an appropriate solution. On the other hand, patients may want to leave the practice wearing their original lenses, in which case they can be reinserted, after the handling session, from the temporary case. This will usually be the case for night therapy patients.

From a medicolegal point of view, it is important to establish the condition of the cornea and the rest of the anterior segment immediately prior to embarking on orthokeratology treatment. To this end the cornea should be examined on the slit lamp using fluorescein, together with a rapid examination of the anterior segment. Given that this will have been done in some depth at the initial visit, this is a purely confirmatory check and need take no longer than a few seconds. Occasionally, a significant (usually corneal) lesion may be found which precludes immediately embarking on night therapy. This is typically due to wearing a torn or damaged soft lens. In these circumstances, the practitioner will need to follow the patient until the cornea recovers and then orthokeratology can begin.

In some practices, the verification of new lenses is performed by skilled technicians. It is important that the practitioner is confident that the new lenses are scrupulously clean prior to placing them on the patient's eyes. It reinforces good hygiene if the lens fitter is seen to clean and rinse the lenses prior to insertion for the first time. The solutions employed are described later in this chapter, but in the event of a polymeric bead cleaner being the

practitioner's choice, it is most important that the lens is thoroughly rinsed prior to insertion and the appropriate wetting agent applied.

In all cases of RGP lens fitting, initial comfort is increased if, after insertion, the patient takes up an inferior gaze position. The patient is instructed to rest the head against the head support (set so that the head is upright, not tilted back). The patient looks down slightly and the lens is placed on to the cornea directly from the fitter's index finger, whilst the upper lid is retracted with the other hand. Patients are then instructed to keep the gaze in the same position and encouraged to look at an appropriately placed object (or their hands). The upper lid is then released and they are instructed to blink gently. It is wise to tell patients who are embarking on daytime wear that they must be careful not to develop any strange blinking habits and consciously to relax the facial muscles to avoid any anomalous mannerisms or appearances.

It is most important to tell patients that the comfort can only improve from now onwards. Over a period of minutes they are encouraged to raise their gaze progressively until they are looking straight ahead. At this time the acuity can be recorded, where appropriate. A quick spherical overrefraction, perhaps using the duochrome chart, is then made to establish that the lenses are correctly powered. This procedure can be particularly rapid in the case of night therapy, where the vision through the lens is obviously of much less importance.

The lens fitting can then be checked. Initially, the degree of movement can be assessed using white diffuse light. Clearly a nonmobile lens at this stage would be unacceptable. Following this, fluorescein is instilled and the fitting pattern evaluated, using cobalt blue light and a barrier filter, as described in Chapter 6. Where the issued lens is identical in specification to the trial lens, clearly there should be no significant difference to the fluorescein pattern. There will be many occasions where the lens fitter has slightly altered the lens specification following careful appraisal of the corneal response trial. This is the moment when the practitioner gets the first opportunity of seeing whether the changes made have improved the fitting pattern further. Often the changes are sufficiently subtle that it is only by inspecting the topographic change map at future aftercare visits that any improvement becomes obvious. Sometimes, particularly in the early days of learning to work with an orthokeratology lens design, the fitting is actually worse following the changes made and the practitioner has to reschedule the lens issue appointment and reorder new lenses.

THE INSTRUCTION SESSION

This is a crucial time for any new contact lens wearer, particularly patients embarking on a somewhat novel and different clinical technique like orthokeratology. They are about to start wearing rigid contact lenses, putting them into and removing them from their eyes. It may be the first time that they have tried to use contact lenses. The care and completeness of the dispensing appointment set the stage for the style of care the patients will exert themselves when wearing lenses.

Sloppy demonstrations suggest that hygiene is unimportant, when everything should point to the need for a rigorous system. Contact lens wearers will often modify their care systems with time and mostly in the direction of less rather than more care.

New contact lens wearers assume some of the responsibilities for the long-term success of contact lens wearing. They need careful training and complete instructions for them to be confident of their own skills and abilities and to understand their ongoing role.

Patients expect:

- training and instruction in the successful use of their lenses and the care system
- advice on the typical normal occurrences to expect
- a source of contact to deal with problems, emergencies, and adverse responses. In the case of overnight orthokeratology, a 24-h pager number is advised
- advice on ongoing care and necessary appointments.

New wearers need:

- self-confidence boosting with instructions on lens insertion and removal
- instruction in the proper care and storage of the lenses, use of solutions, and case hygiene

- clear instructions on the need to follow carefully the care system regimens and advice against changing any part of the system without reference to the practitioner
- a wearing schedule, where daytime wear is being employed
- warning of adaptive symptoms and how to deal with them
- advice on what to do in an emergency and how to obtain professional assistance in cases of difficulty.

A great deal of information is imparted on this occasion and it is useful to have printed instructions which can be given to the patient for future reference. These instructions should cover handling, insertion, and removal of lenses and routine use of the care system. This is reassuring from the patients' point of view as it provides an available source of information and guidance. It is also a source of protection for practitioners should they forget to mention anything and is desirable from a legal standpoint. It is worthwhile having patients sign a part of this booklet to say that they have received and understood instructions in the care and handling of their orthokeratology lenses. Figure 9.6 shows the suggested general advice written information for patients and Figure 9.7 shows the written handling instructions that might be issued. Where daily disposable lenses are being used and where patients have no experience with soft lenses, they will need to be shown how to insert and remove these. Figure 9.8 shows written advice that may be given to augment the practical instruction session.

WEARING SCHEDULES

Adaptation to orthokeratology contact lenses worn during the day is usually necessary and the daily wearing time is therefore gradually increased. Wearing schedules can be variable and the schedule should provide for the fastest passage possible through to complete daily wear, provided that patients are physically and visually comfortable in the process. There is no advantage in slow adaptation if proper safeguards are met. Typically, wearers start with 4 h on the first day, with 2–3 h added daily. Whilst it is often the case that these periods can be split into two sessions at

ADVICE ON CARING FOR YOUR LENSES

Figure 9.6
Suggested general
advice issued to
patients.

- Hands must be clean and free of creams. Alkl traces of soap must be rinsed off. Avoid contamination of the lenses with perfumes, hair spray etc.
- Whilst handling the lenses alway work over a smooth soft surface (hand towel spread over a table). This avoids scratching or losing a lens on the floor.
- If the lens is dropped, do not move until the lens is located. Always lift a dropped lens by wetting a fingertip or suction holder. lanses must not be slid across the table surfaces,
- Never wipe lenses with a handkerchief or other material. If wiping is necessary use only the softest of paper tissues (lint-free)
- To avoid distorting the lenses never leave them near heat and handle very gently. Avoid holding the lenses by the edges.
- Fingernails should be cleaned and kept reasonably short to avoid scratching the eyes.

Hygiene and storage

Absolute cleanliness is essential in the handling and storage of contact lenses. In order to prevent dirt or harmful organisms being transferred to the eye.

The following rules should be observed:

- The lenses should be stored in a disinfecting solution intended for contact lens use. Solutions intended specifically for RGP lenses improve lens wettability and comfort.
- The case should be emptied and fresh solution should be used each day. The lenses should be completely immersed in solution.
- The lenses should not be stored dry as this may affect the curvature of the lens and the wettability of its surface.
- The lenses may normally be inserted direct from the storage solution. This helps the surface wet more easily and forms a protective cushion in the event of the lens being inserted too quickly. If sensitive to the storage solution this can be rinsed off with saline solution and a change of solution discussed with the practitioner.
- Remove lenses, clean with the recommended cleaner and rinse off with saline, prior to placing the lenses in the case with the soaking solution.
- If working over a hand basin be sure to put the plug in.
- Never lick the lenses as harmful organisms can be transferred from themouth to the eye.
- Examine the lenses regularly for scratches and chips and to ensure each lens is being worn in the correct eye.

the beginning and end of the day, in orthokeratology the practitioner must consider how patients are going to correct their sight with the lenses out.

Where patients only have modest degrees of myopia (<2 D), it may be that the period between the two wearing sessions will be spent at work and that they will function perfectly well with uncorrected myopia, replacing the lenses for the journey home. In the instance where the patient has a higher degree of myopia (>2 D) it may be necessary to give patients daily disposable lenses to use in the interval between wearing sessions. The decision on what power to use is similar to that with night therapy. Patients seem perfectly able to decide if they need to increase or decrease the daily disposable power as the days pass and indeed seem to enjoy performing a simple visual test each day to see if they are fully corrected. They will typically choose an object requiring good acuity to visualize, such as the clock on a domestic video recorder.

With night therapy no adaptation is required and patients will wear the lens for their entire sleeping period. This is very convenient for patients, but once again they will need to use daily disposables in the first week or so whilst their myopia is reducing.

Schedules should always be given with the proviso that daily wearing time can be held at the same level for some days or built up more slowly if there are problems. It should be stressed that the lens wear should not be continued if there is persistent discomfort. In these circumstances the practitioner should be contacted.

Where the handling and care instructions are given by a technician, it is worth giving a checklist to work from so that he or she can be certain always to give patients all the instructions they need. A sample list is shown in Figure 9.9.

Night-therapy orthokeratology patients should be given some preservative-free artificial tears

ADVICE ON CARING FOR YOUR LENSES

Figure 9.7 Suggested advice issued to patients on lens handling.

Insertion of RGP lenses

To prevent the right and left lenses being interchanged accidentally, they should be removed from the soaking container and inserted one at a time.

- Place a wetted lens on the tip of the forefinger of one hand where it will be retained.
- Look downwards and using two fingers of the other hand hold the upper lid and eyelashes well clear of the cornea.
- Then use the middle finger of the hand holding the lens to pull down the lower lid by the very edge.
- Keep the head and eyes pointing in the same direction and place the lens gently on the cornea.
- Remove the forefinger, release the lower lid and finally the upper lid.

If the lens slips onto the white of the eye, it may be replaced by lifting one lid beyond the lens and pushing it back on to the cornea with the lid margin using a finger on either side of the lens as a guide. A mirror will aid lens location and this should be held to one side so the eye is looking in the opposite direction from where the lens is positioned. Alternatively a suction holder may be used if one is available.

There may be slight irritation for the first minute or so. In the case of marked irritation, a particle of dust or fluff may have become trapped behind the lens. The lens should be removed, rinsed with sterile saline or storage solution and re-inserted. You should never wear a lens that is provoking irritation of the eye and feel scratchy.

Removal of RGP lenses

Although *Method 1* is the simplest and most commonly used you are advised to practice all three techniques so that should one not work an alternative method can be used.

Method 1

Work over a table and hold the free hand cupped to catch the lens. Bend the head slightly and open the eye as wide as possible, so that both lids are beyond the edges of the lens. Stare straight in front of you and place a finger at the outer edge, separating the lids. Pull the lids towards the direction of of the top of the ear and give a strong blink, when the lens should be ejected from the eye. At first it may stick to the lashes from where it is easily removed.

Method two

Place the forefinger of each hand on the very edge of the upper and lower lid at the inner corner of the eye. Each lid is then slowly stretched around the lens and together. Working over a mirror may be helpful at first, though this should be discarded as soon as possible as it may not be available in an emergency.

Method 3

Look straight ahead into a mirror. Place the forefinger of one hand on the upper lid above the lens and the forefinger of the other hand on the lower lid below the lens. Pull the lids slightly apart to reveal the whole of the lens. Gently press the lids on the eye and move the fingers towards each other. The lens should then come away from the eye and be removed by the two fingers.

Method 4

Using a suction holder. This method should only be used if all else fails. Always check the lens is in place before attempting to use a suction holder. Squeeze the bulb of the moistened suction holder firmly and place the end gently against the dome of the lens. release the pressure on the bulb and slowly withdraw both holder and lens.

to instil on awakening. These help the lens to unbind and move. If the patient attempts to remove a bound lens, epithelial damage can occur and this is prevented by using the drops. Patients should be shown how to loosen up a bound lens after instilling the drop. This involves gently indenting the sclera immediately below the lens, allowing the tears to enter, and enabling the lens to move again. Patients can look in a mirror to confirm that the lens is moving before removing it from the eye.

SCHEDULING AFTERCARE VISITS

When starting out in orthokeratology practice, practitioners are advised to schedule visits more frequently than later, so that they can appreciate the typical time course and learn the nuances of

ADVICE ON CARING FOR YOUR LENSES

Insertion of daily disposable lenses

Daily disposable lenses are intended to be worn on a one-off basis, being discarded after they have been worn. Lens cleaning is not necessary. Simply wash your hands and remove the lens from the blister pack. Never reuse your daily disposible lenses. The insertion of these lenses is as for orthokeratology lenses, except that it is much more difficult to be certain that the lenses are the correct way round. A lens inserted directly from the blister pack may be inside out, but no harm will occur if this is inserted into the eye, it will simply be unstable and feel loose. If this occurs simply remove and invert it. When placed on a dry finger it is possible to determine whether or not the lens is inside out by applying the so-called 'taco test.' Here the lens is pinched between thumb and forefinger and if the edges rill inwards easily and meet, then the lens is the correct way round. If the edges roll outwards it is inverted.

Removal of daily disposible lenses

Method 1
- Hold the upper and lower lids apart as described under lens insertion. This time the mirror may be used in either a vertical or horizontal position
- Turn the head so that you are looking across your nose into the mirror, that is, for the right eye, turn your head to the right so that you are then looking to the left to see in the mirror
- Using the index finger slide the lens off the cornea towards the ear, on to the white of the eye. Keep hold of the upper lid but take away the right hand and turn so that the side of the thumb and forefinger are facing the eye.
- Keeping the head position constant, hold the lids at the corner of the eye apart with the side of the thumb and forefinger and gently pinch the lens off the eye with the thumb and forefinger.

Method 2
Bend the chin into the neck so that you look upwards to see the eye in the mirror. Slide the lens below the cornes and pinch off using thumb and forefinger (or middle finger) as before.
If you have longer fingernails, deep set eyes or smaller than average distance between the lids Methods 1 & 2 may prove more difficult.

Always discard used daily disposable lenses.

ADVICE ON CARING FOR YOUR LENSES

CHECK LIST

Wash your hands

- Show how to remove the lens from the case
- If it is a soft lens demonstrate how to tell if it is inside-out
- Show the patient how to insert the lens
- Show them how to check that the lens is centred on the cornea
- Explain that they must empty and rinse the case after insertion
- Talk about adaptive symptoms they might experience
- Write down the wearing schedule
- Show them how to remove the lens
- Discuss unrolling a stuck lens
- Show them how to clean the lens on removal (unless daily disposable)
- Demonstrate rinsing the cleaner from the lens
- Show them how to place into the case
- Instruct on disinfection
- Instruct on the use of artificial tears on awakening if lenses are worn overnight
- Go through the instruction material with the patient
- Provide the contact number if more advice is needed or in the case of an emergency
- Make an appointment for the first after-care

Figure 9.8 *Suggested advice issued to patients on handling daily disposable lenses.*

Figure 9.9 *Suggested checklist for assistants advising patients on handling of lenses.*

refining the fit to give optimal results. A typical visit schedule is shown in Table 9.2. The super-script a denotes visits that the more experienced practitioner may later only perform if there is an indication, such as when a change to the lens fit has been made at a previous visit.

Table 9.2 Suggested aftercare schedule for orthokeratology patients

Day	Time	Lenses in situ?	Action
0	Any	No	Issue lenses to patient, together with supply of daily disposables where required and literature detailed in Table 9.3
7	a.m. for night therapy. p.m. for day wear	Yes. In order to check for binding	Perform investigations shown in Table 9.3
14[a]	p.m.	Yes	Perform investigations shown in Table 9.3
28	p.m.	Yes for day wear only	Perform investigations shown in Table 9.3 Consider reducing patient to alternate-night wear
60[a]	p.m.	Yes for day wear only	Perform investigations shown in Table 9.3 Consider reducing patient to alternate-night wear
90 (3 months)	a.m. for night therapy. p.m. for day wear	Yes for day wear only	Perform investigations shown in Table 9.3 Consider reducing patient to alternate-night wear
180 (6 months)	a.m. for night therapy. p.m. for day wear	Yes for day wear only	Perform investigations shown in Table 9.3
360 (1 year)	a.m. for night therapy. p.m. for day wear	Yes for day wear only	Perform a full eye examination as well as investigations shown in Table 9.3
Every 6 months	a.m. for night therapy. p.m. for day wear	Yes for day wear only	Perform a full eye examination as well as investigations shown in Table 9.3

[a] Optional visit.

THE FIRST AFTERCARE

As stated above, the scheduling of the first aftercare visit will generally be one week after the first wearing session. However, where the practitioner has made a significant change to the lens fit as a result of the first trial wear, then he may want to treat this as a second trial period and see the patient sooner. Also, where the practitioner has slight reservations as to the quality of the fit or feels that the patient's response needs to be closely investigated then the scheduling of the first visit may be made sooner than normal. For night-therapy patients, the first aftercare will always take place early in the day to ensure that there are no complications arising from overnight wear. Daytime wearers will typically be seen towards the end of the day, when any complications should be more evident.

Patients wearing the lenses during the day should attend the first aftercare with the lenses in situ. For overnight wearers the lenses should also

Table 9.3 Summary of the investigations that should be performed at every aftercare visit

Investigation	Comments
Symptoms and history	Question regarding comfort and condition of the eyes during lens wear
	Quality and stability of vision with daily disposables, where worn
Vision with lenses in situ (day wear only)	Should be excellent unless patient has residual astigmatism
Lens movement and position (night therapy first visit only)	Daytime wearers should always have mobile lenses
	Nighttime wearers should show no lens binding when attending with lenses in situ
	Lens centration should be good
Fluorescein fit (night therapy first visit only)	Should still show classic orthokeratology pattern: if not, patient needs refitting
Unaided vision and refraction	Should show significant improvement and no loss of best corrected visual acuity
Slit-lamp examination	Eye should be white and show no more than grade 2 corneal stain (CCLRU scale). No stain should be present if lenses have been out more than 4 h
Corneal topography	Bull's-eye topographic change map should be present
Lens condition	Look for back surface scratches, blocked fenestrations, and deposition
Decision on continuing suitability	Decide if physiological response is satisfactory and whether fit needs modification

CCLRU, Cornea and Contact Lens Research Unit.

be in place, so that the practitioner can see if the lenses have spontaneously unbound and that there is no significant corneal stain.

The investigations that should be carried out at this and all subsequent aftercare visits are summarized in Table 9.3.

The investigations listed in Table 9.3 will now be considered in more detail.

SYMPTOMS AND HISTORY

Patient education is an important part of orthokeratology. In order to gain valuable information from the patient the practitioner must teach the patient what to look out for and when to look for it.

Any symptoms reported after wear of the trial lens should be reduced with the final dispensed lenses. This should be the case for two reasons. Firstly, a week will have passed, allowing adaptation to occur and secondly, the fitting may have been further improved between the trial lens and the final lens, producing even better results. To elicit symptoms the practitioner should avoid "closed" questions like "Is everything alright?" A better starting point is: "Tell me how you feel about the vision when you remove the lenses," followed by: "Are you aware of the lenses at any

time?" and "How do your eyes look just before you take the lenses out?" Additionally the question: "When did you last sleep in the lenses?" should be asked in case the patient has missed a night's wear. In this case there is little point in examining the patient's cornea as clearly it is unlikely to show any adverse signs. Later on, more closed questions can be used like "What power of disposable lens are you using now?" and "Does the vision vary much during the day?"

Practitioners routinely using night therapy frequently remark how few symptoms patients report to them. Only mild irritation on rising, a definite absence of redness, and a slight increase in dried mucus at the inner canthi are typical observations reported by patients. Additionally, daytime wearers report typical mild symptoms associated with RGP lens wear: foreign-body sensation from time to time, mild 3 and 9 o'clock stain (never seen in nighttime wearers), and occasional lens greasing.

It follows that any extra symptoms or more severe symptoms should be treated seriously by practitioners. The avoidance of any significant complications of contact lens wear should be our primary concern when examining patients at aftercare visits.

Table 9.4 An example of the daily disposable lens powers that might be issued to a −2.50 D myope in the first week of night therapy using single reverse geometry orthokeratology lenses

Day number	Power required a.m.	Power required p.m.
1	−1.75	−2.50
2	−1.50	−2.50
3	−1.25	−2.00
4	−1.25	−1.75
5	−1.00	−1.50
6	−0.75	−1.50
7	−0.50	−1.00

Table 9.5 lists typical normal and abnormal symptoms that may arise in both overnight and daytime orthokeratology. Recognition of abnormal symptoms is vital if complications are to be avoided. Familiarity with the typical range of mild symptoms and signs arising during orthokeratology treatment is essential to enable the practitioner to manage patients conscientiously.

Quality of vision should be assessed both with and without the lenses in situ. In the case of overnight orthokeratology, the quality of vision with the lenses in place is almost irrelevant, but clearly needs to be adequate for patients to find their way about indoors and function normally if they awaken during the night. Obviously, the quality of this aspect of vision is more important for the daytime wearer. Of more interest is the quality of vision on lens removal. This will be both an assessment immediately on lens removal

Table 9.5 Normal and abnormal symptoms that may arise during orthokeratology treatment (modality in parentheses)

Normal symptoms expected during adaptation	Abnormal symptoms
Lens awareness that goes with lens removal	Pain or awareness not eased by removing the lens
Sudden-onset foreign-body sensation in windy conditions eased by allowing reflex tears to pass behind lens or removing lens (daytime wear)	Sudden-onset foreign-body sensation in windy conditions not eased by allowing reflex tears to pass behind lens or removing lens (daytime wear)
Mild reddening of the eyes towards the end of the wearing period, resolved by removing the lens	Marked reddening or reddening not eased by removing the lens
Dry sensation towards the end of the wearing period which resolves on removal of lens	Marked dry sensation or dryness not resolved by removing the lens
Slight sore or puffy feeling to the eyelids improved by removing lens	Obviously red or swollen eyelids or soreness or puffiness not resolved by removing the lens
Slight increase in the amount of "sleep" found at the inner canthus on awakening (night therapy)	Discharge collecting on the eyelids and lashes on awakening (night therapy)
Occasional misting of the vision during the day improved by removing lens and cleaning it or several forced blinks (daytime wear)	Vision mists over shortly after insertion or misting at any time not resolved by removing and cleaning lens (daytime wear)
Imperfect vision through existing spectacles following lens removal (all modalities) or slightly imperfect vision with daily disposable lenses worn during day (night therapy)	Any distortion apparent when examining text at near point without lenses in situ (all modalities)
Lenses immobile on awakening but start to move after a few minutes or after instillation of one drop artificial tears and indenting sclera (night therapy)	Immobile lens not freed by use of scleral indentation and artificial tear instillation or producing pain on removal (night therapy)

and then of the stability of this vision during the day.

Where daily disposables are being worn, patients should be questioned as to the powers in current use and the quality of the vision through them.

VISION WITH LENSES IN SITU

Where lenses are going to be worn during daytime hours, it is most important to ascertain the quality of the visual result and overrefraction in the normal manner. Thus any deficiencies can be corrected to optimize the corrected acuity. The major difference between orthokeratology and conventional RGP lens fitting when considering this subject is the presence of a negative-powered liquid lens between the lens and the cornea. In a conventional alignment RGP fitting, the liquid lens serves to correct solely the front-surface corneal astigmatism. In the case of orthokeratology this is still true, but in addition the tear lens may correct up to 4 D of myopia. This arises because the lenses are fitted flatter than the underlying central cornea. The general clinical rule of thumb applied in these circumstances is that for every 0.1 mm that the lens is flatter than the underlying cornea, there is a tear lens with a power of –0.50 D. This optical effect is predicted by the difference in refractive index between the lens material (typically about 1.47) and the tear film (taken to be 1.336). Thus, depending on how flat the central fitting is, the lens back vertex power will have been reduced accordingly.

Where the patient is wearing the lenses overnight, there is little point in performing an overrefraction since the lens will generally be worn with the eyes closed and a plano lens offers the best equivalent oxygen percentage (EOP) profile. Another advantage of ordering a plano lens is that it can be retained as a future trial lens should a second lens be necessary.

Given that the patients will typically be myopes between –1.00 and –4.00 D, then the negative liquid lens will usually be sufficient to correct the majority of the ametropia, allowing good functional vision. If plano lenses are used, this minimizes lens thicknesses and improves oxygen transmissibility. In normal circumstances

in night therapy practice it is rarely necessary to check the vision and overrefraction with the lenses in place.

LENS MOVEMENT AND POSITION

The next examination that takes place following the symptom and acuity recording is the examination of lens movement using white diffuse light (to reduce reflex lacrimation and afford a better view) and low magnification on the slit-lamp microscope. If the lens has been worn overnight and the patient is seen more than an hour after rising, following instillation of artificial tears on rising, then there will generally be some lens movement. If the lens is bound and a corneal imprint is visible once the lens is manually freed up, then this may be regarded as an unacceptable degree of lens binding, or at least one that requires careful monitoring. Whether or not binding is evident at this visit, all patients must be shown how to look for lens movement and free up the lens by indenting the sclera and using artificial tears. This is described above under wearing schedules.

No lens binding should occur during a daytime trial and, if it does, this must be regarded as an adverse sign. Should this arise, then the practitioner is advised to follow the problem-solving approach set out later in this chapter.

Given that a very typical diameter for an orthokeratology lens is between 10.00 and 11 mm, the amount of movement seen on blink is relatively small. It is of the order of 1.00–1.50 mm. This can be seen at the same time as one is looking for binding. It is relatively easy to judge lens movement amplitude at low magnification, if it is compared to anatomical features such as the pupil border to inferior limbus distance. If the pupil size is 4 mm and the horizontal visible iris diameter is 12 mm, then this distance will be 4 mm, so that a movement of 1 mm will be equal to approximately a quarter of the pupil border to inferior limbus distance.

The direction of movement should always be vertical and an arcuate movement will almost always indicate a lens that is too flat or an eye that has significant against-the-rule astigmatism. The use of the push-up test, where the lids are

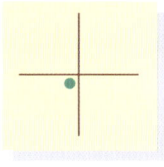

Figure 9.10 Simple means of recording 1.5 mm of inferior temporal decentration of a right lens. The ends of the lines represent the edges of the cornea and the dot the lens center.

separated and the lens is pushed upwards with the lower lid and allowed to fall, is useful for establishing that there is no arcuate movement.

Another observation to be made at this stage is the habitual riding position of the lens. To assess this the patient must have the eye in the primary position, so it may be appropriate to use a fixation target. Centration is typically recorded as the amplitude of decentration from the pupil center in millimeters, together with the direction. For example: 1.5 mm inferotemporal decentration. The use of a simple cross to represent the cornea together with a spot to represent the lens center is a useful means of representing decentration. For example, 1.5 mm inferotemporal decentration in the right eye would be recorded as shown in Figure 9.10.

For daytime wear, this measure of centration is sufficient. The topographic change map usually confirms that the lens is decentered in the manner recorded, in that the zone of flattening is decentered in a similar manner. However, for overnight wear the situation is more complex. The authors

have observed several cases where the centration of the lens at first follow-up was less than ideal, but when the lens is centered on the cornea, the fit was perfect. However, when the topography difference maps were inspected the treatment zones were perfectly centered. This implies that the centration exhibited by a lens in daytime wear can be quite different from that in overnight wear. Presumably this is due to a variation in gravitational forces when lying down, together with the absence of blinking, and the different relationship of the lids to the lens.

Therefore in those patients on night therapy, more attention should be paid to the position of the zone of flattening measured using videokeratoscopy than the apparent lens centration with the eyes open. Figure 9.11 shows a topographical change map for a patient who had a narrow palpebral aperture and on whom trial lenses always rode low when seated in the consulting-room chair. However, the results in terms of the centration of the flattened zone on the cornea indicate that the lens must center correctly with the eyes closed. The fluorescein pattern with the lens manually centered also demonstrated all the correct attributes of an orthokeratology fitting.

FLUORESCEIN FIT ASSESSMENT

It is probably true to say that, providing the topographic response of the cornea is correct and the

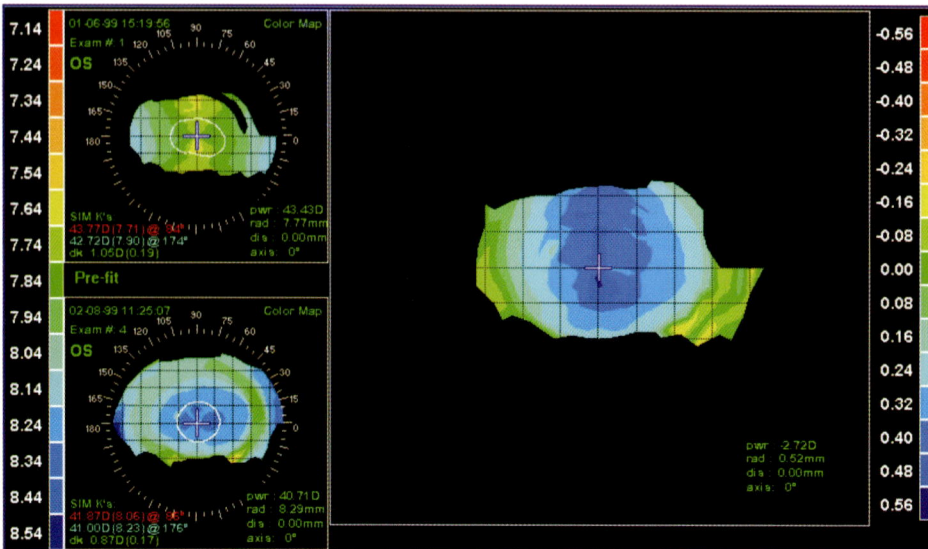

Figure 9.11 Topographical changes in a patient wearing a lens that was consistently decentered in primary gaze with the eyes open, yet produced a perfectly centered zone of flattening. The lens must ride in the correct position during sleep.

cornea shows no adverse response to contact lens wear, then the fluorescein assessment of lens fitting is almost irrelevant. However, the vast majority of practitioners will want to look at the lens in situ at least once, if for no other reason than to ensure that it is not binding. Thus, as already stated, at this first aftercare visit the night therapy patient will generally attend wearing the lenses, allowing this determination to be made. Having the patient attend the practice on at least one occasion wearing the lenses has the further advantage that the cornea can be assessed immediately on lens removal, allowing any staining and edema to be seen that might otherwise have resolved by the time the patient gets to the practice after awakening.

Fluorescein instillation should be left until the movement, centration, and surface wetting of the lens have been assessed in case the extra fluid causes a change in these features. The postwear fluorescein pattern should not differ significantly from that observed on first insertion. The apparent depth of the tear reservoir may be slightly reduced but otherwise the features of the fluorescein pattern are as shown in Chapter 6.

Where this is not the case and the topographic change difference map shows anything other than a bull's-eye response, then the practitioner must resolve the deficiencies of the fit and, if necessary, schedule a retrial with an appropriately modified trial lens or ordered lens.

It is generally easier to inspect the fluorescein fitting at the slit lamp. This has several advantages over the hand-held Burton lamp. Firstly, the patient is already seated at the instrument and all one need do is instill fluorescein and inspect the fitting. Secondly, the use of a barrier filter to enhance the fluorescence is much easier at the slit lamp. Thirdly, the higher magnification afforded by the microscope permits the practitioner to observe more of the subtle indicators of an imperfect fitting, for example, persistent bubbles within the tear reservoir, bubbles at the lens edge, inadequate differentiation between tear reservoir and peripheral bearing zone, no tear flow through the fenestrations. Fourthly, several modern RGP lens materials incorporate an ultraviolet filter that prevents fluorescein from being properly activated. Clearly, nobody should be practicing orthokeratology without a slit lamp, so the use of a separate lamp to inspect the lens fitting is probably unnecessary.

A small quantity of dye is instilled directly from a fluoret (fluorescein-impregnated strip). The strip is wetted firstly with only one drop of sterile saline. Flooding the eye with fluorescein will lead to greater difficulty in analysis of the fit by virtue of front surface fluorescein and the extra tear volume will give a false impression as to the essential balance between the zones of "contact" and clearance. In addition, a large quantity of fluorescein simply does not fluoresce very much. It is more difficult to instill the correct amount of dye from a minim or other form of ready-mixed fluorescein.

Whatever the riding position, the fluorescein pattern should be assessed with the lens held in the centered position with the lids and the fingers. It is impossible to determine the reasons for lens decentration with the lens decentered, since the lens will be resting over peripheral cornea and an asymmetric pattern will result.

As described in Chapter 6, there is now a variety of genuinely different lens designs on the market. However, when correctly fitted, the fluorescein patterns are very similar.

During the assessment of the fluorescein pattern, the practitioner will be able to inspect the fenestrations (if present) for any sign of tear flow through them. During normal blinking, it should be possible to observe the outward flow of fluorescein-laden tears through the fenestrations. This is another sign that lens movement is occurring and that the lens is not bound. It is believed that the fenestrations help reduce the lens to unbind on awakening, after instillation of artificial tears.

POSTREMOVAL VISUAL ASSESSMENT

On removal the unaided vision should be recorded. This is a crucial indication of the efficacy of the procedure in meeting patients' expectations. Depending on the lens type and degree of initial myopia, this change may be marked or relatively minor. One of the rewarding aspects of orthokeratology practice is seeing the satisfaction of patients experiencing improved vision on the removal of their lenses.

Additionally, the refraction on lens removal should be measured together with the corrected acuity. It is not acceptable for there to be any reduction of best-corrected visual acuity. The patient and practitioner may have to accept a little induced against-the-rule astigmatism, particularly in the early stages, as described in Chapter 7, but neither this nor any induced mild peripheral corneal distortion should lead to loss of full visual potential with refraction. If it does, then careful attention to the fit should be made and if necessary the patient discontinued from the procedure.

Corneal examination

At any aftercare visit there should be no significant increase in limbal or bulbar hyperemia, providing a very high-*Dk* material has been used. This is in marked contrast to conventional extended-wear hydrogel lens wear where an increase in limbal hyperemia after overnight wear is almost universal (Holden et al 1986). Hyperemia is best assessed using diffuse illumination at low magnification. Then using direct focal illumination, the cornea is examined for any sign of edema.

If corneal striae or even folds are seen in a patient wearing a high-permeability lens for overnight wear or, even more unlikely, in a daytime-wear patient, then it is evident that the degree of metabolic embarrassment is too much for the cornea concerned. It may be that moving patients to daytime wear would enable sufficient oxygen to pass to the cornea, but if not, it is best to advise patients that orthokeratology is not a viable procedure for them and it should be discontinued.

Corneal microcysts will not be observed after one wearing session as these are a longer-term response to hypoxia. However they have not been observed to date by the authors in any patient at any aftercare visit. Central corneal clouding, as seen in polymethyl methacrylate (PMMA) wearers, should never be seen in overnight orthokeratology patients, as the degree of corneal edema produced is extremely low (see Ch. 3).

If the technique of overnight orthokeratology brings any surprise to the experienced contact lens practitioner, it is the near-total absence of corneal stain following a successful overnight wear. One hour or so after rising, when the patient attends at the practice, there should be no more than grade 1 or 2 (trace or mild on the Cornea and Contact Lens Research Unit (CCLRU) scale) central stain, no 3 and 9 o'clock stain, and only the faintest indication that the lens bound during the night. Figure 9.12 shows the features of a just acceptable corneal response in terms of stain. There is grade 2 nonconfluent stain, which would require careful monitoring by the practitioner. The causes and solutions for corneal staining are dealt with later in the problem-solving section. To improve the visualization of fluorescein stain, the practitioner is recommended to use a Wratten 16 yellow filter, as was used to view the fitting pattern.

Typical adverse responses are evident as grosser degrees of stain, particularly if confluent. Figure 9.13 shows significant confluent stain. Figure 9.14 shows a gross degree of compression stain associated with severe binding, which occurred during a daytime trial. This will usually be associated with limbal desiccation stain, in the approximately "3 and 9" format. When severe binding occurs overnight, there is no limbal stain of this sort since no desiccation occurs. However, if the lens binds off-center, there may be some compression of the bulbar conjunctiva.

Equally, in daytime wearers, there should be only minimal corneal response, although there

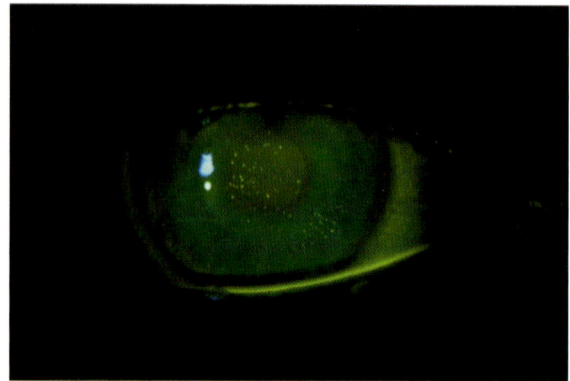

Figure 9.12 Grade 2 nonconfluent stain in a patient immediately following removal of the lens at the first aftercare.

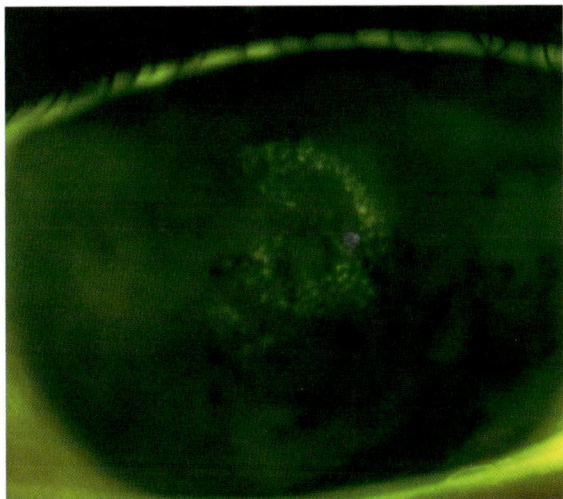

Figure 9.13   Unacceptable confluent grade 3 stain following overnight lens wear (Cornea and Contact Lens Research unit).

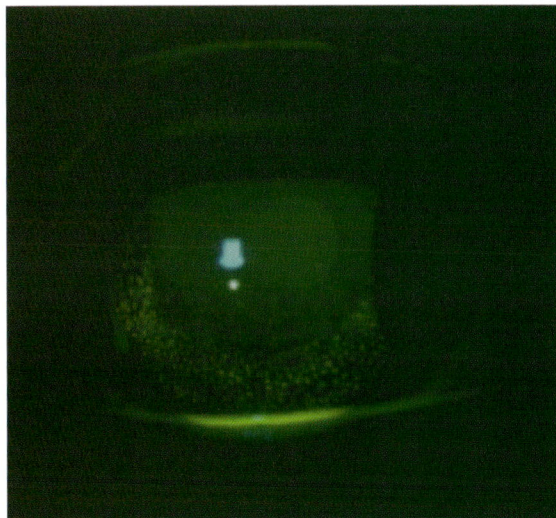

Figure 9.15   Corneal "dimpling" seen on removal of a lens fitted too steeply with a deep tear reservoir.

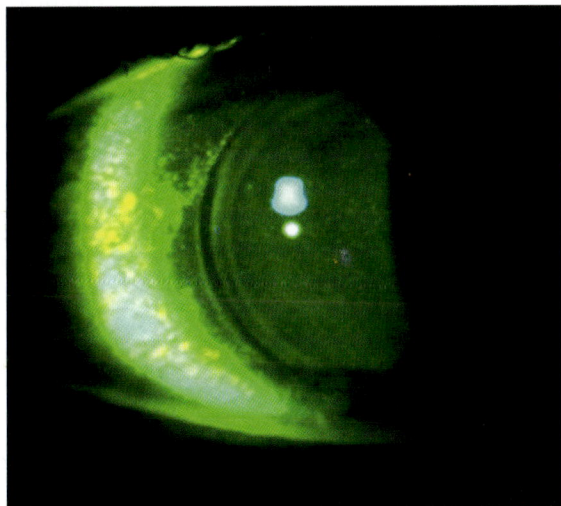

Figure 9.14   Unacceptable degree of corneal compression in a daytime wearer. Note that there is also stain over the limbus representing desiccation of the cornea.

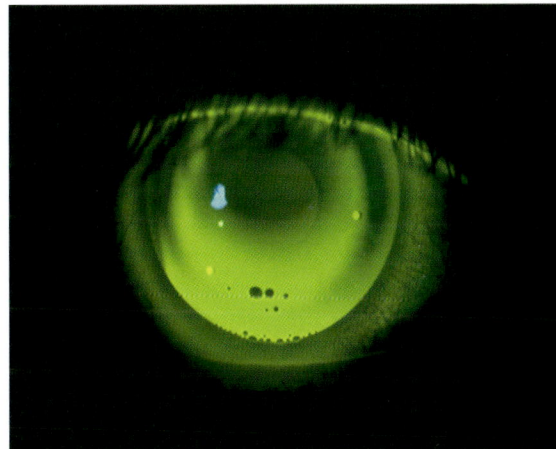

Figure 9.16   Bubble formation occurring under the edge of an excessively flat lens.

may be a little more lid hyperemia due to the greater lid interaction than occurs compared to overnight wear. Unlike an overnight trial, there should be no sign of any corneal compression due to binding, as the lens should remain freely moving at all times.

A common observation following a short period of lens wear is a degree of corneal "dimpling." This occurs because of bubble formation under the lens, typically under the tear reservoir.

Whilst this can be a sign of a steep fit, if the topographic change map indicated that this is not the case, then the situation should be monitored. Clinical experience indicates that this reduces over time. An example of this dimpling is shown in Figure 9.15. A variant of this arises when bubbles form under the lens edge. This is illustrated in Figure 9.16 and usually occurs when the fit is too flat or the edge clearance is excessive. Discussion of a problem-solving strategy for dimpling is given later in this chapter.

Corneal topography changes

Currently, there is no better way of evaluating the technique of orthokeratology than by measuring the shape change in the very tissue that is being altered, i.e., the cornea. Whilst, strictly speaking, all Placido disk-based topographers measure the shape of the tear film, it seems reasonable to suppose that, away from the lids, this will be almost the same as the anterior corneal surface.

The attributes of the ideal instrument for the orthokeratology practitioner have already been discussed in Chapter 2, but careful attention to image capture, editing, and analysis will greatly aid in the correct discrimination of the ideal from the imperfect fit. The objective unbiased nature of topography measurement is a marvellous way to validate the technique of orthokeratology and a calibrated instrument of the appropriate quality should be regarded as part of the essential armoury of the competent orthokeratologist.

It is a well-known fact that the line of sight and the geometrical center of the cornea do not co-incide. Typically, the line of sight is decentered nasally with respect to the center of the cornea. Thus a degree of nasal decentration is by no means a bad thing: the center of the zone of flattening is more likely to be located over the line of sight, which coincides with the center of the eye's entrance pupil (the image of the pupil produced by the cornea). In topographic systems that allow the entrance pupil to be identified (see Ch. 2), it is easy to establish that this has occurred. Where the entrance pupil is not identified, then it is reasonable to assume that the center will typically lie 0.5 mm nasally from the center of the topography map.

As has already been stated, the topography difference map will indicate whether the lens has centered correctly. If there is a continuous ring of mid-peripheral steepening around a zone of flattening which is centered over the middle of the pupil, then a perfect result has been obtained. This aspect of confirming the quality of lens centration is an important one and is not easily done by any other means than sequential topography. In terms of difficulty, the most significant problem that arises in orthokeratology is to ensure that the lens is well-centered.

The analysis of the postwear topography difference map is the same as that set out in Chapter 6, namely the differentiation of the bull's-eye response from central islands and smiley face-type responses.

Clearly, the smaller the treatment zone (see Ch. 7), the more critical is good centration to avoid flare. At aftercare visits, it is crucial that the quality of lens centration, as determined by the topography change map, is thoroughly appraised. At this first visit, it is unlikely that patients will report flare, as the degree of refractive change will generally be modest. However, the practitioner who does not attend to improvement of centration at this visit risks significant problems with poor-quality vision and corneal distortion later.

As has already been described in Chapter 2, the topography plays a vital role in the selection of the first lens by virtue of its ability to measure the apical radius and the eccentricity of the cornea. Clearly, as the cornea changes, so will these values. However, there is no evidence that they are of any value when it comes to refitting the patient with future lenses. This is because of the nature of the topographical change in the cornea. As has already been described in Chapter 7, it has been known for many years that the endpoint of orthokeratology treatment is a spherical cornea.

The posttreatment apical radius and eccentricity data only serve to indicate that the apex of the cornea has flattened and that its eccentricity has changed. The practitioner must carefully inspect the posttrial tangential map to infer what the nature of the topography change is. The endpoint of orthokeratology becomes evident when there is no further refractive change and the central 4–5 mm of the tangential plot is spherical. In addition, the absence of any of the topographical signs of steep or flat fits and the presence of the ideal topographic change indicate that the lens fitting is still optimal. If it is not, then the diligent practitioner will refit until both the fluorescein pattern and the topographical change maps are perfect.

Lens condition

It is unlikely that the lenses will have been damaged by the time of the first aftercare appointment. However, the practitioner is duty-bound to inspect both lenses for scratches, deposits, and blocked fenestrations. This is best done by a combination of two techniques. Firstly, the lens surface is inspected on the slit lamp at medium magnification and using diffuse illumination. Rapid hazing of the surface after blinking may indicate a wetting problem that may be related to poor manufacture or possibly lack of attention to cleaning by the patient. The lenses should be removed, cleaned, and then carefully dried. The clean, dry lens should then be critically inspected either using a loupe or the slit lamp.

A lens is shown in Figure 9.17 that has developed a heavy layer of adherent surface plaque. Figure 9.18 shows a lens that has marked lipid deposition on its surface.

In view of the close proximity of the lens to the corneal surface, any scratches or adherent deposits may give rise to corneal trauma. If the deposits cannot be removed either by using protein remover tablets or by careful cleaning of the lens rear surface using a cotton bud dipped in a contact lens cleaner containing polymeric beads (Boston cleaner), then the lens should be replaced.

Most unlikely at this stage is finding the fenestrations blocked by deposits and other dried ocular secretions. However, this should always be looked for, particularly in a patient who complains of discomfort who was previously a com-

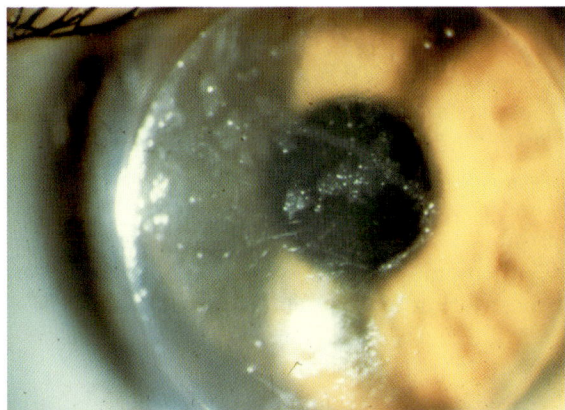

Figure 9.18   Lipoidal deposits on the lens front surface. Courtesy of Pat Caroline.

fortable wearer. The material can be removed by the practitioner by careful use of a cocktail stick and polymeric bead cleaner. Afterwards, the fenestration should be inspected on the slit lamp to ensure that all the material has been removed and that the lens has not been damaged.

Figure 9.19 shows a reverse geometry lens with a blocked fenestration. The debris in the fenestration caused a mild degree of corneal insult which disappeared once it was removed by careful use of a cocktail stick and contact lens cleaner.

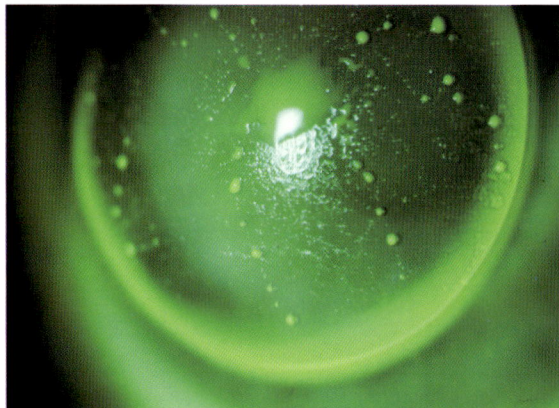

Figure 9.17   Example of a scratched lens with associated protein deposition. Courtesy of Pat Caroline.

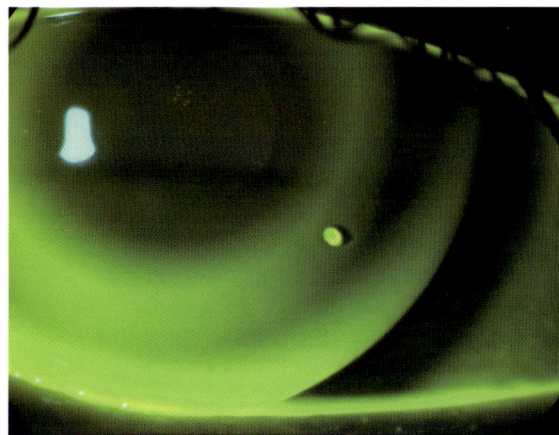

Figure 9.19   A reverse geometry lens with a blocked fenestration. The debris caused a minor degree of corneal insult.

DECISION ON CONTINUING SUITABILITY FOR ORTHOKERATOLOGY TREATMENT

By the end of the first aftercare visit, practitioners will be able to decide if the patient has demonstrated the following:

1. satisfaction with the treatment to date and its effectiveness
2. the appropriate improvement in unaided vision
3. no undesirable response in terms of corneal stain, edema, or distortion
4. the appropriate topographical response.

If this is the case then the patient should continue with lens wear and follow the aftercare schedule set out in Table 9.2. If not then the practitioner must adopt a problem-solving strategy and either modify the fit or discontinue the patient from the treatment plan.

VISUAL CORRECTION DURING THE FIRST WEEK

During the first week, patients on night therapy need to be given some form of daytime vision correction. Their existing spectacles are generally now too strong for comfortable use. This is not the case with myopic children who may have an older pair of spectacles that incorporate a lower correction. Those patients with no suitable spectacles (or those who refuse to wear spectacles) need a vision correction to function normally during the day. The introduction of daily disposable soft lenses has made dealing with the progressively reducing myopia much more straightforward. The problems here are:

- The patient has to learn how to handle what is generally a more challenging type of lens.
- The power required will vary during the day and from day to day.
- The existing daily disposable lenses do not correct astigmatism.
- Patients may like disposable lenses so much they decide against orthokeratology – this happens occasionally!

There is little doubt that patients unused to soft lenses can find daily disposable lenses more difficult to handle initially. The larger diameter, thin substance, and often low modulus of elasticity make them more difficult to insert than an RGP lens. However, with careful instruction it is not a problem. There will be some patients, typically low myopes, who will prefer to do without lenses and tolerate the blur arising from undercorrection of their myopia for the first few days. Others will ask if they can just put in the orthokeratology lenses when they want to see particularly well. This is perfectly acceptable providing the lens has been appropriately powered for their degree of ametropia. But for the vast majority the use of daily disposable soft lenses does not trouble them. It is interesting that several remark how much more comfortable their orthokeratology lenses are than soft lenses. Removal rarely presents a problem.

As described in Chapter 7, the typical dioptric change after the first wearing session with single reverse geometry orthokeratology lenses is approximately 0.75–1.00 D. The practitioner will know from the response trial exactly what change the patient exhibited. Therefore the choice of power for the morning of the first day is relatively straightforward. However, a few hours later regression will have set in and this power will be incorrect. Therefore it is normal practice to give patients a further pair of lenses approximately 0.75 D stronger to use when they notice the distance vision tapering off. Mountford's study using single reverse geometry lenses (Mountford 1998) shows that in the first week of treatment an average of 1.93 D of reduction in apical corneal power (and, by inference, myopia) occurred. This was measured in the morning. Eight hours later, 0.52 D of the apical corneal power had returned. These are average figures, concealing some diversity in individual patient responses. Notwithstanding this, it does give the orthokeratologist some basis for deciding what powers of daily disposable lenses to issue to the patient. Patients seem to enjoy checking their vision at various times during the day and selecting another lens from their selection as appropriate. It is possible to supply patients with a vision chart so that they can assure themselves that their vision is good enough for driving purposes for the country in which they are resident.

To clarify this area, Table 9.4 shows the powers that might be issued during the first week to a patient with 2.50 D of myopia. Several extra lenses of each power are also issued so that patients can "jump up" (or down) the scale if they feel that their progress is falling behind or exceeding that predicted for them.

The approach described above may seem somewhat crude and unscientific. However, in practice it works perfectly well, providing patients understand the difficulty in giving them a completely accurate lens for both eyes for every minute of the day.

When double reverse geometry lenses are being used, the refractive changes will be much more rapid. Clinical experience indicates that approximately 75% of the final refractive change occurs during the first night of lens wear if the lens fit is perfect. Thus the first overnight trial will indicate the appropriate strength of daily disposable lenses to use on the first day. This may be up to 2.50–3.00 D less than the original refraction, assuming a large refractive change was programmed into the lens design. Subsequent changes will be rapid, meaning that it is unlikely that daily disposable lenses will be required after the first few days. Therefore the practitioner may supply an initial lens power based on the overnight trial and a couple of other lens powers between 0.50 and 1.00 D less than this for the second and third days.

The correction of astigmatism in the first week is more problematic. Assuming that patients have been selected for night therapy on the basis that they have no more than 1.50 DC of with-the-rule astigmatism the uncorrected astigmatism does not generally prove to be a problem. As already outlined in Chapter 7 there is a great shortage of good studies in the time course of astigmatic changes in orthokeratology. What can generally be stated is that the reduction in with-the-rule astigmatism lags behind the reduction in myopia and that a 50% reduction in astigmatism up to −1.75 DC occurs (Mountford & Pesudovs 2002). Patients with astigmatism should therefore be advised that the vision through the daily disposable lens will not be perfect in the initial stages.

FURTHER AFTERCARE VISITS

In terms of the scheduling of further visits, the program set out in Table 9.2 is generally appropriate. However, where the practitioner has made an alteration to the lens fit or wishes to keep a close check on an individual patient, then clearly more frequent visits will be scheduled. Once a patient has reached a stable situation and been followed for 6 months with no problems, then routine follow up is advised every 6 months, as set out in Table 9.2.

Orthokeratology treatment should always be tailored to an individual patient and care taken that the ideal topographic and physiological response is maintained. Practitioners new to the procedure are advised to see the treatment intervals set out in Table 9.2 as minima and always err on the side of caution and see a patient more frequently when they feel that this is clinically indicated.

EMERGENCIES

Increasingly, eye-care practitioners work in a more regulated and litigious environment. It is becoming incumbent on contact lens fitters to provide continuing care, not only in normal consulting hours, but also outside them. It is no longer considered satisfactory to say to the patient: "If you have serious problems outside of working hours, then go to the hospital emergency department." The first piece of advice that should be given is: "if in doubt, take them out." The vast majority of contact lens-induced disorders start to improve on removal of the lens. The practitioner should supply a list of what sort of symptoms may be considered normal during the initial few days of wear, and those that are abnormal and should lead to lens removal and the patient seeking advice from the practitioner. A suggested list of such symptoms is given in Table 9.5, together with indications as to how these symptoms may relate to the mode of wear.

In those instances where simple removal of the lenses does not lead to a reduction and then resolution of the symptom, patients need to know how they should contact the practitioner for advice. During consulting hours this will be by telephoning the practice. In the event that the orthokeratology practitioner is not in attendance, most queries can be dealt with by any contact lens practitioner or trained member of staff. However, such nonqualified staff need to be aware of the danger signs associated with contact lens-induced symptoms. These are no different from any other type of contact lens.

These are:

- pain
- discharge
- redness
- poor vision.

Although in most cases a "false alert" will be raised, avoidance of microbial keratitis should be uppermost in any contact lens practitioner's mind. Therefore practitioners must ensure that they are contactable wherever they might be during daylight hours. This may be via mobile telephone or pager. If overseas, a colleague experienced in contact lens management (and ideally orthokeratology) should be asked to provide cover.

When the situation arises outside consulting hours, then patients should have an emergency number to seek guidance. Again, this might be a pager or mobile telephone number. Naturally clear advice in what constitutes an emergency is prudent to avoid unnecessary calls. Increasing pain, blurring of vision, redness, or discharge following lens removal are the signs the patient must be aware of.

Only if contact with the practitioner is impossible should the patient have to resort to attending an emergency department. It is recommended that as well as getting patients to sign a statement of informed consent (detailed in Ch. 5), they be given a card indicating that they wear rigid contact lenses and bearing an emergency out-of-hours number. In several years of issuing patients with such information, the authors have been troubled on only very few occasions.

PROBLEM-SOLVING

Orthokeratology should not be considered a "routine" optometric procedure. The time to achieve the correct fitting response requires considerable experience in the interpretation of sodium fluorescein patterns and a reasonable understanding of corneal topographic changes.

However, of greater importance is the management of fitting complications. Although many of these complications are similar to those observed with conventionally designed RGP lenses, the fact that the design is radically different means that modification of lens parameters requires a different approach. One key difference in both fitting and modification of lens parameters is the manner in which one considers the fit of the lens. Rather than simply think of the lens as being flat or steep with regard to the BOZR, practitioners should consider the relationship between the sag of the lens and the sag of the cornea. The principal reason for using this approach is because the fit of the lens is not primarily controlled by the BOZR as with conventional RGP lenses; the secondary and sometimes tertiary reverse curves also have a significant impact on the fit of the lens.

Previous chapters have dealt with strategies designed to minimize the risk of adverse outcomes with respect to patient selection and trial lens fitting. However, as with all forms of contact lens practice, problems will occur after the lenses have been dispensed. In orthokeratology, these take the form of corneal and conjunctival staining, dimple veiling, contact lens papillary conjunctivitis (CLPC), lack or loss of refractive response, and unwanted corneal distortion and poor visual acuity.

The single most common cause of a poorly performing lens is practitioner misinterpretation of the results of an overnight trial, where the final lens is ordered on the basis of incorrect information. This problem is compounded if the lens is empirically fitted, as the practitioner is then dependent on the laboratory consultant (who has never seen the patient) to resolve the issues. In the authors' opinion, the critical factor in the correct interpretation of a trial wear period is a comprehensive knowledge of topography maps and the information they present. The majority of problems can be resolved simply by doing a trial overnight wear and interpreting the results correctly.

In this chapter, the common causes of the events that occur postlens fitting will be described, as well as the means of rectification.

CORNEAL STAINING

Several types of sodium fluroescein stain may be seen with day wear or overnight orthokeratology. These varied stains have different etiologies and are listed below:

- central stain
- 3 and 9 o'clock staining
- dimpling
- Fischer–Schweitzer polygonal mosaic
- conjunctival stain
- fenestration imprint
- lens binding
- deposit-induced staining.

As with any type of ocular abnormality, practitioners should grade the severity using a standardized scale.

Central staining

With overnight wear, the most common form of staining seen is central superficial punctate erosions (SPE). At most aftercare visits, the patient will have removed their lenses several hours previously. Generally, the degree of staining observed will be very low. It can range from insignificant grade 1 staining to unacceptable grade 2 staining and above. The CCLRU scale is ideal for recording staining changes, as both the severity and location can be recorded.

Localized central staining is shown in Figure 9.20. This is grade 2 staining and is unac-

ceptable. Grade 1 or less staining is clinically insignificant, and is usually totally resolved within an hour of lens removal. The staining can occur at the first aftercare or any time afterwards, and if consistently present indicates that the cause is mechanical, in that the lens back surface is coming into direct and heavy contact with the epithelium. The primary cause for this is a lens that has insufficient apical clearance, or alternatively, too much peripheral clearance, thereby allowing the lens to settle back into direct contact with the corneal surface. The aim of remedying localized central staining would therefore be to increase the sag of the lens to relieve the excessive apical bearing. This can be done by:

1. steepening the BOZR (not possible if the Jessen factor is used)
2. steepening the alignment curve(s)
3. increasing the TD (three-zone lenses)
4. steepening the reverse curve.

In the case of four- and five-zone lenses, the most common approach is to steepen the alignment curve. As shown in Chapter 4, steepening the alignment curve by 0.15 mm (0.75 D) will lead to an increase of 10 μm in lens sag. The Corneal Refractive Therapy (CRT) lens requires that the return zone depth be increased or the cone angle steepened, whilst the BE program requests that the practitioner supply information about the error of the instrument so that corneal sag can be recalculated, leading to changes in the BOZR, reverse curves, and tangent.

In practice, the practitioner will also utilize findings from topography patterns to decide whether the lens is "steep" or "flat". However, in some instances topography can be misleading. For example, in the case of central corneal staining, as shown in Figure 9.20, the reflection of the topography mires can be slightly distorted (often this cannot be discerned by observation of the Placido mires). Because of the subtle distorting effects of the centrally stained area, a topographic pattern that would indicate a "flat" fit could lead to the practitioner making an incorrect decision. Figure 9.21 shows a topographic difference map obtained from a patient who had localized central staining caused by a flat lens. This represents a "fake" central island, and occurs due to the inability of the

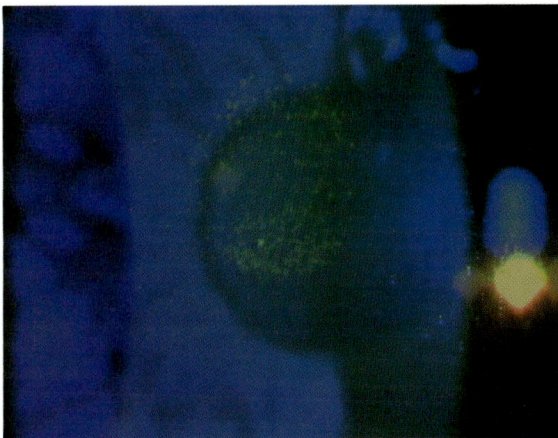

Figure 9.20 Unacceptable grade 2 confluent superficial stain present 2 h after the removal of an orthokeratology lens.

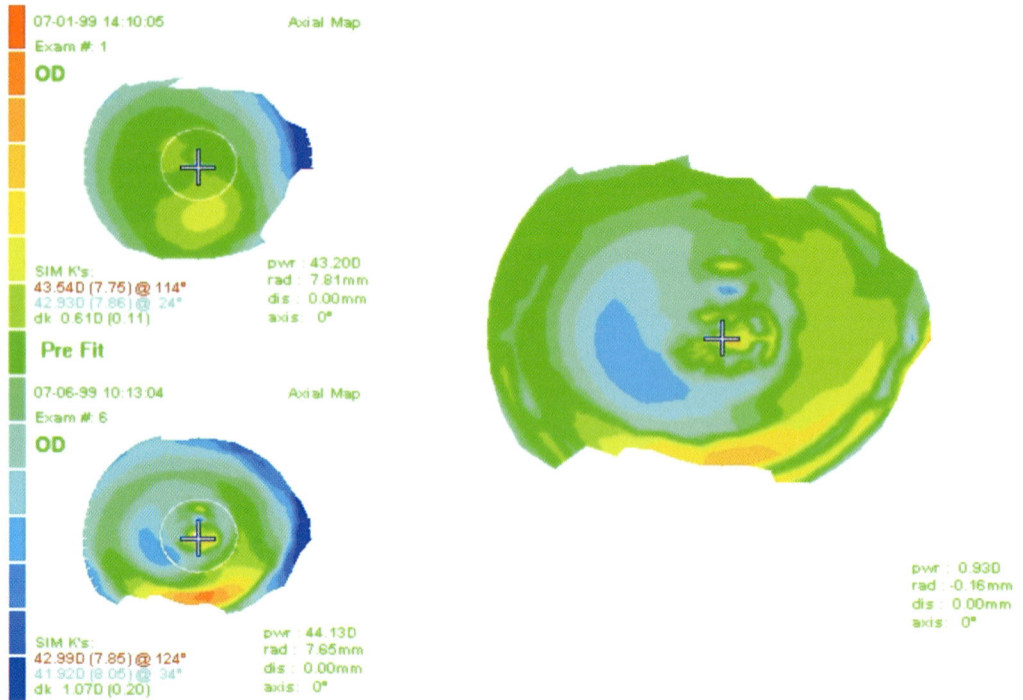

Figure 9.21 The effect of localized corneal superficial punctate erosion stain on topography. It can be seen that the difference map (center right) shows relative central steepening. In fact, the posttrial map (lower left) shows steepening compared to the pretrial map (upper left). This is an artefact arising due to the corneal stain in this region.

instrument's reconstruction algorithm to represent the changes correctly.

Alternatively, gross disruption of the mires will result in a central divot topography map, wherein the "ring jam" occurring as a result of the staining leads to the appearance of gross central flattening (Fig. 9.22). The important differential diagnostic tool in these instances is the tangential subtractive map, which would show the centration of the lens. If the lens was decentered superiorly, it could be considered to be too flat. However, if the lens is well-centered, the cause of the central staining may be due to three other factors: lens binding, surface deposits, or an incorrectly made lens (see later).

Three and 9 o'clock staining

Three and 9 o'clock staining is a complication exclusive to RGP lenses (Fig. 9.23). It occurs as a result of corneal exposure at the nasal and temporal regions at the edge of a contact lens extending to the corneal periphery (Korb & Korb 1970). Principally, the etiology lies in the fact that the cornea does not wet in the 3 and 9 o'clock areas. Reduced corneal wetting is exacerbated by the fact that the lid cannot wet the cornea because of the edge of the contact lens (Fig. 9.24). Thus, excessive edge lift is a major cause of RGP 3 and 9 o'clock staining. However, insufficient edge lift has also been implicated in 3 and 9 o'clock staining in extended RGP wear (Andrasko 1991) as a result of reduced tear flow under the edge of the lens. Most orthokeratology lenses are fitted in order to have an axial edge clearance (AEC) of 70–80 μm and a width of approximately 0.5 mm.

Three and 9 o'clock staining has been shown to be more prevalent with extended wear (Schnider et al 1991). However, it is the authors' experience that, in contrast to previous studies (Schnider et al 1991), modern-day orthokeratology lenses rarely cause 3 and 9 o'clock staining and the staining is never seen in overnight wear, presumably because the lenses are removed on awakening. Another possible explanation may lie in the large-diameter lenses used (generally exceeding 10 mm).

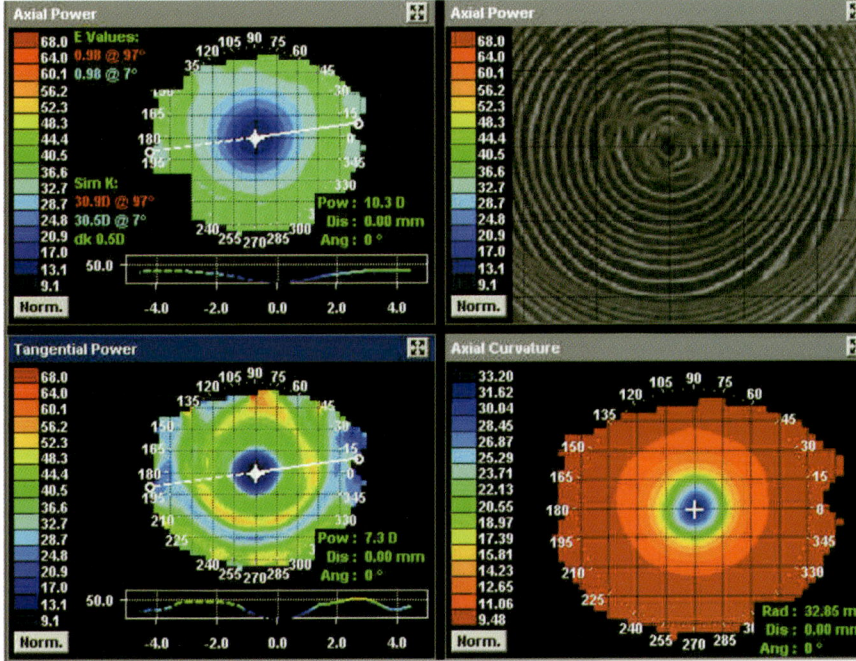

Figure 9.22   A central divot caused by marked central staining and distortion of the topographer mires (seen in the top right-hand image). Note the large false refractive change and the small area over which it occurs, as shown in the tangential map (bottom left-hand image).

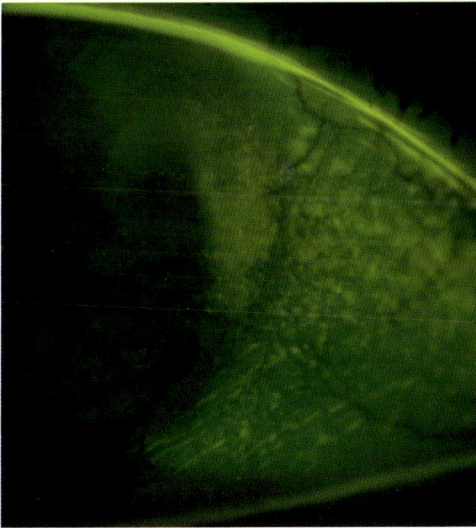

Figure 9.23   Three and 9 o'clock staining in a daytime wearer of small-diameter low-riding orthokeratology lenses.

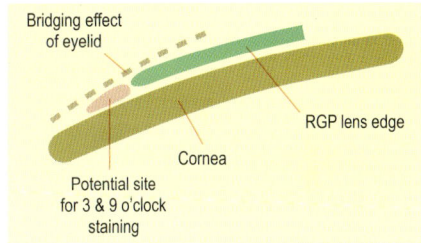

Figure 9.24   The bridging theory is often used to explain the etiology of 3 and 9 o'clock staining. During blinking, the eyelid cannot wet the entire cornea outside the boundary of the contact lens (in the temporal and nasal areas). As a result, drying occurs, leading to localized punctate staining in these areas.

If 3 and 9 o'clock staining occurs in daily wear, then it is recommended that the peripheral curves are altered such that, if there is too much edge lift, it is reduced, and if there is too little, then it is increased in order to increase tear flow. Additionally the practitioner should ensure that lens centration is optimal and low-riding lenses avoided by attention to the fit and the addition of a negative carrier or Korb edge to increase lens–lid interaction.

Dimple staining

Dimple staining is a misnomer. There is no actual staining present, but fluorescein pooling. In order to face the challenge of correcting greater degrees of myopia, manufacturers have altered lens designs by increasing the width or depth of the

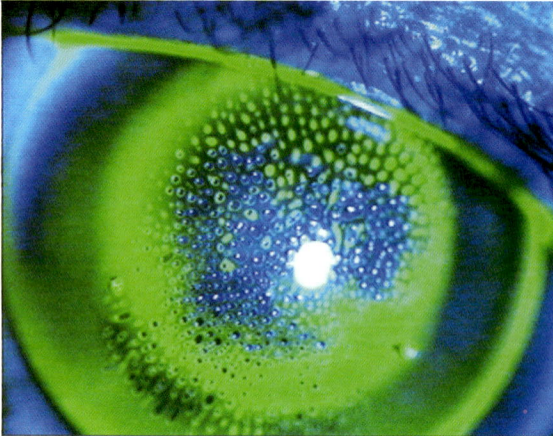

Figure 9.25 Dimple veiling underneath a double reverse geometry lens. Note the large width of the tear reservoir and the degree of dimpling, particularly in the central cornea.

tear reservoir (TR). These factors will often promote bubble formation within the TR. With time (often as little as 30 min) and repetitive blinking, the bubbles break down and froth. These smaller bubbles can spread to encompass the central cornea (Fig. 9.25). This is an unfortunate but completely innocuous complication of advanced orthokeratology. So-called dimple staining or dimple veiling simply represents multiple indentations within the corneal epithelium caused by the bubbles. The staining usually recovers after 1–2 h. Dimple staining prevents the practitioner from recording accurate or valid acuity measurements upon lens removal if the "staining" involves the central cornea. Furthermore, it also prevents accurate corneal topographic measurements from being taken as the "dimples" distort the reflected Placido mires. This degree of dimpling would certainly need to be managed.

In the authors' experience, dimpling may also occur haphazardly as an isolated incident. When dimpling is seen as an isolated incidence, patients should be advised to fill the back surface of the lens with wetting or conditioning solution, as this will usually resolve the problem. The true etiology of dimpling with regards to orthokeratology has not yet been discovered, although it appears that it is likely to be associated with the design of the TR.

All four- and five-zone reverse geometry lenses function optimally with a tear layer thickness (TLT) at the BOZD of between 45 and 65 μm. If the TLT exceeds this amount and approaches 90 μm, bubbles will occur. TLT of this magnitude will occur if a lens design that has fixed parameters is fitted to a high-eccentricity cornea, or where the corneal topographer has underestimated the eccentricity of the cornea, resulting in a "steep" lens fit. If the eccentricity is underestimated, so the apical clearance will be too great and the reverse curve and alignment curves or tangent effectively be too steep. This not only increases the apical clearance, but also the TLT at BOZD, to the extent that the formation of bubbles becomes possible.

Since the apical clearance is excessive, the refractive change will be minimal, although this can be difficult to determine if the dimpling invades the pupil zone. Certainly, the incidence of dimple veiling is greater with orthokeratology lenses compared to conventional rigid designs. The management strategy is to reduce clearance of the lens from the cornea in order to minimize bubble formation. This is usually accomplished by one of the following:

1. Perform a retrial with the next flattest lens in the trial set so that a better match to the eccentricity becomes possible.
2. Cease lens wear and repeat topography.
3. Flatten the alignment curve(s).
4. Flatten the reverse curve(s).

It is not uncommon to have dimple veiling occur on the overnight trial. However, this usually occurs as the trial lens parameters are primarily based on the mean corneal eccentricity, and if the individual eccentricity is higher, the clearance factor or TLT depth at the BOZD will be greater than that of the prescription lens. The bubbles do not usually occur with the correct lens.

Fischer–Schweitzer polygonal mosaic

The Fischer–Schweitzer polygonal mosaic is occasionally noted on lens removal. It comprises fluorescein pooling in a polygonal fashion over the central region of the cornea. Furthermore, there is no break in the corneal epithelial layer (Fig. 9.26). The etiology of the polygonal mosaic

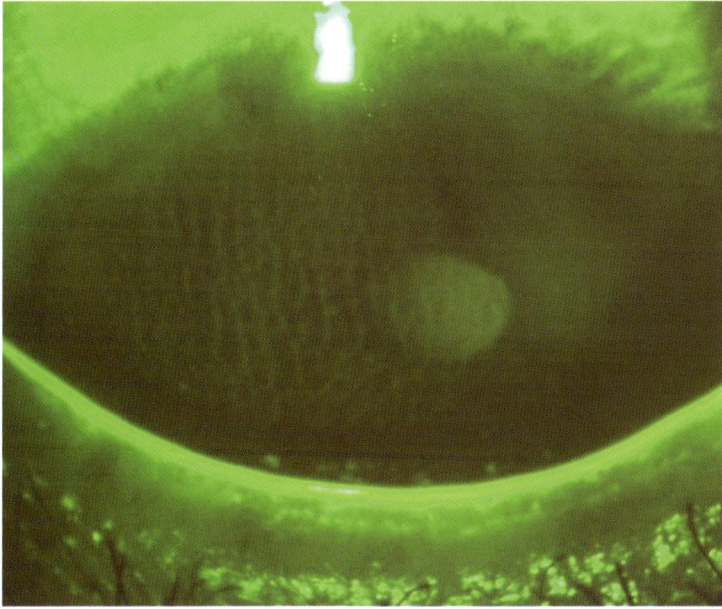

Figure 9.26 Fischer–Schweitzer polygonal mosaic. This is rarely seen following orthokeratology lens wear.

was originally described by Bron et al (1978), who suggested that the fluorescein pattern occurs as a result of external pressure on the cornea causing ridges to form in Bowman's layer. As the external force is removed and Bowman's layer returns to its original shape, grooves form where epithelial cells have been compressed into the ridges. The mosaic effect is usually present for up to 10 min, after which it disappears. The presence of the Fischer–Schweitzer polygonal mosaic is generally considered to be of no clinical significance in orthokeratology patients. It is rarely seen; however, this may be as a result of the fact that most patients are reviewed without lenses in situ following completion of the treatment and additionally the forces acting on the central cornea are modest.

Conjunctival staining

The use of localized central SPE stain in providing evidence of a flat-fitting reverse geometry lens has already been discussed. Inferior conjunctival stain may also provide a clue to the fit of a reverse geometry lens (although it is not as diagnostic a sign as central staining). Inferior conjunctival staining may be present in a steep-fitting lens, a bound lens (Fig. 9.27), or even occasionally

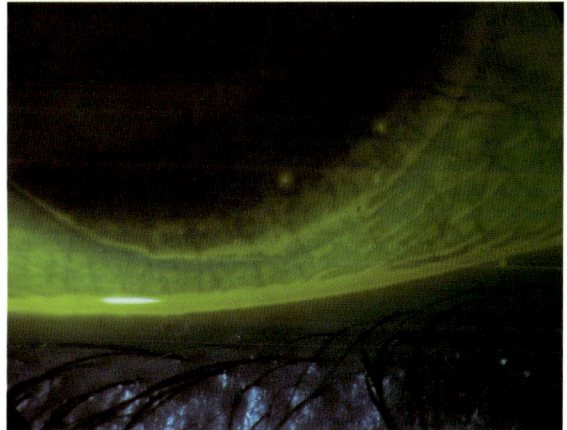

Figure 9.27 Indentation in the inferior limbal conjunctiva arising from a low-riding lens that has bound.

with a flat-fitting lens. Superior conjunctival stain is indicative of a flat-fitting lens.

Lens modification is usually successful in treating the staining. For example, inferior conjunctival stain associated with lens binding would be treated by one of the following:

- Reduce total diameter by 0.5 mm and retrial.
- Try a flatter lens in 0.02 mm steps (remember that small changes in BOZR have a radical effect on the fit of the lens).

Table 9.6 The likely nature of the lens fit with the presence of corneal and conjunctival staining

	Steep	Flat
Central SPE stain		✓
Inferior conjunctival stain	✓	✓
Superior conjunctival stain		✓

SPE, superficial punctate erosion.

- Steepen the alignment curve to improve centration.

Superior corneal staining may also be accompanied with a topographic smiley-face pattern (see Ch. 2, Fig. 2.23A). The accuracy of topographer and lens design will dictate the magnitude of the change in base curve. Generally, increments of 0.02 or 0.05 mm are made when refining lens fit.

Table 9.6 shows the likely causes of conjunctival stain.

Fenestration imprint

Some practitioners feel that fenestrations at the center of the TR reduce the incidence of dimpling (as a way for bubbles to leave) whist others believe that fenestrations may act as an entrance site for bubbles. The fact is that bubbles form under both fenestrated and nonfenestrated lenses. There are also some who believe that fenestrations reduce the likelihood of lens adherence; however, this is an unlikely scenario, as the fenestrations are sealed once the lids are closed over the lens surface. From a purely logical perspective, fenestrations may work to help loosen up a bound lens by allowing enhanced tear exchange with resulting dilution of the mucous layer under the lens. There is much dispute regarding these statements. Moreover, there is no evidence to support or reject the use of fenestrations in orthokeratology. From the authors' experience, if the lens is marginally too steep, fenestrations will exacerbate the problem. The negative pressure under a "steep" lens may *draw* tears through the lens fenestration, and in so doing will also allow

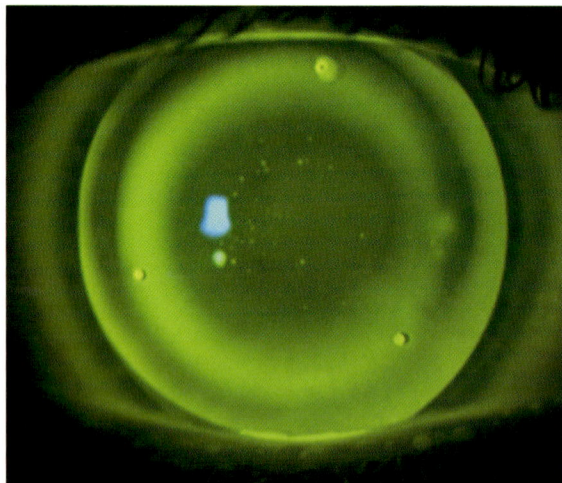

Figure 9.28 Practitioners should note the position of fenestrations prior to removal in case of corneal staining. This figure also illustrates the effect of the fenestration in facilitating the flow of tears out of the fenestration (superior fenestration).

air into the postlens tear film if the TLT is excessive. Thus, the problem may not be the fenestrations, but excessive apical clearance. If fenestrated lenses are the preferred option, always ensure that the trial lenses are also fenestrated, so that easier detection of lens clearance at the BOZD is made by the appearance of bubbles in the postlens tear layer.

Occasionally, one may see a fine local area of staining on the corneal surface on removal of the lens. The practitioner should always make a note of the position of the fenestrations before lens removal as often these areas of staining correspond to the location of the fenestration (Fig. 9.28).

The fenestration should always be placed at the point of maximal tear layer depth of the lens, at the BOZD/reverse curve interface. If staining occurs as a result of the fenestration, the following are the most likely causes:

1. the fenestration is in the incorrect position (on the reverse curve/alignment curve junction)
2. the fenestration is poorly finished
3. the fenestration is clogged with debris.

Corneal staining from fenestrations is a rare occurrence.

Lens binding

During a morning aftercare, slight central staining may occur in a patient who has, until that time, always shown an ideal response to the lens and no staining. This is usually due to an episode of lens binding, and the associated minimal trauma induced by an incorrect attempt at freeing up the lens. Another common cause of this binding-associated staining is the simple act of requiring the patient to present in the morning with the lens in situ. Patients usually report discomfort and mild photophobia and offer the comment that this usually only occurs when they have to wear the lenses into the practice. A simple means of verifying that the staining occurred as a result of the extended period of open-eye wear is to have the patient represent a few days later having removed the lenses at home in the usual manner. If the staining is still present, it is either due to incorrect removal following binding or an incorrect fit.

The etiology and appearance of lens adherence are discussed in Chapter 3. Although most subjects suffer from adherence on waking, most lenses tend to become mobile after a short period of eye opening. The incidence of lens binding following overnight wear with either reverse geometry or standard gas-permeable lenses ranges from 90% to zero, depending on the author and anecdotal reports. Those claiming a zero rate of binding are obviously not assessing the lens fit prior to lens removal, and basing their assessment on patient reports.

The important factor to remember with lens binding is that *alterations to the lens fit do not resolve the problem* (Swarbrick & Holden 1996). Lens binding occurs as a direct result of the alterations to corneal shape and the postlens tear film induced by the lens, and is, in some ways, a patient-dependent phenomenon. Some patients, due to their tear viscosity, are chronic binders, whilst others will have episodic events that appear to be random.

Overnight wear of reverse geometry lenses leads to an increase in viscosity of the tear layer, and this, associated with the molding effect of the lens, increases the viscous adhesion between the lens and the ocular surface. The fluid forces induced by the lenses are modeled in Chapter 10, and it appears that binding *is to be expected* from overnight wear. The majority of lenses will automatically free up following active blinking and induced tear exchange. It is of vital importance that patients should be properly instructed on the correct method of freeing up a bound lens.

All orthokeratology patients should be shown how to loosen bound lenses prior to removal so as not to cause or to minimize any possible epithelial damage. Patients must also be taught the difference in awareness between a bound lens and one that is mobile. Bound lenses are usually quite comfortable, with the main symptom being a feeling of dryness. Mobile lenses, on the other hand, are always a source of mild discomfort to the patient due to the lens movement. Orthokeratology patients never really adapt to the feeling of the lens in the open-eye situation, simply because they never wear them long enough to become adapted. Once the patient can appreciate the difference in sensation between a bound and mobile lens, the technique for removal can be taught. If the lens is mobile when removal is about to occur, no special steps need to be taken. If the lens is bound and immobile, the following procedure should be followed:

1. Instill one or two drops of lens lubricant into the eye and blink a few times.
2. Look upwards, and press gently but firmly against the inferior limbus with the edge of the lower eyelid three times using the index finger.
3. Look downwards and repeat the procedure with the upper lid against the superior limbus.
4. Once the patient becomes aware of the feeling of lens movement, the lens can be safely removed in the usual manner. It is vital that the patient be made aware of the difference in feeling between a free-moving lens and a bound lens. This is usually taught at the trial fit, and then reinforced at the first and second morning aftercare visits.

It is vital to make sure that the patient does not push the edge of the lens with the lid. This will induce a large shear stress that can exacerbate the potential for trauma.

Figure 9.29 shows the sequence of steps required to free up a bound lens.

Once the lens is free, it is not uncommon to see a layer of thick mucus in the postlens tear layer.

This will sometimes stain with fluorescein and give the appearance of staining (Fig. 9.30). If the lens is removed and a lubricant instilled, the "staining" will no longer be present.

Patients who do not have a previous history of lens binding, but present with the signs and symptoms of the condition, should be assessed for any changes in the ocular surface that could lead to increased mucus production or other tear

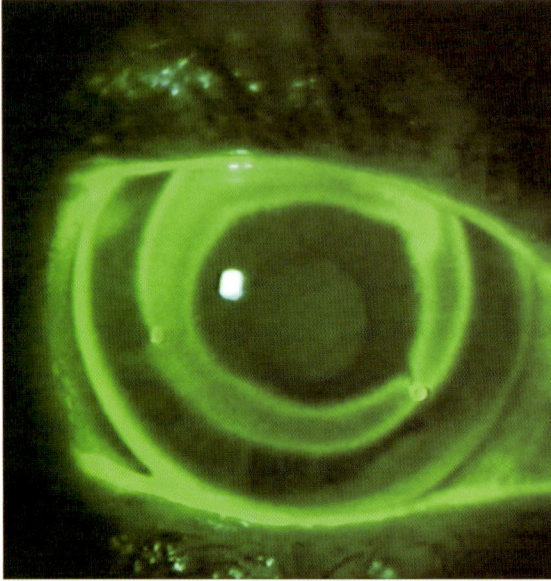

A

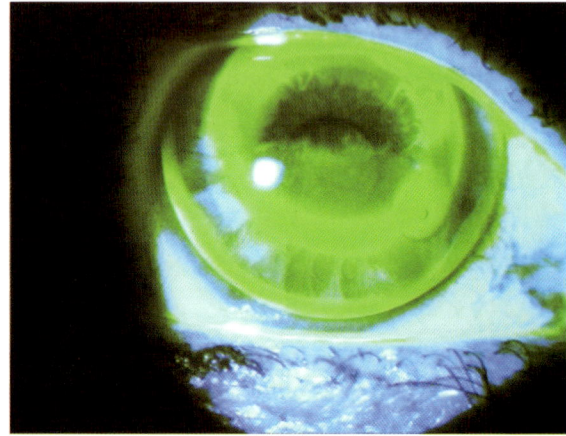

B

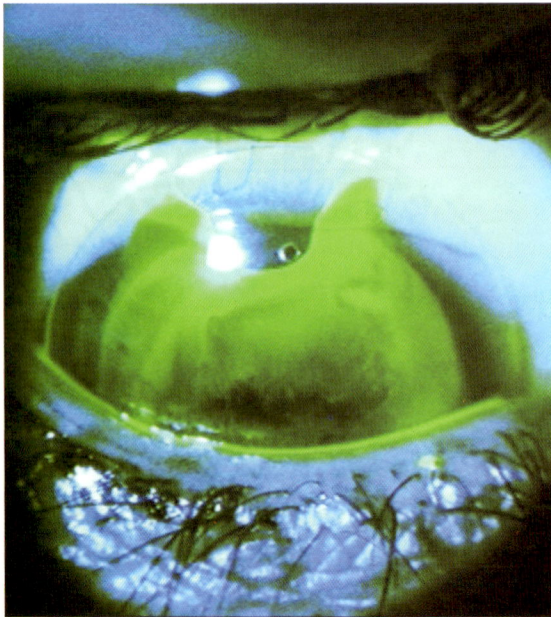

C

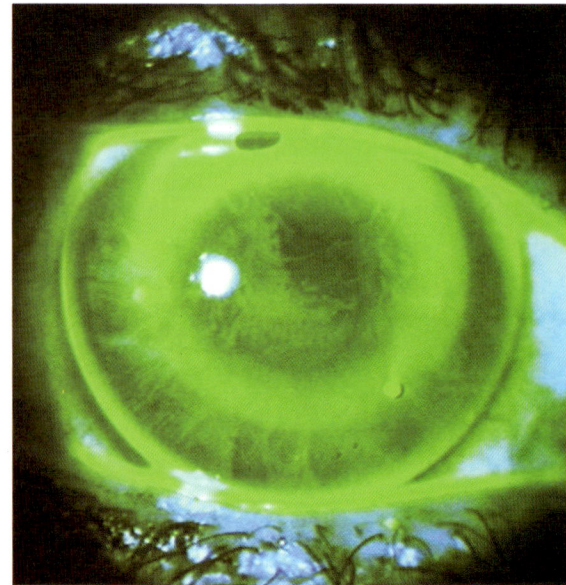

D

Figure 9.29   (A) The sequences of images (A, B, C, and D) show the process of freeing up a bound orthokeratology lens prior to removal. (A) The bound lens with fluorescein leaking in through the fenestrations following the instillation of lens lubricant. Pressure is then applied to the lower limbus through the lid (B) until the surface tension is broken. The same pressure is applied to the superior limbus (C). The lens is finally released (D) with the patient being aware of lens movement. It is now safe to remove using the usual technique. Note the layer of thick mucus under the center of the lens.

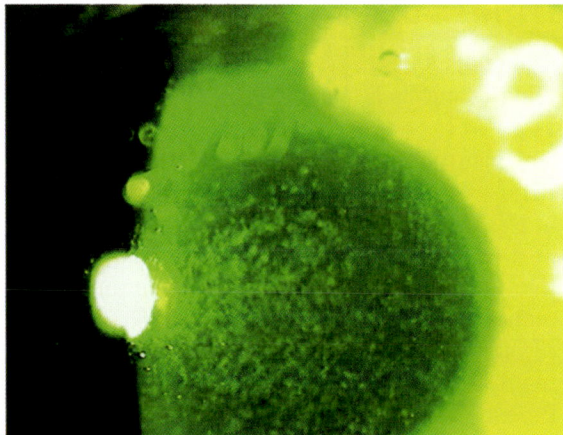

Figure 9.30   A layer of thick mucus is seen that stains with fluorescein. If the lens is removed and a lubricant instilled, the "staining" will no longer be present after a few firm blinks.

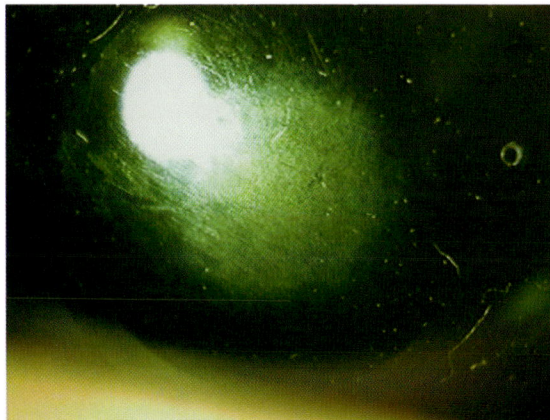

Figure 9.31   Heavy deposit build-up on the back surface of an orthokeratology lens within the optic zone.

abnormalities, and treatment initiated. Also, a heavily coated lens is prone to binding, and the lens must be inspected and cleaned if this is the cause.

In summary, binding should be considered a relatively normal aspect of overnight wear, with a major emphasis placed on the correct removal of the lens.

Surface deposit–induced staining

Central diffuse grade 1 type staining will sometimes occur after 9–12 months of successful lens wear. It is commonly associated with symptoms of blurred vision at night and a loss of retention. This usually results in the lenses being worn on a nightly schedule instead of every second night. The onset of the effect is slow, but usually gets to the stage that it becomes the main motivation for the visit. The single most common cause of this loss of effect is a heavy build-up of deposits in the back optic zone of the lens (Fig. 9.31). It is invariably associated with increased discomfort and corneal staining.

In a personal communication, the late Roger Kame reported that microscopic analysis of the deposits showed them to be a mixture of exfoliated epithelial cells and thick mucus. The average thickness of the films analyzed was 15 μm. This layer of debris has an enormous effect on the mode of action of the lens. The

surface layer on the back of the lens has a dramatic effect on the dynamics of the squeeze film forces, and reduces them to the extent that the cornea does not attain the correct shape following lens wear. The corneal staining often seen in these instances is easily explained when one considers that the apical clearance in orthokeratology is of the order of 5–10 μm. The added thickness of surface deposits of 15 μm will effectively result in contact and thus insult to the corneal epithelium. Corneal staining is resolved by sending the lens back to the laboratory for professional repolishing, or manually cleaning the debris off the lens by using Boston Advanced Cleaner and a cotton bud. This job is best performed by the practitioner as the patient may be too enthusiastic and warp or damage the lens. A thorough clean and polish of the lens is all that is usually required to resolve this type of staining.

CONTACT LENS PAPILLARY CONJUNCTIVITIS

CLPC is a rare complication of orthokeratology lens wear. It is associated with episodes of itching, mucus discharge, and heavily deposited lenses (Fig. 9.32). The treatment regimen is the same as for standard cases of CLPC; special care is taken to reinforce the correct maintenance procedures.

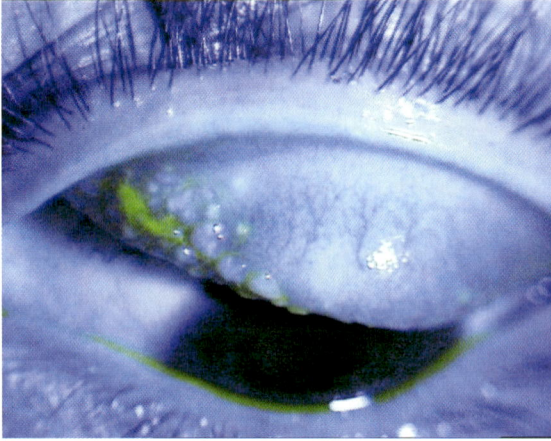

Figure 9.32 A rare case of contact lens–induced papillary conjunctivitis following 1 year of orthokeratology lens wear.

EPITHELIAL IRON DEPOSITION

Cho et al (2002) noted the formation in orthokeratology subjects of incomplete iron rings that occur as a direct result of reverse geometry lens wear. An example is shown in Figure 9.33. The iron deposition is in the same area as the deepest part of the TLT under the lens, and coincides with the area of greatest corneal curvature change. These two factors are the prerequisite for iron ring formation (Barraquer-Sommers et al 1983, Mbekeani & Waring 1998). The ring is *not pathological*, and requires no treatment (Mbekeani & Waring 1998, Probst et al 1999).

Over a 6-month period, the rings become complete, as shown in Figure 9.34. Further studies are currently being performed to assess the incidence

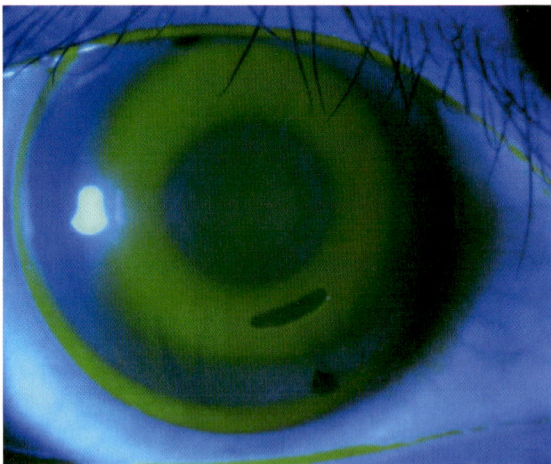

A

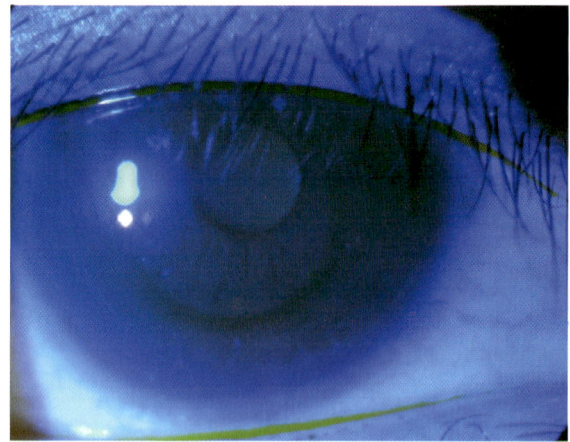

B

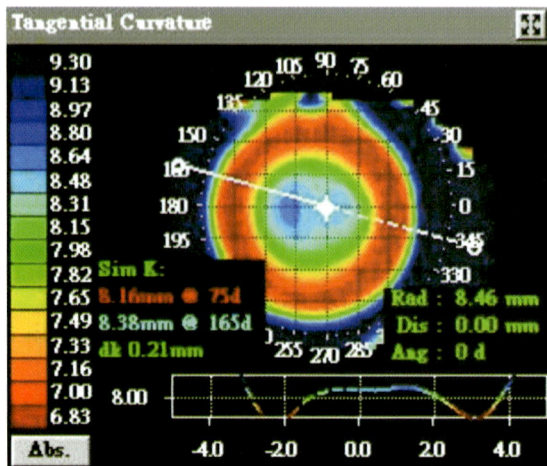

C

Figure 9.33 An incomplete iron ring in a patient who showed ideal topographic and physiological response to orthokeratology lenses. (A) The fluorescein fit; (B) incomplete iron ring; (C) the topography map. The ring coincides with the area of greatest change in corneal curve, and the deepest part of the postlens tear layer. Courtesy of Pauline Cho and Vincent Chui.

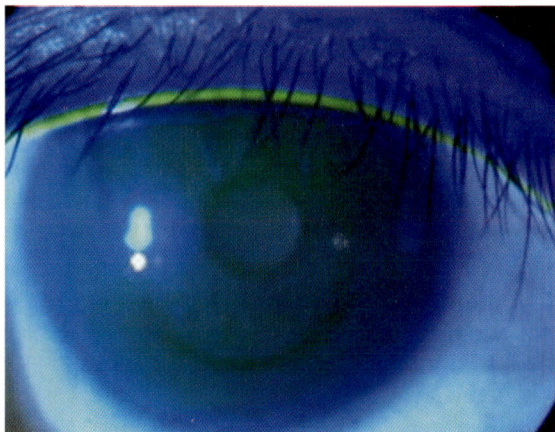

Figure 9.34 A complete iron ring in the patient shown in Figure 9.33 several months later. Courtesy of Pauline Cho and Vincent Chui.

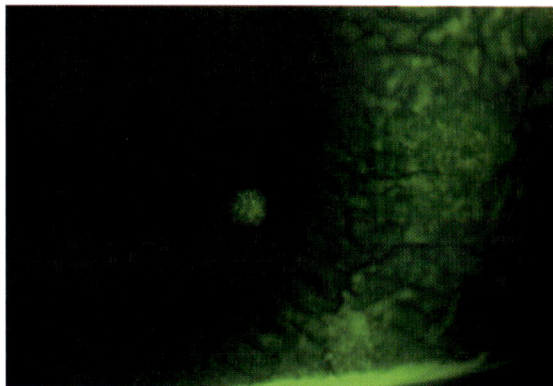

Figure 9.35 A peripheral sterile ulcer in a patient with a lens that bound off-center. No medical intervention was required.

of the rings, and whether cessation of lens wear leads to their disappearance. However, results to date indicate a correlation between higher refractive change and the associated deeper TLT at the BOZD and the appearance and severity of the iron rings. The same ring formation has also been noted by Rah et al (2002) in studies of the CRT and other reverse geometry lenses.

STERILE PERIPHERAL ULCERS

Contact lens-induced sterile infiltrative keratitis (CL-SIK) occurs primarily as a consequence of overnight wear of contact lenses in orthokeratology. It is a rare event and the general etiology is discussed in Chapter 3. Anecdotal evidence (Keddie & Ng 2001) indicates that the problem is more common when lenses of very steep (> 9.00 D) and narrow reverse curves are used and where severe binding occurs. There is no doubt that, as the number of patients wearing reverse geometry lenses for overnight wear increases, the number of these events will rise. At present, it is simply not known whether the cause is related to the lens design, but further research may be able to provide the answers. Treatment is as per the accepted clinical protocols. This will generally involve cessation of lens wear, use of artifical tears, and close monitoring by the practitioner until resolution. The incidence of peripheral infiltrates is rare when the standard reverse

geometry three-, four-, or five-zone lenses are used. Where it is recurrent the patient should be discontinued from the treatment.

Figure 9.35 shows a peripheral ulcer staining with fluorescein in a patient wearing orthokeratology lens that bound severely.

MICROBIAL KERATITIS (MK)

Any practitioner who fits a patient with a lens for overnight wear should be aware of the increased risks of MK involved in the process. The recent experiences in China and Hong Kong show that if proper aftercare or patient compliance is breached and/or inadequate materials used, then this serious complication can occur (for review, see Ch. 3). MK is a serious event. Patients must remove their lenses and seek urgent medical attention.

The importance of using only a material that has an acceptable Dk/t for overnight orthokeratology cannot be stressed enough. At present, these materials include Boston XO, Paragon HDS, and Menicon Z.

LOSS OF THE EFFECT

As stated above, loss of the effect is often associated with the appearance of heavy back surface deposits on the lens. It can also occur if the lens is warped, or simply put in the wrong eye. Polymer

Technology has developed an excellent solution to this problem: in future, all Boston XO materials for orthokeratology use only will be made in yellow and red, with the color denoting either right or left eyes. Warped lenses require replacement. If the problem occurs in one eye only, and the lens is in perfect condition, the cause is far less obvious. In most cases the onset is sudden, and the patient will report poor vision in one eye only over the past week or so.

Topography usually shows decentered distortion, whereas previously the lens had functioned perfectly. The course of events is that the patient realizes that the vision is not optimal and re-inserts the lens the next night in order to resolve the problem. In fact, if the lens did somehow become decentered during the night, then re-inserting it the following night will lead to the lens finding center over the distorted zone, thereby making the distortion worse the next day. The solution to the problem is to cease lens wear until the distortion has settled, and then recommence lens wear. It is therefore vital that the practitioner is able to assess the lens parameters accurately, particularly the BOZR. A radiuscope is a mandatory instrument in orthokeratology practice.

Another factor to consider is the age of the lens. Lenses made out of high-*Dk* materials can have a tendency to steepen or flatten with age. Slight steepening of the BOZR could also include steepening of the other curves in the lens, leading to an increase in the apical clearance and loss of the effect. At present, there have been no concrete recommendations made as to the optimal replacement schedule for orthokeratology lenses, but yearly replacement may be the best way of ensuring consistently well-performing lenses.

There is an assumption that orthokeratology has the ability to retard or prevent the progression of myopia. This has never been proven in a controlled study, so another cause for loss of effect could simply be an increase in the myopia. If, for example, the patient originally had an Rx of −2.50 D, which was fully corrected by the lens, but advanced to 3.00 D underlying myopia, he or she would be effectively undercorrected by the end of the day, leading to the symptoms of blurred vision. The obvious means of determining whether there has been an increase in the myopia is to perform overrefraction over the lens in situ and compare the results to the prior history.

Finally, in rare instances, the procedure simply ceases to be effective. Slit-lamp examination will usually show a "granular" epithelial appearance with minimal or no staining present. In these cases, the most common cause has been found to be poor compliance in that the patient has switched to an inappropriate storage medium, even including tap water! The treatment is to cease lens wear until the corneal appearance returns to normal. Recommencement of lens wear, to date, has resulted in a successful outcome being achieved.

In summary, most problems should be resolved before the lens is dispensed if a correct trial lens wear period has been performed. If lenses are ordered empirically, the procedures set out in Chapter 6 will need to be followed to resolve the difficulties. The majority of problems occurring in orthokeratology are due to incorrect or inaccurate fitting. The other adverse events outlined in this chapter are thankfully rare.

REFERENCES

Andrasko G J (1991) Keeping your eye on edge quality. Contact Lens Spectrum 6: 37–39

Bennett A G (1957) The calibration of keratometers. Optician 151: 557–560

Bron A J, Tripathi R C, Harding J J, Crabbe M J C (1978) Stromal loss in keratoconus. Transactions of the Ophthalmology Society of the UK 98: 393–396

Cho P, Chui W S, Mountford J, Cheung S W (2002) Corneal iron ring associated with orthokeratology lens wear: A case report. Optometry and Vision Science (in press)

Drysdale C V (1900) On a simple direct method of measuring the curvature of small lenses. Transactions of the Optical Society 2: 1–12

Holden B A, Sweeney D F, Swarbrick H, Vannas A, Nilson K T, Efron N (1986) The vascular response to long term extended contact lens wear. Clinical and Experimental Optometry 69: 112–119

Hough D A (1998) Contact lens standards. Contact Lens and Anterior Eye 21 (suppl.): S41–S45

Korb D R, Korb J M E (1970) A study of 3 and 9 o'clock staining after unilateral lens removal. Journal of the American Optometric Association 41: 7

La Hood D The edge shape and comfort of RGP lenses. American Journal of Optometry and Physiological Optics 65: 613–618

Mountford J A (1998) Retention and regression of orthokeratology with time. International Contact Lens Clinic 25: 1–6

Mountford J A, Pesudovs K (2002) An analysis of the changes induced by accelerated orthokeratology. Clinical and Experimental Optometry 85(5): 284–293

Pearson R M (1986) How thick is a contact lens? Transactions of the British Contact Lens Association Conference, pp. 82–86

Picciano S, Andrasko G J (1989) Which factors influence RGP lens comfort? Contact Lens Spectrum 4: 31–33

Port M J A (1987) A new method of edge thickness measurement for rigid lenses. Journal of the British Contact Lens Association 10: 16–20

Probst L E, Almasswary M A, Bell B (1999) Pseudo-Fleischer ring after hyperopic laser in situ keratomileusis. Journal of Cataract and Refractive Surgery 25: 868–870

Rah M J, Barr J T, Bailey M D (2002) Corneal pigmentation in overnight orthokeratology: a case series. Journal of the American Optometric Association 73: 425–434

Schnider C M, Bennett E S, Grohe R M (1991) Rigid extended wear. In: Bennett E S, Weissemann B A (eds) Clinical contact lens practice, vol. 56. Philadelphia, JP Lippincott, pp. 1–14

Swarbrick H A, Holden B A (1966) Effects of lens parameter variation on rigid gas-permeable lens adherence. Optometry and Vision Science 73: 144

Chapter **10**

A model of forces acting in orthokeratology

John Mountford

CHAPTER CONTENTS

Introduction 269
The forces affecting a contact lens on the
    eye 271
Lid force 271
Surface tension 272
Squeeze film forces 273
Finite element analysis 274
A model of the squeeze film force and lid force
    interaction 277
Modeled force and corneal shape changes 284
Corneal sphericalization 284
Forces causing bull's-eye plots 287
Forces causing smiley faces 287
Central islands 290
Astigmatism 291
Static state molding 295
Conclusions 298
A hypothetical question 299
Acknowledgments 299
References 299

INTRODUCTION

"What you've got here is an engineering problem. If you keep thinking like an optometrist instead of an engineer, you'll never work it out." This statement was made to the author by Tony Matthews, a fluids engineer and a total orthokeratology failure. Roger Tabb had always proposed that the underlying factors governing orthokeratology were hydraulic in nature. These two, an engineer, and an optometrist with an engineering background, are ultimately responsible for the development of this chapter.

Orthokeratology lenses "work" by altering the shape of the cornea. But what is the nature of the work? Various terms have been used to describe the change in corneal shape due to lens wear, mainly corneal molding, corneal bending, and corneal sphericalization, but none has ever been subjected to mathematical modeling. The history of corneal molding with contact lenses goes back a long way, with Pearson (1989) citing Kalt as proposing that contact lenses could be used to reshape and contain the progression of keratoconus by "molding" the cornea into a more regular surface.

Many early contact lens practitioners noted the flattening of the cornea following microlens wear (Bier 1956, Morrison 1958, Jessen 1962) whilst others noted corneal steepening with steep lens fittings (Bronstein 1957, Black 1960, Carney 1975a).

Jessen proposed the molding theory, in that the cornea could be molded to the shape of the lens, leading to the development of what is now called the Jessen factor, in that a 1.00 D refractive change could be induced by fitting the lens 1.00 D flatter than K_f. However, paradoxically, corneal flattening could also be induced by fitting lenses steeper than the cornea (Paige 1971, Nolan 1972, Coon 1982, 1984), leading to the development of the "corneal sphericalization" model. Research had shown a tendency for the cornea to become less aspheric during rigid lens wear (Carney 1975b, Kerns 1977, Freeman 1978, Hovding 1983), leading Kerns to note that the limit of orthokeratology was reached when corneal asphericity became zero.

Kerns (1978) also speculated that intraocular pressure or ocular rigidity could play a role in determining the outcome of orthokeratology, but this has subsequently been shown not to be the case (Carkeet et al 1995, Joe et al 1996).

The "hydraulic" model was proposed by Dickinson (1957) and expanded and refined by Tabb (Coon 1982). Roger Tabb had initially trained as an engineer and applied fluid hydraulic theory to the design of contact lenses. The lens was fitted with apical clearance and the back optic zone constructed to contain 70% of the tear volume under the lens. The peripheral zones of the lens were then modified to alter the tear volume under the lens as the cornea changed shape. Tabb postulated that corneal shape altered in response to the variations in fluid force under the lens, resulting in sphericalization as the fluid forces equalized.

Coon (1984) noted central corneal thinning in his orthokeratology group, and proposed that the change in thickness could have a bearing on the refractive change.

Swarbrick et al (1998) have shown that the refractive changes occurring from orthokeratology treatment are in fact associated with central epithelial thinning, and mid-stromal thickening. Central thinning has also been found by Nichols et al (2000) and Soni & Nguyen (2002). The cornea appears to change due to this central thinning, mid-stromal thickening, and as yet unverified bending. These effects are shown in Figure 10.1.

"Molding" is sometimes confused with the term "casting." Casting occurs when a liquid is poured into a mold which, when set, takes on the exact shape of the mold. True molding, in an engineering sense, is the use of positive or negative force (and heat) to form a material into a

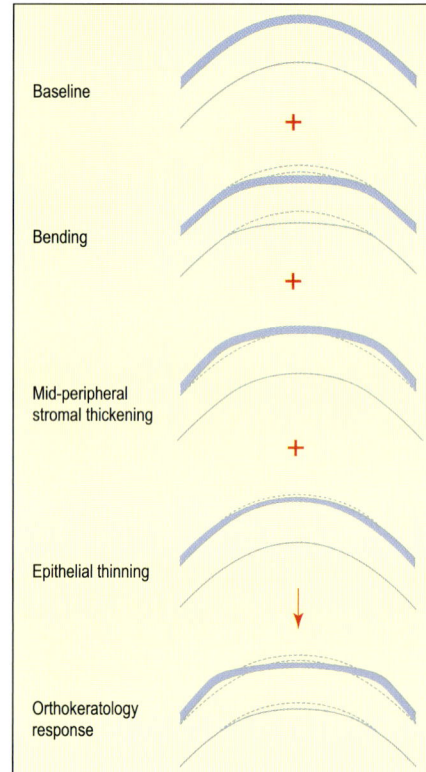

Figure 10.1 Schematic illustrating different models of corneal shape changes, including epithelial thinning, stromal thickening and bending. Courtesy of Julia Mainstone and Leo Carney.

specific shape. The shape of the final product may vary from that of the mold depending on the physical and chemical characteristics of the material to be molded. Viscoelastic solids like the cornea, for example, may require a mold that does not relate to the final shape, due to the effect of the mold on the viscoelastic nature and memory of the material.

Put simply, molding involves either "sucking" or "blowing" a material into the shape required. An example of blowing is the forced injection of foam to form a surfboard, whilst sucking is used to create vacuum-molded products. Orthokeratology, as will be shown, probably involves a form of vacuum molding, as well as a unique form that does not exist elsewhere: "fluid jacket molding."

However, it is the underlying forces of the lid and tear layer under and around the lens that have the greatest influence on the effect that lenses have on corneal shape. In order to understand fully why reverse geometry lenses "work" the way they do, there must be a basic analysis of the forces involved. The literature is relatively rich in this area, with the majority of the work being done by engineers who were interested in the complex forces at work.

The aim of this chapter is to investigate the underlying forces that occur in the contact lens/cornea relationship. Corneal molding can be modeled in two totally separate ways, either by squeeze film force (fluid jacket molding) or hydrostatic pressure (vacuum molding). These will be considered one after the other and the way in which they match clinical observations will be considered. Additionally, the inherent limitations of the procedure will be considered in the light of the insights gained from these models.

THE FORCES AFFECTING A CONTACT LENS ON THE EYE

The most complete work concerning this complex area has been done by Hayashi (1977). Tommy Hayashi was an engineer until he studied optometry at UC Berkeley and came under the influence of Irving Fatt, a fellow engineer. His PhD thesis, "Mechanics of contact lens motion," applied engineering terms, both theoretical and experimental, to the forces governing lens behavior. He defined the forces acting on a contact lens as:

1. gravity
2. lid force
3. surface tension
4. tear layer (fluid) forces.

Gravity acts through the center of the lens mass towards the earth's center. The effects of gravity are dependent on the mass of the lens, with greater lens mass resulting in a low-riding lens. The net effect of gravity and the specific gravity of lens materials, however, are small when compared to the greater effects of lid tension, surface tension, and the postlens tear layer forces (Carney et al 1996a, b). As a result, the effects of gravity will be disregarded in the development of the reverse geometry model, except in the section dealing with hydrostatic pressures.

LID FORCE

During open-eye contact lens wear, the lid is one of the major forces affecting the lens. However, during closed-eye wear, as occurs with overnight orthokeratology, the effects are less significant. Early research into the action of the lids on the eye concluded that lid forces were quite large, as they were associated with a corresponding retropulsion of the globe back into the orbit (Miller 1967, Doane 1980, 1981).

However, Evinger et al (1984) showed that the lids did not force the globe back into the socket, but in effect, there was a co-contraction of the extraocular muscles that coincided with the rate of the blink. This was later verified by Collewijn et al (1985), Riggs et al (1985) and Collins et al (1992).

Moller (1954) measured the intraorbital pressure as a direct result of blinking by the use of a modified Tybjaerg–Hansen manometer. His results showed very small (10 mm H_2O) changes associated with gentle blinking, rising to a maximum of 50 mm H_2O with forced blinking. Lydon & Tait (1988) measured the globe displacement and the force applied to cause it and concluded that the lid force, under normal conditions, was insufficient to disrupt the normal corneal surface. The relationship between displacement and force is:

$$y = 3.84e^{-2} x \ (r = 0.87)$$

where y is force applied, and x is displacement.

Therefore, for the development of this model, the following assumptions can be made:

1. The lid force, by itself, is insufficient to cause corneal shape change.
2. If a contact lens of nominal center thickness (0.25 mm) is placed on the eye, the increase in lid tension caused by the thickness of the lens becomes the force of the lid on the lens.
3. The thickness of the lens does not cause globe displacement into the orbit.
4. The force of the lid under this situation acts over the surface area of the lens.
5. Using the Lydon–Tait model, the degree of the lid force would be similar to the force required to change globe displacement by 0.25 mm.

The calculated lid force, using this model, over a lens with a common chord of contact with the cornea of 9.40 mm, is 68×10^{-7} Nm². The lid force is "compressive" or positive force. The analogy to this force, in optometric terms, is that it roughly equates to 0.5 mmHg.

SURFACE TENSION

Surface tension is the force that exists around the edge of the lens. Kikkawa (1970) showed that the tear meniscus at the edge of the lens, and in contact with air, produced a large negative or tension force that exerted control over lens adherence to the corneal surface and lens centration. The force was determined by the radius of curvature of the tear layer formed between the edge of the lens and the corneal surface. This work was expanded by Hayashi (1977) and Hayashi & Fatt (1980), who concluded that the forces acting on a contact lens to maintain centration could only exist in a quasistatic state, and were controlled by the surface tension forces around the lens edge, gravity, and the reaction force due to pressure in the postlens tear film. They calculated that the surface tension around the edge of the lens was of the order of −2000 Pa.

However, surface tension forces require a liquid/air interface in order to be present (Miller 1963, Greber & Dybbs 1972). A model of open-eye reverse geometry lens wear would therefore require the inclusion of these effects, but these conditions do not exist in the closed-eye state, where the lens can be considered to be immersed in a lake of tears, with no air/liquid interface present. Swarbrick & Alharbi (unpublished) have shown a distinct difference in the response rate of eyes under open- and closed-eye situations, with the open-eye state causing greater and more rapid changes to vision, refraction, and corneal shape. The difference between the two states is thought to be due to the presence of surface tension forces around the lens during open-eye wear, and its absence during closed-eye wear. Also, the open-eye state is in effect a dynamic state, where the influence of blinking, lens movement (both up and down and towards the ocular surface), and gravity all combine to accelerate the effect seen with overnight wear. The open-eye state is a complex system when compared to the closed-eye state. It may indeed produce a faster result, but there are insufficient experimental data available in order to assess the differences between the shortcomings of daily wear and those of overnight wear.

Experienced orthokeratologists prefer night therapy over daily wear due to the following anecdotal factors:

1. The effects appear to be better maintained than that achieved with daily wear.
2. Reverse geometry lenses are not "ideal" for daily wear due to the rapid binding that occurs as the cornea changes shape.
3. Far less adaptation is required for overnight wear than daily wear.
4. Dust, wind, and symptoms of "dryness" no longer occur with overnight wear.
5. Patients find night therapy more effective and appealing.

The effect of blinking on the forces measured under contact lenses was studied by Weiss et al (1975) and Gan-Mor et al (1979). They constructed an elaborate model eye, with a tear pump and lid motion, and measured the pressures under the lens with different lens designs. The results can be summarized as:

1. The pressure levels on an eye are up to 20 times higher with a rigid lens in place than without one.
2. The pressures induced by rigid lenses are sensitive to change in the base curve fitting relationship, with "flat" lenses causing an increase in pressure 10 times greater than the no-lens situation, "on-K" lenses 12 times greater, and "steep" lenses 15 times greater.
3. The pressure on the astigmatic cornea is greater than that on the spherical cornea.

However, in developing the model, they used Miller's values for lid force, and this has been shown to be an order of magnitude greater than those that actually occur. Nevertheless, the trends shown by Gan-Mor et al would still be present, but to a smaller degree. Current orthokeratology treatment is usually restricted to overnight therapy due to its practical benefits over daytime wear of the lenses. Future research may indeed show that daytime wear of a limited period could produce the same results seen with overnight wear, but at present, this is not the case. The model outlined in the sections to follow will therefore be limited to the closed-eye situation, which only involves the interactions of lid force and squeeze film forces, or alternatively, the static system of "vacuum molding."

SQUEEZE FILM FORCES

Hayashi (1977) was the first to construct a model tear layer profile of a spherical lens on an aspheric cornea. The tear layer profile is parabolic, and could be modeled using a simple "slider" analogy. This is based on the assumption that, if the liquid gap between two surfaces is many times smaller in value than the total length of the surface, the forces are similar to those existing between two parallel surfaces separated by a liquid layer. For example, if the tear layer under a contact lens is assumed to be 10 μm, and the diameter 10 mm, the length-to-thickness ratio is 1 : 1000.

This principle was expanded by Allaire & Flack (1980), who developed a model of the squeeze film forces acting in the tear layer assuming a parabolic two-dimensional tear layer designed to mimic a lens on an astigmatic cornea.

The maximum pressure under the lens is given as:

$$P_{peak} = 4.5(\mu\,VD^2/h_0^3)$$

where μ is tear viscosity, V the velocity of the lens towards the ocular surface, D the lens diameter, and h_0 the maximum tear layer depth.

Conway (1982) expanded this formula to include the calculation of the pressure under a rotationally symmetric aspheric surface with a spherical contact lens in place. The formula for maximum pressure (P_{max}) is;

$$P_{max} = \frac{3\,\mu VD^2 \times (2-\alpha)}{8h_0^3\,(1-\alpha)^2}$$

where μ is tear viscosity, V lens velocity towards the eye, D lens diameter (mm) and h_0 maximum tear layer depth. The term α refers to the "steepness factor" and is equal to $(h_0 - h)/h_0$, where h is minimum tear layer thickness.

By integration of the pressure over the area of the lens, the maximum force (F) is given as:

$$F = (3\,\pi\mu\,VD^4)/\{32(1-\alpha)^2\,h_0^3\}$$

Conway's formula for the rotationally symmetric model gives pressure values of exactly one-half those of the two-dimensional model of Allaire & Flack (1980). In both cases, the prime determinant of the pressure and force is the α value, or the relationship between the maximum and minimum tear layer thickness (TLT). If $\alpha = 0$, the tear layer profile is parallel, and the force equal in all directions. However, if α is 1, the whole formula is redundant, *and no squeeze film force is generated*. An α value of 1 occurs if the minimum TLT is zero. When this occurs, the above formula is reduced to zero, with no squeeze film force present. This is the simple reason why all reverse geometry lenses theoretically need to be fitted with some degree of apical clearance.

Hayashi has shown that, if a lens with zero apical tear thickness is placed on the cornea, the lack of a squeeze film force allows the lid to manipulate the lens position until a situation is reached where there is a tear layer present. This occurs when the lens decenters, usually superiorly, until the squeeze force is balanced by the surface tension forces around the lens so that a quasistatic state reemerges.

Orthokeratology lenses that are theoretically fitted with less than zero apical clearance make the assumption that the lens will compress the cornea, thereby changing its shape. In other words, the cornea is "molded" to the shape of the lens purely due to the effect of compression from the lens against the corneal surface, somewhat like pressing your finger into putty. Does this happen?

Carney & Clarke (1972) studied the effects of prolonged applanation tonometry (direct compression) on the cornea with corneal topography. They applied a tonometer probe with varying forces against the cornea for up to 5 min and found no measurable change in corneal contour using the autocollimating photokeratoscope. Any small corneal distortions totally resolved in 8 s. They concluded that direct compression alone was insufficient to cause corneal flattening.

However, Sridharan (2001) found statistically significant changes in corneal shape following 10 min of reverse geometry lens wear that took up to 1 h to return to baseline levels. It therefore

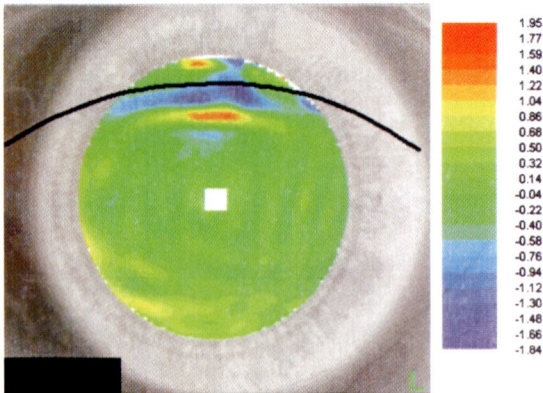

Figure 10.2 Topography map of superior corneal flattening and adjacent corneal steepening from upper lid pressure. Courtesy of Michael Collins.

appears that there is more than simple compression at work.

Beuhren et al (2001) studied the effects of lid pressure on corneal topography. A well-defined area of corneal flattening associated with an area of adjacent steepening occurred at the position of the upper lid (Fig. 10.2). The lid position is shown in Fig. 10.3. The tear film creates a tear wedge at the lid margin that, due to its high curvature, exerts a surface tension (negative) force on the cornea adjacent to the area of compressive force from the lid. The result appears to be a displacement of corneal tissue. The epithelium is an order of magnitude lower in Young's modulus than the stroma, and is sensitive to tangential stress (Kwok 1991). The combination of compression and

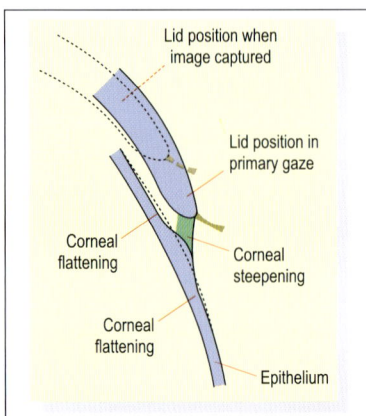

Figure 10.3
The upper lid is shown in the normal and elevated position. In the normal position, there is compression by the lid, and tension from the tear wedge formed at the lid margin. Courtesy of Michael Collins.

tension sets up a tangential stress in the epithelium that induces these changes.

All squeeze film forces are negative or tension forces, and pull the lens towards the eye. The total force acting on a cornea/lens system under the closed-eye state can therefore be expressed as:

Force = lid force (+ve) + squeeze film force (−ve)

This has been commonly referred to as the "push–pull" mechanism.

In effect, reverse geometry lenses "work" by applying both compressive and tension forces at different sites across the corneal surface. These areas of compression and tension set up the tangential stresses required in order to make the epithelium "flow" (for want of a better word) like a Newtonian fluid in order to cause equalization of the forces. Neither compression nor tension by themselves is sufficient to instigate the changes: there must be an initial inequality of forces across the surface to initiate the changes. When the cornea changes, it results in a loss of central epithelial thickness in the order of 20 μm maximum (Swarbrick & Alharbi 2001), but not in a change in cellular volume.

As shown by Greenbery & Hill (1976), the basal epithelial layers lose height, but this is compensated for by an increase in width. In the context of orthokeratology treatment, the corneal epithelium is a constant, somewhat like the law of the conservation of corneal power: it cannot be created or destroyed, just redistributed. This is the basic underlying limit of the process. The epithelium can be "pushed around," but it cannot be added to, nor subtracted from. There is a constancy of volume and surface area. This constancy has its limits of change.

FINITE ELEMENT ANALYSIS

Finite analysis is the reduction of complex surfaces to "finite elements" that interact with each other when forces or stresses are applied. This is then used to determine the effects of forces and loads on everything from car bumper bars to aeroplanes in order to optimize the design of the structure. It is at the forefront of engineering modeling of what happens to structures when loads or forces are applied to them. It is far beyond the parameters of this chapter to delve into this advanced science, but it has been used to study the effects of contact lenses on the cornea.

Pye (1996) applied the finite element method to study the stress effects of contact lenses on the cornea. The model simulated eyelid force applied to the cornea under three conditions: no lens, an alignment fit, and a Contex OK-3. In all cases, the tear layer was included as an incompressible solid with no shear strength. The effects of lid force in the no-lens situation are shown in Figure 10.4. Greater compressive forces occur in the posterior cornea than the anterior at the corneal apex. At approximately 1.8 mm from center, the compressive forces are equal at all layers, and then reverse, so that the compressive forces are greater in the anterior cornea than the posterior cornea. This pattern continues out to the limbus. When an alignment lens is placed on the eye, there is a dramatic change in the stress distribution (Fig. 10.5). The compressive force is greater in the anterior layers at the apex. There is some fluctuation in the stress until a point 2.0 mm from center is reached. The compressive force for all layers then remains constant to a distance of approximately 3.00 mm from the apex, where the anterior layers develop more compressive stress

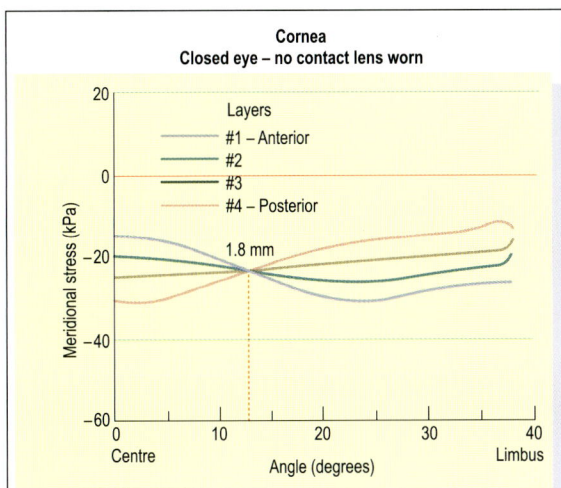

Figure 10.5.   The stress induced by an alignment fitting lens. Note the difference from the no-lens situation. Courtesy of David Pye.

than the posterior layers, and this then continues out to the limbus.

The addition of the OK-3 to the surface does not appear to change the compression centrally to any significant degree, indicating that the flat back optic zone radius (BOZR) has no greater effect than the alignment BOZR. However, the meridional stresses become constant and equal for all layers between 1.80 and 3.40 mm from

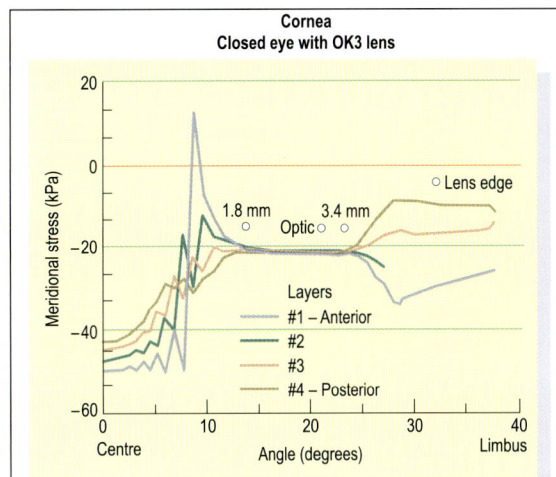

Figure 10.4   Finite element analysis of the stresses on the closed eye with no lens. The stress reverses at approximately 1.80 mm from center. Courtesy of David Pye.

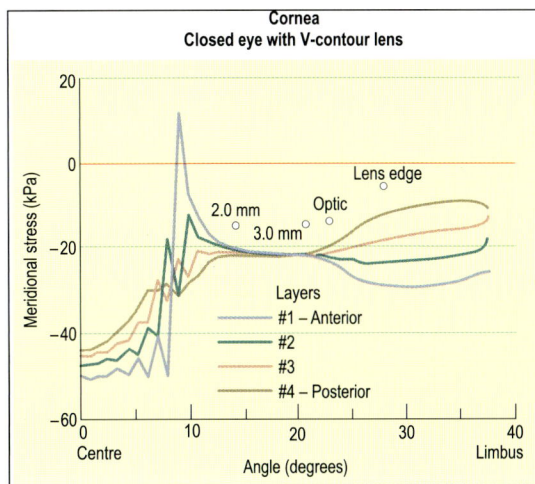

Figure 10.6   The effect of an OK-3 reverse geometry lens on the eye. There is an increase in the stress between the alignment lens and the OK-3 in the area that corresponds with the back optic zone diameter. Courtesy of David Pye.

center, which is a 60% greater surface area effect than that of the alignment lens (Fig. 10.6). The gradient of change from the 3.40 mm zone to the limbus is greater than that of the alignment lens, although the values become approximately equal at the limbus.

Pye concludes that the manner by which the reverse geometry lens may alter corneal shape is due to either one or both of the following factors:

1. The tear layer trapped between the back surface of the lens and the corneal surface exerts an effect that keeps the cornea in a constant compressive stress in all layers. This may prevent the cornea from maintaining its normal shape in the 1.80–3.40 mm area. This

also corresponds to the deepest part of the postlens tear layer, and the area of corneal shape change seen with the lens.

2. The gradient of change in meridional stress outside the 3.40 mm area from the corneal center is greater than the no-lens or alignment lens conditions. The steep gradient may act as a "driving force" to the corneal shape changes seen with reverse geometry wear.

The model was extended by Howard (2000), who manipulated the viscosity of the tear layer under the lens and also added a measurement of the displacement of the cornea caused by the induced stress of the lens. The model predicted that an applied load to the corneal apex would result in "downwards" deflection of the surface associated with an "upwards and outwards" dis-

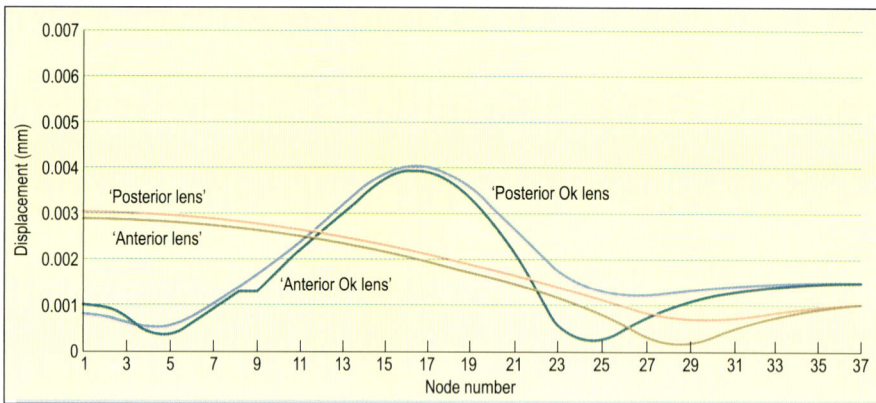

Figure 10.7 The displacement induced by the stress of an OK–3. Note the central backward displacement, and the forward displacement at the back optic zone diameter. Courtesy of Michael Howard.

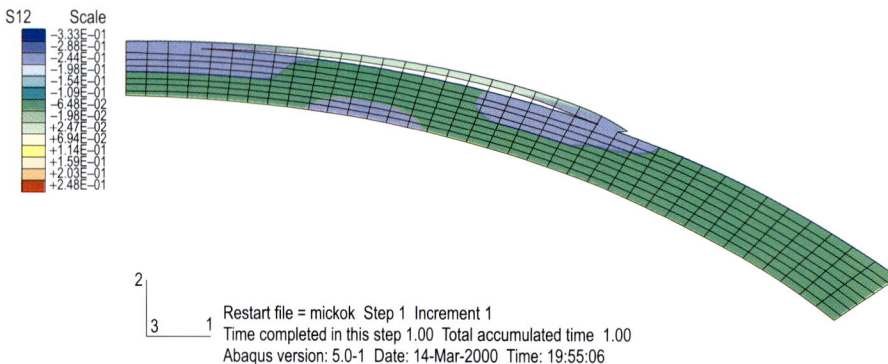

Figure 10.8 The stress on the anterior and posterior cornea. Compression exists anteriorly at the apex and near the edge of the lens. The posterior stromal stress occurs in the area of the reverse curve. Courtesy of Michael Howard.

placement of the cornea in the mid-periphery. The mid-peripheral deflection was due to the hydraulic forces acting on the surface. The displacement of corneal tissue by both a modeled alignment and OK-3 lens is shown in Figure 10.7. The stresses acting on the cornea are shown in Figure 10.8. Note the compression centrally and at the edge of the lens and the tension on the posterior surface of the cornea at the optic zone/reverse curve junction.

The lid forces that were applied in each model differed dramatically, with the Pye model applying 3.9 kPa, and the Howard model only 0.46 Pa. However, both of these models do give some good information on the likely stress effects of the lens on the cornea. The modeled displacements do reflect what is currently known with respect to central corneal thinning and mid-peripheral thickening, and are reflected in the postwear topography plots of treated eyes. Future advances in the application of the finite element method may add more information on the exact interaction of the lens/cornea/tear layer system. Howard, like Pye, found that the overall flattening effects of the OK-3 lens were not any more significant than those produced by the standard contact lens model. However, the negative forces produced in the tear layer under the reverse geometry lens, which reach a maximum at the optic zone/reverse curve border, caused significantly greater changes in the mid-periphery.

A MODEL OF THE SQUEEZE FILM FORCE AND LID FORCE INTERACTION

The following model takes the squeeze film force formulas developed by Conway and adds them to the modeled lid force as defined by Lydon & Tait (1988). It must be stressed that this is a purely hypothetical model. However, the intention is to demonstrate graphically the forces under the lens, and then vary the lens design and assess the change in the model. A further extension will be to try to use the model to explain some of the observed outcomes of orthokeratology lens wear.

The concept of the squeeze film force model is shown in Figure 10.9. The lens approaches the surface of the eye due to the force of the lid, and is separated from the cornea by a tear layer. The

squeeze action creates negative force under the lens, with the escape channel being the difference in shape between the horizontal and vertical meridians. This is a quasistatic state, in that some movement of the lens towards the surface of the eye is occurring. Both the Allaire & Flack and Conway models assume this to be in the order of 0.1 μm/s. As the movement of the lens towards the eye decreases, the viscosity of the tears increases.

Figure 10.10 shows the tear layer profiles of a trio of alignment lenses fitted according to sag philosophy to a cornea of R_0 7.80 mm and eccentricity of 0.50. The back optic zone diameter

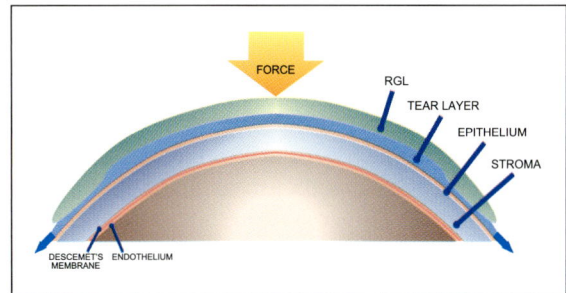

Figure 10.9   A model of the squeeze film force. The lens approaches the eye by the force of the lid through a liquid tear layer. The squeeze film escape channel is due to the difference between the flat and steep meridian. RGL, reverse geometry lens. Courtesy of Christina Eglund, Polymer Technology Corporation.

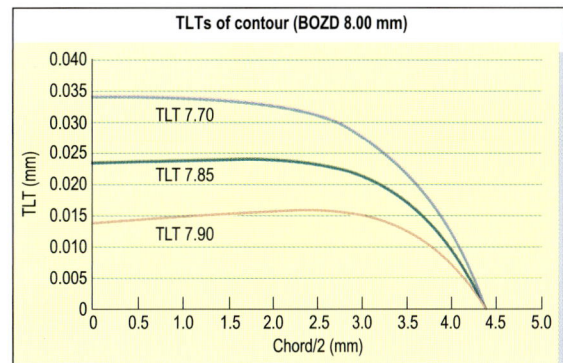

Figure 10.10   The tear layer profile of a group of spherical back optic zone radius lenses on a typical aspheric cornea. The flat lens (7.90 mm) shows less apical clearance than the ideal (7.85 mm) or steep (7.70 mm) lens. TLT, tear layer thickness.

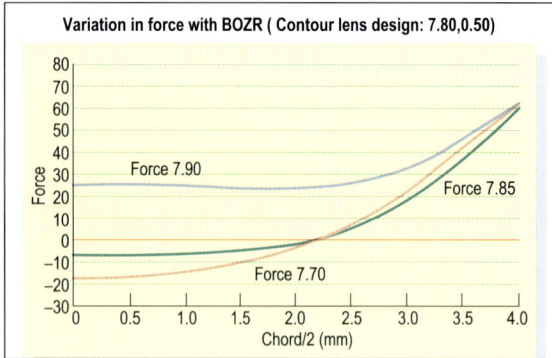

Figure 10.11   The force distribution under the three lenses. The steep lens shows negative (tension) centrally, whilst the ideal fit shows little force centrally, and the flat lens shows central compression.

(BOZD) is 8.00 mm and the periphery is a tangent. The profile extends to the edge of the BOZD. The "ideal" fit, 7.85 mm BOZR, shows approximately 25 μm of apical clearance, whilst the "steep" lens has 35 μm and the "flat" lens 15 μm. This is an accurate reflection of what is observed in clinical practice. The next step is to calculate the combined lid and squeeze film forces and observe what happens. The result is shown in Figure 10.11. Note that the 7.90 mm BOZR lens applies greater positive force centrally than the other two lenses.

As the BOZR of the lens is steepened, the force under the center of the lens becomes more negative, reflecting the clinical adage that steep lenses steepen the cornea by negative or suction force. The force at the edge of the BOZD is positive, and equals the lid force. In the open-eye situation, this positive force is balanced by the surface tension force around the edge of the lens. "Flat"-fitting lenses show greater central compression than do steep lenses, but they also show relative negative tension forces at the BOZD. Optometrists have always understood that flat lenses flatten the cornea by applying compressive force to the surface, and that steep lenses steepen the cornea due to the presence of negative or suction forces under the lens. The modeled forces reflect what is seen in practice.

The values for the force are $Nm^2 \times 10^{-7}$, and this is the unit of measurement used for all successive force graphs.

The tear layer profile of a four-zone reverse geometry lens is shown in Figure 10.12. The lens has approximately 5 μm of apical clearance with a BOZR fitted 3.50 D flatter than K_f. The alignment curve has 10 μm of clearance at the reverse curve/alignment curve junction, and comes into contact with the cornea at its outer edge.

The force graph for the same lens is shown in Figure 10.13. Note that the central area is positive or compression force, but this rapidly changes to tension or negative force at the edge of the BOZD. The force then becomes positive again at the beginning of the alignment curve. Reim (1998) has termed this type of lens construction "dual compression" design, and the force distribution confirms the statement.

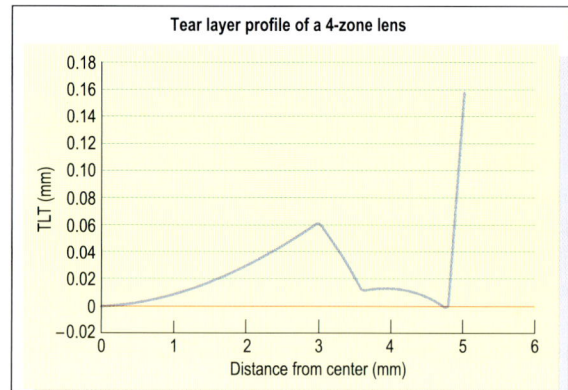

Figure 10.12   The tear layer profile of a four-zone lens showing 5 μm of apical clearance. TLT, tear layer thickness.

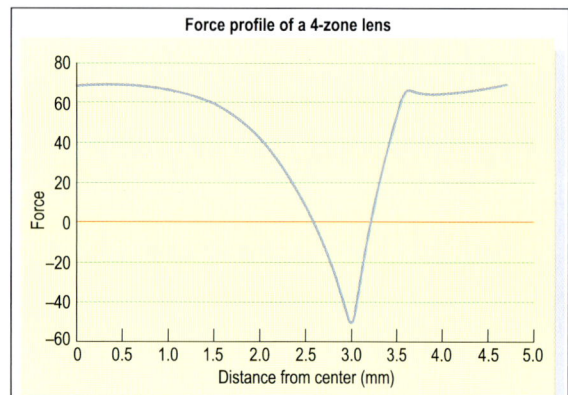

Figure 10.13   The force distribution under the same lens as Figure 10.12. The central force (compression) is positive, while the negative force (tension) reaches a maximum at the back optic zone diameter.

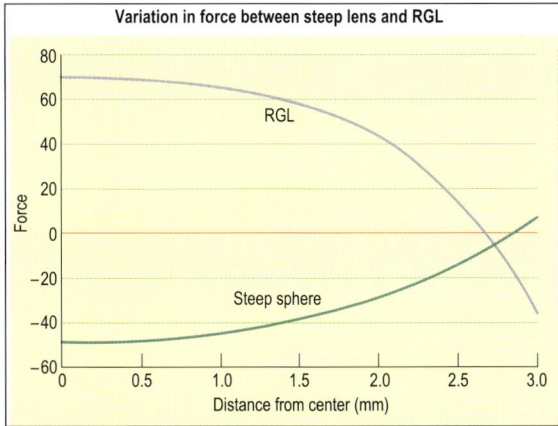

Figure 10.14   The force under a steep lens and a reverse geometry lens (RGL). Both lenses are approximately 3.00 D steeper or flatter than K. Note that the flat lens shows central compression and the steep lens central tension.

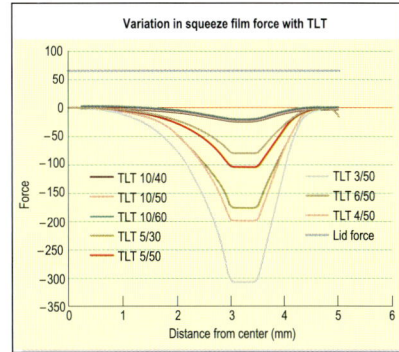

Figure 10.15   The squeeze film forces under a group of varying tear layer profile lenses. The squeeze film force is always negative. The lid force is positive. Note that the squeeze force varies with changes to the tear layer thickness (TLT) centrally and at the edge of the back optic zone diameter. The lens shown is a BE.

The difference between a very steep (3.00 D steeper than K_f) spherical lens and a reverse geometry lens (3.00 D flatter than K_f) over the BOZD is shown in Figure 10.14. Note that they are total opposites. The "steep" lens generates substantial negative force centrally whilst the RGL generates only positive force. However, the important thing to note is that there is a *change* in the forces acting across the corneal surface. The "steep" lens has negative or tension force centrally and positive force peripherally, whilst the "flat" lens has compressive force centrally and negative force peripherally. It is the differential between the areas of positive and negative forces that determines the tangential stress across the corneal surface. This is dependent on the TLT under the lens which, in turn, is responsible for the squeeze film force. The squeeze film force is dependent on the difference between the maximum and minimum TLT (α factor), so a logical next step is to calculate the difference in force on the lens for differing TLTs. This is shown in Figure 10.15.

The squeeze film force varies with the change in thickness of the tear layer, either with increasing or decreasing thickness at the edge of the BOZD, or with alterations to the apical clearance. Note that the lid force (blue line) is constant over

the lens surface. The lid force is positive, and the squeeze film force negative.

This indicates that the variation of the effect seen with the lenses could be due to the change in relative negative force at the BOZD rather then the central compressive force from the lids, which remains relatively constant, as the degree of force centrally is very low.

There are two methods of altering the TLT: keeping the apical clearance constant and altering the depth of the tear layer at the BOZD, or, conversely, keeping the TLT at the BOZD constant, and changing the apical clearance.

In practical optometric terms, the first option is the Jessen factor. Here we change the BOZR as a means of controlling the refractive change. If the BOZR is flatter than the flat-K, the degree of flattening controls the depth of the tear layer at the edge of the BOZD.

This is shown in Figure 10.16, where a four-zone lens is fitted 2.00, 3.00, and 4.00 D flatter than K on the model eye with an apical radius (R_0) of 7.80 mm and an eccentricity of 0.50. The apical clearance is assumed to be 10 μm in each case. Note that, as the BOZR is flattened, the negative force at the BOZD increases. However, the difference between the lens fitted 4.00 D flatter than K_f is very small when compared to the 3.00 D lens. The effect of flattening the BOZR to increase the TLT at the BOZD increases the α

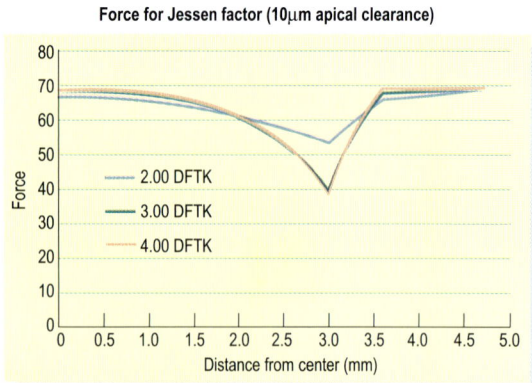

Figure 10.16 The forces generated by a four-zone lens fitted according to the Jessen factor. The apical clearance is assumed to be 10 μm. Note that there is little difference between the 3.00 D and 4.00 D change lens.

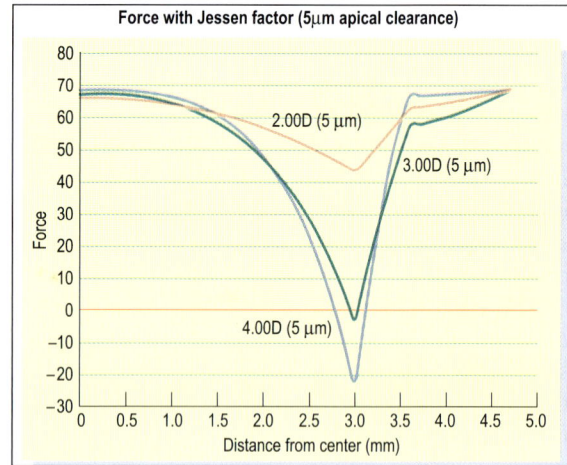

Figure 10.17 The forces under a four-zone lens with the apical clearance decreased to 5 μm. Note the marked increase in tension at the back optic zone diameter (BOZD). The central compression remains unaltered. Once again, there is little difference between the 3.00 D and 4.00 D lens. The apical clearance is fixed, and the tear layer thickness at the BOZD variable with the back optic zone radius.

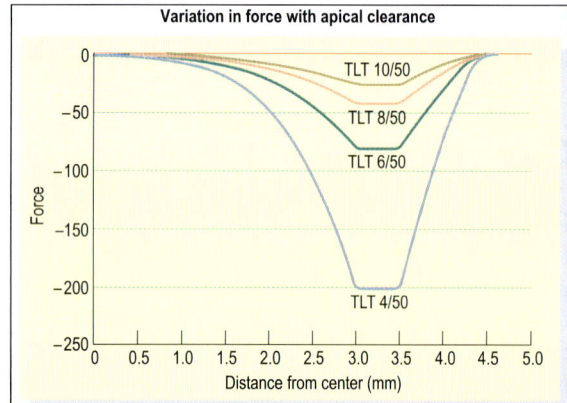

Figure 10.18 The variation in force produced under BE lenses by altering the apical clearance while keeping the tear layer thickness (TLT) at the back optic zone diameter (BOZD) constant. Note that the central compression is unaltered, and that only the force at the edge of the BOZD changes.

factor. Also, the value of h_0 increases, leading to a situation in the Conway formula where increased flattening of the BOZR does not produce a change in the overall force. In the example above, the apical clearance is assumed to be 10 μm. However, what if it were less?

The difference in force with a change in apical clearance while keeping all other factors constant is shown in Figure 10.17. The simple act of changing the apical clearance from 10 to 5 μm causes a major change in the squeeze film force for the same eye and lens design. The force for a 4.00 D refractive change is now a maximum of -20×10^{-7} Nm² compared to $+40 \times 10^{-7}$ Nm² for the greater apical clearance. Therefore it appears that the Jessen factor works by altering the squeeze force by changing the difference between the tear layer at the apex and the BOZD. It is more effective if the apical clearance is reduced. The limit is approximately 4.50 D flatter than K_f, as any greater flattening increases the h_0 to the stage where it has a negative impact on the force. Interestingly enough, Reim (1998) states that the limit of effectiveness for the Dreimlens occurs when the BOZR is approximately 4.75 D flatter than K_f.

The effect that keeping the TLT constant at the BOZD and changing the apical clearance exerts on the force is shown in Figure 10.18. This is the method behind the BE lens design and fitting phi-

losophy. The tension force changes depending on the level of apical clearance. An apical clearance of 1 μm, for example, generates over -2000×10^{-7} Nm² of force at the edge of the BOZD.

However, the compressive force does not vary with changes to the negative or tension force with the exception that the diameter over which it acts is reduced as the negative force increases. This also occurs with the Jessen factor method of fitting, in that the greater the generation of negative force (and thereby, theoretically, the refractive change), the smaller the area of positive compression.

The clinical implication of this is immediately obvious: the greater the refractive change, the smaller the treatment zone (T×Z) diameter and the greater the tension force generated by the tear film, the smaller the area of action of the compression zone. The relationship between the compression zone and the T×Z diameter requires further investigation.

The finite element analysis shows that the compressive effect of the BOZR is of little concern with respect to the stress induced on the cornea. The above model supports the finding, and shows that the real initiator of the shape change is the change in squeeze film force generated by alterations to tear film thickness. In effect, all lenses produce the same degree of compression, but the tension varies with the tear layer profile. This change can be initiated by either flattening the BOZR whilst keeping the apical clearance constant (Jessen factor) or by keeping the tear layer at the BOZD constant and changing the apical clearance (BE). Orthokeratology does not compress the eye into a flatter shape, but rather tends to "suck" the mid-peripheral areas outwards.

However, changes to TLT come at a price, and that is accuracy. Chapter 4 gives the simple rule for fitting reverse geometry lenses:

Lens sag = corneal sag + TLT

The entire premise of fitting lenses according to sag philosophy is that a more accurate fitting relationship between the lens and the cornea than that possible with keratometry will occur. As stated previously in this book, orthokeratology lenses are fitted for an outcome, and not judged solely on the appearance of the fluorescein pattern. The result aimed for is dependent on the accuracy of the fit, particularly with respect to the apical clearance that is the prime factor in controlling the squeeze film forces under the lens. The

difference between the central compressive force and the negative tension force at the BOZD sets up the tangential stress that causes the epithelium to change. If, according to the model, the apical clearance varies, so will the tangential stress and so, theoretically, will the corneal shape change.

This then leads to a few other interesting scenarios with the model. What happens if the original topography data are incorrect or the lens manufacture is incorrect?

An example will be used to show the effect of instrument error (Fig. 10.19). Assuming that the corneal eccentricity on which the lens design is based is 0.50, but the "real" eccentricity value varies, then topography over- or underestimation of the eccentricity will affect the apical clearance values and hence the force.

If the "true" eccentricity is greater than that used to design the lens, then the original data overestimate the sag and the lens will have "excessive" apical clearance. This decreases the force difference under the lens, as shown by the pink and grey lines. Even greater underestimations of the eccentricity lead to less squeeze film force differentials with a correspondingly low corneal change. In extreme cases, central islands occur (see later). If the "true" eccentricity is less

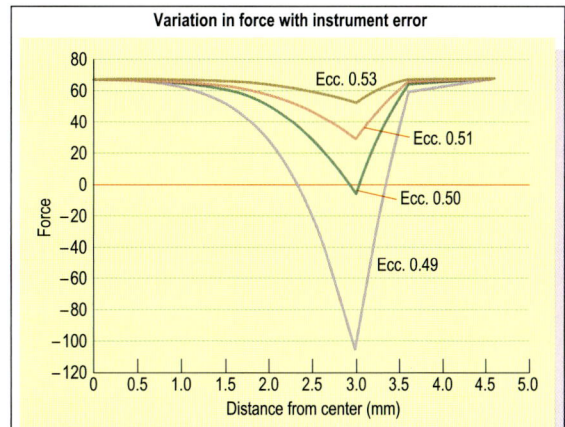

Figure 10.19 The effect of instrument error in calculating corneal eccentricity. Assuming the true eccentricity is 0.50, then if the error produces a lens with less apical clearance, the tension is increased. The opposite occurs if the eccentricity is overestimated against the actual value, resulting in increased apical clearance and less tension.

than that given by the instrument, the sag of the lens will be less than that required, leading to less apical clearance. If the true eccentricity were 0.49, or as little as 0.01 difference from that given by topography, there is a marked increase in the force differences between the center and the BOZD (blue line). Greater underestimations of the eccentricity values lead to zero apical clearance and lens decentration.

The variation in force caused by instrument error raises an interesting question. If the required lens is represented by the green line, but error causes the force represented by the pink line and a less than optimal refractive change, could it explain the concept of "poor or slow responder?" Alternatively, if a lens that produced the blue line were fitted instead of the optimal lens, would this be classed as a "fast or good responder"? This interesting concept will be discussed in greater detail later.

Let it now be assumed that the topography data are perfect, and the lens designed from it is made to the highest standards. The commonly accepted standard of reproducibility for computer numeric-controlled (CNC) lathes is in the order of ± 0.01 mm or ± 2 μm in sag. What effect does this have on the modeled force?

The result of an error of ± 2 μm steeper or flatter than ideal is shown in Figure 10.20. A lens that is 2 μm flatter than required produces a greater force than either the ideal lens or the 2 μm steeper lens.

The difference in force between the two is considerable, and could help to explain some of the variation in responses when a patient is supplied with a "duplicate" lens that either performs better than the original or worse. Also, the difference could explain why some patients are classified as "good responders" whilst others are rated as being "poor responders." In those cases of higher refractive change where the apical clearance becomes critical, this level of error can lead to either over- or undercorrection. Once again, the question of accuracy in fitting comes into the equation. This reaches its zenith when the difference between "what is mathematically perfect" is compared to "what is actually produced." In the examples shown above, the computer program used to produce the lens

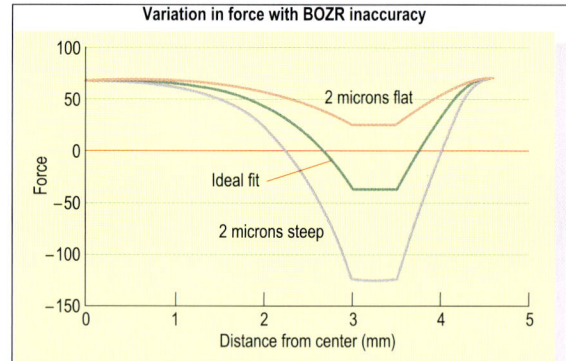

Figure 10.20   The effect of manufacturing error on the squeeze film force. If the final lens is 2.00 μm too steep (grey line), the force is decreased, and increased if the lens is 2.00 μm too flat (blue line) in sag.

prescriptions is set to three decimal places, in that if a specific tear layer profile is desired, the program then calculates out the exact curves required to fulfill that requirement. This is not reproducible in reality, so there is an inherent error present, even in the model.

The theoretical differences between the "calculated lens" (lens 1) where the accuracy is three decimal places, and the manufactured lens (lens 2), where "rounding off" takes place, is shown in Figure 10.21. There is a marked difference between the two, indicating that the simple expedient of rounding off can have an impact on

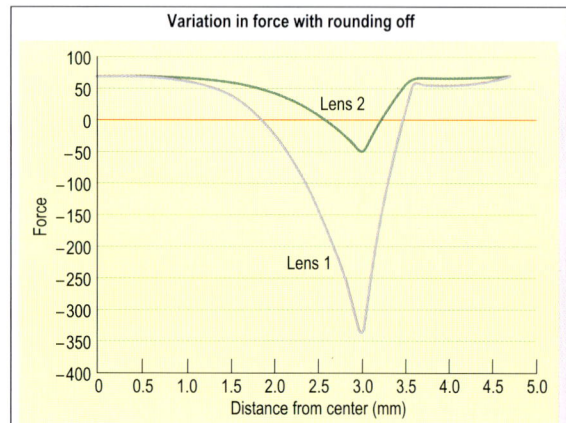

Figure 10.21   The effect of "rounding off" can also have an effect on the force generated under the lens. This can reach significant levels when small apical clearances of 5 μm or less are required.

the results achieved with the lens. In the example, the "calculated lens" has the parameters 8.039:6.00/6.665:7.20/7.673:8.40, whilst the manufactured lens is rounded off to 8.04:6.00/6.66:7.20/7.67:8.40. However, in other cases of modeled changes due to rounding off, there is very little effect. In those cases where the rounding off has a minimal impact on the values, the manufactured lens will cause the same forces as the modeled lens. However, the fact that rounding off does have an effect in certain cases is yet another example of the sometimes unpredictable nature of the process.

A simple rule may be to ensure that the rounding off compensates for any change in sag at the common chord of contact by altering either the reverse curve or alignment curve in order to maintain sagittal equivalency. The differences between the two only become important when very small apical clearances of less than 5.00 μm are required. As stated previously, an apical clearance of 1 μm will theoretically generate a tension force of −2000 Pa at the edge of the BOZD. This is an impossible task, as the limit of manufacturing tolerance at the 95% confidence level is ± 4 μm. Also, the TLT is normally approximately 3 μm and the lens is assumed to rest on the tear layer.

The limit of the squeeze film force is therefore set by some boundary conditions in that the theoretically possible minimal apical clearance is in the order of 3 μm whilst the maximum that will cause a difference in relative force between the center and the BOZD is approximately 20 μm. The model would therefore indicate that the "window" in which orthokeratology can be effective is between apical clearance values of 4 and 20 μm. This is shown by the difference in force generated by a four-zone lens fitted 4.50 D flatter than K_f (0.50 D compression factor) with 5 μm of apical clearance. If the apical clearance is increased to 20 μm, the force differential between compression and tension is negligible (Fig. 10.22).

The force profiles of two different lens designs are shown in Figure 10.23. Both lenses were calculated using the best standard of lens manufacture possible, and the closest-fitting sag match allowing for apical clearance. The graph shows the force developed under a Dreimlens and a BE lens

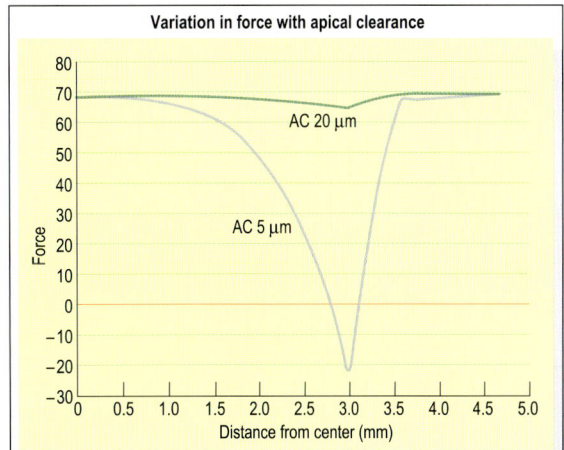

Figure 10.22   A four-zone lens is shown with the relative limits of the squeeze film force and apical clearance. The minimum apical clearance is between 4 and 5 μm, whilst the maximum appears to be approximately 20 μm before there is little or no tension developed at the edge of the optic zone (back optic zone diameter). AC, alignment curve.

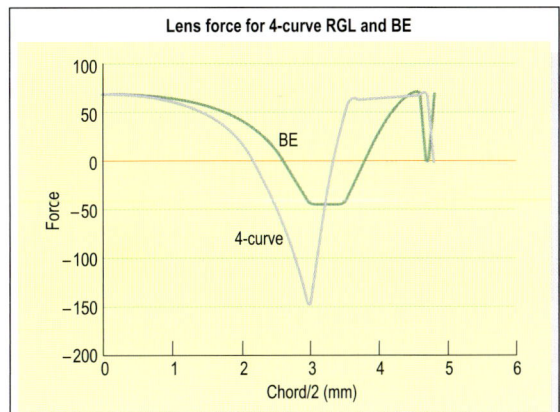

Figure 10.23   The difference in squeeze film force between two different designs, the four-curve design (Dreimlens) and the BE, for the same expected refractive change. The Dreimlens is a "dual compression" design, whereas the BE is based on maximizing the tangential stress across the corneal surface.

for a cornea requiring a 3.00 D refractive change. Note that the force difference between the center and the BOZD is different, and that the compression gradient in the periphery is totally different. The main difference between the designs is the intersection of the compression zone from positive to the negative tension area. This could theoretically result in a difference in T×Z diameters between the designs. Also, the Dreimlens is a "dual compression" lens, whilst the BE is designed under the assumption that the tangential stress is maximized and then extended over a larger area.

The modeled forces under the lens show the sensitivity of the system to changes in the tear layer profile, with particular reference to the apical clearance. The important thing to note is that the values generated by the model are *purely relative*, and are not absolute values. However, it is the *trend* that accuracy is essential in fitting that is of major importance. The α value gives an independent method of assessing the difference between the "calculated" and actual apical clearance of a lens, and can be used as a method of refining the lens fit.

In developing the model, the same assumptions about the velocity of the lens towards the corneal surface and tear viscosity made by both Allaire & Flack (1980) and Conway (1982) were used. In theory, as the velocity of the lens decreases, the viscosity of the tears increases. Conway points out that the inclusion of the α factor is vital, and that all other parameters are basically independent of it. The force will also change depending on the lens diameter and the modeled lid force.

In this model, the force is proportional to the thickness of the lens, so some variation in thickness will lead to a variation in the force. If the lens center thickness is decreased to 0.15 mm, the lid force changes from $68 \times$ to 52×10^{-7} Nm², whilst an increase in center thickness to 0.30 mm would increase the force to 81×10^{-7} Nm². Alterations to the lid force would simply alter the central compressive force, with no real difference to the tension force at the edge of the optic zone or BOZD (Fig. 10.24). However, the tangential stress exerted on the surface is a derivative of the difference between the maximums of the compression and tension values. The slope of the tangential stress would therefore be affected by alteration to lens center thickness, with a hypothesized decreased effect with thinner lenses and an increased effect with thicker lenses. The limitation to this is the *Dk/t* of the lens. There is little point

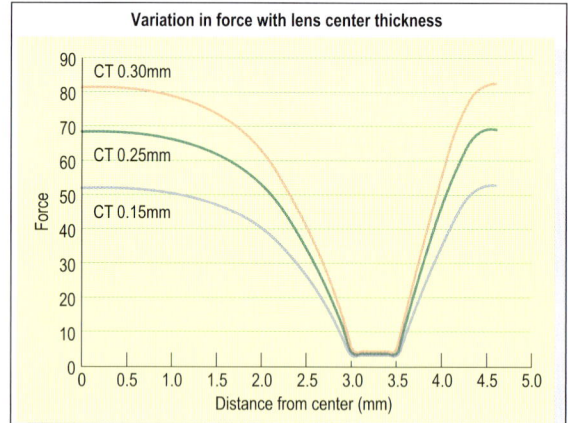

Figure 10.24 The effect of altering the central thickness of the lens. If the central thickness is increased, the central compression also increases. Decreasing the central thickness decreases the central compression, but neither affects the tension at the edge of the back optic zone diameter. The limit is really set by the reverse curve, which determines the overall central thickness of the lens.

in making the lens thicker if the result is an increased risk of edema.

MODELED FORCE AND CORNEAL SHAPE CHANGES

The test of a model is to compare the theoretical results with those that occur in practice. The following section compares the calculated force distribution under the lens to the results seen clinically to ascertain the value of the model. The scenarios are: corneal sphericalization, bull's-eye plots, smiley faces, central islands, and the mystery of astigmatism.

CORNEAL SPHERICALIZATION

One of the simple basic laws of fluid hydraulics and physics is that nature is always seeking equilibrium. The forces beneath a reverse geometry lens in a quasistatic state are not in equilibrium. Compressive forces exist centrally with relative tension forces at the edge of the BOZD. The tear layer itself is an incompressible fluid, but the cornea is not. As a result, the tangential stress

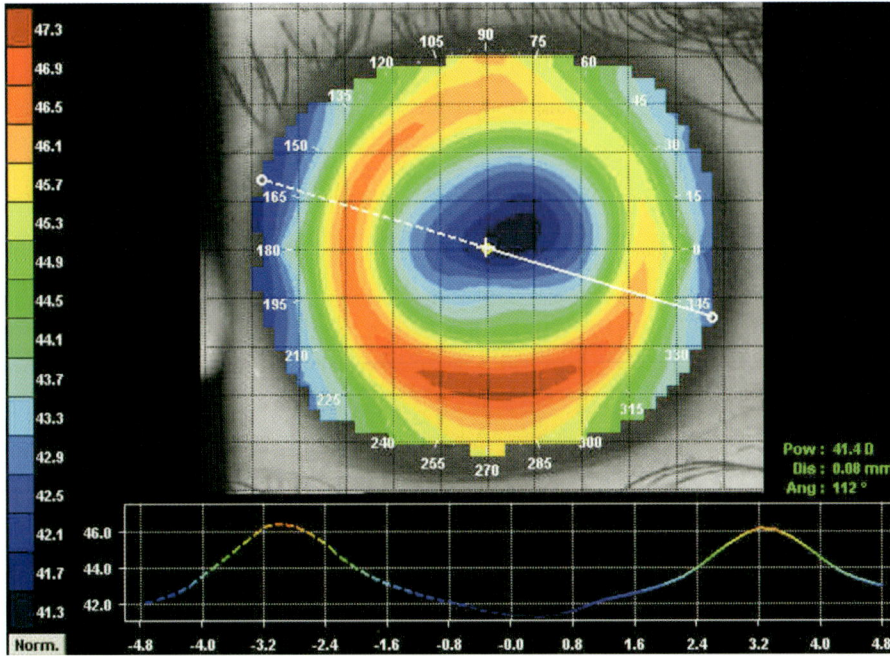

Figure 10.25   Bull's-eye postwear topography plot showing areas of isodioptric change and areas of equal sphericalization. The greatest change should always occur at the apex of the cornea.

across the corneal surface initiates surface shape changes such that the cornea is altered until a state of equilibrium of force exists in the postlens tear layer. Areas of disparate force will always find equilibrium over the smallest possible surface area. The smallest surface area is a sphere (Kwok 1984).

In theory the central cornea will alter shape until a spherical surface exists over the diameter required for equalization to occur. Since the initial corneal shape is aspheric, the equalization will occur over discrete zones (Fig. 10.25).

The corneal shape change is associated with central epithelial thinning and mid-peripheral stromal thickening (Swarbrick et al 1998, Swarbrick & Alharbi 2001). There is little or no change in the extreme periphery (Mountford 1997, Lui & Edwards 2000).

Therefore, as the cornea changes shape, the apical clearance increases as the epithelium thins, and the depth of the tear layer at the BOZD decreases as the stroma thickens. This can be modeled using Noack's relationship between corneal radius change and asphericity. The modeled lens is placed on the initial cornea (R_0 7.80, 0.50 eccentricity), and then the baseline corneal data altered to include the R_0 and eccen-

tricity changes as the cornea alters from a prolate geometry to a sphere. The maximum central corneal thickness change is assumed to be 20 μm, so at the start the lens will have a calculated apical clearance of 5 μm, increasing to a

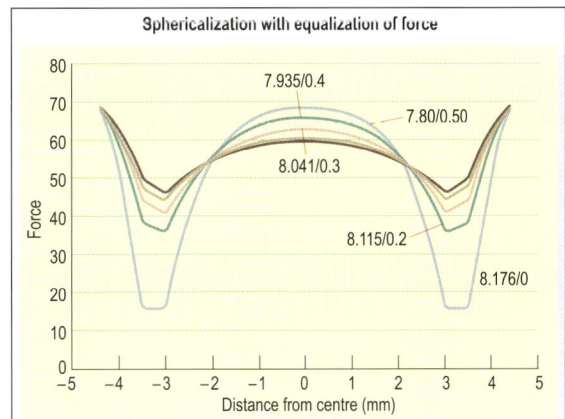

Figure 10.26   The equalization of force occurring under the lens as the cornea changes from a prolate ellipse to a sphere following the Noack model. Note the drop in central compression and the decrease in tension at the edge of the optic zone (back optic zone diameter). In theory, the final line should be virtually straight. This graph can also explain why the same lens works on the altered eye shape, and the effects of regression (see text).

maximum of 25 µm by the stage sphericalization is reached.

The change in the force is shown in Figure 10.26. As the cornea alters shape, there is a decrease in central compression and also in tension at the edge of the BOZD, leading to virtual equalization at sphericalization. The limitation of the model in this instance is due to the inability to determine correctly the volume of the torus generated in the postwear cornea at the BOZD (red ring in Fig. 10.25). If this were possible, the postwear force line would theoretically be a straight line.

The graph answers an interesting question. A reverse geometry lens is designed and fitted to the prefit cornea, based on the rules of sag fitting. It then proceeds to alter the shape of the cornea dramatically. The question that follows is: why does the same lens still work on the altered corneal shape?

For example, the changes occurring with the first overnight wear rarely cause a total reduction in myopia, and the lens needs to be worn every night until the full change is achieved. In Figure 10.26, the initial force exerted on the lens is the dark blue line. Assuming that the cornea changes shape such that the force becomes the light blue line after the first overnight wear period, then total refractive change has not occurred. The lens is not worn during the day, so the cornea regresses to the pink line. That night, on insertion, the instigating force is now the pink line and not the red. Once again, the cornea is altered in the quest for equalization of force, and progressively reaches the goal. When regression occurs, the force generated by the lens on the altered

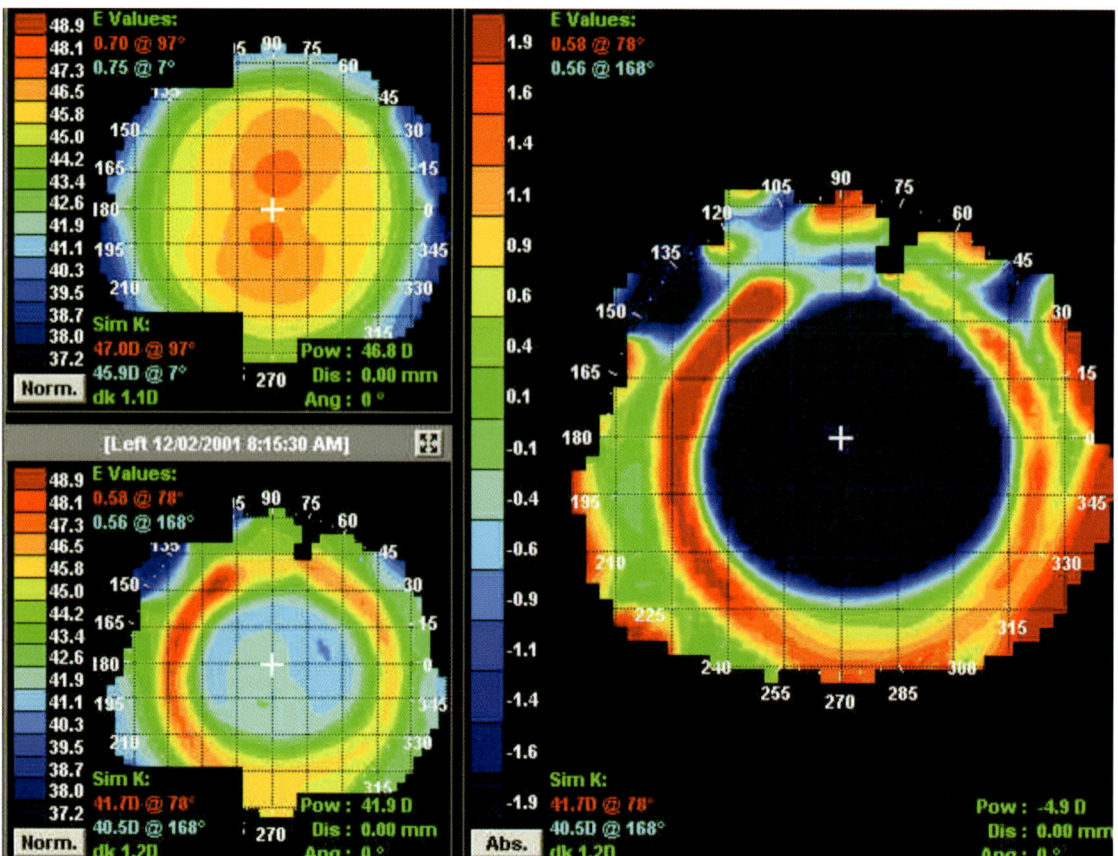

Figure 10.27 A classic bull's eye plot showing a 4.90 D change at the corneal apex. Note that the postwear cornea is spherical centrally.

corneal shape will fall somewhere between the initial and equalized states. This cascade of events is totally dependent on the lens being the correct fit in the first instance, and also that a bull's-eye postwear topography plot occurs.

FORCES CAUSING BULL'S-EYE PLOTS

The requirements for a bull's-eye response are simple: optimized redistribution of force and centration. Figure 10.27 shows the change in corneal topography for a 4.50 D myope, with initial corneal data of R_0 7.20 mm and eccentricity 0.75. The refractive change achieved was 4.90 D with a final R_0 of 8.05 mm and an eccentricity of zero. It should be pointed out that the postwear eccentricity values in the top left-hand side of the lower left plot are totally erroneous. As has been shown by Lui & Edwards (2000), the elliptical model of corneal shape breaks down following reverse geometry lens wear. Also, Tang et al (2000) have shown the inability of corneal topographers to record bicurve and oblate surfaces accurately. An eccentricity value of 0.56 is given for the surface, whilst the axial map shows a spherical surface centrally. In an attempt to overcome the limitations of the torus, the postwear topography data were used to create a "best-fit" asphere and the initial lens placed on the surface. The tear layer profile was then calculated followed by the force. The change in force for this eye is shown in Figure 10.28. Note that in the initial phase the force is centered on the cornea apex (point zero on the x-axis). Following lens wear, equalization of force occurs. The "red ring" that appears as an area of corneal steepening is aligned with the area of maximum tension under the lens.

The model shows that, for a bull's eye to occur, the force must be well-centered, meaning that the lens fit is optimal. In order for this to occur, the data on which the lens is calculated must be accurate, and this is dependent on the accuracy of the topography data and the refinements made following the overnight trial.

However, the fit is less than optimal in some cases, resulting in either a smiley-face or central island postwear plot.

FORCES CAUSING SMILEY FACES

Clinical experience indicates that a smiley-face topographic response is caused by a flat lens that decenters, usually superiorly. This is a commonly accepted fact by all orthokeratology lens designers and fitters. The remedial action required to correct a smiley face is the same for all lens designs: steepen the fit. Placed in the context of

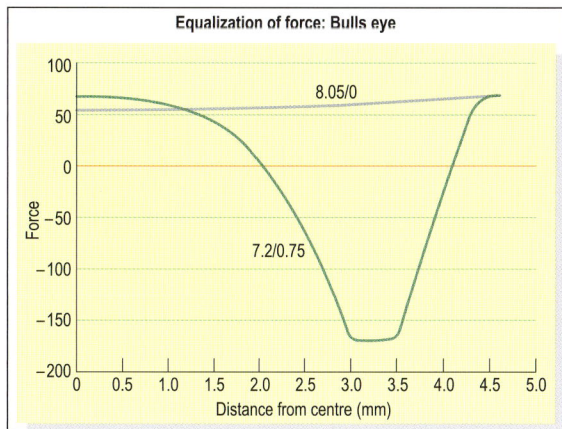

Figure 10.28   The prefit and postwear topographical data from the eye in Figure 10.27 were used to generate the difference in squeeze film force. The final force is equalized across the surface. Complex surface shape analysis of the final corneal curves was used to generate the "final" tear layer profile on which the force was calculated. Bull's-eye plots occur due to ideal lens fit and distribution of force.

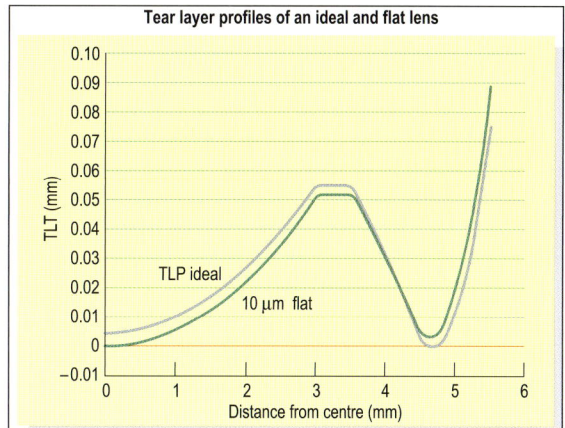

Figure 10.29   The ideal tear layer profile of a BE lens and one that is fitted 10 μm too flat. The flat lens shows central touch, and clearance at the tangent zone. This usually causes superior decentration.

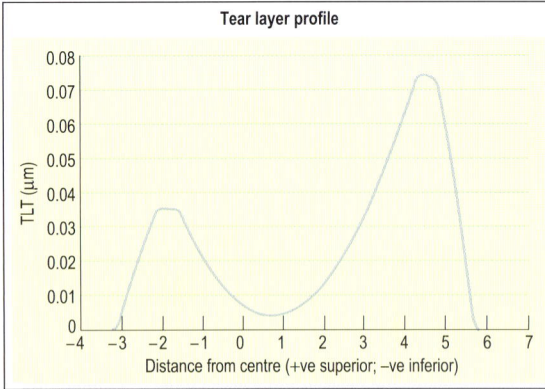

Figure 10.30 The tear layer profile of the vertical meridian of a lens fitted 10 μm too flat. The lens has decentered 1.00 mm superiorly until an apical clearance of approximately 5.00 μm exists. Note that the tear layer thickness is deeper superiorly than inferiorly.

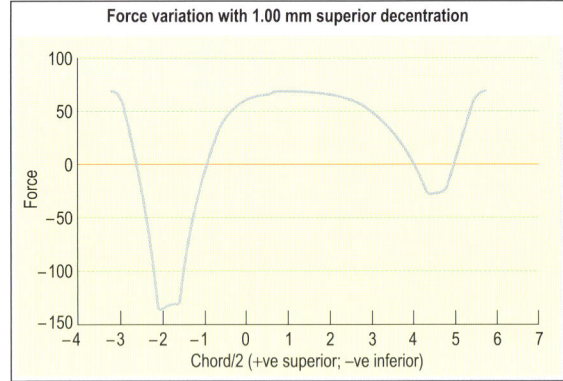

Figure 10.31 The squeeze force generated by the flat lens shows greater tension inferiorly. The compression zone is superior to the corneal apex.

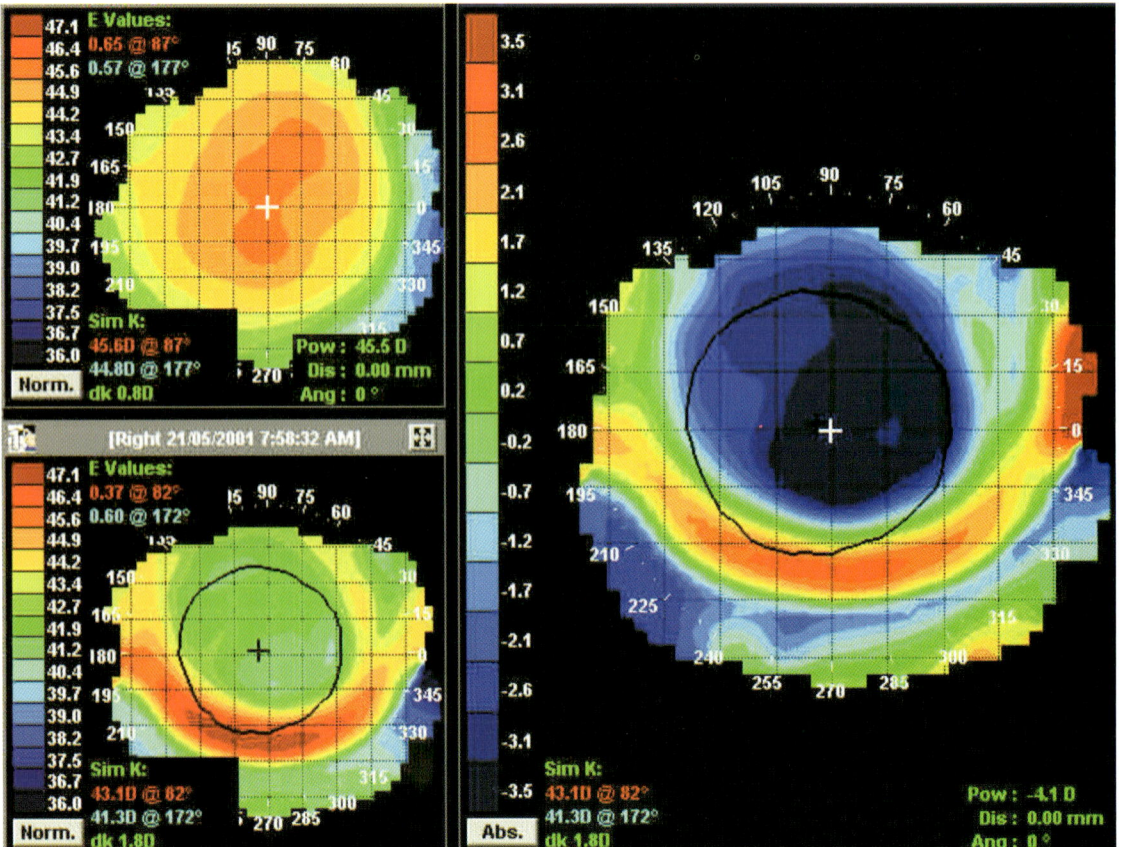

Figure 10.32 A smiley-face postwear topography plot. Note that the flattened zone is aligned with the compression zone in Figure 10.31. The area of maximum tension inferiorly aligns with the red crescent of the smile.

sag philosophy, this simply means that the sag of the lens was initially less than that of the cornea, and is rectified by increasing the sag of the lens by alterations to either the alignment curves or reverse curve. An "ideal" tear layer profile (blue line) and one due to a lens fitted 10 μm too "flat" is shown in Figure 10.29. Note that the flat lens touches at the apex and has clearance at the normal point of contact in the periphery. Under these conditions, a squeeze film force does not exist, so the lid moves the lens until a tear layer that forms a squeeze film is produced (Hayashi 1977).

The tear layer of the lens with 1 mm superior decentration is shown in Figure 10.30. A small (5 μm) clearance is present, with the superior area showing a deeper tear layer at the edge of the BOZD than the inferior. The force generated is shown in Figure 10.31. Note that the area of compression is decentered superiorly and that the tension force is greater in the inferior section. The superior area shows less tension than the inferior, which is contrary to what would normally be expected, as the tear layer is deeper superiorly than inferiorly. This is due to the boundary conditions placed on the α factor, in that there is an upper limit of TLT that will occur before the force decreases. In this instance, the maximum tension developed at 4.2 mm superiorly is -26×10^{-7} Nm^2, compared to -134×10^{-7} Nm^2 at 2.00 mm inferiorly. A smiley-face postwear plot is shown in Figure 10.32.

It is interesting to note that the superior area of flattening on the map is in the same position as the compression zone in the force graph. Also, the red "smile" of steepening occurs at a point

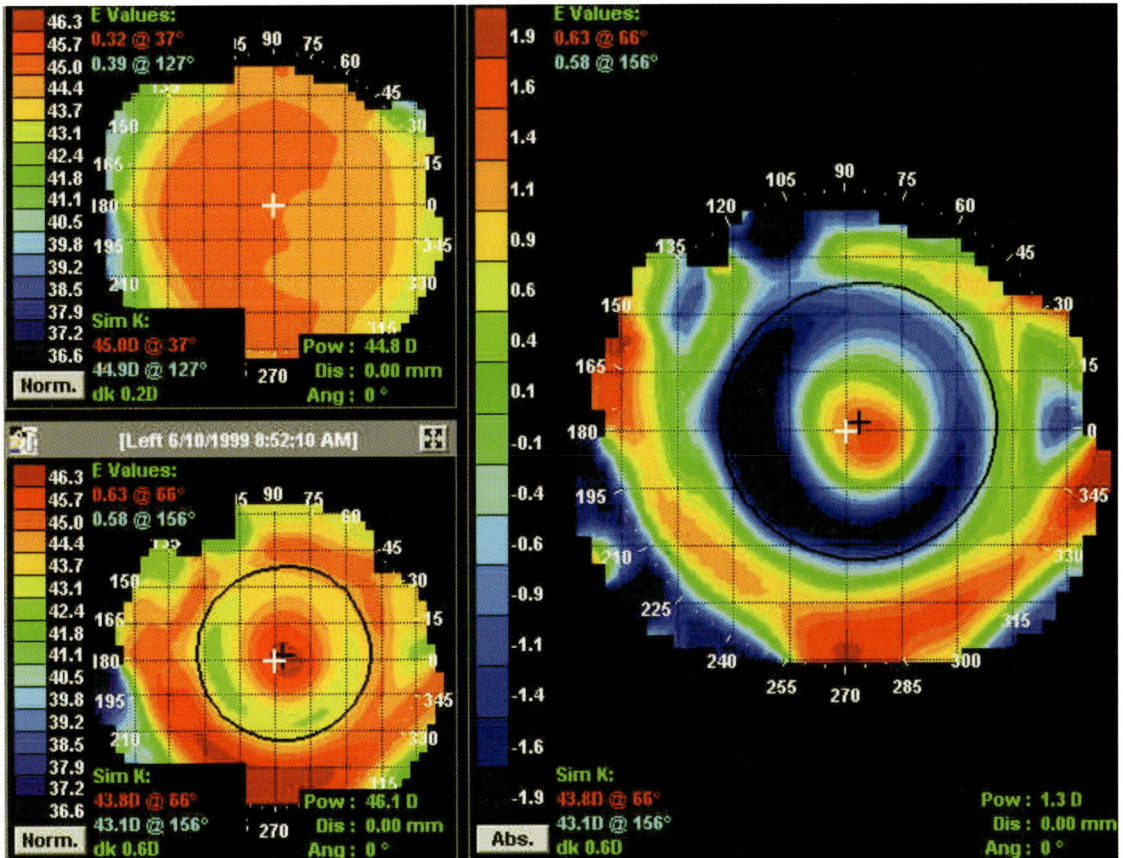

Figure 10.33   A central island postwear plot. Note the apical steepening surrounded by a moat of flattening. The centration is perfect.

2.00 mm inferiorly, which corresponds to the area of greatest tension on the force graph. The model therefore indicates that smiley faces are caused by an inequality of the squeeze film forces between the superior and inferior cornea that is produced when a lens of insufficient apical clearance is decentered by the lid.

CENTRAL ISLANDS

Central islands are caused by steep lenses that exhibit excessive apical clearance, or alternatively, lenses that have a tight alignment curve that causes "peripheral compression." However, as has been shown before, if the apical clearance is excessive, the squeeze film force differential under the lens is minimal, and there is little change in corneal shape. Central islands cause marked changes in corneal shape but with an accompanying decrease in corrected vision due to the central distortion (Fig. 10.33). Note the excellent centration and the steeper central zone surrounded by a "moat" of increased corneal flattening followed by the red ring of steepening. What type of squeeze film force could create this?

Modeling central islands requires some rethinking of the tear layer distribution under the lens. The Conway model assumes an axis-symmetrical surface, with a slight difference between the meridians to act as an escape mechanism for the fluid. In clinical terms, the escape channel becomes either a small degree of with-the-rule astigmatism or, in purely aspheric surfaces, the difference in eccentricity between the flat and steep meridian, and the difference between the horizontal and vertical corneal diameter. The model is based on the assumption that the minimum TLT occurs at the corneal apex, and that greater degrees of clearance at the lens periphery do not affect the α function. In cases where the apical clearance is excessive, the alignment curve is tight, resulting in "seal-off" in the flat meridian. In these cases, the minimum TLT occurs at the periphery of the lens, and not centrally. In effect, the squeeze film force is reversed. The maximum TLT is still present at the edge of the BOZD, but the minimum occurs at a point along the alignment curve in the steep meridian or vertical corneal diameter. The α function is

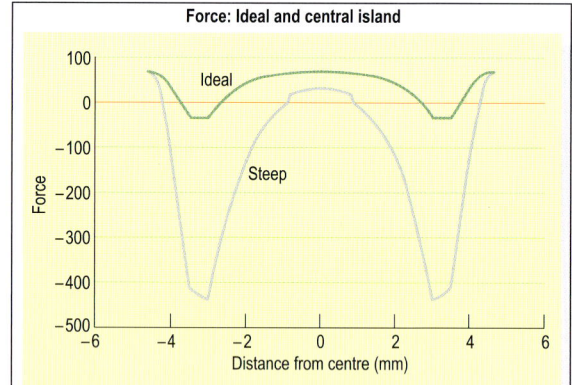

Figure 10.34 The squeeze force of an ideal fit compared to that which causes a central island response. Note the drop in central compression, and the marked increase in tension at the back optic zone diameter.

then determined by these two values, with the apical clearance becoming just another area of force.

The force distribution of an ideal-fitting lens and a lens fitted 20 μm too steep on a cornea with a difference of 0.05 between the horizontal and vertical eccentricity is shown in Figure 10.34. Note that the central zone over an approximate chord of 2.00 mm shows a marked drop in central compression, and is surrounded by a zone of marked tension. The peripheral compression does not differ from that of the ideal-fitting lens. Another point of interest is the slight sudden change in force at the 2.00 mm central zone. This is a complex system. The immediate assumption would be that, since the squeeze forces are "reversed," the stress acts towards the center instead of away from it, thereby causing the steepened island. In the case of a bull's eye and a smiley face the area of paracentral steepening coincides with the point of maximum tension under the lens. This is also the case with the central island, but the exact mechanism that causes the steep central area is difficult to understand. The effect could simply be due to the relative drop in central compression combined with the marked increase in tension near the edge of the BOZD resolving to a tangential stress that tends to act towards the center.

The major problem with both central islands and smiley faces is that the model currently only gives the force distribution at the *initial* phase of the fitting, and not the postwear picture following any equilibrium that may occur. This is primarily due to the difficulties in properly and accurately measuring the postwear corneal curvature changes. Hopefully, further study and development will resolve some of the outstanding issues.

ASTIGMATISM

As shown in Chapter 7, astigmatism presents some interesting complications to orthokeratology treatment. The results are not only dependent on the initial degree of astigmatism, but also on the type of astigmatism with respect to the topography. If central bowtie astigmatism exists, the likely reduction is approximately 50% (Mountford & Pesudovs 2002). Limbus-to-limbus astigmatism, however, appears to be worsened by reverse geometry lens wear due to an inability to "push" the astigmatism out past the pupil zone. The enigma of larger degrees of against-the-rule astigmatism remains just that: an enigma.

The following section shows the squeeze film force model that occurs in both central bowtie and limbus-to-limbus astigmatism.

Figure 10.35 is a simple case of 0.75 D with-the-rule astigmatism with an initial refraction of $-2.00/-0.75 \times 180$. The apical radius is 7.40 mm with eccentricities of 0.56 horizontally and 0.65 vertically (Q values appear on the maps). The forces along the steep and flat meridian generated

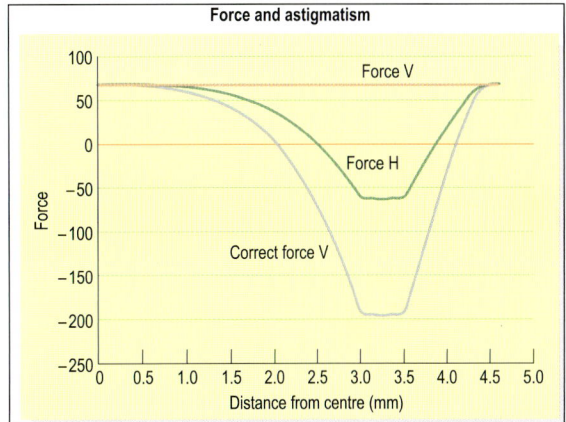

Figure 10.36   The squeeze force for the horizontal meridian and the vertical meridian. The lower eccentricity of the flat meridian means that the lens will be relatively steep in the vertical, leading to compression, but no tension force. The force required to correct the refractive error of the vertical meridian is also shown. This would require a novel lens design.

Figure 10.35   A case of simple central bowtie astigmatism of 0.75 D. Note that the horizontal eccentricity is 0.32, whilst the vertical is 0.43.

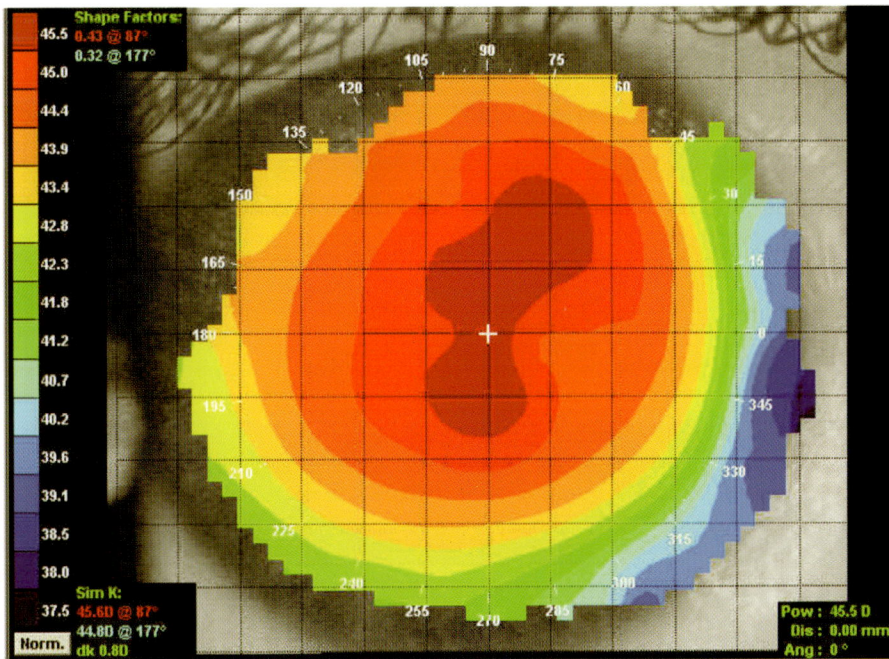

by the lens are shown in Figure 10.36. Note that the difference in the vertical meridian results in no relative tension at the edge of the BOZD of the lens. Equalization of force will result in this case, but there will be less of an effect vertically than horizontally. The force required to sphericalize the vertical meridian is also shown in Figure 10.36. This would require a novel lens construction, with the parameters based on the need for force differentiation in the two meridians. It will not be a toric lens, as the limitations are based on the apical clearance required in the vertical meridian, with the horizontal meridian parameters requiring modification due to the force differentials in apical clearance.

Figure 10.37 shows the effect of a spherical lens on a cornea with simple central astigmatism.

Note that there has been a reduction in the astigmatism, but only over the central 2.00 mm chord. There is no change in astigmatism at the keratometer chord. A lens designed on the force model would, in theory, create greater flattening in the vertical meridian, with a resultant oval treatment zone.

Limbus-to-limbus astigmatism presents an entirely different scenario. A topography map of this complex type of astigmatism is shown in Figure 10.38. Note that, in contrast to the simple central bowtie astigmatism, the astigmatism appears to extend to the peripheral cornea. The apical radius is 7.72 mm, with an eccentricity of 0.68 horizontally, and only 0.15 vertically. The refraction is –2.00/–2.50 × 10. When a spherical lens is fitted to this type of eye, there is an

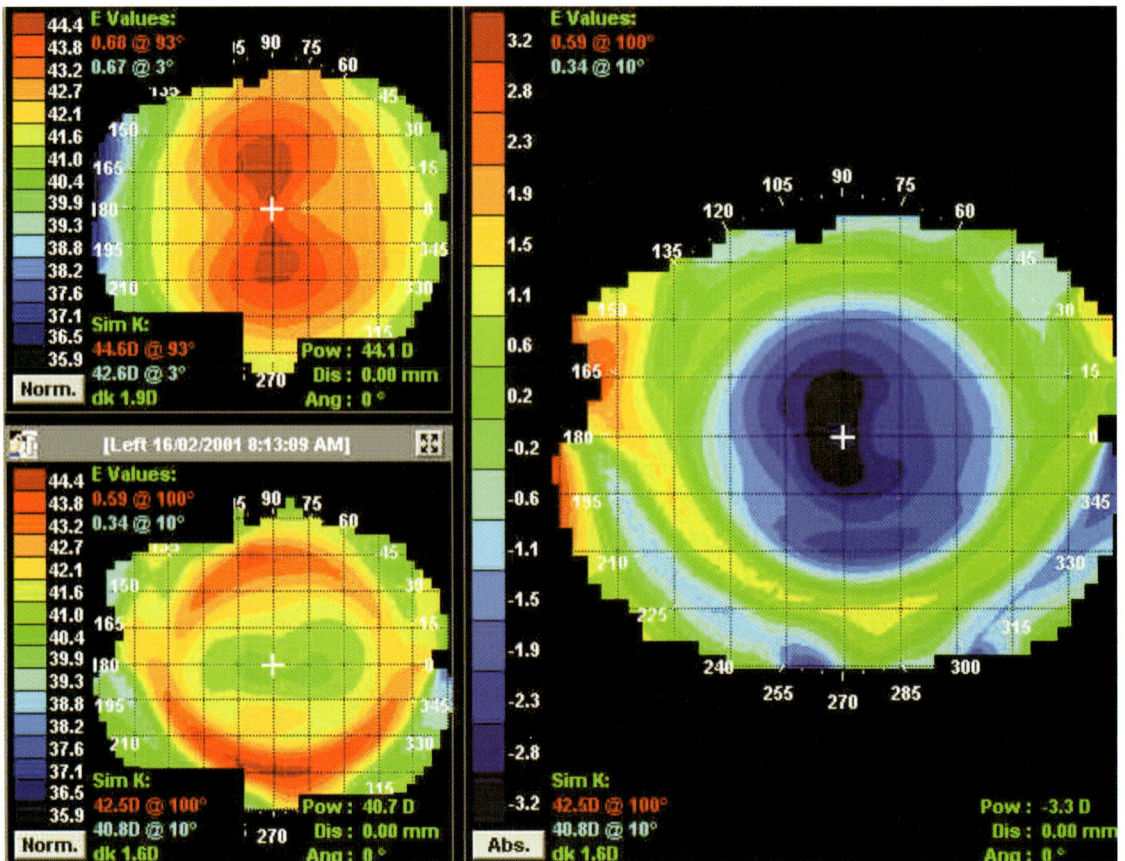

Figure 10.37   A subtractive map of a simple 1.75 D with-the-rule bowtie astigmatism. There is some flattening of the vertical meridian over the central 2.00 mm chord, leading to a reduction of 0.75 D in the refractive astigmatism. There is virtually no change at the keratometer chord of 3.00 mm.

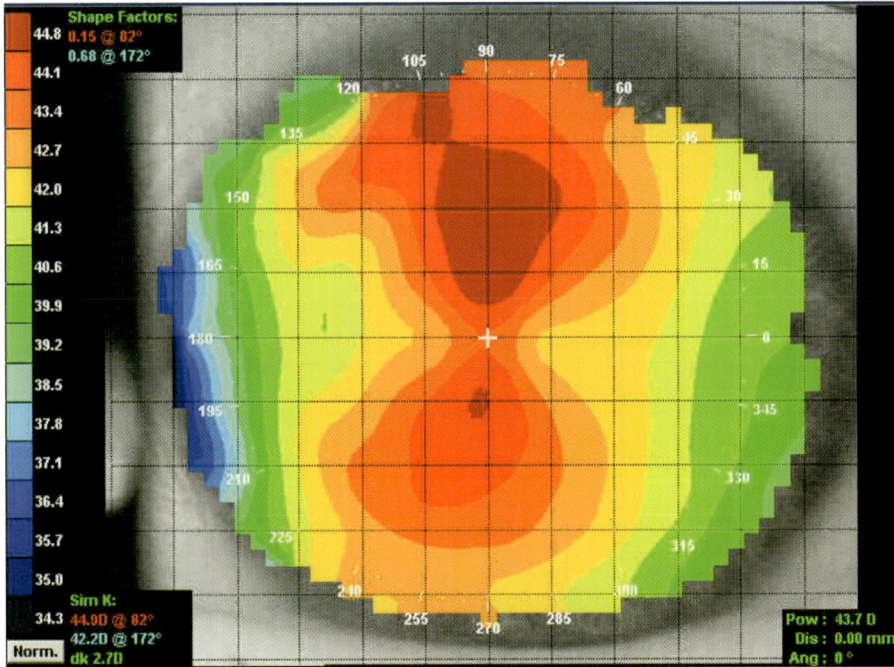

Figure 10.38 Complex limbus–to–limbus astigmatism. Note the differences between the eccentricities in the horizontal (0.68) and vertical (0.15) meridians.

increase in the postwear astigmatism (Fig. 10.39). The reason appears to be an inability to "push" the astigmatism out past the pupil zone. The force produced by a spherical lens on the cornea is shown in Figure 10.40.

If the Conway model is used, the force generated in the vertical meridian is zero, due to the absence of apical clearance resulting in an α value of 1. However, this type of astigmatism fulfills the requirements of the parabolic two-dimensional model of Allaire & Flack (1980), which would once again result in zero force along the vertical meridian, but approximately double the force of the Conway model in the horizontal meridian. This would cause an increased flattening of the horizontal meridian past that required, leading to a hypermetropic horizontal meridian, with an increased astigmatism vertically. The postwear refraction of the patient shown in Figure 10.39 was +1.00/−3.50 × 180.

The model shows that, for astigmatism to be effectively reduced, novel reverse geometry lens designs are required. Mountford & Pesudovs (2002) have shown that, for orthokeratology to reduce totally astigmatism of up to 2.00 D, the "effectiveness" of the lenses would need to be

increased by approximately 80% using Alpins analysis. The lack of efficacy of spherical lenses on astigmatic corneas could be due to the relative lack of a tension force in the steep meridian, which could only be rectified by the use of novel designs. Experiments with the Fargo and BE lenses are currently under way in order to develop these novel astigmatic designs. However, work to date seems to indicate that the level of accuracy that is currently possible for lens manufacture is less than that required to produce lenses that are effective for limbus-to-limbus astigmatism. It would therefore be prudent to exclude those presenting with noncentral astigmatism from orthokeratology for the foreseeable future.

To summarize, the quasistatic model combines the effects of lid forces and the squeeze film forces under the lens. The lids are assumed to be closed, thereby avoiding the effects of surface tension forces. In order for the model to work, some degree of apical clearance must be present, with the lens resting on the peripheral cornea. The escape channel for the squeeze force is the presence of mild with-the-rule astigmatism, or simply the difference between the horizontal and vertical

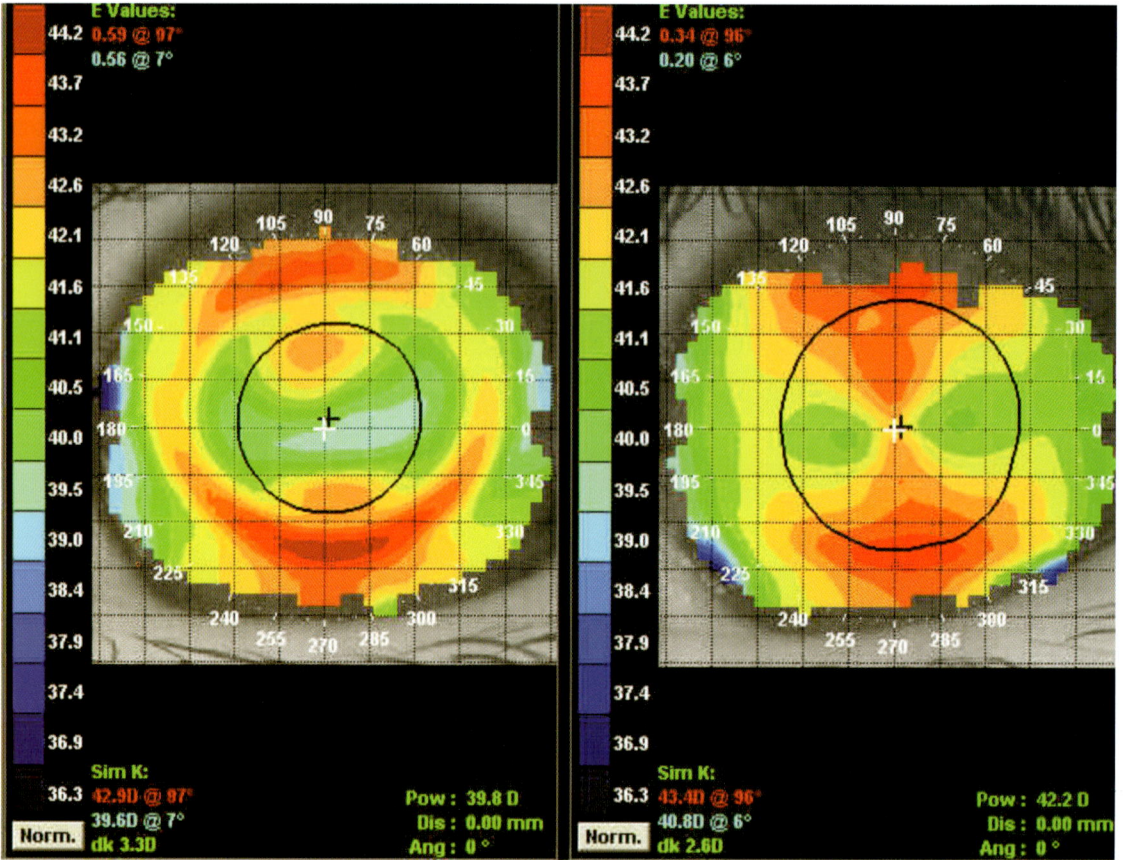

Figure 10.39   Pre- and postorthokeratology topography plots of limbus-to-limbus astigmatism. In effect, the astigmatism is increased. The prefitting plot is on the right.

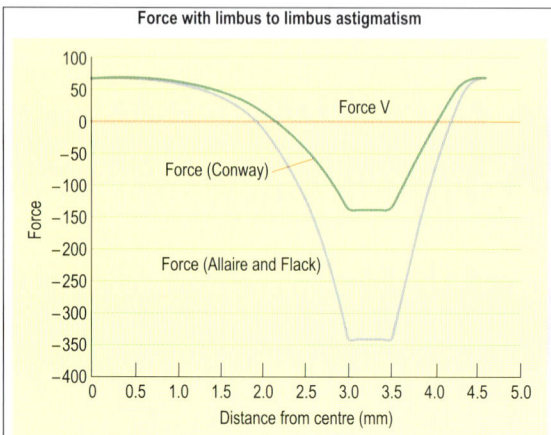

Figure 10.40   Squeeze force of limbus-to-limbus astigmatism. There is no force generated in the vertical meridian. The force generated by the Conway and Allaire & Flack models are shown (see text).

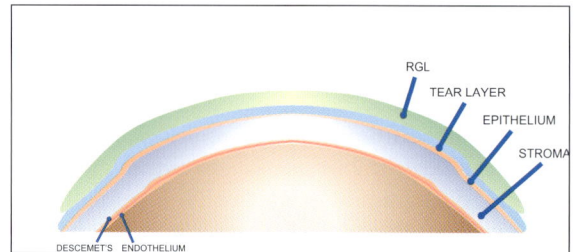

Figure 10.41   The lens–eye relationship where the lens is fitted with greater than zero apical clearance. The squeeze film force causes corneal sphericalization, with an increase in apical clearance due to epithelial thinning, and decreased clearance at the back optic zone diameter, leading to an "equalization" of the tear layer thickness under the lens.

corneal diameter in the case of a nonastigmatic aspheric surface. The back surface geometry of the lens causes positive compressive force centrally, and negative tension force at the edge of the BOZD. The difference in force induces tangential stress across the corneal surface, forcing the cornea to change shape. The shape change ceases when there is equalization of force in the postlens tear film. This occurs over a spherical surface area, which can be related to the refractive change. The shape change is associated with corneal epithelial thinning centrally leading to an *increase* in the apical clearance as the changes occur. The apical clearance reaches a maximum when sphericalization occurs. The peripheral stroma (at the BOZD) is thought to increase in thickness by approximately the same amount as the epithelium thins, leading to a *reduction* in TLT in this area. The equalization of force is therefore accompanied by an "equalization" of the TLT under the lens (Fig. 10.41).

The major determining factor in the squeeze film model is the α factor, that links maximum to minimum TLT. The model shows an increase in squeeze film force (tension) if the base curve (BOZR) of the lens is flattened with respect to the corneal surface. This is analogous to the Jessen factor, where flattening the BOZR leads to an increase in the TLT at the optic zone (BOZD). However, the effect is markedly increased if the apical clearance is decreased. The second alternative, the constant tear layer method, keeps the clearance at the BOZD constant irrespective of corneal shape and alters the apical clearance. This produces even greater tension values at the BOZD, and increases the tangential stress on the surface.

The forces are extremely sensitive to changes in apical clearance, which means that accuracy in fitting is absolutely essential. Orthokeratology with reverse geometry lenses appears, from the model, to have a boundary condition limit of between 3 and 25 μm of apical clearance, and a maximum TLT of approximately 65 μm at the BOZD. The model can adequately explain the sphericalization of the cornea due to force equalization, and gives interesting insight into the initial conditions that cause smiley-face, central island and astigmatic changes. Further research and analysis of the model are required.

STATIC STATE MOLDING

The quasistatic-state model described above makes the assumption that the lens is moving, albeit very slowly, towards the surface of the eye following lid closure. In this case, there are no surface tension factors at work, as the lens is assumed to be bathed in a lake of tears under the lid. However, the other method of assessing the forces at work is to assume that there is no motion involved, and that a totally static state exists. The forces then change from those of a squeeze film to those of hydrostatic pressures, where the pressure acting on the surface is proportional to the depth of the fluid at any given point. The formula for hydrostatic pressure is:

$$P = \rho g h$$

where P is pressure, ρ viscosity, g gravity, and h the height of the tear film above the corneal surface.

The pressures produced in a static state are much smaller than those produced in the quasistatic state. The quasistatic state also requires the presence of apical clearance in order for the squeeze film forces to exist. Many of the currently available lens designs are fitted with an apical clearance of zero, or in some cases less than zero with some degree of peripheral clearance.

Theoretically, this should result in lens decentration until a situation arises where some form of apical clearance exists in order to create squeeze film forces. However, the reverse curve that is present in reverse geometry lenses means that there is some degree of freedom of movement in this area. The deeper tear layer at the edge of the BOZD produces negative pressures that can help maintain some control over centration, even with the lack of apical clearance. This is especially true if the surface tension forces around the lens edge are taken into account.

The surface tension forces are considerable, being approximately –2000 Pa (Hayashi & Fatt 1980), and will work to pull the lens towards the surface of the eye (Fig. 10.42A). In this example, a surface of known apical radius and elevation is fitted with a reverse geometry lens of 4 μm apical clearance, and peripheral contact at a chord of 9.35 mm. Note that the surface tension force, as

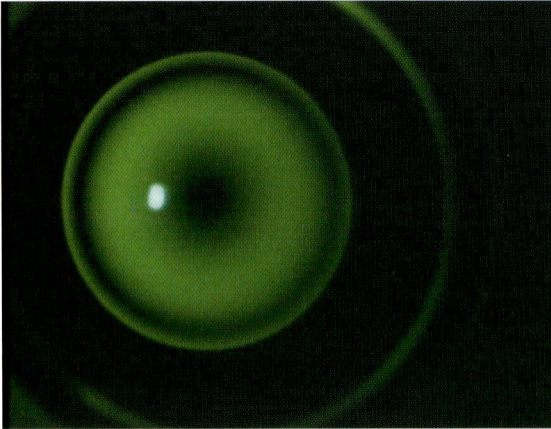
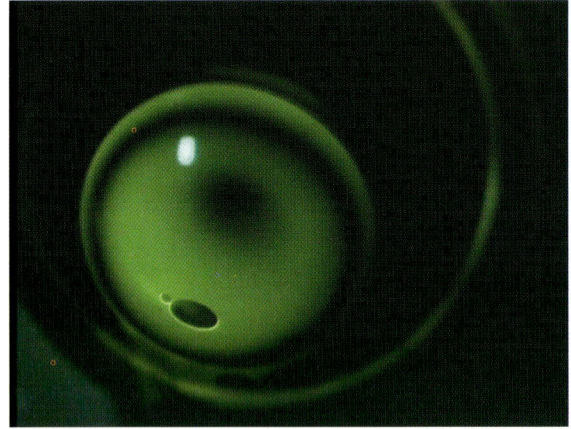

A   B

Figure 10.42   (A) A lens with 4.00 μm apical clearance fitted to a known model aspheric surface. Surface tension around the lens edge and the negative pressure in the reverse curve zone keep the lens on center against the effects of lens mass and gravity. (B) The apical clearance is decreased and the peripheral clearance increased to approximately 20 μm. The surface tension can no longer control centration, so gravity causes the lens to decenter.

well as the reverse curve tear layer, maintains centration against the effects of gravity. If the angular value of the tear wedge at the lens edge is 90° or greater, the surface tension no longer works. In this situation, the mass of the lens exceeds the surface tension force, and gravity will make the lens drop. If the edge lift of a lens or the clearance of the lens from the corneal surface exceeds a certain boundary condition, centration becomes impossible. Figure 10.42B shows a lens with approximately 20 μm of peripheral clearance and apical touch. The surface tension is unable to maintain centration against the forces of lens mass and gravity and the lens decenters. The critical mass of the lens, according to Hayashi & Fatt (1980) is approximately 20 mg.

Therefore, if a lens is to be fitted with an apical clearance of less than zero, the surface tension force becomes dominant in controlling lens centration *prior to lid closure*. This is a vital fact to remember if the preferred fitting philosophy is "apical bearing." The trial lens should show good centration without lid involvement. This is simply achieved by placing the lens on the eye and allowing a few blinks until tear mixing is complete. The lids are then held away from the lens and the centration noted. If the lens immediately drops low, the edge clearance or surface clearance from the corneal surface is excessive,

allowing lens mass and gravity to overcome the surface tension forces. This can be rectified by decreasing the peripheral clearance of the lens by steepening either the reverse curve or the alignment curve. If the lens remains relatively well-centered, the lids should be allowed to cover the lens. The patient is then asked to keep the lids closed for 10–15 seconds, and then open them. The lens position immediately on eye opening will be the "resting position" when the lids are closed. If the lens rides too high, the alignment curve is too flat, and if it is decentered inferiorly, too steep. Reim (1998) notes through clinical experience that the ideal quasistatic resting position for the lens prior to lid closure is slight inferior decentration of approximately 0.50 mm.

Once the lids are closed, the quasistatic state ceases as there is no apical clearance under the lens, and theoretically, no movement of the lens towards the ocular surface. The static state pressures then take over.

Figure 10.43 shows the lids closed over the lens. Note that there is zero apical clearance and peripheral clearance at the alignment zone. The lid drapes over the lens until it comes into contact with the ocular surface again. This area forms a tear wedge between the lid and the ocular surface. The tear layer profile is shown in Figure 10.44A. Note that the depth of the tears

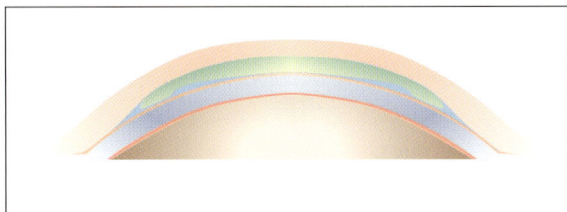

Figure 10.43 The situation that arises when the lid covers the reverse geometry lens on the eye.

outside the lens is much greater than that in the reverse zone under the lens. The hydrostatic pressure is directly related to the depth of the tear layer. This is modeled in Figure 10.44B. The negative pressure generated in the tear layer outside the edge of the lens is much greater than that which occurs under the lens. The pressure under the lens is relatively positive compared to that outside the lens.

This pressure gradient must attempt to find equalization, so fluid will move out from under the lens towards the peripheral wedge formed by the lid and lens. The aqueous phase of the tear layer will move first due to its lower viscosity when compared to the mucous phase. This creates a relative vacuum under the lens, which the epithelium will move to fill. As the tear layer increases in viscosity, the pressure increases. In effect, the cornea is "molded" to the back surface

of the lens (Fig. 10.45). The limit of the process is determined by the mucous layer between the lens and the cornea.

This is a classic form of vacuum molding, and shows why the Jessen factor works so well as a means of corneal molding. The variation in results is due, once again, to the accuracy of the lens fit. Both the reverse and alignment curves must satisfy sagittal equivalency in order for the "mold" to work correctly. If the reverse curve and

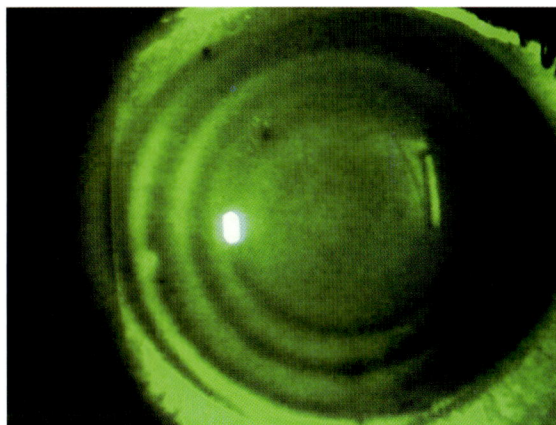

Figure 10.45 The result of hydrostatic "vacuum molding." The cornea is molded to the back surface shape of the lens. The imprint of the lens on the cornea is shown. Note the lack of any corneal staining.

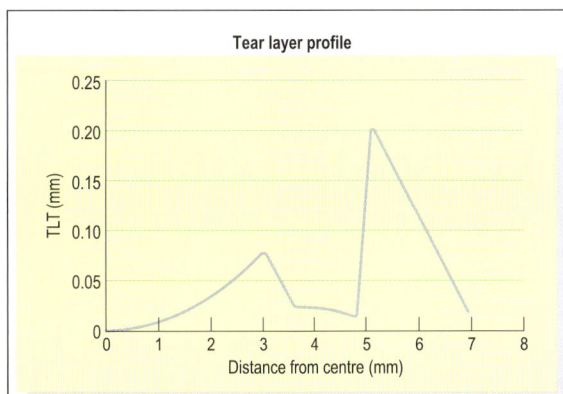

A

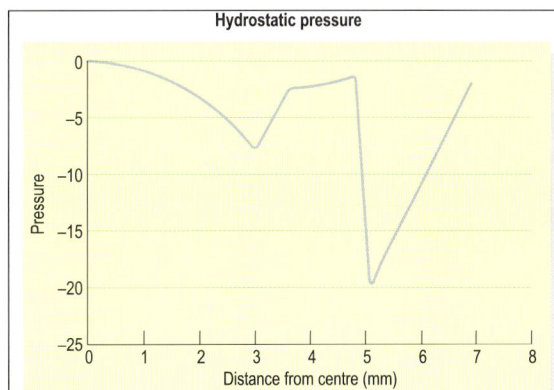

B

Figure 10.44 (A) This graph shows the tear layer profile of the lens under the closed lid. There is a marked increase in the tear layer thickness (TLT) at the lens edge due to the lens thickness and lid interaction. The apical clearance is zero, and there is approximately 10 μm of clearance at the edge of the alignment curve. (B) The hydrostatic force generated under the lens in the static state is shown. The marked increase in negative pressure outside the edge of the lens generates the pressure gradient needed for molding to occur. Pressure values are Pa × 10^{-2}.

apical clearance are inaccurate, or based on false assumptions about the corneal shape, the cornea cannot accurately mold to the base curve, thereby affecting the refractive change. The surface area matching between lens and cornea as described by Jim Day therefore makes perfect logical and mathematical sense if this form of molding is to be used. The other factors that will therefore determine the success of the mold are the thickness of the lens edge and the edge clearance. If the lens edge is too thin and tapered, the pressure in the tear wedge created outside the lens by the lid is decreased with respect to the tear layer under the lens at the edge of the optic zone and could result in a less than optimal response.

Also, the viscosity of the tear layer plays an important role, not only in the preclosure quasistatic state, but also in the static state. The centration effect of the surface tension is increased if the viscosity of the liquid covering the ocular surface is increased. Therefore, mild cases of decentration could be assisted by the use of a viscous coupling agent between the lens and the eye. This would also theoretically increase the hydrostatic pressure in the closed-eye environment.

The same limitations with respect to astigmatism apply in this model, in that the differential in pressure in the steep meridian may be insufficient to cause a change. The same basic mechanisms are at work to produce smiley faces, whilst central islands are still somewhat difficult to explain. Sphericalization occurs due to the spherical shape of the lens surface. Equalization of pressure, however, does not occur, as the area outside the lens will always have a greater negative pressure than that under the lens.

The critical factor once again is the accuracy of the lens fit, and, especially in this model, the clearance of the lens at the alignment curve.

The concepts of a quasistatic and static state may at first appear difficult to understand. A static state assumes that everything is in an absolute state of rest, whilst the quasistatic state assumes that there is some movement, albeit minimal, of the lens towards the ocular surface following lid closure. The two conditions are not mutually exclusive in this case: the initial phase may be quasistatic followed by a static phase. Both models help explain the cause-and-effect

relationship in orthokeratology, and may help in the design of future lenses for astigmatic correction and in the control of T×Z diameters.

CONCLUSIONS

Corneal molding can be modeled in two totally separate ways, either by squeeze film force (fluid jacket molding) or hydrostatic pressure (vacuum molding). In squeeze film force molding, the effect is corneal sphericalization and a movement of the cornea away from the lens. The opposite occurs with hydrostatic "vacuum" molding, where the lens is molded to the back surface geometry of the lens, leading to a reduction in clearance between the two surfaces. In both cases, lens binding occurs due to increased tear viscosity. This must therefore be accepted as a normal part of the process, and attention directed to the correct loosening-up of the lens.

If the forces and pressures under the lens can be controlled, then lens design variations that can increase effective T×Z diameters and correct astigmatism become possible. All that is required is a very high degree of accuracy in lens design, fitting, and manufacture. The keratometer is simply not up to this task, and neither is fitting by fluorescein pattern analysis.

Topographical fitting, followed by postwear topography assessment, led to strategies that alter the lens in order to rectify any problems. Alterations in lens fit change the forces and pressures involved. Control the forces and pressures, and the corneal shape changes are controlled. The only thing unpredictable about orthokeratology is then the effect of instrument error and fitting.

However, it must be clearly stated that the molding models outlined above are purely that: models. The values of the forces and pressures are only relative and not actual values. However, the trends that the model shows with respect to lens and instrument error, as well as the insights as to the underlying conditions that cause bull's-eye, smiley-face, and central island plots are intriguing. The future extensions to the model include the resolution of the tangential stresses across the surface, and the resolving of the surface tension forces at the lens edge.

What the models do show is that orthokeratology is far more complex than a simple "flatter than K" fitting philosophy. Simplistic solutions to complex problems result in errors, and, in the case of orthokeratology, a low first-fit success rate and a degree of unpredictability in the procedure. Orthokeratology is complex, not simple. It is the epitome of rigid lens fitting, purely because such a high degree of accuracy in all aspects of lens design and fitting is required. Optometry would benefit by having engineers help resolve some of these problems.

A HYPOTHETICAL QUESTION

The refractive changes that occur with reverse geometry lens wear can be accounted for by the change in epithelial thickness. However, there also seems to be a thickening of the stroma in the mid-periphery near the edge of the optic zone of the lens. This is where the major tension force is at work. The epithelium is not a viscoelastic solid, whereas the stroma is. Hypothetically, then, could the stromal changes have some control on the regression of the effect? Clinical experience shows that the majority of patients can happily drop down to every second night's wear, and over the long term, even less. Is this retention of the effect due in some way to changes in the viscoelastic memory of the mid-peripheral stroma, and, if so, is there a definite tangential stress or tension force required to bring about a change in the corneal

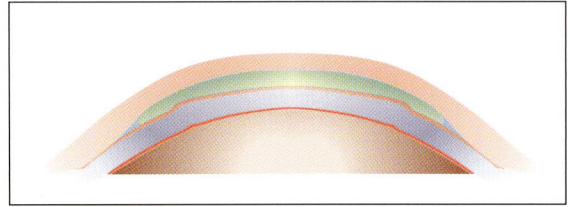

Figure 10.46 The effect of "vacuum molding." The cornea is "drawn up" into the back surface of the lens, resulting in minimal clearance between the two. Courtesy of Christina Eglund, Polymer Technology Corporation.

elastic memory? Conversely, could the regression be explained purely in terms of epithelial cell movement? If so, why do some corneas retain the effect longer than others?

ACKNOWLEDGMENTS

The author wishes to thank sincerely the individuals who helped with the production of this chapter. Firstly, Don Noack, who forced me to relearn algebra and construct the spreadsheets that were used to model the forces. Secondly, Tony Matthews and Roger Tabb, who started the engineering outlook, and finally, Professor Douglas Hargreaves BE (Mech), MSc, PhD, Fuch Chair in Tribology, School of Mechanical, Manufacturing and Medical Engineering, Queensland University of Technology, for great insights into fluid hydraulics, and for checking the veracity of the model.

REFERENCES

Allaire P E, Flack R P (1980) Squeeze forces in contact lenses with a steep base curvature radius. American Journal of Optometry and Physiological Optics 57(4): 219–227

Beuhren T, Collins M J, Iskander D R, Davis B, Lingelbach B (2001) The stability of corneal topography in the post-blink interval. Cornea 20: 826–833

Bier N (1956) The contour lens. Journal of the American Optometric Association 28: 394–396

Black C J (1960) Ocular, anatomical and physiological changes due to contact lenses. Illinois Medical Journal 118: 279–281

Bronstein L (1957) Symptomology of corneal type lenses. Contacto 1: 31–35

Carkeet N L, Mountford J, Carney L G (1995) Predicting success with orthokeratology lens wear: a retrospective analysis of ocular characteristics. Optometry and Vision Science 72: 829–898

Carney L G (1975a) Refractive error and VA changes during contact lens wear. Contact Lens Journal 5: 28–34

Carney L G (1975b) Corneal topographical changes during contact lens wear. Contact Lens Journal 5: 5–16

Carney L G, Clarke B A (1972) Experimental deformation of the in vivo cornea. American Journal of Optometry and Archives of the American Academy of Optics 49(1): 28–34

Carney L G, Mainstone J C, Quinn T G et al (1996a) Rigid centration: effects of lens design and material density. International Contact Lens Clinic 23: 6–1

Carney L G, Mainstone J C, Carkeet A et al (1996b) The influence of centre of gravity and lens mass on rigid lens dynamics. CLAO Journal 22: 195–204

Collewijn H, Van Der Steen J, Steinman R M (1985) Human eye movements associated with blinks and prolonged eye closure. Journal of Neurophysiology 54: 11

Collins M J et al (1992) The synkinesis between the antero-posterior eye position and lid fissure width. Clinical and Experimental Optometry 75(2): 38–41

Conway H D (1982) Effects of base curvature on squeeze pressures in contact lenses. American Journal of Optometry and Physiological Optics 59(92): 152–154

Coon L (1982) Orthokeratology: part 1 – Historical perspectives. Journal of the American Optometric Association 55: 187–195

Coon L (1984) Orthokeratology: part 2. Evaluating the Tabb method. Journal of the American Optometric Association 55: 409–418

Dickinson F (1957) The value of microlenses in the progression of myopia. Optician 133: 263–272

Doane M G (1980) Interaction of eyelids and tears and the dynamics of the normal human eyeblink. American Journal of Ophthalmology 89: 507

Doane M G (1981) Blinking and the mechanics of the lacrimal drainage. Survey of Ophthalmology 88: 844

Evinger C, Shaw M D, Peck C K, Manning K A, Baker R (1984) Blinking and associated eye movements in humans, guinea pigs and rabbits. Journal of Neurophysiology 52: 323

Freeman R A (1978) Predicting stable changes in orthokeratology. Contact Lens Forum 3(1): 21–31

Gan-Mor S, Dybbs A, Greber I (1979) Pressure measurements on model corneas due to hard and soft lenses. Case Western Reserve University Report FTAS/TR-141

Greber I, Dybbs A (1972) Fluid dynamic analysis of contact lens motion. Case Western Reserve University Report FTAS/TR-72-81

Greenbery M H, Hill R (1976) The pressure response to contact lenses. Contact Lens Forum July: 49–53

Hayashi T (1977) Mechanics of contact lens motion. PhD thesis. School of Optometry, UC Berkeley

Hayashi T, Fatt I (1980) Forces retaining a contact lens on the eye. American Journal of Optometry and Physiological Optics 57(8): 485–507

Hovding P (1983) Variation of central corneal curvature during the first year of contact lens wear. Acta Ophthalmologica 61: 117–118

Howard M (2000) Sight correction using accelerated orthokeratology lenses. Honours Project. Department of Civil Engineering, University of Dundee

Jessen G N (1962) Orthofocus techniques. Contacto 6: 200–204

Joe J J, Marsden H J, Edrington T B (1996) The relationship between corneal eccentricity and improvement in visual acuity with orthokeratology. Journal of the American Optometric Association 67: 87–97

Kerns R L (1977) Research in orthokeratology. Part V. Recovery aspects. Journal of the American Optometric Association 48: 345–359

Kerns R L (1978) Research in orthokeratology. Part VIII. Results, conclusions and examination of techniques.

Journal of the American Optometric Association 49: 308–314

Kikkawa Y (1970) The mechanism of contact lens adherence and centralization. American Journal of Optometry and Archives of the American Academy of Optometry 47(4): 275–281

Kwok L S (1984) Calculation and application of the anterior surface area of a model human cornea. Journal of Theoretical Biology 108: 295–313

Kwok L S (1991) Hydroelastic deformation of rabbit corneal epithelium by intraocular pressure, ARVO abstracts. Investigative Ophthalmology and Vision Science 32: 888

Lui W O, Edwards M H (2000) Orthokeratology in low myopia. Part 2: Corneal topographic changes and safety over 100 days. Contact Lens and Anterior Eye 23(3): 90–99

Lydon D, Tait A (1988) Lid pressure: its measurement and probable effects on the shape and form of the cornea-rigid contact lens system. Journal of the British Contact Lens Association 11(1): 11–22

Miller D (1963) An analysis of the physical forces applied to a contact lens. Archives of Ophthalmology 70(6): 823–829

Miller D (1967) Pressure of the lid on the eye. Archives of Ophthalmology 78: 328–330

Moller P M (1954) Tissue pressure in the orbit. Acta Ophthalmologica 32: 597

Morrison R J (1958) Observations on contact lenses and progression of myopia. Contacto 2: 20–25

Mountford J A (1997) An analysis of the changes in corneal shape and refractive error induced by accelerated orthokeratology. International Contact Lens Clinic 24: 128–143

Mountford J A, Pesudovs K (2002) An analysis of the astigmatic changes induced by accelerated orthokeratology. Clinical and Experimental Optometry 85(5): 284–293

Nichols J J, Marsich M M, Nguyen M, Barr J T, Bullimore M A (2000) Overnight orthokeratology. Optometry and Vision Science 77: 252–259

Nolan J A (1972) Orthokeratology with steep lenses. Contacto 16: 31–37

Paige N (1971) The plus lens increment. A system of myopia control and reduction. Contacto 15: 28–29

Pearson R M (1989) Kalt, keratoconus and the contact lens. Optometry and Vision Science 66: 643–646

Pye D C (1996) The finite element method and orthokeratology. University of New South Wales (inhouse publication)

Reim T (1998) Dreimlens instruction manual. Dreimlens International Pty Ltd (inhouse publication)

Riggs L A, Kelly J P, Manning K A, Moore R K (1985) Blink related eye movements. Investigative Ophthalmology and Vision Science 28: 334

Soni P, Nguyen T (2002) Which corneal parameter, anterior corneal curvature, posterior corneal curvature or corneal thickness is most sensitive to acute changes with reverse geometry orthokeratology lenses? ARVO abstracts 3086. Investigative Ophthalmology and Visual Science

Sridharan R (2001) Response and regression of the cornea with short-term orthokeratology lens wear. Masters thesis. University of New South Wales, Sydney, Australia

Swarbrick H A, Wong G, O'Leary D J (1998) Corneal response to orthokeratology. Optometry and Vision Science 75: 791–799

Tang W, Collins M, Carney L C, Davis B (2000) The accuracy and precision performance of four videokeratoscopes in measuring test surfaces. Optometry and Vision Science 77(9): 483–491

Weiss B, Dybbs A, Greber I (1975) Experiments on a model corneal contact lens system. Case Western Reserve University Report FIAS/TR-112

Chapter 11

The future

John Mountford

CHAPTER CONTENTS

Introduction 303
Educational standards 304
Topography 305
Unanswered questions 306
Conclusions 309
References 309

INTRODUCTION

The making of predictions for those involved in areas of constant change can be a dangerous occupation (Edwards & Hough 2001, Efron 2001), so the author has decided to "play it safe" and not make any predictions regarding the future directions of orthokeratology. However, there are a lot of unanswered questions, and these need to be looked at with controlled research. The aim of this chapter is to investigate and highlight some of these areas as well as other areas in orthokeratology practice that need improvement.

Traditional orthokeratology suffered from an excess of enthusiasm, leading to exaggerated claims of efficacy that were not borne out by controlled research. These results led to a general rejection of the procedure by the optometric community, which has taken 20 years, further research and development, and improved technology to negate. However, some forms of marketing never let the truth get in the way of a good story, with the result that the mistakes of the past could be repeated. This has already begun, with totally unsubstantiated claims of large refractive corrections, which, when taken in the context of the limits of the procedure as outlined in this book, would require an exceptionally high degree of accuracy in lens fitting and manufacture. Also, the large refractive claims made would automatically, if they did occur, lead to such a small treatment zone diameter that there would be a huge negative impact on the quality of unaided vision. It seems paradoxical that the lens is fitted by simply providing the company with keratometry readings and the refractive change required. The method of controlling these types of claims is to subject them to peer review, and also to provide a high degree of education to those practitioners wishing to become involved in the care of orthokeratology patients.

EDUCATIONAL STANDARDS

The *minimum* requirement for those who practice orthokeratology is a recognized qualification in ophthalmology, optometry, or contact lens-based opticianry, together with a solid background and experience in fitting rigid gas-permeable (RGP) lenses.

Furthermore, an accredited program of education that is orthokeratology-specific should be undertaken before access to the lenses is granted. The Food and Drug Administration has set training courses in fitting the Corneal Refractive Therapy (CRT), and presumably all other reverse geometry lenses, as a prerequisite to the active use of the lenses. Following the outbreak of ulcerative keratitis in China and Hong Kong, the government withdrew the lenses from the market (in China) until the manufacturers fulfilled requirements that the materials met safety standards for overnight wear and production, and that there was an accepted educational platform in place for practitioners involved in fitting the lenses.

It therefore seems logical to insist that completion of an independently accredited course be mandatory before a practitioner gains access to the lenses or fitting them.

An educational program in orthokeratology should not be construed as simply a description of the fitting philosophy of a particular lens. Ideally, such a course would also include instruction in areas such as:

1. the results of controlled research carried out on the effects of orthokeratology, with particular emphasis on the factors that determine suitability for the procedure
2. the physiological requirements for overnight wear, and its associated pathophysiology
3. the use and interpretation of corneal topography

4. a description of the lens design and fitting philosophy
5. lens modification strategies to optimize the fit and response
6. adverse events and their management
7. "hands-on" practical sessions, including an overnight trial and assessment of the results the next day.

The exact curriculum will, of course, be determined by those given the task of setting educational standards, but the important thing is that some form of standard be accepted and implemented.

Another factor that was reported at the time of the China scare was that some of the lenses were made from material that was simply not acceptable for overnight wear. The patient, as well as the practitioner, must be certain that the material from which the lenses have been made has not been substituted with an inferior product. In the USA, Polymer Technology Corporation, as part of a settlement made with the patent holders of orthokeratology lenses, is paying a royalty on each lens made. In order to track the lenses, they are being made in two colors, red and yellow, that will *only* be used to make reverse geometry lenses. This idea has exceptional merit, and should be used worldwide as a means of assuring both patient and practitioner that they do have the correct material. It could be clearly stated in the literature given to patients that orthokeratology lenses *must* be a specific color.

A greater problem occurs in trying to get laboratories to restrict the supply of lenses to those who have completed a course of instruction in their use. Both Polymer Technology and Paragon have a responsibility to control material supply to manufacturers who do not meet either production or educational standards. As stated above, the course should not be allowed to proceed unless it has been granted independent accreditation. The International College of Orthokeratology, which was established at the Global Orthokeratology Symposium in Toronto in August 2002, is the logical body to oversee educational standards. It has representatives from 26 countries, a high proportion of whom are independent academics. The individual lens designers and manufacturers are not, and should not be, in positions of influence in this body. It is imperative that it maintains total independence from them. Helen Swarbrick of the Cornea and Contact Lens Research Unit (CCLRU) is presently the president of the body, and will present the results of the agreement on educational standards at the next conference.

The second factor to consider is the standard of instrumentation. As outlined throughout this book, the authors consider the routine use of corneal topography to be a "minimum standard" in the care of patients undergoing orthokeratology. The sole use of keratometry should be considered to be unethical, as it is incapable of providing the information essential for fitting and aftercare.

The discussion on standards of education is not based on legal precedents, but there is an inescapable moral and ethical argument that cannot be discounted. Orthokeratology is doomed to legislative interference if incidents similar to those which occurred in China and Hong Kong occur elsewhere, and the only way of preventing that is to have strict educational standards.

TOPOGRAPHY

The authors of this book have no financial interest in, or financial ties to, any topographer manufacturer.

All topographers are not created equal. The simple possession of a topographer does not automatically mean that it is suitable for use in orthokeratology. In fact, most of the currently available topographers are not particularly "ortho-k-friendly." They were designed for refractive surgeons, with contact lens fitting added as an afterthought. However, topographer makers should realize that the refractive surgery market is saturated, and that orthokeratology presents an opportunity to expand the market for their instruments. Having said that, there are requirements for orthokeratology that are simply not available in the majority of instruments.

The basic requirements of a topographer have been set out in Chapter 2, but the following list is an outline of the orthokeratology-specific features that should be developed and incorporated into

the topographer to make it more appealing to the practitioner.

1. The values for R_0 and eccentricity (e), asphericity (Q), and shape factor (p) should be easily accessible and identified by the use of the accepted notations (p, e, and Q).
2. The e, Q, and p values should be available for both the flat and steep meridians. This will be vital in the future for designing lenses to correct astigmatism. The chord over which the asphericity is measured should be variable.
3. The elevation values at specific chords should be easily available.
4. The instrument must be repeatable, and supply, in tabular form, a statistical analysis of repeated readings (Edwards & Hough 2001). At present, the only instrument that offers this feature is the Medmont E300 (Medmont, Melbourne, Australia).
5. The arc-step reconstruction algorithm must be smoothed as vertex normal is reached. The "errors" of smoothing are minimal to the errors that occur when it is not done. For example, in those cases where the central 1.00 mm chord is not smoothed, the postwear topography plots will commonly show what appear to be central islands. The author spent a lot of money replacing lenses that apparently caused central islands only to find that they were, in reality, "glitches" caused by the confusion that arrives as tangent normal approaches 90° and R_0 approaches infinity. Smoothing the central data negates this confusion, and is a desirable compromise.
6. The topographer should have the ability to interface with the particular lens fitting software. Paragon has achieved integration of the CRT software with most of the currently available topographers, and the WAVE software is integrated with the Keratron. However, the fitting is usually based on a single reading, and, as has been shown previously, this can lead to errors. If topography is to be properly integrated, the suggestions of Hough & Edwards (2000) must be incorporated.
7. The instrument reconstruction algorithm should be able to reconstruct the postorthokeratology corneal shape accurately and

provide valid elevation data. This is essential if a lens does not quite reach the refractive change required. The ability to cause greater refractive changes whilst simultaneously modifying the treatment zone (TxZ) may require fitting a specially designed second lens. The lens parameters would then be calculated from the data of the altered corneal shape. At present, this is not possible due to the inability of topographers to measure oblate surfaces accurately (Tang et al 2000).

8. The subtractive refractive power map should automatically measure the TxZ diameter.
9. Ideally, the topographer should also display aberration maps. This is already available with the Keratograph topographer. Also, a program that integrates with most of the currently available topographers and uses the data to generate Zernike maps is available from CT View (www.sarverassociates.com). This then gives the practitioner and researcher the ability to assess the quality of the unaided vision objectively. Also, Beuhren et al (2001) have shown that the incorporation of wavefront analysis can be used to correct for image tilt. If separate topography maps are performed (subtractive maps, for example), the assumption is that fixation and apex detection are identical to the original capture. This is not the case, resulting in some degree of tilt between maps. This in turn leads to inaccuracies in the subtractive difference maps.
10. The instrument and its software must be simple and user-friendly. The hardware must be dependable. A large database storage capacity is essential.
11. The practitioner must be able to observe the patient's alignment, fixation stability, and the position of eyelash, brow, and nose shadows before image capture takes place.

Some corneal topographers are simply not suitable for orthokeratology. They lack either the accuracy and repeatability of other instruments or some of the essential requirements such as subtractive axial, tangential, and refractive power maps and the derivation of apical radius and the eccentricity of the flat meridian. Practitioners should carefully assess the instrument prior to purchase, and make sure it meets the correct requirements.

UNANSWERED QUESTIONS

There are still a lot of mysteries in orthokeratology. The following section deals with these gray areas, and the author is indebted to the following academics for their helpful suggestions of topics for future research: John Mark Jackson, Marjorie Rah, Helen Swarbrick, Ed Bennett, Joe Barr, Pauline Cho, Harue Marsden, Nathan Efron, and Milton Hom.

Efficacy and predictability

The ultimate test of the efficacy of ortho-k, as I trust you appreciate, is a large-scale, randomized, placebo-controlled, double-masked study of what is anecdotally considered to be the ultimate ortho-k lens. The problem is, of course, that the ortho-k community keeps changing its mind about what is the best lens, based on accumulated anecdotal evidence . . . i.e. clinical hunches leading to other clinical hunches. The only way forward into the future is for the procedure to be properly validated by the type of study described above. Failing that, ortho-k will always remain a possible technique for the future . . . (N Efron personal communication).

The previous statement was made by Nathan Efron, and is basically correct. The study described above *is necessary* particularly as the currently accepted standard for assessing the efficacy of a procedure is the evidence-based model. The author does, however, strongly disagree with the statement that the refinement of the designs is purely based on "hunches leading to other clinical hunches." In reality, the changes usually occurred as a result of the application of a specific model based on a mathematical fitting correlation between the lens and the corneal shape, trials of the model followed by statistical analysis of the results, and then modification of the model to overcome the inadequacies of the design. The application of topography-based fitting, and the mathematical formulae described in this book did not occur through hunches: they have been an accepted part of the theory of contact lens design and fitting for over 20 years (Bibby 1976, Atkinson 1984, Young 1998).

However, Efron (2001) does raise the important point of independent validation, and this should be a priority in research areas. The difficulty is funding such a large-scale project. The other area of orthokeratology that is still in need of concentrated work is that of predictability. This is a vitally important area. The practitioner must be able to determine accurately the likely change in refraction possible before undertaking a course of treatment in order to rule out those subjects who will not achieve the ideal outcome of emmetropia or slight overcorrection and good-quality high- and low-contrast vision. The predictive value of the initial corneal eccentricity has been reported in this book, with both the Mountford and Noack model and the Day surface area model. Also, both the Mountford and El Hage et al (1999) studies found a similar relationship between corneal shape change and refractive change.

However, neither study was designed to meet the highest standards of experimentation and controls, as both were retrospective studies on an admittedly successful group of patients. What the studies did show was that, in the case of ideal responders, a correlation between the two factors existed. To date neither study has been repeated, and therefore lack independent corroboration. Similarly, those who use the Jessen factor do not have independent published proof of the accuracy of the underlying assumption. The data, when analyzed, show large variations and a relatively poor correlation coefficient. The issue of a valid and repeatable predictive tool is a necessary project.

Visual acuity

The studies on visual acuity to date have reported on the change in high- and, in some cases, low-contrast vision, but without any reference to the quality or otherwise of the postwear topography. Future research should try to correlate the topography outcomes to the unaided visual acuity, as well as the aberrations induced in the altered corneal shape and its effect on the quality of vision. The results may then lead to modifications in lens design that could improve the visual outcomes. Tang (2001) has suggested adopting a standard protocol of which optotypes are best suited to determining the quality of unaided vision following the procedure (see Ch. 7).

Astigmatism

Vickers (2000) makes the classic statement: "the one good thing about being an optometrist is being able to talk about astigmatism without understanding what it is." The basic understanding is that astigmatism represents two different radii separated by an axis difference of 90°. Topographical interpretations of the "appearance" of astigmatism confuse the issue even further. For example, the appearance of astigmatism differs markedly between axial and tangential maps. Theoretically, tangential maps are superior at showing fine local changes in curvature, but the axial map representation of astigmatism is more representative of what we "think" it "should" look like. The immediate question (and this is important when trying to design lenses that correct astigmatism) is which elevation should the lens fit be based on: the steep or flat meridian, and is there a difference in elevation for different types of astigmatism? Also, how does the degree of astigmatism affect R_0? Areas that may be fertile grounds for investigation are the differences in eccentricity along the two principal meridians, but this is somewhat limited at present, as the basic research of evaluating the accuracy of topography data for astigmatic values has not been performed.

To date, only Jackson et al (2002) and Mountford & Pesudovs (2002) have published the results of the effects of orthokeratology on astigmatism. The results raised more questions than they answered. For example, it has been a long-held clinical anecdote that reverse geometry lenses do not perform well on significant degrees (>0.75 D) of against-the-rule astigmatism. Why? Also, why does limbus-to-limbus astigmatism respond so poorly, and why is there such a large variation in outcomes with different patients? When astigmatism is reduced with spherical lenses, the reduction is in the order of 50%, and then only over the central 2.00 mm chord, and the predictability of the final axis is poor. The model of forces acting in orthokeratology gives some insights into these problems, but requires much more analysis before any clinical applications occur.

There is no doubt that the efficacious reduction of astigmatism will require novel lens designs. However, until the underlying effect of spherical lenses on astigmatism is better understood, the attempts at correction with more adventurous designs will remain somewhat hit and miss. The work of Kwok (1984) on the surface area of astigmatic surfaces could hold promise in this area.

What changes and why?

At first glance, this seems to be a relatively simple question to answer: the cornea changes shape, and thereby refraction due to the influence of the lens. However, the refractive changes are due to epithelial thinning and perhaps some form of corneal bending, but the exact cause of this is still in the realms of modeled speculation. The forces modeled in Chapter 10 are purely that, models, and require controlled experimentation to validate the concepts. Why do the effects last for up to 4 days in some individuals, yet others need to wear the lenses every night in order to maintain clear vision for all the waking hours? The variations in regression are not related to the magnitude of the induced changes (Soni & Horner 1993, Mountford 1998), and tend to suggest that a viscoelastic effect is at work. This would therefore indicate a stromal involvement.

However, as has been shown in studies of extended-wear RGP lenses (Ren et al 2002), there is a decrease in epithelial surface cell exfoliation with time. Does this have a correlation with overnight orthokeratology lens wear and the stability of the refractive change, or does the absence of the lens during the daytime influence the changes?

These are areas of great interest, as being able to understand fully the interaction of the forces involved and the corneal response to them at all levels will lead to greater control of the outcomes with orthokeratology.

Myopia control

This was the most commonly mentioned area of interest to most of the academics approached for their thoughts on the future directions of orthokeratology research. The impetus behind it is probably due to the strongly held beliefs of some practitioners that their clinical experience supports the theory. However, there is simply no proof to support the anecdotal reports, so controlled studies must be performed to arrive at the truth. If orthokeratology were shown to be effective at controlling the rate of progression of myopia, the impact, especially in Asian countries, would be enormous. The question then arises as to how long (years?) would the lenses need to be worn in order for the effect to be maintained or stabilized, and what would happen if lens wear ceased? Would the myopia simply progress to the stage it would have reached if intervention had not occurred, or would the reductions be maintained? These questions will take years to answer properly, and in the end, the whole concept depends on orthokeratology lens wear having an effect on the eyes' axial length.

Accuracy of fit and different designs

There are obvious contradictions in orthokeratology with respect to the fitting philosophies used by different designs. The basic approach is simply to supply the laboratory with the relevant keratometry readings and spectacle prescription and the lens will be manufactured. The opposite viewpoint is that the efficacy of the procedure, especially with respect to the first-fit success rate, is totally dependent on accurate topography-based fitting and the correct interpretation of trial wear periods. Can they both be correct?

The simple approach relies on patient reports of quality of vision, whereas the complex approach treats this as only one part of the picture, in that the quality of the vision is intimately related to the quality of the postwear topography, and that other factors, such as TxZ diameter, low-contrast vision, and refraction, all combine to set the standard of success or failure. The assessment of both techniques using wavefront analysis and other objective methods of determining unaided vision may eventually give the answers. At present, most of the designs appear to give the same refractive results, but the differences in visual quality, first-fit success rates, and time required for a satisfactory result are unknown. However, a common problem is the relatively small T×Zs possible with higher refractive errors and the incidence of flare and haloes at night. Research is also required to determine if design modifications can be made that will lead to an increase in effective T×Z diameter.

Long-term patient acceptance and satisfaction

Will orthokeratology patients wear their lenses for years? What will the drop-out rate be in the long term, and what term of lens wear defines the success or otherwise of the procedure? Early indi-cations are that new orthokeratology patients rate the process highly, yet 30% still complain of poor night vision and flare. The true success of the procedure may not be known for years, but the simple fact that it has survived for 40 years, with relatively modest results, does indicate that there is a high demand for a nonsurgical means of vision correction.

CONCLUSIONS

As stated in Chapter 1, orthokeratology "belongs" to optometry. However, it alone cannot answer some of the questions asked above. It will require the help of ophthalmologists, anatomists, physiologists, engineers, and other scientists. More complex questions will be raised as the simpler ones are answered. Orthokeratology is complex, not simple.

REFERENCES

Atkinson T C O (1984) A re-appraisal of the concept of fitting rigid hard lenses by the tear layer and edge clearance technique. Journal of the British Contact Lens Association 7: 106–110

Beuhren T, Collins M J, Iskander D R, Davis B, Lingelbach B (2001) The stability of corneal topography in the post-blink interval. Cornea 20: 826–833

Bibby M M (1976) Computer assisted photokeratoscopy and contact lens design. Optician 171(4423): 37–44; 171(4424): 11–17; 171(4426): 15–17

Edwards K, Hough T (2001) Fear and loathing in Surfers' Paradise: on the demise of rigid contact lenses – a critique. Optometry Today October 19, 16–19

Efron N (2001) Contact lens practice and a very soft option. Clinical and Experimental Optometry 83(5): 243–245

El Hage S G, Leach N E, Shahin R (1999) Controlled kerato-reformation (CKR): an alternative to refractive surgery. Practical Optometry 10(6): 230–235

Hough T, Edwards K (1999) The reproducibility of videokeratoscope measurements as applied to the human cornea. Contact Lens and Anterior Eye 22: 91–99

Jackson J M, Rah M J, Jones L A, Bailey M D, Marsden H, Barr J T (2002) Analysis of refractive error changes in overnight orthokeratology using power vectors. ARVO abstract. Investigative Ophthalmology and Visual Science

Kwok S (1984) Calculation and application of the anterior surface area of the model human cornea. Journal of Biology 108: 295–313

Mountford J A (1998) Retention and regression of orthokeratology with time. International Contact Lens Clinics 25: 60–64

Mountford J A, Pesudovs K (2002) An analysis of the changes in astigmatism with accelerated orthokeratology. Clinical and Experimental Optometry 85(5): 284–293

Ren D H, Yamamoto K, Iadage P M et al (2002) Adaptive effects of 30-night wear of hyper O_2 transmissible lenses on bacterial binding and corneal epithelium. Ophthalmology 109: 27–39

Soni P S, Horner D J (1993) Orthokeratology. In: Bennett E, Weissman B (eds) Clinical contact lens practice. Philadelphia, J B Lippincott, ch. 49

Tang W (2001) The relationship between corneal topography and visual performance. PhD thesis. Centre for Eye Research, Queensland University of Technology, Brisbane, Australia

Tang W, Collins M J, Carney L, Davis B (2000) The accuracy and precision performance of four videokeratoscopes in measuring test surfaces. Optometry and Vision Science 77: 483–491

Vickers M (2000) Chairside: the 10 great things about being an optometrist. Review Optometry October: 12

Young G (1998) The effect of rigid lens design on fluorescein fit. Contact Lens and Anterior Eye 21(2): 41–46

Index

3D surface reconstruction, computer-assisted videokeratography 30

A

abnormal symptoms, orthokeratology treatment 244
academics 4–5
Acanthamoeba, RGP lenses 62–4
accuracy
    corneal topography 18
    EyeSys Corneal Analysis System 43–4
    of fit, future 308–9
    sag fitting accuracy 104–6, 232–3
ACP *see* apical corneal power
aftercare 240–54
    continuing suitability decision 252
    emergencies 253–4
    first 242–3
    fluorescein fit assessment 246–7
    lens movement 245–6
    lens position 245–6
    postremoval visual assessment 247–51
    problem-solving 254
    scheduling 240–2
    symptoms and history 243–5
    visual correction, first week 252–3
age of lenses 266
aims, this book's 12–13
algorithms
    computer-assisted videokeratography 29–33
    corneal profile reconstruction 31–3
alignment curve variations, reverse geometry lenses 86

alignment peripheral curves
    construction 88–104
    design 88–104
    reverse geometry lenses 88–104
Alpins method, astigmatism 185–6
anatomical classification, corneal topography 34
anatomical factors, patient selection 118–26
apical corneal power (ACP) 188–90
    refractive changes 180
apical radius, refractive changes 207–10
aspheric mold
    BOZR 96–102
    reverse geometry lenses 80–1
asphericity
    corneal changes 207–10
    refractive changes 207–10
astigmatism
    Alpins method 185–6
    complications 291–5
    corneal shape changes 291–5
    corneal topography 186–8
    future 307–8
    limbus-to-limbus 119–20, 291–5
    orthokeratology 185–6
    patient selection 114–17
    wedge 119–20
ATLAS 20, 24

B

back optic zone diameter (BOZD) 6
    reverse geometry lenses 72–80, 83–106
    TxZ 123
back optic zone radius (BOZR) 2–3, 6
    Dreimlens 96–102

El Hage aspheric mold 96–102
empirical fitting 141
measurement 229–30
refractive changes 98–102
reverse geometry lenses 69–106
sag fitting accuracy 104–6, 232–3
trial lens fitting 147–51
verification 228–9
back peripheral zone diameter (BPZD), measurement 231–2
back vertex power (BVP), verification 228–9
band magnifier 231
BE lens (Mountford and Noack)
    anterior corneal power 198
    fluorescein pattern analysis 153–6
    reverse geometry lenses 85–6
    trial set 151
BE software 220–4
binding, lens 261–3
bleb response
    endothelium 55–6
    RGP lenses 55–6
blocked fenestration 251
BOZD *see* back optic zone diameter
BOZR *see* back optic zone radius
BPD$_1$ (first back peripheral diameter) 6
BPR$_1$ (first back peripheral radius) 6
BPR$_2$ (second back peripheral radius) 6
BPR$_3$ (third back peripheral radius) 6
BPR$_4$ (fourth back peripheral radius) 7
BPZD *see* back peripheral zone diameter
bridging theory, three and 9 o'clock staining 257
bubble formation 249

bull's eye 9
  forces causing 285–7
  topography-based fitting 162–4,
    165, 172
BVP (back vertex power), verification
    228–9

C

calibration method, computer-assisted
    videokeratography 31
care and maintenance
  lens care advice 238–40
  trial lenses 151–2
  see also aftercare
central island 9–11
  empirical fitting 143
  fake 164–6
  forces causing 289–91
  topography-based fitting 164–8
central staining 255–6, 257
central touch zone 8
CKR lens, fluorescein pattern analysis
    152
CL-MIK see contact lens-induced
    microbial infiltrative keratitis
CL-SIK see contact lens-induced sterile
    infiltrative keratitis
classification, corneal topography 34
clearance factor 8–9
  reverse geometry lenses 79
CLPC see contact lens papillary
    conjunctivitis
computer-assisted videokeratography
    19–24
  algorithms 29–33
  design factors 24–9
  focusing systems 26–9
  image editing 26–7
  MasterVue dual-camera system
    26–7
  rasterstereography 27–9
  reference points 25–6
  scanning slit topography 27–9
  working distance 24–5
computer programmers 5
computerized modeling
  BE software 220–4
  constant lamellar length model
    207–10
  EZM calculator 211, 213
  EZM software (Gelflex) 213
  Free Choice OK software 217–20
  kappa function 205–7, 209
  lens design/fitting software 212–24
  lens fitting 205–25
  Ortho Tool 2000; 212, 215–17

outcomes 205–25
  refractive changes 207–10
  software 212–24
  sphere/oblate corneal shape
    210–12
  surface area 205–7
  WAVE software 213–15
cone angles 9
conjunctival staining 259–60
consent, informed, patient selection
    134–6
constant lamellar length model,
    computerized modeling
    207–10
constant-surface-area concept
  four-and five-zone lenses 103–4
  reverse geometry lenses 103–4
contact lens-induced microbial
    infiltrative keratitis (CL-MIK),
    RGP lenses 62–4
contact lens-induced sterile
    infiltrative keratitis (CL-SIK)
    265
  RGP lenses 61–2
contact lens papillary conjunctivitis
    (CLPC) 263–4
Contex lenses 2–3
  difference maps 41, 42
  finite element analysis 274–7
  fluorescein pattern analysis 152–4,
    158
  reverse geometry lenses 75–80
  trial set 151
continuous targets, computer-assisted
    videokeratography 30
contraindications, patient selection
    127–9, 130
corneal changes 175–203, 250
  asphericity 207–10
corneal compression 249
corneal dimpling 249
corneal dystrophies, patient selection
    128
corneal eccentricity
  calculating 281
  patient selection 120–2
corneal edema
  patient selection 128
  RGP lenses 50–1, 54–5
corneal elevation 8
corneal examination 248–9
corneal power displays,
    computer-assisted
    videokeratography 33–44
corneal profile reconstruction
  algorithms 31–3
  computer-assisted
    videokeratography 31–3

Corneal Refractive Therapy (CRT)
    3–4
  lens, reverse geometry lenses
    84–5
corneal sag 8
corneal shape changes 284–95
  astigmatism 291–5
  bull's eye causes 285–7
  central island causes 289–91
  corneal sphericalization 284–7
  models 270
  retention 188–90
  smiley face causes 287–90
  stability 188–90
  topography 250, 270
corneal sphericalization 284–7
corneal staining 197–8, 255–63
corneal thickness 194–7
corneal topography 17–47
  accuracy 18
  anatomical classification 34
  astigmatism 186–8
  changes 250, 270
  classification 34
  historical overview 18–19
  patient selection 118–20
  qualitative descriptors 34–9
  quantitative descriptors 39–40
  refractive changes 178–81
  use of 40
CRT see Corneal Refractive Therapy

D

data resolution, computer-assisted
    videokeratography 30–1
day therapy 130–2
delivery, lens 236–8
design factors, computer-assisted
    videokeratography 24–9
design variables, reverse geometry
    lenses 69–107
diameter gages 112, 231–2
diameters measurement 231–2
Dicon CT 200; 20, 24
difference maps, computer-assisted
    videokeratography 40–3
dimensional tolerances 236
dimple staining 257–8
Dreimlens
  BOZR 96–8
  fluorescein pattern analysis
    153–8
  reverse geometry lenses 81–3
  tear layer profile 90
  trial set 150
dry eye, patient selection 128–9

E

eccentricity, corneal 120–2, 281
edge profile inspection 234
educational standards, future 304–5
efficacy, future 306–7
El Hage aspheric mold
 BOZR 96–102
 reverse geometry lenses 80–1
elevation maps, computer-assisted
 videokeratography 37–8
emergencies, aftercare 253–4
empirical fitting
 BOZR 141
 methods 141
 recommendations 140
 cf. trial lens fitting 147
endothelium
 bleb response 55–6
 polymegathism 56–9
 RGP lenses 55–9
epithelial iron deposition 264–5
epithelial microcysts, RGP lenses 52–4,
 248
Euclid Emerald
 fluorescein pattern analysis 152
 trial set 151
Euclid ET-800; 20, 103–4
Eye-Map EH-290; 20
EyeSys Corneal Analysis System 20,
 24
 accuracy 43–4
 sagittal maps 34–6
EZM calculator, computerized
 modeling 211, 213
EZM software (Gelflex) 213

F

Fargo lens 103–4
 fluorescein pattern analysis
 153–8
fenestration imprint 260
finite element analysis, forces affecting
 lenses 274–7
first back peripheral diameter (BPD$_1$) 6
first back peripheral radius (BPR$_1$) 6
Fischer-Schweitzer polygonal mosaic
 258–9
fitting
 empirical 140–7
 philosophies, reverse geometry
 lenses 69–107
 principles, reverse geometry lenses
 70
 trial lens 139–74

fluid jacket molding *see* squeeze film
 forces
fluorescein fit assessment 246–7
fluorescein pattern analysis, trial lens
 fitting 152–8
focimeters 112, 229
focusing systems, computer-assisted
 videokeratography 26–9
Fontana lens 2
forces affecting lenses 271–84
 finite element analysis 274–7
 lid force 271–2
 squeeze film forces 273–4, 277–84
 surface tension 272–3
formulae, lens construction, reverse
 geometry lenses 72–4
four-and five-zone lenses
 constant-surface-area concept
 103–4
 reverse geometry lenses 80–6
 tear layer profile 92
fourth back peripheral radius (BPR$_4$) 7
Free Choice OK software 217–20
future 303–9
 accuracy of fit 308–9
 astigmatism 307–8
 educational standards 304–5
 efficacy 306–7
 long-term acceptance 309
 myopia control 308
 predictability 306–7
 topography 305–6
 unanswered questions 306–9
 VA 307

G

Gaussian maps, computer-assisted
 videokeratography 36–7
Gelflex EZM lens, trial set 151
Gelflex VMC lens, reverse geometry
 lenses 83–4, 213
general principles, orthokeratology
 1–16

H

high-order polynomial descriptors,
 corneal topography 40
history, orthokeratology 1–16
horizontal visible iris diameter
 (HVID) 124–6
 refractive changes 207–10
hydraulic model 270
hygiene 236–8
hypoxia, RGP lenses 50–1

I

image editing, computer-assisted
 videokeratography 26–7
information, patient, patient selection
 132–4
informed consent, patient selection
 134–6
instruction session 238
instrumentation standards 110–12
International Orthokeratology Society,
 first meeting 14–16
iron deposition, epithelial 264–5

J

Jessen's factor 8, 269–70
 reverse geometry lenses 92–4

K

kappa function, computerized
 modeling 205–7, 209
keratoconus, patient selection 127–8
Keratograph/CTK corneal
 topographer 21
keratometry 122
 changes 176–8, 179–81
keratoscopes 111–12
Keratron 21, 24, 43
KR-8000P 21

L

lens adherence, RGP lenses 60–1
lens binding 261–3
lens care advice 238–40
 see also aftercare
lens condition 250–1
lens delivery 236–8
lens design/fitting software,
 computerized modeling
 212–24
lens fitting, computerized modeling
 205–25
lens movement 245–6
lens position 245–6
lens sag 8
 measurement 232–3
lid force, forces affecting lenses 271–2
lid position/tension, patient selection
 126
limbus-to-limbus astigmatism 119–20,
 291–5
lipoidal deposits 251

long-term acceptance, future 309
long-term changes 200
loss of the effect 265–6

M

marginal dry eye, patient selection
    128–9
MasterVue dual-camera system,
    computer-assisted
    videokeratography 26–7
materials companies 5–6
mean curvature maps,
    computer-assisted
    videokeratography 36–7
measurement
    BOZR 229–30
    BPZD 231–2
    corneal topography 17–47
    diameters 231–2
    lens sag 232–3
    peripheral radii 230–1
    power 229
Medmont E300; 22
meridional skew, computer-assisted
    videokeratography 30
microbial infection, RGP lenses 62–4
microbial keratitis (MK) 265
microcysts 52–4, 248
microscopes 111, 229–30
MK see microbial keratitis
modeling, computerized see
    computerized modeling
Mountford-Noack lens sag gage 232–3
multiple-arc technique, computer-
    assisted videokeratography
    32–3
Munnerlyn's formula 98–102, 122–3
myopia control, future 308
myopia, patient selection 113–14

N

night therapy 12, 130–2
Nightmove lens, fluorescein pattern
    analysis 153
noninfectious ocular inflammation,
    RGP lenses 61–2
normal symptoms, orthokeratology
    treatment 244

O

objectives, this book's 12–13
oblate/sphere corneal shape,
    computerized modeling 210–12

occupational factors, patient selection
    126–7
one-step curve fitting,
    computer-assisted
    videokeratography 31–2
Orbscan II; 22, 29
Ortho Tool 2000; 212, 215–17
orthokeratology
    astigmatism 185–6
    defining 1
    general principles 1–16
    history 1–16
outcomes, computerized modeling
    205–25
oxygen transmissibility, RGP lenses
    50–1

P

PAR CTS 22–3, 28–9
Paragon CRT lens
    fluorescein pattern analysis 153
    reverse geometry lenses 84–5
    trial set 150–1
patient satisfaction 200–1, 309
patient selection 109–38
    anatomical factors 118–26
    astigmatism 114–17
    consent, informed 134–6
    contraindications 127–9, 130
    corneal dystrophies 128
    corneal eccentricity 120–2
    corneal edema 128
    corneal topography 118–20
    dry eye 128–9
    factors affecting 112–30
    information, patient 132–4
    informed consent 134–6
    instrumentation 110–12
    keratoconus 127–8
    lid position/tension 126
    marginal dry eye 128–9
    myopia 113–14
    occupational factors 126–7
    physiological factors 127–9
    PMMA lenses 117
    psychological factors 129–30
    pupil diameter 122–6
    recreational factors 126–7
    refractive factors 112–8
    RGP lenses 117–18
    standards,
        practice/instrumentation
        110–12
    unstable refractive errors 117–18
    VA 112–13
peripheral radii, measurement 230–1

physiological factors, patient selection
    127–9
physiological signs, RGP lenses 51
Placido disk 18
PMMA lenses see polymethyl
    methacrylate lenses
polymegathism
    endothelium 56–9
    RGP lenses 56–9
polymethyl methacrylate (PMMA)
    lenses, patient selection 117
postorthokeratology topography
    181–5
postremoval visual assessment 247–51
power measurement 229
practice, standards 110–12
practitioners 2–4
predictability, future 306–7
protein deposition 251
Pseudomonas aeruginosa, RGP lenses 64
psychological factors, patient
    selection 129–30
pupil diameter, patient selection
    122–6

Q

qualitative descriptors, corneal
    topography 34–9
quantitative descriptors, corneal
    topography 39–40

R

R&R lens, trial set 151
radial keratotomy (RK), mean
    curvature maps 36, 37
radiuscope 112
    BOZR 229–30
rasterstereography, computer-assisted
    videokeratography 27–9
recreational factors, patient selection
    126–7
reference points, computer-assisted
    videokeratography 25–6
refractive changes 175–203
    ACP 180
    apical radius 207–10
    asphericity 207–10
    BOZR 98–102
    computerized modeling 207–10
    corneal topography 178–81
    HVID 207–10
    reverse geometry lenses 190–2
refractive errors, unstable, patient
    selection 117–18

refractive factors, patient selection 112–18
Reinhart Reeves lens, fluorescein pattern analysis 153
research 4–5
retention, corneal shape changes 188–90
reverse geometry lenses
    alignment curve variations 86
    alignment peripheral curves 88–104
    aspheric mold 80–1, 96–102
    background 75
    BE lens (Mountford and Noack) 85–6
    blocked fenestration 251
    BOZD 72–80, 83–106
    BOZR 69–106
    clearance factor 79
    constant-surface-area concept 103–4
    Contex OK series 75–80
    CRT lens 84–5
    design variables 69–107
    Dreimlens 81–3
    El Hage aspheric mold 80–1, 96–102
    empirical fitting 140–7
    fitting philosophies 69–107
    fitting principles 70
    formulae, lens construction 72–4
    four-and five-zone lenses 80–6
    history 75
    Jessen's factor 92–4
    Munnerlyn's formula 98–102
    Paragon CRT lens 84–5
    peripheral curve design 74–5
    refractive changes 190–2
    sag fitting accuracy 104–6
    sag philosophy 70–2, 77
    Scioptic EZM (Gelflex VMC) lens 83–4, 213
    short-term changes 198–200
    tangential peripheries 86–8
    three-zone lenses 75–80
    WAVE lens 84
rigid gas-permeable (RGP) lenses
    Acanthamoeba 62–4
    bleb response 55–6
    CL-SIK 61–2
    complications, clinical 60–4
    complications summary 58–9
    corneal edema 50–1, 54–5
    day therapy 130–2
    dimensional tolerances 236
    endothelium 55–9
    epithelial microcysts 52–4, 248
    extended wear 49–67
    hypoxia 50–1
    lens adherence 60–1

night therapy 130–2
noninfectious ocular inflammation 61–2
overnight wear 49–67
oxygen transmissibility 50–1
patient selection 117–18
physiological signs 51
polymegathism 56–9
Pseudomonas aeruginosa 64
stroma 54–5
tear composition 51
tonicity/pH 51–9
ring jam 11–12

S

sag
    corneal 8
    lens 8, 232–3
sag fitting accuracy
    BOZR 104–6, 232–3
    reverse geometry lenses 104–6
sag philosophy, reverse geometry lenses 70–2, 77
sagittal maps, computer-assisted videokeratography 33, 34–6, 41, 42
SAI *see* surface asymmetry index
satisfaction, patient 200–1, 309
scanning slit topography, computer-assisted videokeratography 27–9
schedules, wearing 238–40
Scioptic EZM (Gelflex VMC) lens, reverse geometry lenses 83–4, 213
scratched lens 251
second back peripheral radius (BPR$_2$) 6
short-term changes, reverse geometry lenses 198–200
smiley face 9, 10, 11
    empirical fitting 142
    forces causing 287–90
    topography-based fitting 164–7, 172
software, lens design/fitting 212–24
sphere/oblate corneal shape, computerized modeling 210–12
squeeze film forces 273–4, 277–84
SRI *see* surface regularity index
stability, corneal shape changes 188–90
staining *see* central staining; conjunctival staining; corneal staining; fluorescein fit

assessment; fluorescein pattern analysis
standards
    educational standards 304–5
    instrumentation 110–12
    practice 110–12
static state molding 295–8
stroma, RGP lenses 54–5
surface area, computerized modeling 205–7
surface asymmetry index (SAI) 38–9
surface deposit-induced staining 263
surface quality 234–6
surface regularity index (SRI) 38–9
surface tension, forces affecting lenses 272–3
symptoms and history
    abnormal symptoms 244
    aftercare 243–5
    normal symptoms 244
systems, computer-assisted videokeratography 19–24

T

tangential maps, computer-assisted videokeratography 33, 36
tangential peripheries
    construction 86–8
    design 86–8
    reverse geometry lenses 86–8
tear composition, RGP lenses 51
tear layer profile
    Dreimlens 90
    four-and five-zone lenses 92
tear reservoir 7–8
terminology 6
test charts 112
thickness gages 112, 233–4
third back peripheral radius (BPR$_3$) 6
three and 9 o'clock staining 256–7
three-zone lenses, reverse geometry lenses 75–80
tinting 235
TMS-2N (TOMEY) 23, 24
tolerances, dimensional 236
tonicity/pH, RGP lenses 51–9
topography-based fitting
    assessment, post-trial 162–8
    bull's eye 162–4, 165, 172
    refining the fit 171–3
    smiley face 164–7, 172
    trial lens fitting 158–68
topography, corneal *see* corneal topography

topography, future 305–6
topography, postorthokeratology *see*
    postorthokeratology
    topography
treatment zone diameter (TxZ) 11,
    122–6
trial lens fitting 139–74
    BOZR 147–51
    care and maintenance 151–2
    cf. empirical fitting 147
    fluorescein pattern analysis
        152–8
    postwear results 168–71
    topography-based fitting
        158–68
    trial lens sets 147–51
TxZ *see* treatment zone diameter

U

unanswered questions, future 306–9
unstable refractive errors, patient
    selection 117–18

V

V-gage 231
VA *see* visual acuity
vacuum molding 297–9
verification 228–9
videokeratography, computer-assisted
        see computer-assisted
        videokeratography
videokeratoscopy, principles 29–31

visual acuity (VA) 192–4
    future 307
    patient selection 112–13
visual assessment, postremoval
    247–51
visual correction, first week 252–3

W

WAVE lens, reverse geometry lenses
    84
WAVE software 213–15
wearing schedules 238–40
wedge astigmatism 119–20
working distance, computer-assisted
        videokeratography 24–5